CONDITIONING EXERCISES

CONDITIONING EXERCISES

Exercises to improve body form and function / Third edition

VERMON S. BARNEY, R.P.T., P.E.D.

Superintendent of Schools, Garfield County, Utah; previously Associate Professor, College of Physical Education, Brigham Young University, Provo, Utah

CYNTHA C. HIRST, M.S.

Assistant Professor, College of Physical Education, Brigham Young University, Provo, Utah

CLAYNE R. JENSEN, P.E.D.

Professor and Assistant Dean, College of Physical Education, Brigham Young University, Provo, Utah

With 191 illustrations

THE C. V. MOSBY COMPANY

Saint Louis 1972

Preface

Hardly a month passes without an exercise program being featured in one of the popular magazines. Exercise tips occur regularly in newspapers, and many national and local television channels frequently carry such programs to help listeners improve their condition.

These programs are usually attractively presented with lovely models, fancy equipment, booklet offers, and health fad information. A few of them have some scientific basis, but many of the programs are prepared and presented by persons who lack professional backgrounds to design and conduct them. As a result, many of the programs are less effective than they ought to be.

While teaching courses in conditioning and body mechanics to college students and adult groups, we observed that the students compiled their own exercise manuals composed of clippings from newspapers and magazines. This practice resulted in collections of exercise descriptions that were incomplete and that were not organized scientifically into progressions. The need for a suitable exercise textbook became apparent.

As library sources were examined, it became evident that no book already written would sufficiently meet the needs of class members. Therefore we believed that a book was needed which would provide the following:

1. Sufficient scientific information about the effects of exercise on the human body
2. Well-planned, progressive exercises for all parts of the body
3. Material on the modern approach to posture
4. Basic principles of body mechanics
5. Techniques of relaxation
6. An outlined exercise program that could easily be followed

This book is designed to fill the above needs.

We express appreciation to the models, Kathleen Creer, Frances Roylance, Carolyn Jensen, Dan Staples, Linda Hatch, and Fred Gagen, who gave freely of their time, to Allie Howe for her technical assistance, and to Frank Hirst for his expert photography.

V. S. B.
C. C. H.
C. R. J.

Contents

CONDITIONING EXERCISES

Chapter 1
Why exercise?

Because of increased mechanization, a higher percentage of professional workers, more emphasis on academic training of youth and adults, and greater mobilization, many people have slipped into a pattern of sedentary living, wherein they fail to participate in regular vigorous activity. As people live this sedentary pattern, their muscles lose their normal tone. Eventually this leads to inefficiency, loss of physical vigor, poor posture, and in some cases discomfort.

Muscle groups most susceptible to loss of muscle tone and disfigurement are the abdominal muscles, the upper back extensors, and the shoulder adductors. Let us look at a particular example to see what may happen to these muscle groups. Consider a man who is active in school athletics and after graduation from college becomes an athletic coach. His job presents one of the best opportunities for keeping in good condition, but he chooses to fall in line with the usual practice of teaching activity—that of talking and not of demonstrating and participating. Eventually, we see the following picture: a man overweight because his habits of eating are essentially the same as when he lived an active life. He consumes more calories than are needed for his now sedentary job; hence he gradually becomes *just plain fat*. We see a man with abdominal ptosis because he has eliminated vigorous activities that require trunk flexion and help retain muscle tone of the abdominal wall. He performs most of his work behind a desk—preparing for teaching, correcting papers, and so forth. This assumed posture contributes to a forward neck tilt, rounded shoulders, and a sunken chest. This condition results from certain muscles becoming tight as a result of poor postural positions, while the opposing muscles become overstretched. The muscles which are in a shortened position become contracted in this position. Over

1

a period of time, this postural attitude becomes fixed and remains so until corrected by the restretching of shortened muscles and the strengthening of the weakened, overstretched muscles.

Other examples similar to this one could be given for dentists, stenographers, factory workers, medical doctors, white-collar workers, and numerous people of other occupations. Similarly, some youngsters spend too much time sitting, watching, and listening and too little time playing or working vigorously. The example of the coach could apply to any individual who fails to participate regularly in an adequate amount of activity.

Exercise programs have proved valuable in helping many people develop and maintain a satisfactory level of muscular fitness. By emphasizing specific exercises the following may be accomplished:

1. Correct or prevent postural deviations.
2. Help control body weight.
3. Change the shape and contour of the body.
4. Increase muscular strength, endurance, and tone.
5. Improve cardiovascular endurance and general physical vigor.
6. Improve flexibility.
7. Increase neuromuscular coordinations.
8. Relieve tension and improve ability to relax voluntarily.

Once the individual has learned the correct methods of performing the different exercises, he may conveniently carry on the program in the privacy of his own home. Such a program requires little space and equipment, and it is practical in terms of time required. Specific exercises are valuable to people of various ages and are, therefore, useful during a large portion of one's life.

What actually happens to the human body as a result of regular vigorous physical activity? Which systems are affected and to what extent? What are the differences between the functioning of these systems in well-conditioned (physically fit) and poorly conditioned individuals?

Through measurements and controlled observations, evidence has been produced that regular vigorous physical activity will result in specific changes in the different systems of the body, especially the muscular, circulatory, and respiratory systems. Other systems are affected by activity, but to a lesser extent. The following brief explanations clarify the effects on these systems as a result of activity.

CHANGES IN THE MUSCLES

Regular vigorous activity can result in more efficient use of muscles, can eliminate extraneous movements, and can increase the efficiency of the muscle contractions. Following are specific changes that occur as a result of vigorous exercise.

Increased strength and efficiency

Regular exercises against heavy resistance cause an increase in the diameter of the individual muscle fibers. This results in stronger muscle fibers. Increased strength means that fewer fibers need to contract in order to apply a given amount of tension. This results in improved efficiency of the muscle and increased muscular endurance. If there is excessive fat within the muscle, exercise may cause the total muscle to reduce in size due to decreased fatty tissue, while the muscle fibers increase in size and strength.

Increased number of capillaries

Regular vigorous activity also increases the number of capillaries in the muscle fibers. This allows better circulation of blood, which, in turn, increases muscular endurance because endurance is dependent upon blood supply to the acting muscles.

Reduction of fat

Fatty tissue within the muscle causes friction between the muscle layers and thereby reduces the speed and efficiency of the muscle contraction. Regular exercise decreases the fat within the muscle and thus increases the efficiency of the contractions.

Increased tone

Skeletal muscles normally display a firmness, slight tension, and correct shape that result from a condition known as muscle tone. Muscle tone is essential to good posture and to properly shaped muscles. Regular exercise is necessary for the development and maintenance of good muscle tone.

CHANGES IN THE CIRCULATORY SYSTEM

Regular vigorous exercise will bring about several favorable changes in the circulatory system. Some of these are as follows:

1. The heart rate at rest becomes slower because the heart muscles grow stronger and the blood output per heart beat (stroke volume) becomes greater.
2. Following vigorous exercise, the heart rate returns to normal more quickly because the heart muscles are stronger and the blood output is greater.
3. The circulation of blood (venous return) is improved because of improved muscle tone and the improvement of the respiratory action.
4. The number of capillaries being increased in the exercised muscles causes increased circulation of blood in those muscles.
5. The return of blood pressure to normal following vigorous exercise occurs more readily.

6. The capacity of the blood to carry oxygen and waste products to and from the cells is increased.

CHANGES IN THE BREATHING MECHANISM

Repeated periods of deep breathing which accompany vigorous exercise may produce changes in the respiratory system. Deep breathing stretches the lung tissues and thereby increases their capacity. Vigorous exercise also strengthens the diaphragm, which in turn may increase the volume intake of the lungs. The improved efficiency of the respiratory system resulting from vigorous exercise is manifested by a greater absorption of oxygen per liter of ventilation.

OVERLOADING IS ESSENTIAL

In order to systematically increase the functional ability of any body system, overload must be successively applied to that system. To increase the strength of muscles, they must be contracted repeatedly against resistance heavier than that to which they are accustomed. By this process the muscles are "overloaded." To increase muscular endurance, the muscles should be overloaded in terms of the number of repetitions of contraction against a given resistance. To improve the effectiveness of the circulatory and respiratory systems, overload must be applied to them.

ABUSE OF INACTIVITY

Ample evidence indicates that extensive inactivity has detrimental effects on the human body.

The circulatory system deteriorates

Spencer* points out that excessive inactivity has a deteriorating effect on the circulatory system. By studying normal individuals who were immobilized by casting the entire body, he learned the following facts:

1. During prolonged inactivity the skeletal muscles lose their tone, which in turn reduces the amount of venous flow to the heart, because the pumping action of the skeletal muscles is important for the maintenance of the force needed to return blood to the heart.
2. During inactivity the expansion of the thoracic cage is lessened because of loss of muscle tone in the muscles causing respiration. This also reduces the venous flow of blood.

Spencer also noted other less significant adverse effects of inactivity on the circulation of blood. A return to normal activity reversed all of the adverse effects.

*Spencer, William A.: Physiological considerations in rehabilitation, The Physical Therapy Review 34:61, Feb. 1954.

Bone atrophy develops

Dock, in his study "The Evil Sequelae of Complete Bed Rest," points out that bone atrophy is not infrequent in subjects submitted to bed rest.* Ghormley substantiates the evidence of bone atrophy from prolonged bed rest and states that this condition should be regarded as pathologic.†

The cause of bone atrophy is believed to be due to demineralization of the bone. Even though an individual receives an adequate amount of calcium and phosphorus in his daily diet, bone atrophy is still evidenced during inactivity. Apparently the body requires a normal amount of activity to utilize its supply of calcium and phosphorus. The demineralization of bone due to inactivity is well substantiated by research, and the atrophy apparently varies with the degree of inactivity.

The changes in the bone that take place during inactivity can be corrected by resuming normal activity. This is pointed out by Powers in his comparative study of 100 patients who were allowed to walk on the first day after major operations and an equal number of patients who remained in bed for the traditional period of 10 to 15 days after operations of the same type and magnitude. The results of the study showed that demineralization of bone was entirely obliterated through exercise.‡

Atrophy of muscles occurs

The wasting away of muscle tissue is evidenced by casting an extremity during a simple fracture. On removal of the cast after a short period there is a dramatic decrease in muscle mass. This wasting away of muscle, known as muscle atrophy, has also been observed in studies on inactive normal subjects where no healing or repair of tissue is required. A study by Spencer showed that there was a definite decrease of muscle mass and of muscle strength in the immobilized body parts during inactivity. Return to normal activity reversed these effects.§ Ghormley also showed definite evidence of changes in muscle resulting from inactivity.† Thus, it is evident that certain changes in muscle tissue resulting from inactivity are undesirable but can be corrected by resumption of normal vigorous activities.

Only a few years ago it was routine practice for a new mother to be confined to the hospital for a period of ten days. Today, a mother enters the hospital for child delivery, and within three days (provided that there are no complications) she is out of bed, caring for herself and, in many hospi-

---

*Dock, William: The evil sequelae of complete bed rest, Journal of American Medical Association **125**:1083, Aug. 1944.

†Ghormley, R. K.: The abuse of bed rest in orthopedic surgery, Journal of American Medical Association **125**:1085, Aug. 1944.

‡Powers, John H.: Abuse of bed rest as a therapeutic measure in surgery, Journal of American Medical Association **125**:1079, Aug. 1944.

§Spencer, William A.: Physiological considerations in rehabilitation, The Physical Therapy Review **34**:61, Feb. 1954.

tals, for the child. Within five days she is usually released from the hospital to perform modified activities of daily living.

Evidence shows that in treating patients with complications such as heart disease, rheumatic fever, surgery, or fractures, excessive inactivity has actually caused undesirable effects.

In a study of 38 men who participated in a reconditioning program following rheumatic fever, Karpovich lists the following results. The delay in beginning a reconditioning program was decreased from 77.3 days to 16.2 days without causing an increase in the incidence of cardiac damage during 6 to 12 months of observation.[*]

Such studies merely confirm Powers' warning, "Rest as a therapeutic measure is fraught with hazard."[†] He discovered that participation in early activity after operations was, in many respects, beneficial to the total recovery of the patient.

Complications of inactivity have also been pointed out by Dock. "Bone atrophy, muscle wasting, and vasomotor instability," he says, "are not infrequent in subjects submitted to bed rest; backache, constipation, and other similar disabilities may appear during bed rest and persist for some time."[‡]

Therefore, it can be said that evidence strongly indicates that unnecessary excessive inactivity is harmful to both body form and function.

FACTS ABOUT FATIGUE

If a person performs muscular exercise to a point that the muscles seem to become exhausted, he experiences what is known as neuromuscular fatigue. This type of fatigue may be defined as a decrease in ability to do muscular work due to work itself. Neuromuscular fatigue is attributed to one or a combination of three conditions: (1) accumulation of acid waste products which decrease the irritability of the muscle, (2) depletion of the stored fuel (oxygen) supply in the muscle, and (3) failure or partial failure in the neuromuscular (nerve-muscle) junction at the motor end plate.[§] Probably the most significant factor contributing to this type of fatigue is inadequate circulation of blood through the muscles or, in other words, the inability of the circulatory system to supply oxygen and to remove waste products from the working muscles.

It should be noted that the person in poor physical condition is much

---

[*]Karpovich, Peter V., Merritt, P. S., Stoll, C. Q., and Weiss, R. A.: Physical reconditioning after rheumatic fever, Journal of American Medical Association 130:1199, Apr. 1946.
[†]From Powers, John H.: Abuse of bed rest as a therapeutic measure in surgery, Journal of American Medical Association 125:1079, Aug. 1944.
[‡]From Dock, William: The evil sequelae of complete bed rest, Journal of American Medical Association 125:1083, Aug. 1944.
[§]Morehouse, L. E., and Miller, A. T.: Physiology of exercise, St. Louis, 1967, The C. V. Mosby Co.

more susceptible to fatigue than is the highly trained person. Good physical condition is essentially an opponent of fatigue.

MUSCLE SORENESS AND STIFFNESS

The only ways to prevent a muscle from becoming sore and stiff are (1) never to overexert the muscle and (2) to keep the muscle in peak condition constantly. Of course, this is not possible in the case of every muscle; therefore, almost everyone has experienced muscle soreness and stiffness at one time or another. However, an individual can avoid excessive muscle discomfort by following some commonsense rules. *First,* each conditioning period should start with light exercises and gradually work into more vigorous movements. In other words, loosen up before making any all-out efforts. *Second,* start with light conditioning and gradually over a period of days build up to heavier conditioning routines. Continue this building up process until the desired level is reached. *Third,* keep the exercise level rather consistent. Do not be sporadic, working hard this week and then laying off next week. Decide the activity level that is best for you and then stick with it.

Unless the muscle fibers are actually injured (ruptured or torn), the best treatment for soreness and stiffness is a light, smooth type of exercise. This type of exercise hastens the circulatory removal of metabolic waste products from the muscle and thus reinstates it to normalcy. Massage and application of heat may also prove helpful.

RULES OF EXERCISE WISDOM

In order to gain maximum benefit from an exercise program and at the same time to suffer minimum discomfort, the performer should follow these rules.

1. *Find a comfortable and stable position.* When placing the body in the correct exercising position, strive for comfort and adequate stability in order to prevent (a) overstress on any muscle or joint that may result in injury and (b) undue pressure on bony areas that may become bruised and tender.
2. *Use smooth motions.* All exercise motions in a conditioning program should be smooth, rather than jerky and sporadic. Smooth motion will help to reduce injury to muscle fibers which causes undue soreness and stiffness.
3. *Prevent overdosage.* Too much exercise at one time results in unnecessary soreness and also general fatigue and physical discomfort. The exercise load should start at a low level and increase steadily as the conditioning of the body increases. The overload, beyond what the body is accustomed to, should always be gradual.
4. *Keep the exercise period short.* If the exercise program is well or-

ganized in the correct sequence, there is no need to make the period excessively long.

5. *Exercise regularly.* The purpose of an exercise program cannot be accomplished by exercising this week and laying off next week. The program must be continuous.

6. *Make the exercise periods fun, rather than drudgery.* Look upon them with a jovial attitude and let them refresh and recreate the mind and spirit as well as the body.

Chapter 2
Designing programs to fill specific needs

Most people prefer and need a general conditioning program that builds muscle tone, stimulates functioning of the different organic systems, and generally improves the vitality and well-being of the individual. But it should be recognized that exercises may be especially selected to accomplish more specific purposes. For instance, one individual may wish to follow a program which emphasizes the development of strength, another may want to alter the shape and contour of the body, and still another may follow a program especially prescribed for corrective or therapeutic purposes.

BUILDING STRENGTH

Muscular strength is the ability of a muscle to resist force or to move against force. Strength is basic to all vigorous motor performances, and some leading physical educators claim it is the most important single item in performance.

Light resistance for many repetitions builds muscle endurance and has little effect on muscle strength, whereas exercise against heavy resistance for fewer repetitions builds strength. All vigorous work and play activities provide heavy resistance against the contractions of the acting muscles and result in some increased strength and endurance. If a person wants to strengthen certain muscle groups at a very rapid rate, he should perform specific exercises against heavy resistance. The resistance should become progressively heavier as the acting muscles are strengthened. Such a program is referred to as a "progressive resistance" exercise program.

The necessary resistance against which a muscle contracts may be furnished by several methods: (1) weight training, in which the muscles contract against movable weights, (2) pull-ups or other exercises where the muscles contract against the weight of the body, or (3) contractions against a stationary object, such as a fixed bar. Whatever source of resistance is used, the performer must remember that, in order to build strength rapidly, he must apply heavy resistance (near maximum) over a low number of exercise repetitions (six to ten).

INCREASING MUSCULAR ENDURANCE

Endurance is the ability to resist fatigue or to recover quickly after fatigue. Endurance may also be defined as the ability to sustain prolonged activity. It is necessary for a sustained effort at a high level of performance. Among the several factors that influence endurance are strength, skill, fat, oxygen supply, and waste products.

Strength

A load easily carried by strong muscles may exhaust weaker ones; therefore, muscle endurance is dependent upon strength. As strength is increased, endurance is also increased.

Skill

Experiments show that unskilled performers use several times more energy to perform particular tasks than do skilled individuals. Therefore, as an individual improves skill in movement, he also increases endurance for activities involving those movements.

Fat

Fatty tissue in and around the muscles adds weight resistance to a particular movement and also provides friction between the muscle layers, causing a braking action within the muscle itself. Furthermore, fat requires a constant supply of blood. Therefore, excess fatty tissue limits endurance in three ways.

Oxygen supply and waste products

Endurance is further limited by the amount of oxygen debt that the individual can tolerate, the amount of lactic acid that can be tolerated, and the ability of the body to free the muscles of accumulated carbon dioxide. Therefore, endurance is directly dependent upon the ability of the circulatory and respiratory systems to supply energy to and carry waste from the working muscles. Hence, endurance calls for efficiency of the circulatory and respiratory systems.

Endurance can be increased through participation in regular vigorous exercise because such exercise can be selected (1) to improve strength, (2) to reduce fatty tissue, (3) to increase the capacity of the circulatory and respiratory systems, and (4) to improve skill in body movements.

In order to increase endurance without emphasizing strength and without adding muscle bulk, light exercises should be selected and repeated a high number of times. To build both strength and endurance, select heavy exercises which can be repeated only a few times in succession. For information on specific exercises to improve muscle strength, endurance, and tone, see Chapter 4.

INCREASING CARDIOVASCULAR ENDURANCE

Cardiovascular endurance refers to the ability of the circulatory system to provide oxygen to the cells to support the oxidative energy schemes of the body and to remove the waste products of metabolism. The primary objective of cardiovascular endurance training is to improve the circulation of blood to the working muscles and thus increase the delivery of oxygen to the cells. Cardiovascular endurance training can be divided into two main categories, aerobic training and anaerobic training. Aerobic training involves the systems that supply oxygen to the cells of the body, whereas anaerobic training involves the energy mechanisms that supply energy without the presence of oxygen. The ability of the body to supply the cells with oxygen (aerobic capacity) is the key to cardiovascular endurance.

Aerobic training

In order to develop aerobic endurance, the circulatory system must be worked beyond its accustomed level (overload). This can be done by continuous hard work for long periods of time, as in cross-country running (or jogging), long-distance swimming, or cross-country skiing. However, a better method for developing this kind of endurance is known as interval training. This technique consists of a series of work bouts with short rest intervals between bouts. In order for this kind of training to continue to be effective over a period of time, the intensity must be increased as endurance is gained, so that overload will continue to be applied. This can be done by altering one or more of four different variables: (1) the number of work bouts can be increased, (2) the length of each bout can be increased, (3) the intensity of each bout can be increased, and (4) the rest periods between bouts can be shortened.

It is recommended that the work bouts be *3 to 5 minutes* in length, with light activity or rest between bouts. The number of bouts, the intensity of each bout, and the amount of rest between bouts should be geared to the fitness level of the particular person.

The heart rate should be used as a criterion for determining the optimal training load. It should be maintained at a rate within ten beats of maximum heart rate during each of the 3- to 5-minute work bouts. If less than optimal rate of increase in aerobic endurance is desired, the heart rate does not need to be maintained within ten beats of maximum, but it is important to recognize that the work bouts must be vigorous enough to stimulate a significant increase in heart rate.

In summary, it should be said that running and swimming are the best

activities for developing aerobic endurance. Endurance will develop at
at optimal rate as a result of doing a sufficient number of successive bouts
3 to 5 minutes in length, with short rest periods between bouts, where
the work bouts are intensive enough to cause the heart rate to be maintained within ten beats of maximal rate. Furthermore, aerobic endurance
can be developed at less than optimal rate by doing bouts of work that
are less intense and therefore do not maintain the heart rate within ten
beats of maximal. Also, aerobic endurance can be developed at a reasonable but less than optimal rate, by doing continuous work over an extended period of time at less than maximum intensity, such as jogging
or long-distance swimming.

Anaerobic training

Anaerobic endurance refers to the effectiveness of the processes of the
body that provide energy for muscular contraction in the absence of oxygen,
or, in other words, when sufficient oxygen is not available to the cells.
This kind of endurance is accomplished best by repeated short bouts of
maximal effort, followed by brief rest periods between bouts. Extremely
high levels of lactic acid are found in the blood following four or five work
bouts of this type, indicating great use of anaerobic mechanisms in the cells.

Well-trained athletes are typically able to tolerate much higher lactate
levels than untrained athletes. This indicates that anaerobic training would
be of great value to athletes involved in vigorous short-duration activities.
It is important that the work periods for anaerobic training not be too
short. Research indicates that 10 to 15 seconds of vigorous work does not
increase lactate levels a significant amount, and thus would have little,
if any, effect upon anaerobic endurance. Successive vigorous work bouts
of about *1 minute* in length are the most effective for this type of endurance.

ALTERING THE BODY SHAPE AND CONTOUR

Within certain limitations placed on them by hereditary factors, body
shape and contour can be changed through an exercise program. This is
done in several ways. (1) By use of specific exercises, certain muscles
can be strengthened while antagonistic muscles are stretched, thus changing the body posture. For example, rounded shoulders can be corrected
by strengthening the overstretched and weakened muscles of the upper
back and stretching the tightened muscles across the chest. (2) Exercise
improves the tone of weak and sagging muscles and thereby improves the
contour of specific areas of the body, such as the abdomen, buttocks, hips,
calves, and thighs. (3) Specific exercises can help remove deposits of fat in
areas where it is unbecoming to body contour. Also, a regular exercise program will serve as a preventative measure against formation of fat deposits.

Although body proportions may be changed significantly through exercise, it must be recognized that exercise is not a panacea. It will not turn

heavy bones into light bones, change heavy muscles into long slender muscles, or give slender hips to one with a broad pelvic bony structure. It must be recognized that the contribution which exercise can make to body shape and contour is limited not only by one's desire and effort, but also by one's capacity for improvement.

For those who are accustomed to a sedentary existence, a general physical conditioning program will improve the shape and contour of the whole body by adding muscle tone and reducing fatty tissue. In order to improve the contour of specific areas of the body, appropriate exercises should be especially selected for that purpose.

GAINING AND LOSING WEIGHT

Overweight and underweight are dependent upon the relationship between calorie intake and daily calorie requirements. If the intake is greater than the requirement (calories burned), the result will be an increase in weight. If the daily requirement surpasses the intake, a loss in weight will occur. An increase in amount of daily physical activity increases the catabolic processes and aids in weight reduction.

The daily calorie requirement of an active adult male may range from 3,000 to 8,000 calories, depending upon his size, physical condition, and amount of daily vigorous activity which he performs. People who enter into a vigorous activity program may increase their food intake and still not gain weight. One must remember that when activity is reduced, food intake must also be reduced if normal body weight is to be maintained.

The best way to control body weight is to combine an adequate amount of regular activity with a diet that provides the amount of calories required for your level of activity. Weight reduction is possible by simply reducing food intake without performing vigorous physical activity. But this approach results in untoned, sagging muscles which cause undesirable body contours.

It is possible for most people to lose weight at a healthy rate by doing some type of moderate or vigorous exercise for only one-half hour a day. A person may burn as much as 500 to 800 calories in only one-half hour of swimming, dancing, fast walking, cycling, tennis, or other such moderately active sports. Of course, in order to lose weight by this method, food intake must not be increased.

Underweight individuals may use exercise to gain weight. Moderate exercise may stimulate one's appetite so that his increased calorie intake exceeds the calories burned as a result of the exercise. This would result in increased body weight.

There is a direct relationship between muscle strength and the thickness of the muscle. This means that generally increased strength results in increased muscle mass. Therefore, strength-building activities may result in increased body weight. However, this is not always true because the increased muscle mass may be offset by a loss of fatty tissue in and around the muscle. It can be concluded that, in most cases, body weight can be either increased or decreased by the correct combination of exercise and diet control.

INCREASING FLEXIBILITY

Inadequate flexibility is one of the most frequent causes of improper movement. Flexibility is indicated by the range of motion in specific joints. In turn, the range of motion in a particular joint is dependent upon (1) the length of ligaments and other tissues surrounding the joint, (2) the length and extensibility of those muscles and tendons that are antagonistic to flexion of the joint, (3) excessive amounts of muscle and fat that may limit complete movement in the joint, and (4) the bony structure in the joint itself.

Excessive inactivity causes muscles, tendons, and ligaments to lose their normal amount of extensibility. Inactivity may also contribute to accumulation of excessive amounts of body fat, which may further restrict body flexibility.

In most cases, flexibility in specific areas of the body can be increased by a significant amount with stretching exercises. Specific exercises can be employed to stretch muscles and tendons and to extend the ligaments surrounding the joint. Also, regular vigorous exercise combined with diet control can remove fat deposits that restrict the range of motion. For information on exercises used to increase flexibility of specific body parts, see Chapter 3.

PLANNING AND DIRECTING A PROGRAM

Regardless of the specific purposes of an exercise program, it should contain certain qualities. Those who prescribe or direct exercise programs should be aware of these qualities.

1. The program should consist of regular exercise sessions, preferably every second day, at the least, and each session should be long enough to complete an effective program without haste.
2. Each individual should emphasize those exercises which best meet his particular need.
3. The program should include progressions within each exercise, progressions within the exercise series, and progressions within the exercise program as a whole.
4. In order to reduce soreness and possible injury, necessary precautions for each specific exercise should be practiced.
5. Exercise descriptions and instructions must be specific and clear in order that the exercise will be performed correctly, thus accomplishing the purpose for which it was selected.

6. The program should contain ample exercises of each kind to allow for variety within the program. New exercises add freshness to an otherwise dull routine.

In directing exercise sessions for groups or in teaching physical conditioning courses, the leader should be well acquainted with the following guides:

1. Plan each lesson well from beginning to end.
2. Be sure you understand each exercise and its specific purpose.
3. Remember that all students need not work on the same progression at the same time.
4. Do not allow the cadence to become monotonous.
5. Be enthusiastic while directing the program and keep it moving at a good rate.
6. Make clear to the students the specific objectives of each exercise.
7. Include in each exercise session some stretching, some overall conditioning, some relaxation exercises, plus exercises to meet the specific needs of each participant.
8. Remember physical conditioning is a slow process. Do not become discouraged when results are not readily apparent.

A SUGGESTED GENERAL CONDITIONING ROUTINE

A general conditioning routine should include the following four types of exercises:

1. The first part of each day's lesson should include the stretching exercises. These exercises are designed to help prepare the body and the mind for action and can reduce muscle soreness by a considerable amount.
2. Strengthening and muscle-toning exercises for specific muscle groups are a second requirement in a conditioning program. These include exercises for all parts of the body. Start with the first progression of exercises for the abdominal muscles, shoulder, neck, and chest muscles, back muscles, hip and leg muscles, and foot muscles.
3. The overall conditioning exercises will come third. These are vigorous, total-body exercises which stimulate the functioning of the muscles and the various supporting systems.
4. The relaxation exercises should be performed during the last part of the exercise period. These can be alternated with the body mechanics and posture work. Each should be introduced early enough to allow time for the learning of the exercises, so that they can become a part of the exercise program and a part of the daily life of the individual involved.

SUGGESTED EXERCISE PROGRAM

First week daily program

Stretching	Strengthening	Slenderizing and general conditioning	Relaxing

Hamstrings and muscles of the lower back
Exercise 1
Exercise 2
	Muscles of the
	A. Abdomen
	  Exercise 18
	  Exercise 21
	B. Shoulders
	  Exercise 41
	  or
	  Exercise 42
	  or
	  Exercise 43
	  or
	  Exercise 44
	C. Chest
	  Exercise 50
	  Exercise 51
	  Exercise 52
	D. Back and neck
	  Exercise 53
	E. Hips and legs
	  Exercise 63
		A. Hips
		  Exercise 70
		B. Total body fitness
		  Exercise 71
		C. Waist
		  Exercise 72
			Back
			Lying with deep breathing

SUGGESTED EXERCISE PROGRAM—cont'd

Second week daily program

Stretching	Strengthening	Slenderizing and general conditioning	Relaxing
Hamstrings and muscles of the lower back	Muscles of the		
Exercise 2	A. Abdomen	A. Waist	Back
Exercise 4	Exercise 19	Exercise 74	Lying with
Exercise 5	Exercise 20	B. Total body fitness	deep
	Exercise 22	Exercise 71	breathing
	Exercise 24	3 min. walk/run	
	B. Shoulders		
	Exercise 42		
	or		
	Exercise 43		
	or		
	Exercise 44		
	or		
	Exercise 45		
	C. Chest		
	Exercise 50		
	Exercise 51		
	Exercise 52		
	D. Back		
	Exercise 54		
	Exercise 59		
	E. Hips		
	Exercise 64		
	Exercise 65		
	F. Feet		
	Exercise 66		

SUGGESTED EXERCISE PROGRAM—cont'd

Third week daily program

Stretching	Strengthening	Slenderizing and general conditioning	Relaxing
Hamstrings and muscles of the lower back	Muscles of the		
Exercise 1	A. Abdomen	A. Waist	Exercise 88
Exercise 2	Exercise 23	Exercise 72	
Exercise 4	Exercise 25	Exercise 74	
	Exercise 32	Exercise 79	
	Exercise 39	B. Hips	
	B. Shoulders	Exercise 75	
	Exercise 45	C. Total body fitness	
	or	5 min. walk/run	
	Exercise 46		
	Exercise 47		
	C. Back		
	Exercise 55		
	Exercise 56		
	Exercise 60		
	D. Hips		
	Exercise 64		
	Exercise 65		
	E. Feet		
	Exercise 66		
	Exercise 67		

SUGGESTED EXERCISE PROGRAM—cont'd
Fourth week daily program

Stretching	Strengthening	Slenderizing and general conditioning	Relaxing
Hamstrings and muscles of the lower back	Muscles of the A. Abdomen	A. Waist	Exercise 88
Exercise 5	Exercise 26	Exercise 72	
Exercise 7	Exercise 34	Exercise 76	
Exercise 9	Exercise 39	Exercise 79	
Exercise 10	B. Shoulders	B. Hips	
	Exercise 46	Exercise 70	
	C. Upper back	C. Total body fitness	
	Exercise 57	Exercise 71	
	Exercise 61	5 min. walk/run	
	D. Feet		
	Exercise 68		
	Exercise 69		

Chapter 3
Exercises to improve flexibility

There is no set standard as to the desirable amount of flexibility that an individual should possess. This is dependent upon a person's age, structural and muscular build, and the activities in which he desires to participate. Some activities such as dancing, gymnastics, and tumbling require a greater amount of flexibility by the participants than do softball, basketball, or fencing. It is important, however, that an individual develop sufficient flexibility to allow him to follow his normal daily living routine without undue muscular strain. This daily living must include his working, playing, and resting activities. One of the most frequent causes of improper movement is poor flexibility. When ungainly movement is observed, flexibility is one of the first things to be checked.

FLEXIBILITY MEASURES

Various methods of determining a "normal" range of motion may be used by the student to help himself or by the teacher to help his students evaluate flexibility (Figs. 1 to 5). It should be remembered that these ranges are desirable but not essential for everyone to attain. As mentioned previously, the age and body-build of the person must be considered when evaluating flexibility.

STRETCHING EXERCISES

The exercises in this section are designed to increase flexibility. These exercises must be progressive in nature, meaning the force exerted must be increased gradually and the duration of the held position must be progressively lengthened with each practice session.

Throughout this section of exercises, precaution should be taken to avoid bobbing. Doing the exercise smoothly each exercise period at the individual's own maximum level will more quickly and less painfully increase flexibility

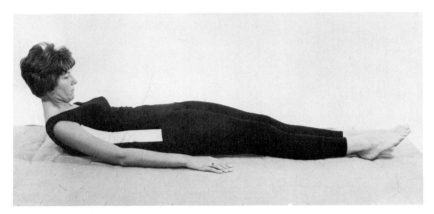

Fig. 1. Normal range of motion in the cervical region. Normal flexibility of the posterior neck muscles allows the chin to be flexed on the upper chest.

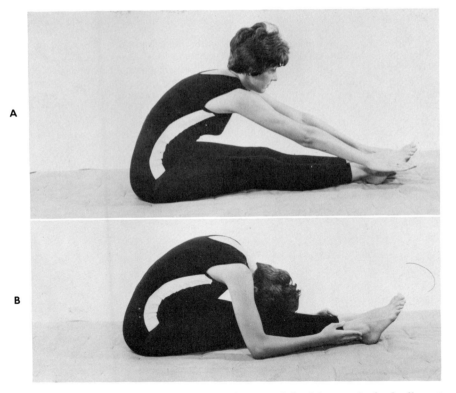

Fig. 2. A, Normal range of motion in the back. Normal flexibility in the back allows it to be flexed to 135 degrees in an adult when the legs are straight. **B,** Normal range of motion in a child allows the back to be flexed until the head touches the knees.

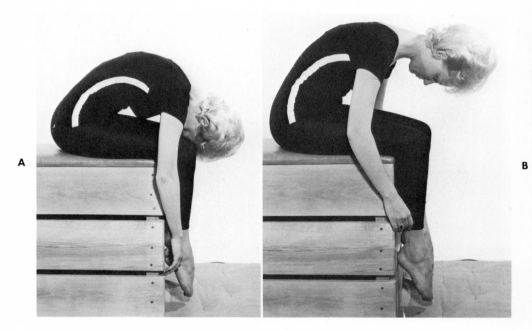

Fig. 3. A, Normal range of motion in the back with the knees bent. When the knees are bent, the tightness which might be caused from the hamstring muscles is eliminated. Here the back can be flexed to 135 degrees. **B,** Slight restriction of motion in the back. This restriction of motion might be due to ligamentous shortening from aging (over 50 years) or from lack of physical conditioning. This type of tightness is normal in aging but can be kept to a minimum with proper physical conditioning.

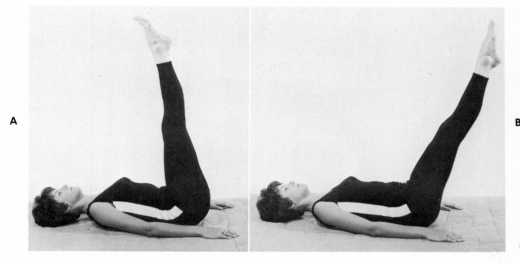

Fig. 4. A, Normal flexibility of the hamstring muscles allows straight leg raising from a back lying position to 90 degrees. **B,** Slight restriction of motion caused by tight hamstring muscles.

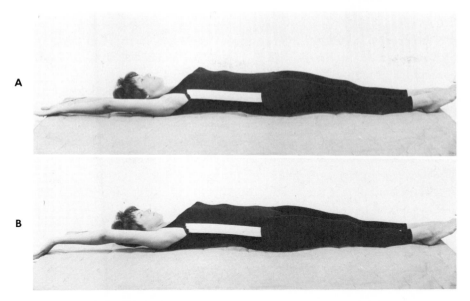

Fig. 5. **A,** Normal flexibility of the chest muscles (pectoralis major). When there is no spasm or tightness of these muscles, the arm can be abducted and flexed to 180 degrees. **B,** Slight restriction of motion in the anterior chest muscles.

than if the individual bobs and pulls the muscles and then experiences muscular soreness.

Note that the term *stretch pain* is used in each exercise. Stretch pain is that pain felt during the exercise that increases as the force is intensified and as the duration of the exercise is lengthened.

Exercises 1 through 17 follow.

Exercise 1

Purpose. To stretch the hamstring and low back extensor muscles.

Starting position. Stand with the feet 3 to 4 inches apart and parallel to each other (Fig. 6, *A*).

Movement. Bend forward from the waist and keep the knees straight. Reach toward the floor as far as possible. Let the arms, trunk, and head hang freely (Fig. 6, *B*). Stretch until the stretch pain is felt. Hold the position 3 to 5 seconds. Return to the starting position.

Progression. Do the exercise three times and increase one time every other exercise period until five.

Precautions. Keep the knees straight throughout the movement. Do not use a bobbing motion. Do not overstretch.

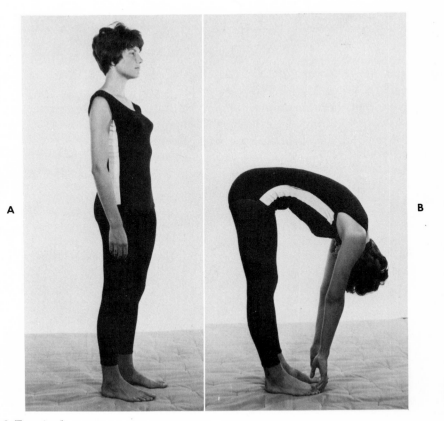

A   B

Fig. 6. Exercise 1.

Exercise 2

Purpose. To stretch the hamstring, low back extensor, and rotator muscles, and the iliotibial band.

Starting position. Stand, cross the right leg over the left leg and assume a position of stability. Place the right hand on the left shoulder and place the left arm across the small of the back (Fig. 7, *A*).

Movement. Bend forward from the waist and keep the left knee stabilized with the right leg. Let the head and trunk hang freely. Rotate in the direction of the right leg (Fig. 7, *B*). Stretch until a stretch pain is felt. Hold the position 3 to 5 seconds and return to the starting position. Do alternately.

Progression. Do the exercise three times to each side and increase one time every other exercise period until five.

Precautions. Be sure the base of support is wide enough to maintain balance. Keep the left leg straight. Do not use a jerking or bobbing motion.

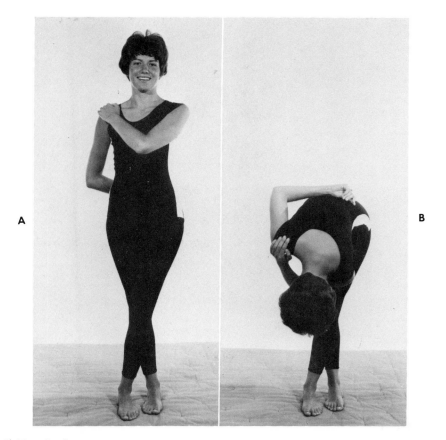

A   B

Fig. 7. Exercise 2.

Exercise 3

Purpose. To stretch the hamstring, low back extensor, and rotator muscles.

Starting position. Stand at the side of a table or bench at approximately crotch level. Place the leg nearest table on top of table and let the opposite leg hang freely.

Movement. From this position, bend forward at the waist and let the head hang freely. Reach toward the outside of the foot of the extended leg (Fig. 8). Stretch until a stretch pain is felt. Hold the position 3 to 5 seconds and return to starting position.

Progression. Do the exercise three times to each side and increase one time every other exercise period until five.

Precautions. Keep the extended leg straight. Do not use a jerking or bobbing motion.

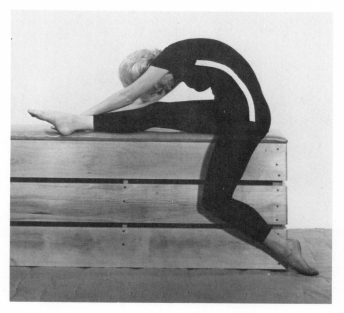

Fig. 8. Exercise 3.

Exercise 4

Purpose. To stretch the hamstring muscles.

Starting position. Sit with the legs extended and the arms outstretched (Fig. 9, *A*).

Movement. Bend forward from the waist and attempt to reach beyond the toes (Fig. 9, *B*). Stretch until a stretch pain is felt. Hold the position 3 to 5 seconds and return to the starting position.

Progression. Do the exercise three times and increase one time every other exercise period until five.

Precautions. Do not let the knees bend during the stretch. Do not use a bobbing motion.

A 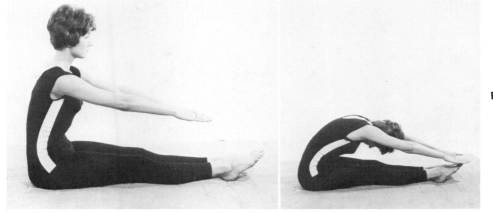 B

Fig. 9. Exercise 4.

Exercise 5

Purpose. To stretch the back extensor muscles.

Starting position. Sit in a tailor position with the arms folded across the chest (Fig. 10, *A*).

Movement. Roll the chin on the chest and in a curling motion attempt to touch the forehead to the knees (Fig. 10, *B*). Hold this position for 3 to 5 seconds and return to starting position.

Progression. Do the exercise three times and increase one time every other exercise period until five.

Precautions. Keep the knees level throughout the movement. Do not use a bobbing motion. Do not overstretch. Do not raise the hips from the mat.

A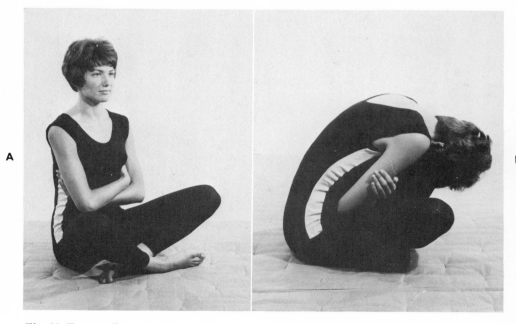B

Fig. 10. Exercise 5.

Exercise 6

Purpose. To stretch the rotator muscles of the back.

Starting position. Sit in a straight back chair with the hips pushed back as far as possible; keep the legs parallel to each other and about 3 to 4 inches apart and the feet flat on the floor. Maintain this position throughout the movement (Fig. 11, *A*).

Movement. Reach the left arm around behind the body and grasp the right side frame of the chair back. Reach the right arm across the body and grasp the left side frame of the chair back. Rotate the trunk, chest, and head to the left as far as possible. While holding the chair with the right hand, release the left hand and place the thumb and index finger along the base of the right side of the chin on the right. Keep elbow in a horizontal position. Apply a slight pressure with the hand until a very slight stretch pain is felt through the neck and entire back (Fig. 11, *B*). Hold from 3 to 5 seconds. Alternate to each side.

Progression. Do the exercise three times each exercise period.

Precautions. Maintain the hips as described in the starting position. Do not lift or rotate the hips or legs during the stretch.

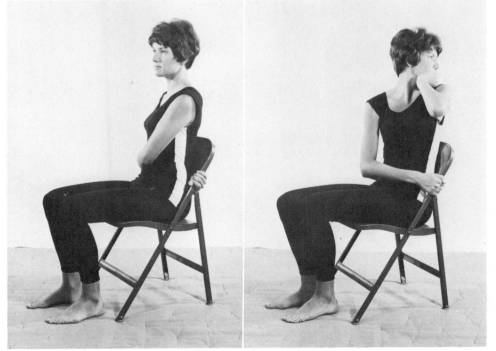

Fig. 11. Exercise 6.

Exercise 7

Purpose. To stretch the rotator muscles of the lower back and the ligaments of the pelvic girdle.

Starting position. Lie on the back with the arms at side (Fig. 12, *A*).

Movement. Extend one leg vertically to an angle of 90 degrees (Fig. 12, *A*). Let the leg hang inward (Fig. 12, *B*) until a slight stretch pain is felt in the lower back. Maintain this position 5 seconds and return to starting position.

Progression. Do the exercise three times each exercise period.

Precautions. Keep the knees straight and the legs extended throughout the movement. Do not raise the trunk off the mat.

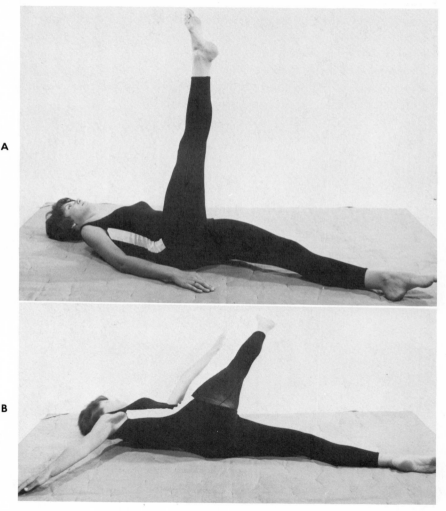

A

B

Fig. 12. Exercise 7.

Exercise 8

Purpose. To stretch the rotator muscles of the lower back and the ligaments of the pelvic girdle.

Starting position. Lie on the back with the arms at shoulder level.

Movement. Raise one leg to a vertical position, keeping the knee extended. The opposite leg should be flat on the floor and in an extended position. Keep the shoulders, arms, and back on the mat. Reach toward the opposite hand with raised leg (Fig. 13). Stretch until a stretch pain is felt. Hold 3 to 5 seconds and return to starting position.

Progression. Do the exercise three times with each leg each exercise period.

Precautions. Keep the knees straight and the legs extended throughout the movement. Do not raise the trunk off the mat.

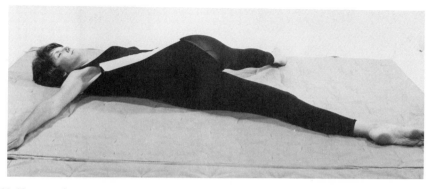

Fig. 13. Exercise 8.

Exercise 9

Purpose. To stretch the hip extensor and flexor muscles.

Starting position. Lie on the back.

Movement. Bring the right knee to the chest and grasp the leg just below the knee (Fig. 14). Pull the knee toward the chest until a stretch pain is felt. Hold position 5 seconds and return to starting position.

Progression. Do the exercise five times with each leg each exercise period.

Precautions. Keep extended leg straight. Do not use a bobbing motion.

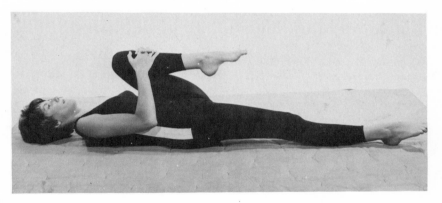

Fig. 14. Exercise 9.

Exercise 10

Purpose. To stretch the low back and hip extensor muscles.

Starting position. Lie on the back.

Movement. Bring the knees to the chest and grasp the legs just below the knees. Pull the knees toward the axillae, keeping the trunk on the mat (Fig. 15). Hold the position 5 seconds and return to the starting position.

Progression. Do the exercise five times and increase one time every other day until twenty-five.

Precautions. Be sure the knees are brought out toward the axillae and not straight to the chest. Do not use a bobbing motion.

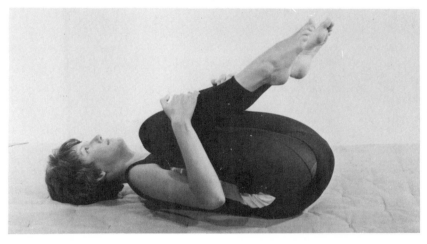

Fig. 15. Exercise 10.

Exercise 11

Purpose. To stretch the hip flexor and extensor muscles.

Starting position. Lie on the back on a table with the buttocks at the edge of the table.

Movement. Bring the right leg to the chest and grasp it with laced fingers just below the knee (Fig. 16). Let the opposite leg hang freely over the edge of the table. Hold the position until stretch pain is felt and then hold position for an additional 10 seconds.

Progression. Do the exercise alternately three times to each side and increase one time each side each exercise period until ten.

Precautions. Be sure the leg hangs freely over the edge of the table. Completely relax to ensure stretch. Be sure the knees are brought out toward the axillae and not straight to the chest. Do not use a bobbing motion and stretch only one leg at a time.

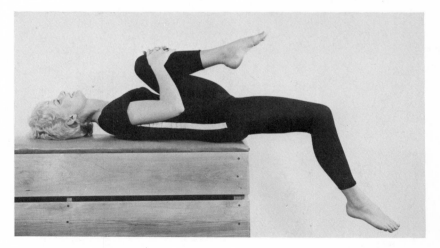

Fig. 16. Exercise 11.

Exercise 12

Purpose. To stretch the muscles and ligaments of the pelvic and hip regions.

Starting position. Stand with heels and toes together about 18 inches from and sidewise to a wall. Place one elbow against the wall at shoulder level, with the forearm and hand resting on the wall, the heel of the opposite hand placed on the upper position of the buttocks, and the shoulders kept in line with the elbow and perpendicular to the wall. Do not allow the shoulders to shift forward. Keep the knees completely extended (Fig. 17, *A*).

Movement. Contract the abdominal and gluteal muscles strongly while shifting the hips slightly forward and inward toward the wall. This movement is aided by pressure on the buttocks with the heel of the hand (Fig. 17, *B*).

Progression. Do the exercise three times to each side each exercise period.

Precautions. Keep the knees straight and the body in alignment. Push forward and toward the wall.

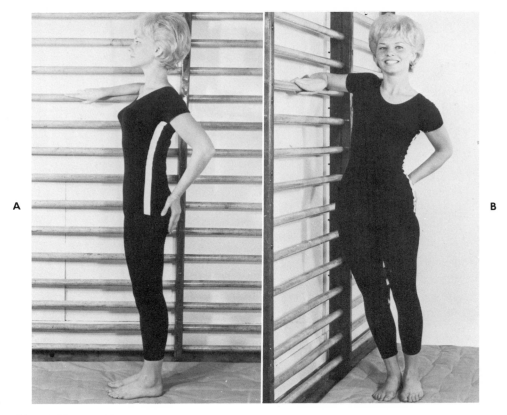

A   B

Fig. 17. Exercise 12.

Exercise 13

>*Purpose.* To stretch the anterior chest muscles.
>
>*Starting position.* Stand facing a corner or a door frame.
>
>*Movement.* Walk through the door or into the corner (Fig. 18, *A*). Place hands on the wall or door frame at shoulder level. Keeping the body in good alignment, walk until a stretch pain is felt (Fig. 18, *B*). Hold the position 3 to 5 seconds.
>
>*Progression.* Do the exercise three times and increase one time every other exercise period until five.
>
>*Precautions.* Keep the body in good standing posture throughout.
>
>NOTE: Exercise should also be done with the arms extended 45 degrees upward (Fig. 18, *C*).

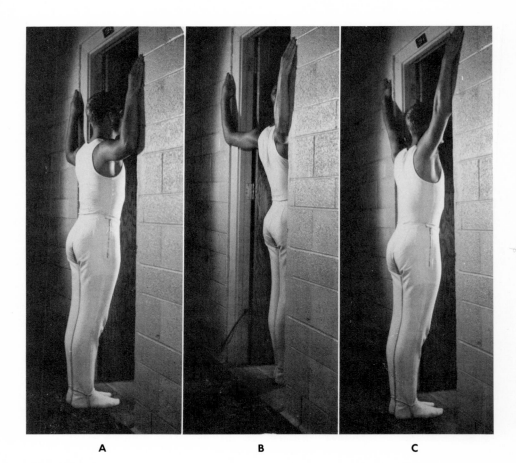

A   B   C

Fig. 18. Exercise 13.

Exercise 14

 Purpose. To stretch the spinal ligaments and back and chest muscles.

 Starting position. Hang from stall bars or other apparatus. Grasp the stall bars with the palms forward and the back to the stall bars.

 Movement. Hang and maintain this position to tolerance (Fig. 19).

 Progression. Do the exercise three times daily.

 Precautions. Lower the body weight by placing the feet on the stall bar and rest in this position between repetitions.

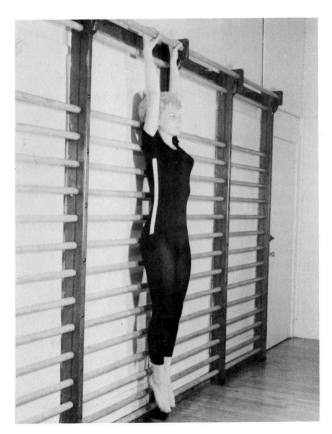

Fig. 19. Exercise 14.

Exercise 15

Purpose. To stretch the heel cords and ankle extensor muscles.

Starting position. Stand and face the stall bars or wall approximately an arm's length from the wall with the knees straight. Keep the feet 3 to 4 inches apart and flat on the floor and the body in alignment (Fig. 20, A).

Movement. Lean forward, catching the body weight with the hands. Keep the head, shoulders, hips, chest, and ankles in alignment. Bend the elbows slowly until stretch pain is felt behind the knees and in the calf of the leg (Fig. 20, B). Hold 3 to 5 seconds and return to the starting position.

Progression. Do the exercise three times to start and increase one time each week until five.

Precautions. Keep the leg straight and the heels on the floor. Do not bend at the hips or knees.

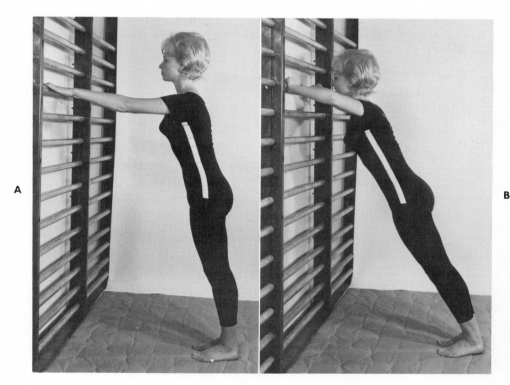

A   B

Fig. 20. Exercise 15.

Exercise 16

Purpose. To stretch the low back muscles and the sacroiliac ligaments.

Starting position. Sit in a chair with the hips back in the chair, the feet flat on the floor and parallel to each other.

Movement. Interlock the arms and bend forward from the waist. Keep the hips in the chair at all times. Curl the head, shoulders, and back toward the floor, with the knees spread apart so that the interlocked arms will pass between the knees. Bend forward until a stretch pain is felt in the low back (Fig. 21). Hold the position 3 to 5 seconds and then return to the starting position.

Progression. Do the exercise five times and increase two times each exercise period until twenty-five.

Precautions. Keep the hips well back in the seat of the chair at all times. Keep the feet flat on the floor and parallel to each other.

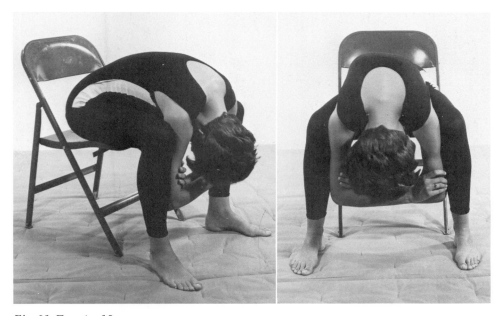

Fig. 21. Exercise 16.

Exercise 17

Purpose. To stretch the soleus (back of lower leg) muscle.

Starting position. Stand and face the wall or doorway approximately 24 inches away from it. Lean forward until the hands rest on the stall bars or wall. Keep the heels on the floor.

Movement. Cross the right lower leg over the left calf at about midcalf level (Fig. 22, A). Bend the knee approximately 15 degrees. Lean forward until a stretch pain is felt in the calf of the leg. Hold the position 5 seconds (Fig. 22, B). Return to the starting position.

Progression. Do the exercise three times and increase one time every other day until five.

Precautions. Keep the trunk, pelvis, and feet in proper alignment throughout movement. Keep the heels on floor. Do not bend the knee of the weight-bearing leg. Do not arch the back or tilt the pelvis.

A 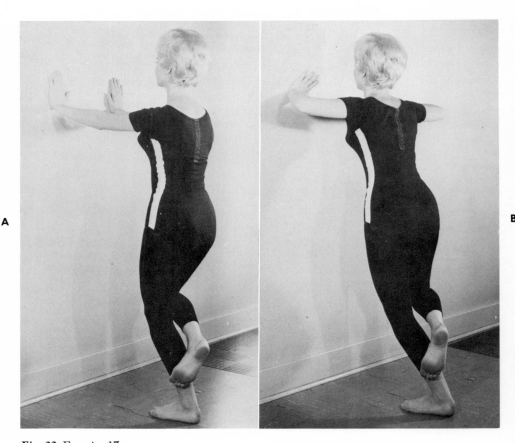 B

Fig. 22. Exercise 17.

Chapter 4
Exercises to build muscular strength, endurance, and tone

Exercises that are designed to increase strength and endurance and to develop muscle tone compose a large part of most exercise programs. This is understandable when the importance of these factors to posture and physical performance is understood. *Strength*, the ability to apply force against resistance, is increased as the resistance against the muscles being used is increased. Strength in a certain amount is needed in all phases of sports, dancing, gymnastics, and aquatics. It is an essential part of housework, gardening, child care, and numerous other vocations. Many persons in professions that require little strength involve themselves in avocations that require great strength—mountain climbing, skiing, hiking, and so forth.

Muscle endurance is the ability of the muscles to resist fatigue—or to continue to contract after prolonged activity. Certain kinds of activity rely heavily on endurance, depending upon the duration and intensity of the activity.

Muscle tone is a characteristic of firmness and slight tension which results from a sustained contraction of a few of the muscle fibers. A muscle with good tone feels firm and yet is not hard or lumpy.

Strength, endurance, and good muscle tone are all essential to the maintenance of an erect standing posture, good sitting posture, and smooth walking, running, and working movements. Strength, endurance, and tone can be developed and maintained through regular and diligent participation in sports activities or in an exercise program. Participation in either program—sports or exercises—must be regular and not a momentary whim of eagerness or a sporadic need for "getting some exercise." During an exercise program, the exercises must become progressively more difficult and last for longer durations of time or be performed against additional weight resistance.

The exercises in this section are grouped as follows:

1. Exercises for toning and strengthening the abdominal wall.
2. Exercises for strengthening the muscles of the shoulder girdle, neck, and chest.
3. Exercises for strengthening the muscles of the back.
4. Exercises for strengthening the muscles of the hips and legs.
5. Exercises for strengthening the muscles of the feet.

It should be kept in mind that when strength is increased endurance also increases.

EXERCISES FOR THE ABDOMINAL WALL

The exercises contained in this section deal with the muscles of the abdominal region. The action of these muscles is varied. The direction of the *rectus abdominis* muscle is vertical, the *external* and *internal oblique* muscles are at an angle, and the *transversus abdominis* muscle is horizontal. Exercises for the abdominal area need to include types for each direction these muscles take. Therefore, there is no one abdominal exercise. When performing these exercises, the participant should take care to maintain the recommended position, to observe the progressions, and to adhere to the precautions indicated in the exercise description.

The need for exercises for the abdominal area arises very often because of poor pelvic posture and a sagging abdominal wall.

Exercises 18 through 40 follow.

Exercise 18

Purpose. To develop tone in the abdominal muscles.

Starting position. Lie on the back with the legs extended and the arms at the side (Fig. 23).

Movement. Tilt the pelvis and attempt to flatten the back on the mat by contracting the muscles of the lower abdominal wall. Hold the position 5 seconds, relax, and return to the starting position.

Progression. Do the exercise five times and increase one time every other exercise period until ten.

Precautions. Do not attempt to perform this motion by simply compressing the abdominal wall. Do not hold the breath. Do not bend the knees during the contraction.

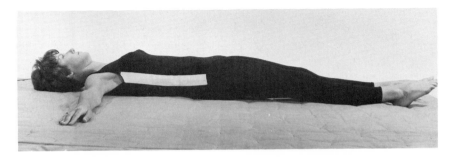

Fig. 23. Exercise 18.

Exercise 19

Purpose. To develop tone in the abdominal muscles.

Starting position. Lie on the back with the heels placed at the buttocks and the knees bent (Fig. 24).

Movement. Flatten the back to the floor and tilt the pelvis posteriorly by contracting the lower abdominal muscles.

Progression. Do the exercise five times and increase one time every other exercise period until ten.

Precautions. Do not attempt to perform this motion by simply compressing the abdominal wall. Do not hold the breath.

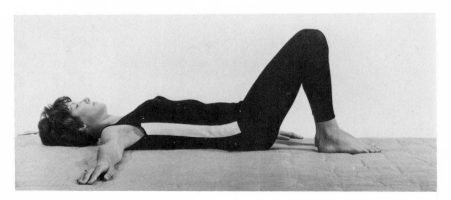

Fig. 24. Exercise 19.

Exercise 20

Purpose. To strengthen the hip and trunk rotator muscles.

Starting position. Lie on the back with the legs extended and the arms extended over the head. Stabilize the entire body by keeping the legs, back, hips, arms, and head flat on the mat.

Movement. Attempt to roll to the right and hold the position 5 seconds and then attempt to roll to the left and hold 5 seconds (Fig. 25).

Progression. Do the exercise five times and increase one time every other exercise period until ten.

Precautions. Be sure that arms, head, back, hips, and legs are not lifted from the mat. The only movement which occurs is tightening of the transversus abdominis muscles and a slight rotation movement of the lower abdominal wall.

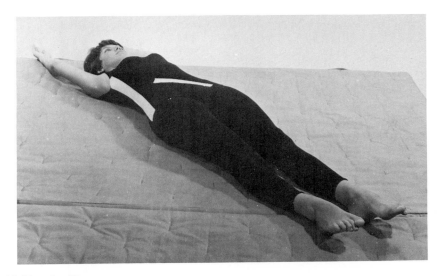

Fig. 25. Exercise 20.

Exercise 21

> *Purpose.* To strengthen the abdominal wall.
>
> *Starting position.* Kneel on the hands and knees with the knees 3 to 4 inches apart. The knees should be directly under the hips and the arms should be under the shoulders. The abdominal wall is relaxed so that the back is arched.
>
> *Movement.* Drop the head, contract the abdominal muscles, vigorously contract the gluteal muscles, and hump the lower back (Fig. 26). Hold this position 3 to 5 seconds. Relax and return to the starting position.
>
> *Progression.* Do the exercise five times, increase one time every exercise period until ten, and then continue throughout the exercise program.
>
> *Precautions.* Do not assume a tense position. When starting this movement, be sure the head is relaxed completely and not extended. Be sure to extend the head when returning to the starting position. Do not hold the breath.

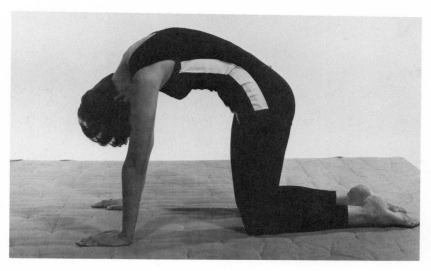

Fig. 26. Exercise 21.

Exercise 22

Purpose. To develop tone in the transversus abdominis muscles.

Starting position. Kneel on the hands and knees, with the knees 3 to 4 inches apart and directly under the hips; the arms should be under the shoulders. Let the abdominal wall relax so that the back is arched.

Movement. Drop the head and contract the abdominal muscles. Vigorously contract the gluteal muscles and hump the lower back, using a rocking movement back over the hips as the muscles are contracted. Completely relax and raise the head, letting the abdominal wall relax and rocking the body back over the shoulders (Fig. 27).

Progression. Do the exercise five times, increase one time every exercise period until ten, and then continue throughout the exercise program.

Precautions. Do not assume a tense position. When starting this movement, be sure the neck is relaxed completely. Also be sure to extend the head when returning to the starting position. Do not hold the breath.

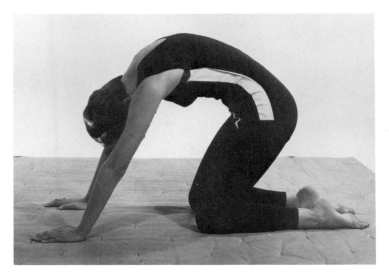

Fig. 27. Exercise 22.

Exercise 23

Purpose. To develop tóne in the abdominal muscles.

Starting position. Kneel on the hands and knees, with the trunk horizontal. The arms should be directly under the shoulders and the knees directly under the hips (Fig. 28, *A*).

Movement. Swing the trunk forward over the shoulders, bend the elbows, and lower the chest to the floor. Then extend the arms, lower the head, and extend and arch the lower part of the back, reaching forward with the chest and head. Roll the pelvis under and let the head drop. Shift the weight back over the hips. Come to a position as high as possible (Fig. 28, *B*). Hold the position 5 seconds; then relax the abdominal wall. Bring the head up and let the back arch. Assume the starting position.

Progression. Do the exercise five times. Increase one time every exercise period until ten and then do ten repeatedly throughout the duration of the exercise program.

Precautions. Keep the legs under the hips throughout the exercise. Do not use the arms and hands to move the trunk back over the hips.

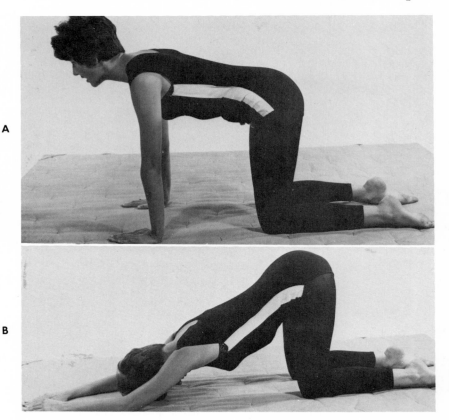

A

B

Fig. 28. Exercise 23.

Exercise 24

Purpose. To strengthen the rectus abdominis muscle.

Starting position. Lie on the back with the arms at the sides and the legs outstretched (Fig. 29, A).

Movement. Tilt the pelvis to flatten the lower back to the floor. Curl the head and shoulders until the shoulders clear the mat (Fig. 29, B). Hold the position 5 seconds and then uncurl to the starting position.

Progression. Do the exercise three times during the first exercise period, five times the second period, seven times the third period, and ten times the second week.

Precautions. Do not use a jerking or pendulum motion to attain the described position. Be sure that the pelvis does not tilt anteriorly (do not arch the back). Eliminate rotation and do not hold the breath. If unable to attain this position, curl as far as possible and hold the maximum shortened position 5 seconds.

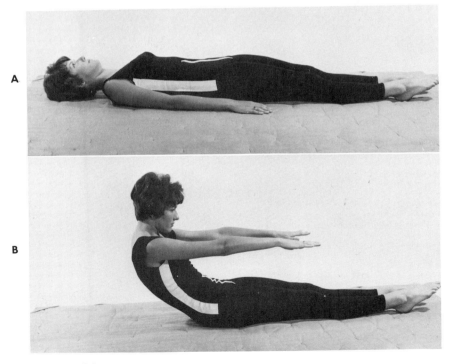

Fig. 29. Exercise 24.

Exercise 25

Purpose. To strengthen the rectus abdominis muscle.

Starting position. Lie on the back with the arms at the sides and the legs outstretched.

Movement. Tilt the pelvis to flatten the lower back to the floor. In position, reach the hands toward the toes and curl the head, shoulders and back while rising to a sitting position (Fig. 30). Return slowly to the starting position.

Progression. Do the exercise five times the first exercise period, seven times the second period, and ten times the third period.

Precautions. This exercise is a progression from Exercise 24 and should not be attempted until ten repetitions of Exercise 24 can be done. Do not allow a jerking or pendulum motion while attaining the described position. Be sure the pelvis does not tilt anteriorly (do not arch the back). Eliminate rotation and do not hold the breath.

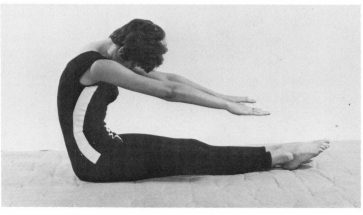

Fig. 30. Exercise 25.

Exercise 26

Purpose. To strengthen the rectus abdominis muscle.

Starting position. Lie on the back with the arms folded across the chest and the legs outstretched.

Movement. Tilt the pelvis to flatten the lower back to the floor. In position with the arms folded across the chest, reach toward the toes, curl the head, shoulders, and back, and come to a sitting position (Fig. 31). Return slowly to the starting position.

Progression. Do the exercise five times the first exercise period, seven times the second period, and ten times the third period.

Precautions. Do not allow a jerking or pendulum motion while attaining the described position. Be sure that the pelvis does not tilt anteriorly (do not arch back). Eliminate rotation and do not hold the breath. If unable to attain this position, curl as far as possible and hold the maximum shortened position 5 seconds. This exercise is a progression from Exercise 25 and should not be attempted until ten repetitions of Exercise 25 can be done.

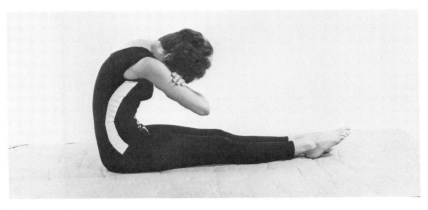

Fig. 31. Exercise 26.

Exercise 27

Purpose. To strengthen the rectus abdominis muscle.

Starting position. Lie on the back with the legs extended and the fingers laced behind the head.

Movement. Tilt the pelvis to flatten the lower back. Curl the head, shoulders, and back and come to a sitting position (Fig. 32). Uncurl to the starting position.

Progression. Do the exercise five times the first exercise period, seven times the second period, and ten times the third period.

Precautions. Do not allow a jerking or pendulum motion while attaining described position. Be sure the pelvis does not tilt anteriorly (do not arch the back). Eliminate rotation and do not hold the breath. If unable to attain this position, curl as far as possible and hold the maximum shortened position 5 seconds. This exercise is a progression from Exercise 26 and should not be attempted until ten repetitions of Exercise 26 can be done.

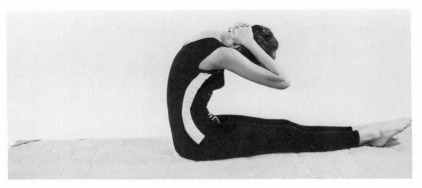

Fig. 32. Exercise 27.

Exercise 28

Purpose. To strengthen the rectus abdominis muscle.

Starting position. Lie on the back, with the knees flexed, the heels to the buttocks, and the arms at the side (Fig. 33, *A*).

Movement. Curl to a sitting position (Fig. 33, *B* and *C*).

Progression. Do the exercise five times the first exercise period, seven times the second period, and ten times the third period.

Precautions. Do not allow a jerking or pendulum motion while attaining the described position. Be sure that the pelvis does not tilt anteriorly (do not arch the back) (Fig. 33, *D*). Eliminate rotation and do not hold the breath. If unable to attain this position, curl as far as possible and hold the maximum shortened position 5 seconds. This exercise is a progression from Exercise 27 and should not be attempted until ten repetitions of Exercise 27 can be done. A partner can stabilize the legs by placing one hand on the knees and one hand on the feet.

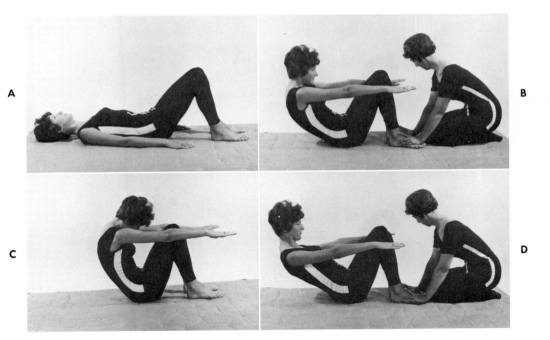

Fig. 33. Exercise 28.

Exercise 29

Purpose. To strengthen the rectus abdominis muscle.

Starting position. Lie on the back with the knees flexed, the heels to the buttocks, and the arms folded across the chest.

Movement. Curl to a sitting position (Fig. 34).

Progression. Do the exercise five times the first exercise period, seven times the second period, and ten times the third period.

Precautions. Do not allow a jerking or pendulum motion while attaining described position. Be sure that the pelvis does not tilt anteriorly (do not arch the back). Eliminate rotation and do not hold the breath. If unable to attain this position, curl as far as possible and hold the maximum shortened position 5 seconds. This exercise is a progression from Exercise 28 and should not be attempted until ten repetitions of Exercise 28 can be done. A partner can stabilize the legs by placing one hand on the knees and one hand on the feet.

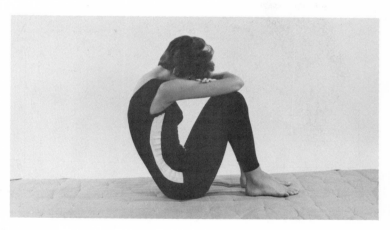

Fig. 34. Exercise 29.

Exercise 30

Purpose. To strengthen the rectus abdominis muscle.

Starting position. Lie on the back, with the fingers laced behind the head and the heels to the buttocks.

Movement. Curl to a sitting position (Fig. 35). Uncurl and return to starting position.

Progression. Do the exercise five times the first exercise period, seven times the second period, and ten times the third period.

Precautions. Do not allow a jerking or pendulum motion while attaining the described position. Be sure that the pelvis does not tilt anteriorly (do not arch the back). Eliminate rotation; do not hold the breath. If unable to attain this position, curl as far as possible and hold the maximum shortened position 5 seconds. This exercise is a progression from Exercise 29 and should not be attempted until ten repetitions of Exercise 29 can be done. A partner can stabilize the legs by placing one hand on the feet and one hand on the knees.

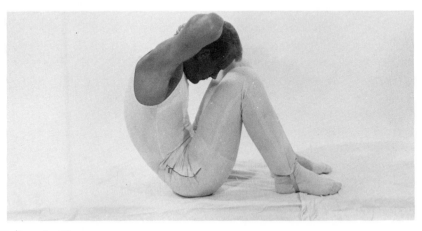

Fig. 35. Exercise 30.

Exercise 31

Purpose. To develop tone in the lateral abdominal muscles.

Starting position. Lie on the back, with the legs straight and the arms folded across the chest (Fig. 36, A).

Movement. Without raising the hips, rotate the trunk, reaching with the right elbow toward the mat on the left side (Fig. 36, B). Hold the position 3 seconds and return to the starting position. Do exercise alternately (Fig. 36, C).

Progression. Do the exercise five times the first exercise period, seven times the second period, and ten times the third period.

Precautions. Be sure that the trunk rotates and that the motion is not merely one of rolling to the side. Keep the arms folded close to the chest and make sure that the opposite elbow is not used as a prop to assist in the motion. The head and opposite shoulder should be slightly off the mat. The head should always be in the same plane of motion as the trunk.

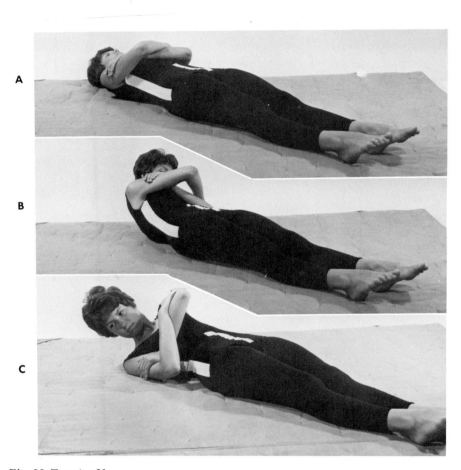

A

B

C

Fig. 36. Exercise 31.

Exercise 32

Purpose. To develop tone in the lateral abdominal muscles.

Starting position. Lie on the back, with one arm folded across the chest at the level of the sternum (Fig. 37, A).

Movement. Reaching toward the inside of the opposite knee, curl the head, shoulders, and back and come to a partial sitting position, reaching only to the inside of the opposite knee (Fig. 37, B). Derotate and uncurl to the starting position. Do exercise alternately.

Progression. Do the exercise three times the first exercise period, five times the second period, seven times the third period, and ten times the second week.

Precautions. Do not allow a jerking motion and make sure that the head, shoulders, and back curl off mat. Do not arch the back or tilt the pelvis forward. If unable to come to this position, come to the maximum position and hold 5 seconds. This exercise is a progression from Exercise 31 and should not be attempted until ten repetitions of Exercise 31 can be done.

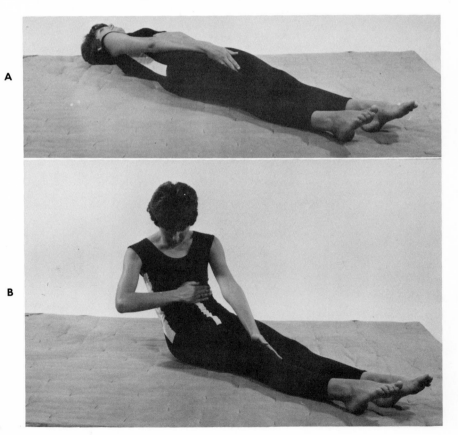

A

B

Fig. 37. Exercise 32.

Exercise 33

Purpose. To develop the muscle tone of the lateral abdominal muscles.

Starting position. Lie on the back, with one arm folded across the chest at the level of the sternum.

Movement. Reaching toward the outside of the opposite knee, curl the head, shoulders, and back, and come to a sitting position, reaching to the outside of the opposite knee (Fig. 38). Derotate and uncurl to the starting position. This exercise should be done in a rotating manner, and the rotation should be initiated at the beginning of the movement and not at the end of the sit-up. Do exercise alternately.

Progression. Do the exercise five times the first exercise period, seven times the second period, and ten times the third period.

Precautions. Be sure that the trunk rotates and that the motion is not merely one of rolling to the side. Keep the arms folded close to the chest and make sure that the opposite elbow is not used as a prop to assist in the motion. The head and opposite shoulder should be slightly off the mat. The head should always be in the same plane of motion as the trunk. This exercise is a progression from Exercise 32 and should not be attempted until ten repetitions of Exercise 32 can be done.

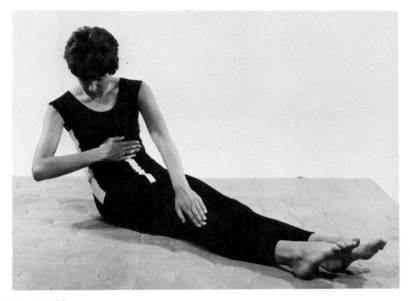

Fig. 38. Exercise 33.

Exercise 34

Purpose. To develop the muscle tone of the lateral abdominal muscles.

Starting position. Lie on the back, with the arms folded across the chest and the legs outstretched (Fig. 39, A).

Movement. Tilt the pelvis to flatten the lower back to the floor and curl the head, shoulders, and back while moving to a sitting position, with one elbow reaching to the opposite knee (Fig. 39, B). Derotate and uncurl to the starting position. Do exercise alternately (Fig. 39, C).

Progression. Do the exercise five times the first exercise period, seven times the second period, and ten times the third period.

Precautions. Be sure that the trunk rotates and that the motion is not merely one of rolling to the side. Keep the arms close to the chest and make sure that the opposite elbow is not used as a prop to assist in the motion. The head and opposite shoulder should be slightly off the mat. The head should always be in the same plane of motion as the trunk. This exercise is a progression from Exercise 33 and should not be attempted until ten repetitions of Exercise 33 can be done.

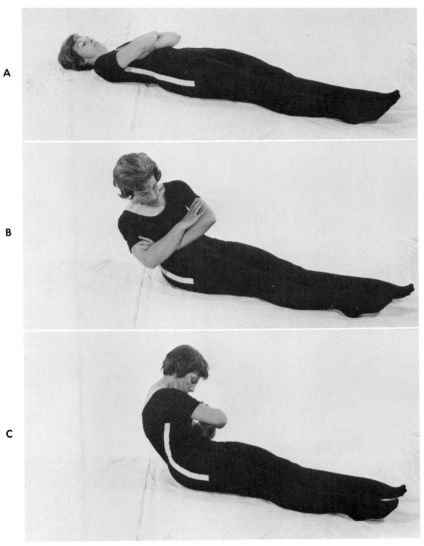

A

B

C

Fig. 39. Exercise 34.

Exercise 35

Purpose. To develop the muscle tone of the lateral abdominal muscles.

Starting position. Lie on the back, with the fingers laced behind the neck and the legs extended (Fig. 40, *A*).

Movement. Reach to the opposite knee with the opposite elbow (Fig. 40, *B*). Derotate and uncurl to the starting position. Do exercise alternately (Fig. 40, *C*).

Progression. Do the exercise five times the first exercise period, seven times the second period, and ten times the third period.

Precautions. Be sure that the trunk rotates and that the motion is not merely one of rolling to the side. Make sure that the opposite elbow is not used as a prop to assist in the motion. The head and opposite shoulder should be slightly off the mat. The head should always be in the same plane of motion as the trunk. This exercise is a progression from Exercise 34 and should not be attempted until ten repetitions of Exercise 34 can be done.

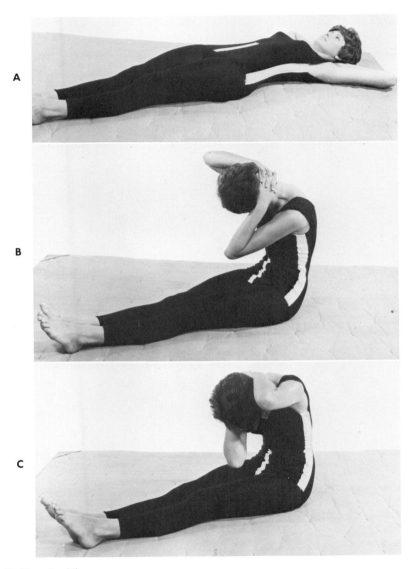

A

B

C

Fig. 40. Exercise 35.

Exercise 36

> *Purpose.* To develop the muscle tone of the lateral abdominal muscles.
>
> *Starting position.* Lie on the back, with the knees flexed.
>
> *Movement.* Extend both arms and reach toward the outside of the right thigh (Fig. 41). Return to the starting position. Do alternately.
>
> *Progression.* Do five repetitions the first exercise period, seven repetitions the second period, and ten repetitions the third period.
>
> *Precautions.* Be sure that the trunk rotates and that the motion is not merely one of rolling to the side. The head and opposite shoulder should be slightly off the mat. The head should always be in the same plane of motion as the trunk. This exercise is a progression from Exercise 35 and should not be attempted until ten repetitions of Exercise 35 can be done. A partner may stabilize the legs by placing one hand on the knees and one hand on the feet.

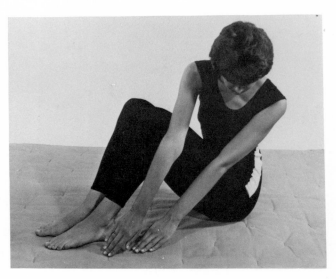

Fig. 41. Exercise 36.

Exercise 37

Purpose. To develop the muscle tone of the lateral abdominal muscles.

Starting position. Lie on the back, with the arms folded across the chest and the heels to the buttocks.

Movement. Curl to a sitting position and touch the right knee with the opposite elbow (Fig. 42). Do alternately.

Progression. Do the exercise five times the first exercise period, seven times the second period, and ten times the third period.

Precautions. Be sure that the trunk rotates and that the motion is not merely one of rolling to the side. Keep the arms folded close to the chest and make sure that the opposite elbow is not used as a prop to assist in the motion. The head and opposite shoulder should be slightly off the mat. The head should always be in the same plane of motion as the trunk. This exercise is a progression from Exercise 36 and should not be attempted until ten repetitions of Exercise 36 can be done. A partner may stabilize the legs by placing one hand on the knees and one hand on the feet.

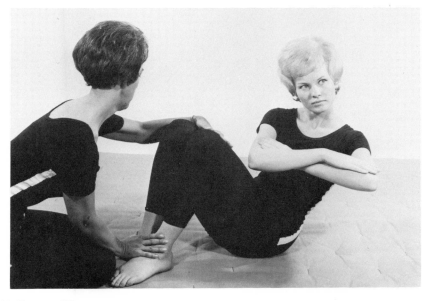

Fig. 42. Exercise 37.

Exercise 38

Purpose. To develop the muscle tone of the lateral abdominal muscles.

Starting position. Lie on the back, with the fingers laced behind the head and the heels to the buttocks.

Movement. Reach toward the outside of the opposite knee. Return to the starting position. Do alternately (Fig. 43, *A* and *B*).

Progression. Do the exercise five times the first exercise period, seven times the second period, and ten times the third period.

Precautions. Eliminate jerking motions; make sure that the motion is performed in a curling fashion. Do not arch the back. Rotation should be initiated at the beginning of the upward movement and derotation should be initiated at the start of the return movement. A partner may stabilize the legs by placing one hand on the knees and one hand on the feet.

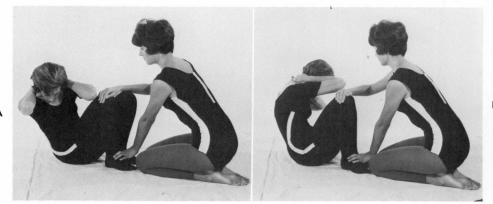

Fig. 43. Exercise 38.

Exercise 39

Purpose. To strengthen the hip flexor and lower abdominal muscles.

Starting position. Lie on the back, with the arms extended at the sides and the legs outstretched (Fig. 44, A).

Movement. Tilt the pelvis and lower the back flat on the mat. Bring the heels to the buttocks and pull the knees to the chest as far as possible (Fig. 44, B to D). Lower the feet to the floor close to the buttocks and extend the legs.

Progression. Do the exercise three times the first exercise period, five times the second period, seven times the third period, and ten times the second week.

Precautions. This exercise should not be attempted until the second progression of the curling sit-up is accomplished.

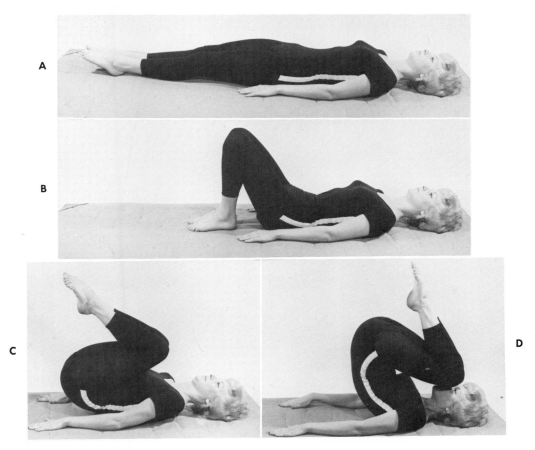

Fig. 44. Exercise 39.

Exercise 40

Purpose. To strengthen the lower abdominal muscles.

Starting position. Lie on the back, with the arms at shoulder level and perpendicular to the trunk.

Movement. Bring the heels along the floor toward the buttocks and curl the knees to the chest, thus lifting the pelvis off the mat. Rotating the pelvis to the left, lower the knees slowly to the left, almost touching the floor over the left shoulder. In this position, lower the pelvis and at the same time derotate to the starting position. Do alternately (Fig. 45, A and B).

Progression. Do the exercise five times the first exercise period, seven times the second period, and ten times the third period.

Precautions. Do not allow jerking motions to raise the pelvis off the mat. Be sure that the movement is a rotation movement instead of a mere rolling of the body from side to side.

A 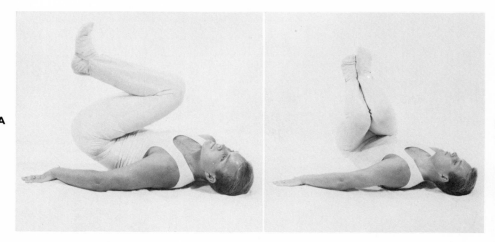 B

Fig. 45. Exercise 40.

EXERCISES FOR MUSCLES OF THE SHOULDER GIRDLE, NECK, AND CHEST

The area of the shoulder girdle includes the muscles that surround the shoulder area, both anteriorly and posteriorly, and those muscles of the shoulder that raise and lower the arm. These muscles tend to lose their tone quickly and can result in postural problems such as rounded shoulders or forward head tilt. These muscles do respond readily to exercise and regain normal action more quickly than do some other muscle groups.

We are living in a round shouldered society. Our daily work and play activities force us into a round shouldered posture. For example, assume the positions used while doing housework—washing dishes—vacuuming—dusting—all are done with shoulders forward. Even yard work demands rounded shoulders—working with power lawn mower, raking and shoveling. Mothers have even more forces working against them. Try to love and cuddle a child with square, pushed back shoulders.

Many professions force people into the round shouldered posture—scientists, photographers, computer operators, and even some athletes. The waiting position in tennis and volleyball, the approach in bowling, infield position in softball, swimming, skiing, basketball, and other sports force the participants into a round shouldered posture. This problem can be corrected by regular participation in activities that strengthen and tone the muscles in the back of the shoulder, such as formal ballet training, fencing, archery, back crawl stroke, and selected formal exercises.

Exercises 41 through 49 follow.

Exercise 41

Purpose. To develop tone and to strengthen the shoulder adductor muscles.

Starting position. Lie facedown, with the arms at the side and the head to the side (Fig. 46, A).

Movement. Place the shoulder blades together, using a smooth, even motion; contract the muscles vigorously (Fig. 46, B). Hold the position 5 seconds, slowly relax the shoulder muscles, and return to the starting position.

Progression. Do the exercise five times the first exercise period, seven times the second period, and ten times the third period.

Precautions. Move the shoulder blades toward each other and eliminate up-and-down movements.

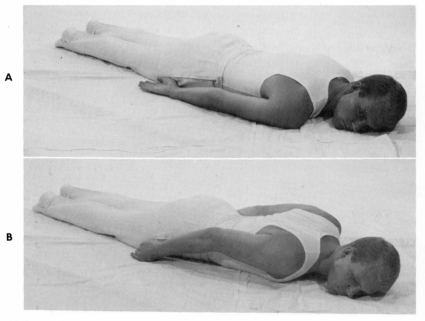

Fig. 46. Exercise 41.

Exercise 42

Purpose. To develop tone and strength in the shoulder adductor muscles.

Starting position. Lie facedown, with the arms at shoulder level, the head to the side, and the elbows bent to 90 degrees.

Movement. Bring the shoulder blades together and lift the arms from the mat. Hold the position 3 to 5 seconds. Return slowly to the starting position (Fig. 47).

Progression. Do the exercise five times the first exercise period, seven times the second period, and ten times the third period.

Precautions. Maintain the initial arm position throughout the movement and keep the wrists the same level as the elbows. Eliminate internal and external rotation. This exercise is a progression from Exercise 41 and should not be attempted until ten repetitions of Exercise 41 can be done.

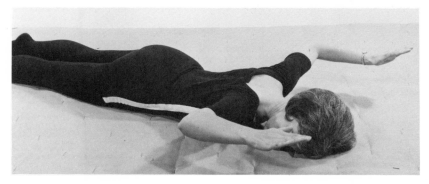

Fig. 47. Exercise 42.

Exercise 43

Purpose. To develop muscle tone and to strengthen the shoulder adductor muscles.

Starting position. Lie facedown, with the arms outstretched at shoulder level.

Movement. Bring the shoulder blades together, raise the arms off the mat as far as possible, and return slowly to starting position (Fig. 48).

Progression. Do the exercise five times the first exercise period, seven times the second period, and ten times the third period.

Precautions. Keep the arms at shoulder level throughout the movement. Do not allow the arms to rotate in either direction during the movement. This exercise is a progression from Exercise 42 and should not be attempted until ten repetitions of Exercise 42 can be done.

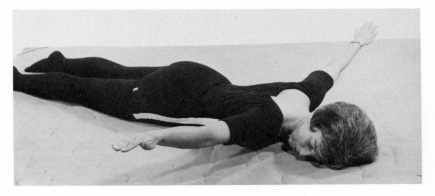

Fig. 48. Exercise 43.

Exercise 44

Purpose. To strengthen the posterior depressor muscles of the shoulder girdle.

Starting position. Lie facedown, with the arms outstretched over the head and in midposition at 45 degrees.

Movement. Raise the arms off the mat as far as possible and keep the elbows straight. Hold 5 seconds and return to the starting position (Fig. 49).

Progression. Do exercise five times the first exercise period, seven times the second period, and ten times the third period.

Precautions. Do not bend the elbows. The face should be at the side. Do not bridge the neck in an attempt to perform this motion. This exercise is a progression of Exercise 43 and should not be done until ten repetitions of Exercise 43 can be done.

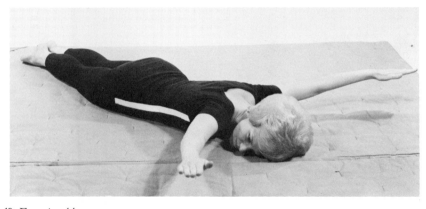

Fig. 49. Exercise 44.

Exercise 45

Purpose. To strengthen the posterior depressor muscles of the shoulder girdle.

Starting position. Lie facedown, with the arms outstretched over the head at approximately 30 degrees abduction.

Movement. Raise the arms off the mat as far as possible and keep the elbows straight. Hold 5 seconds and return to the starting position (Fig. 50).

Progression. Do the exercise five times the first exercise period, seven times the second period, and ten times the third period.

Precautions. Do not bend the elbows. The face should be at the side. Do not bridge the neck in an attempt to perform this motion. This exercise is a progression from Exercise 44 and should not be attempted until ten repetitions of Exercise 44 can be done.

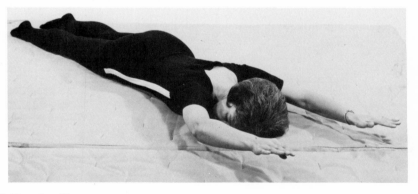

Fig. 50. Exercise 45.

Exercise 46

Purpose. To strengthen the posterior depressor muscles of the shoulder girdle.

Starting position. Lie facedown, with the arms outstretched and extended over the head.

Movement. Raise the arms off the mat as far as possible above the head and keep the elbows straight (Fig. 51). Hold 5 seconds and return to the starting position.

Progression. Do the exercise five times the first exercise period, seven times the second period, and ten times the third period.

Precautions. Do not bend the elbows. The face should be at the side. Do not bridge the neck in an attempt to perform this motion. This exercise is a progression from Exercise 45 and should not be attempted until ten repetitions of Exercise 45 can be done.

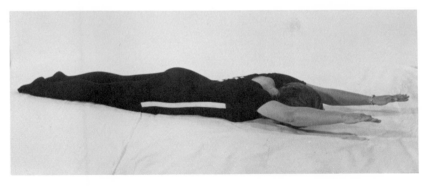

Fig. 51. Exercise 46.

Exercise 47

Purpose. To strengthen the muscles of the upper arm and the shoulder girdle.

Starting position. Stand facing the stall bars or a door frame approximately arm's length away. Lean forward and grasp the stall bars or place the hands on the wall at approximately shoulder level.

Movement. Bending the elbows only, lower the body to the stall bars or into the door space to chest level. Push the body back to the original starting position by extending the arms (Fig. 52, *A*).

Progression. Do the exercise three times the first exercise period, five times the second period, and ten times the third period. Every third exercise period, move down 6 inches below the starting level. Progressively do this until the exercise can be done at waist level. Then a low table should be used to perform this same exercise (Fig. 52, *B* and *C*). The heels are allowed to raise from the floor during the exercise at table level. Do the exercise in this position until ten repetitions can be done easily. Then move to a position between two chairs. Repeat this exercise until ten repetitions can be done. Then progress to a normal leaning rest position and increase three times the second period, five times the third period, seven times the fourth period, and ten times the fifth period (Fig. 52, *D* and *E*). The leaning rest position for women should be with the knees on the floor. For men, a normal leaning rest position would be with the knees extended and the weight on the toes.

Precautions. Be sure that proper body alignment is maintained throughout movement: head, shoulders, hips, knees, and ankles should be in alignment. Keep the elbows at shoulder level.

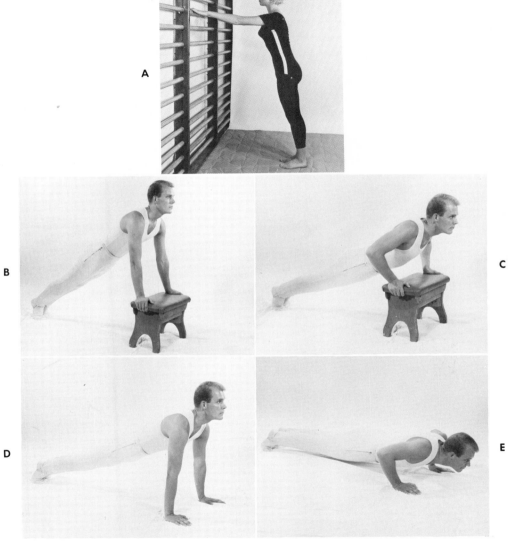

Fig. 52. Exercise 47.

Exercise 48

Purpose. To strengthen the muscles of the arm, shoulder girdle, and wrist.

Starting position. Use a two-arm support on parallel bars (Fig. 53, *A*).

Movement. Keeping the body in a vertical position, bend the arms at the elbows and lower the body until the elbows form a 90 degree angle (Fig. 53, *B*). Return to the starting position.

Progression. Do the exercise one time the first exercise period and increase one time each subsequent exercise period.

Precautions. Keep the elbows above the bar. Lower the body slowly and maintain your grip.

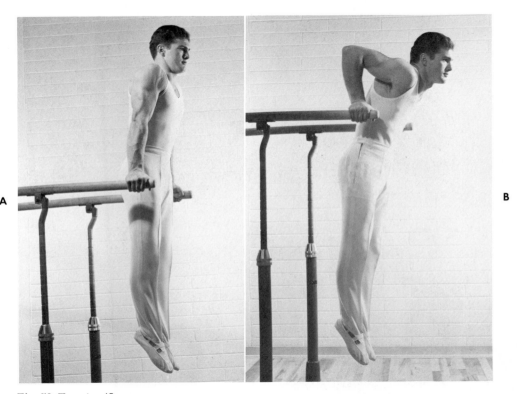

Fig. 53. Exercise 48.

Exercise 49

Purpose. To strengthen the muscles of the arm, shoulder girdle, and wrist.

Starting position. Use a two-arm hanging position (Fig. 54, *A*) (modified hanging position for women, Fig. 54, *B*).

Movement. Pull the body upward until the elbows form a 90 degree angle (Fig. 54, *C* and *D*). Return to the starting position.

Progression. Do the exercise three times the first exercise period, five times the second period, seven times the third period, and ten times each period following.

Precautions. Eliminate all trunk and leg movements and swinging movements.

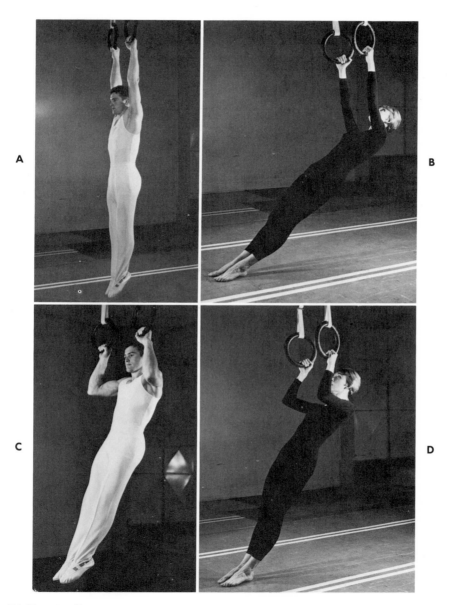

Fig. 54. Exercise 49.

EXERCISES FOR THE ANTERIOR CHEST MUSCLES

The exercises in this section are specifically selected to increase the tone of the anterior chest muscles. The exercises are isometric in nature, which means that there is little or no movement as the muscle contracts against resistance.

Exercise 50

Purpose. To strengthen and tone the middle portion of the pectoralis major muscles (chest muscles).

Starting position. Sit in a tailor position.

Movement. Elevate the arms to shoulder level with the heels of the hands facing each other. Bending the elbows to 90 degrees and compressing the heels of the hands, maintain this position. Push the left arm to the right, forcibly resisting this movement with the right arm. Do alternately to each side (Fig. 55).

Progression. Do the exercise five times to each side. Each repetition should require about 10 seconds.

Precautions. The trunk should not be rotated during this movement. Movement should occur only at the shoulder level. Avoid movement at the hips.

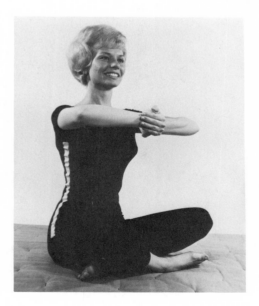

Fig. 55. Exercise 50.

Exercise 51

Purpose. To strengthen and tone the upper portion of the pectoralis major muscles.

Starting position. Sit in a tailor position and elevate the arms to approximately head level (Fig. 56).

Movement. Push the hands forcibly together until a strong contraction is felt in the upper part of the anterior chest muscles. Hold this position for approximately 5 seconds. Release pressure and then relax.

Progression. Do the exercise five times.

Precautions. Maintain the trunk and body in proper alignment, as described in the starting position.

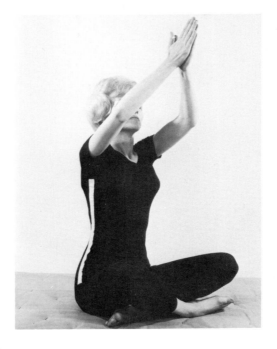

Fig. 56. Exercise 51.

Exercise 52

Purpose. To strengthen and tone the lower portion of the pectoralis major muscle.

Starting position. Sit in a tailor position. Extend the arms and bring the hands together between the knees (Fig. 57).

Movement. Compress the hands together as forcibly as possible, maintaining the arms in the starting position. Hold the position 7 to 8 seconds and relax. Keep the elbows bent at approximately 30 degrees.

Progression. Do the exercise five times.

Precautions. Apply constant pressure. Avoid bobbing movements.

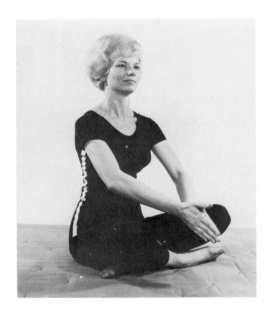

Fig. 57. Exercise 52.

EXERCISES FOR MUSCLES OF THE BACK AND NECK

There are limited activities in regular daily living that provide movement for strengthening the muscles of the upper back and neck. Formal and regular exercise sessions should, therefore, be planned to include strengthening these muscles. Care must be taken to isolate the muscle action during the performance of these exercises in order to avoid placing an unnecessary strain on the lower back muscles.

Exercise 53

Purpose. To strengthen the upper back extensor muscles.

Starting position. Lie facedown, with the arms at the sides (Fig. 58, *A*).

Movement. Place the shoulder blades together and extend or raise the head and chest off the mat. Hold the position 3 seconds and return to the starting position (Fig. 58, *B*).

Progression. Do the exercise three times the first exercise period, five times the second period, seven times the third period, and ten times the second week.

Precautions. Do not allow jerking motions. Be sure that the movement is straight or symmetrical and eliminate rotation. Exercises 53, 54, and 55 could possibly aggravate low back problems.

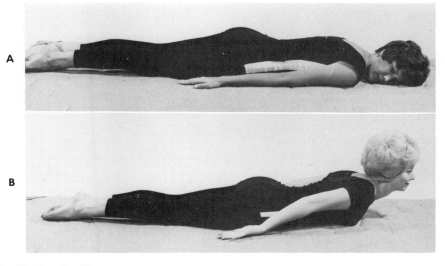

Fig. 58. Exercise 53.

Exercise 54

Purpose. To strengthen the back extensor and shoulder adductor muscles.

Starting position.   Lie facedown, with the hands clasped in the small of the back (Fig. 59, *A*).

Movement. Extend the arms toward the feet, bring the shoulder blades together, and raise the head and shoulders off the mat (Fig. 59, *B*). Hold 3 to 5 seconds and return to the starting position.

Progression. Do the exercise three times the first exercise period, five times the second period, seven times the third period, and ten times the second week.

Precautions. Do not allow jerking motions. Be sure that the movement is straight and symmetrical. Eliminate rotation. This exercise is a progression from Exercise 53 and should not be attempted until ten repetitions of Exercise 53 can be done.

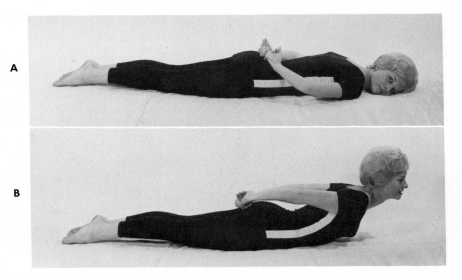

Fig. 59. Exercise 54.

Exercise 55

Purpose. To strengthen the back extensor muscles.

Starting position. Lie facedown, with the fingers laced behind the head (Fig. 60, *A*).

Movement. Raise the elbows off the mat, bring the shoulder blades together, and raise the head and chest off the mat (Fig. 60, *B*). Hold 3 to 5 seconds and return to the starting position.

Progression. Do the exercise five times the first exercise period, seven times the second period, and ten times the third period.

Precautions. Do not allow jerking motions. Be sure that the movement is straight or symmetrical. Eliminate rotation. This exercise is a progression from Exercise 54 and should not be attempted until ten repetitions of Exercise 54 can be done.

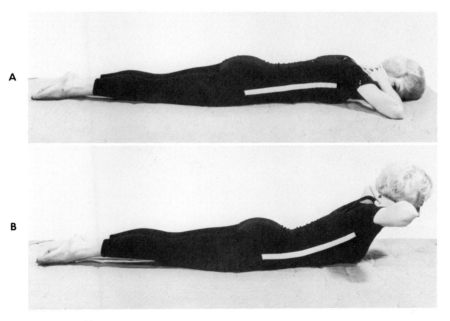

Fig. 60. Exercise 55.

Exercise 56

Purpose. To strengthen the upper back extensor muscles.

Starting position. Kneel and sit on the heels with the knees spread apart and the arms at the sides. Bend forward from the hips. Place the forehead on the mat, reaching forward as far as possible without raising the heels (Fig. 61, *A*).

Movement. Bring the shoulder blades together and extend the neck and the back as high as possible to the horizontal position without moving at the hips. Hold the position 3 to 5 seconds and return to the starting position (Fig. 61, *B*).

Progression. Do the exercise three times the first exercise period, five times the second period, seven times the third period, and ten times the second week.

Precautions. Do not extend beyond the horizontal position, as this will cause movement in the lower back instead of in the upper back. Movement should be initiated from the neck through the upper back and not from the lower back (Fig. 61, *C* and *D*).

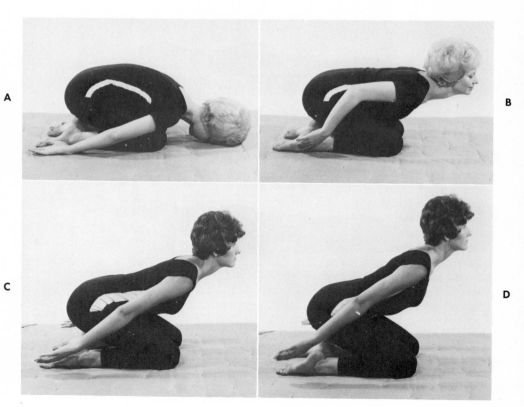

Fig. 61. Exercise 56.

Exercise 57

Purpose. To strengthen the upper back extensor muscles.

Starting position. Kneel and sit on the heels with the knees spread apart and the hands clasped in the small of the back and bend forward from the hips. Place the forehead on the mat and reach forward as far as possible without raising the heels (Fig. 62, *A*).

Movement. Extend the arms, reaching toward the buttocks. Hold the position 3 to 5 seconds and return to starting position (Fig. 62, *B*).

Progression. Do the exercise five times the first exercise period, seven times the second period, and ten times the third period.

Precautions. Do not extend beyond the horizontal position, as this will cause movement in the lower back instead of in the upper back. Movement should be initiated from the neck through the upper back and not from the lower back. This exercise is a progression from Exercise 56 and should not be attempted until ten repetitions of Exercise 56 can be done.

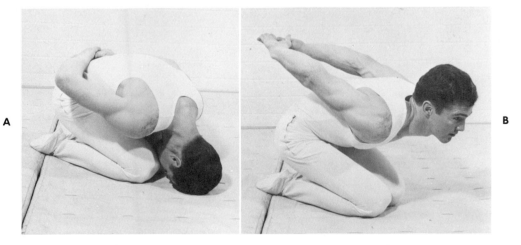

A   B

Fig. 62. Exercise 57.

Exercise 58

Purpose. To strengthen the upper back extensor muscles.

Starting position. Kneel and sit on the heels, with the knees spread apart and the fingers laced behind the head. Bend forward from the hips. Place the forehead on the mat, reaching forward as far as possible without raising the heels (Fig. 63, *A*).

Movement. Extend the arms, reaching toward the buttocks. Raise the elbows and bring the shoulder blades together (Fig. 63, *B*). Hold the position 3 to 5 seconds and return to the starting position.

Progression. Do the exercise five times the first exercise period, seven times the second period, and ten times the third period.

Precautions. Do not extend beyond the horizontal position, as this will cause movement in the lower back instead of in the upper back. Movement should be initiated from the neck through the upper back and not from the lower back. This exercise is a progression from Exercise 57 and should not be attempted until ten repetitions of Exercise 57 can be done.

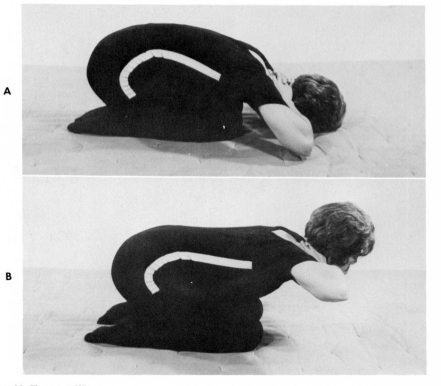

Fig. 63. Exercise 58.

Exercise 59

Purpose. To strengthen the back extensor muscles and rotator muscles of the spine.

Starting position. Lie facedown, with the arms to the sides and the legs extended.

Movement. Place the shoulder blades together. Raise the head and chest off the mat and rotate the upper body to the right from the beginning of the movement (Fig. 64). Hold the position 3 to 5 seconds and return to the starting position, derotating through the return movement. Repeat the exercise to the left.

Progression. Do the exercise three times the first exercise period, five times the second period, seven times the third period, and ten times the second week.

Precautions. Avoid jerking motions. Be sure that the shoulder initiates the movement. Rotation should be initiated at the beginning of the movement and not after the head and chest are off the mat.

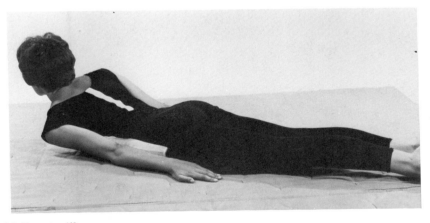

Fig. 64. Exercise 59.

Exercise 60

Purpose. To strengthen the back extensor muscles and rotator muscles of the spine.

Starting position. Lie facedown, with the legs extended and the arms clasped in the small of the back and extended toward the heels.

Movement. Place the shoulder blades together. Raise the head off the mat and then rotate to the right. Raise the trunk off the mat as far as possible (Fig. 65). Hold the position 3 to 5 seconds. Return to the starting position, derotating throughout the return movement. Repeat the exercise to the left.

Progression. Do the exercise three times the first exercise period, five times the second period, seven times the third period, and ten times the second week.

Precautions. Avoid jerking motions. Be sure that the shoulder initiates the movement. Rotation should be initiated at the beginning of the movement and not after the head and chest are off the mat.

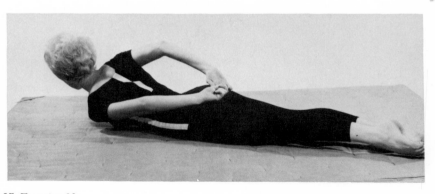

Fig. 65. Exercise 60.

Exercise 61

Purpose. To strengthen the back extensor muscles and rotator muscles of the spine.

Starting position. Lie facedown, with the fingers laced behind the neck and the legs in an extended position.

Movement. Raise the head, chest, and trunk off the mat and rotate the upper body to the right as far as possible (Fig. 66). Hold the position 5 seconds. Return to the starting position, derotating throughout the return movement. Repeat the exercise to the left.

Progression. Do the exercise three times the first exercise period, five times the second period, seven times the third period, and ten times the second week.

Precautions. Be sure that the head is in proper alignment with the trunk throughout the movement. Avoid lateral flexion of the trunk. Do not allow jerking or pendular motions to extend or rotate the trunk.

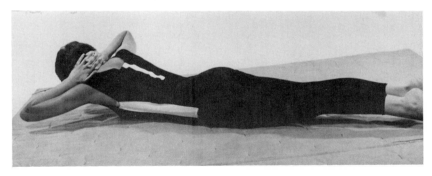

Fig. 66. Exercise 61.

Exercise 62

Purpose. To increase strength in the back extensor muscles and the rotator muscles of the spine.

Starting position. Have a partner stabilize the feet at the ankles. Lie facedown, with the arms extended over the head and the legs extended.

Movement. Raise the arms, head, and trunk off the mat and rotate the upper body to the right as far as possible (Fig. 67, *A*). Hold the position 5 seconds. Derotate, returning to the starting position. Repeat the exercise to the left (Fig. 67, *B*).

Progression. Do the exercise three times the first exercise period, five times the second period, seven times the third period, and ten times the second week.

Precautions. Be sure that the arms, head, and trunk remain in the same plane throughout the motion. Avoid lateral flexion of the trunk. Do not allow jerking motions.

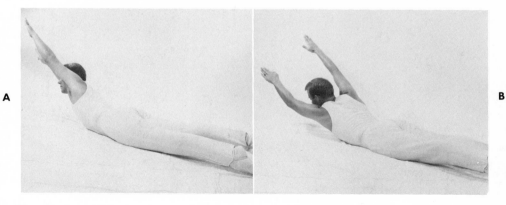

Fig. 67. Exercise 62.

EXERCISES FOR MUSCLES OF THE HIP AND LEG

Because the muscles of the buttock area are difficult to strengthen, care must be taken to isolate the muscle action by avoiding substitution of other related muscle groups. Keeping the pelvis on the floor or mat during the exercise performance is one way of maintaining proper body alignment during these exercises. The strengthening of these muscles is essential to the maintenance of good posture and to the practice of correct walking and running movements.

Exercise 63

Purpose. To strengthen the hip extensor muscles.

Starting position. Lie facedown, with the arms at the sides and the legs extended.

Movement. Raise the leg as high as possible without raising the pelvis off the mat (Fig. 68, A). Return to the starting position. Alternate with each leg.

Progression. Do the exercise three times the first exercise period, five times the second period, seven times the third period, and ten times the second week. When able to do ten repetitions easily, hold the position 3 to 5 seconds each time.

Precautions. Keep the pelvis on the mat at all times. Do not arch the lower back. Keep the face and chest on the mat (Fig. 68, B).

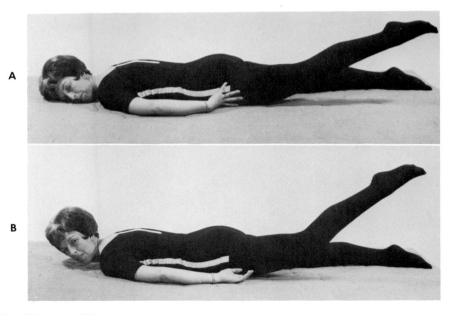

A

B

Fig. 68. Exercise 63.

Exercise 64

Purpose. To strengthen the hip extensor muscles.

Starting position. Lie facedown, with the arms at the sides, the right knee flexed to 90 degrees, and the left leg extended (Fig. 69, *A*).

Movement. Raise the right leg off the mat as high as possible without violating precautions (Fig. 69, *B*). Return to the starting position. Do alternately.

Progression. Do the exercise three times the first exercise period, five times the second period, seven times the third period, and ten times the second week.

Precautions. Keep the pelvis flat on the mat at all times. Do not use the lower back extensor muscles in place of the hip extensor or gluteal muscles.

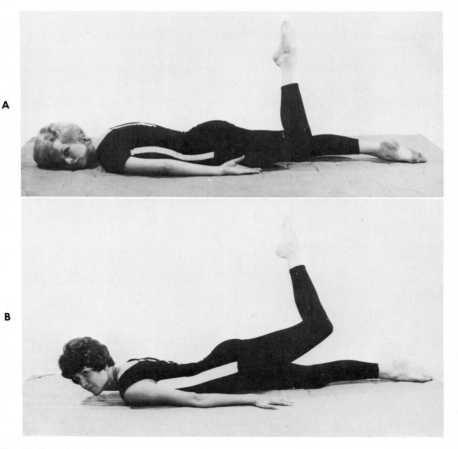

Fig. 69. Exercise 64.

Exercise 65

Purpose. To strengthen the abductor and adductor muscles of the hip.

Starting position. Lie on the right side and place the right hand on the left shoulder, with the arm perpendicular to the body. Place the left arm in a forward extended position, with the palm on the mat. Keep the head, shoulders, hips, knees, and ankles in straight alignment (Fig. 70, *A* and *B*).

Movement. Raise the left leg as high as possible and then raise the right leg up to meet the left leg (Fig. 70, *C*). Return both legs to the starting position.

Progression. Do the exercise three times the first exercise period, five times the second period, seven times the third period, and ten times the second week. When able to do ten repetitions easily, hold the position for 3 seconds each time. Then increase the duration of the hold to 5 seconds.

Precautions. Be sure that the body maintains proper alignment throughout exercise. If this alignment is difficult to maintain, turn the legs inward and extend them until proper alignment is attained. The abdominal wall should remain flat throughout the exercise, and the buttocks should not protrude (Fig. 70, *D* and *E*).

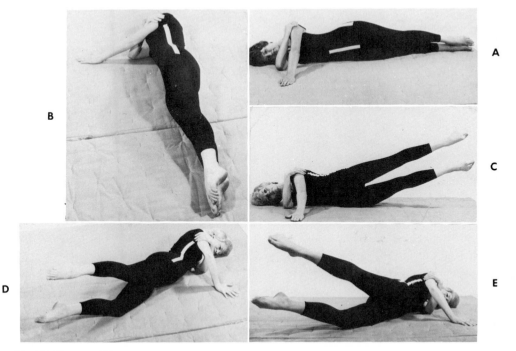

Fig. 70. Exercise 65.

EXERCISES FOR MUSCLES OF THE FEET

Exercises for strengthening of the muscles of the feet are corrective in nature. However, the muscles of the feet can be strengthened, and thus the need for corrective therapy may be prevented.

Exercise 66

Purpose. To strengthen the muscles of the feet.

Starting position. Sit on a bench without the weight on the feet, with marbles in front of the toes and a cup behind the opposite heel.

Movement. Grasp the marbles with the toes. Turn the forepart of the foot and drop the marbles into the cup (Fig. 71, *A* and *B*).

Progression. Use ten marbles throughout.

Precautions. Allow no movement in the hips. Keep all the action in the foot and lower leg.

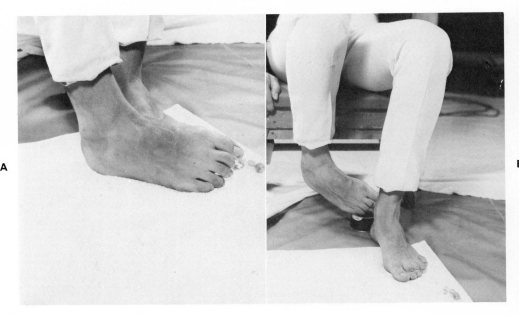

A   B

Fig. 71. Exercise 66.

Exercise 67

Purpose. To strengthen the muscles of the feet.

Starting position. Sit on a bench with the feet placed on a towel (Fig. 72).

Movement. With the feet parallel on the towel, gather the towel under the feet with the toes.

Progression. Do ten times each exercise session.

Precaution. Keep the heels on floor and gather the towel with the toes.

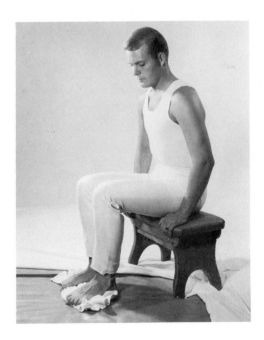

Fig. 72. Exercise 67.

Exercise 68

Purpose. To strengthen the muscles of the feet.
Starting position. Stand on a block or step with the toes extended.
Movement. Bend the toes down over edge of the block or step (Fig. 73).
Progression. Do ten times each exercise session.
Precaution. Keep the heels on the board.

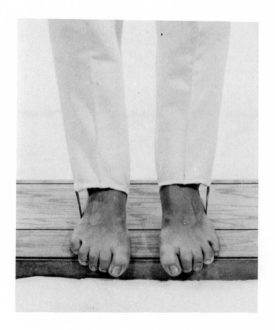

Fig. 73. Exercise 68.

Exercise 69

> *Purpose.* To strengthen the muscles of the feet.
> *Starting position.* Stand with the weight on the outside edge of the feet and with the toes gripped.
> *Movement.* Walk forward (Fig. 74).
> *Progression.* Take ten steps forward with each foot.
> *Precaution.* Maintain good standing and walking posture.

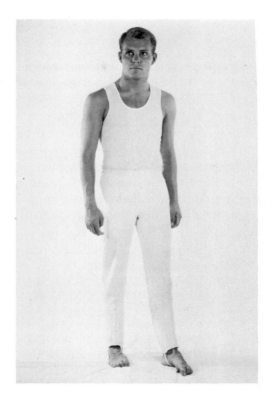

Fig. 74. Exercise 69.

Chapter 5
Exercises to improve
body contour

All of the exercises in the previous chapters will contribute to improved contour of certain parts of the body because they contribute to strength, endurance, and tone of the muscles and to the reduction of fatty deposits in the exercised areas. But the exercises in this particular chapter are especially selected to slenderize or reshape the areas of the body where reshaping is often most desired, with emphasis on the midsection, hips, and thighs. These exercises will cause sagging muscles, especially in the waist and hip regions, to become firm and tight. The increased strength, endurance, and tone resulting from these exercises may also improve posture and body carriage. Furthermore, these exercises will help to prevent fat from accumulating in areas of the body where fat is unbecoming. Several of the exercises in this chapter are also the type that will increase general physical fitness if done with sufficient vigor.

Exercise 70 (hip walking)

Purpose. To localize muscle action primarily to the hip and thigh area in an attempt to slenderize.

Starting position. Sit with legs and arms extended and body in proper alignment (Fig. 75, A).

Movement. Maintaining the legs in straight position and the arms at shoulder level and extended, shift the weight to the right hip and pull the left hip and leg forward. Shift the weight to the left hip and pull the right hip and leg forward (Fig. 75, B). Repeat this movement alternately forward and backward.

Progression. Start by doing five walking motions to the front and five to the back. Increase one time every exercise period until ten. After ten repetitions can be done easily and correctly, the cadence of exercise should then be increased. To begin, the cadence of exercise should be five every 2 seconds, or five walking motions forward and backward should be completed within 5 seconds. The cadence of the exercise should be increased every other exercise period until ten walking motions forward and ten walking motions backward can be completed within one period of 5 seconds. This exercise should be continued for a period of 15 seconds.

Precautions. Be sure that the movement is forward and backward and not from side to side.

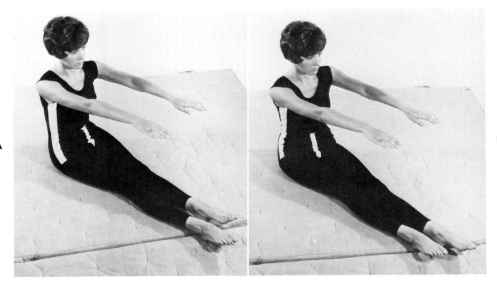

A B

Fig. 75. Exercise 70.

Exercise 71 (side straddle)

Purpose. To develop general physical fitness.

Starting position. A functional standing position is used (Fig. 76, A).

Movement. Jump into the air, landing in a side straddle position, with the arms extended over the head and the feet approximately 18 to 24 inches apart. Jump into the air and return to the starting position (Fig. 76, B).

Progression. Start with ten and increase three times every exercise period until tolerance.

Precautions. This exercise is a reciprocal type of motion and should be done smoothly and rhythmically to a cadence of approximately one jump per second.

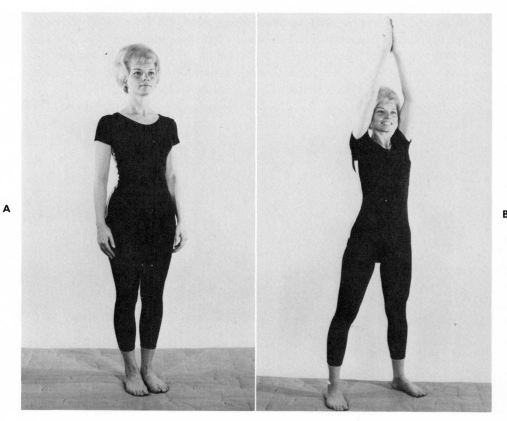

Fig. 76. Exercise 71.

Exercise 72 (bicycling)

Purpose. To slenderize the hip and thigh areas.

Starting position. Lie on back with the knees flexed to the chest and the pelvis lifted off the mat and supported with the hands on the pelvis (Fig. 77, *A*).

Movement. Alternately extend the knee and the hip in an arc of motion equivalent to approximately an 8-inch circle. Then flex the hip and the knee in the same manner. This motion should be done to a count of approximately two movements per second (Fig. 77, *B* and *C*).

Progression. Do twenty repetitions three times with a half-minute rest between each. Increase every third exercise period according to tolerance.

Precautions. Be sure this movement is performed in a bicycling type of motion. Do not bend the knees to the point at which the heel hits the buttocks. Make sure that hip motion is used, not just knee motion.

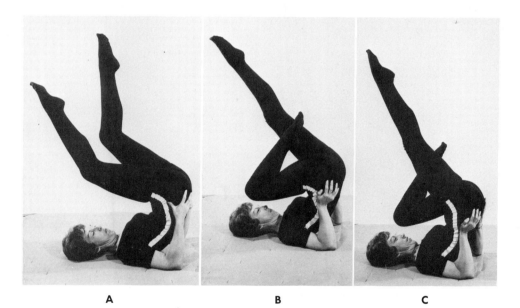

A   B   C

Fig. 77. Exercise 72.

Exercise 73 (running in place)

Purpose. To provide general muscular conditioning and to slenderize the waist and midriff areas.

Starting position. Stand with the hands on the hips.

Movement. Run in place, lifting the knees toward the chest as high as possible (Fig. 78). Running should be done as fast as possible.

Progression. Start running in place for 10 seconds with the first exercise period. Increase 5 seconds after every third workout period until tolerance. Both the speed and length of the exercise period should be done progressively.

Precautions. Maintain a fairly erect standing position with the trunk and bring the knees to the chest. Avoid leaning backward.

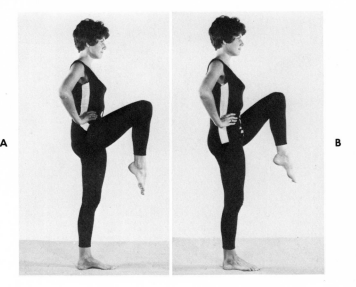

A   B

Fig. 78. Exercise 73.

Exercise 74

Purpose. To slenderize the waist and midriff area.

Starting position. Stand with the legs spread apart in a side stride position and the hands on the hips (Fig. 79, *A*).

Movement. This exercise should be done to a cadence count. On count one, rotate the trunk and bend forward and reach with the right hand to the outside of the left foot. On count two, return to the starting position. On count three, reach with the left hand to the outside of the right foot. On count four return to the starting position (Fig. 79, *B*).

Progression. Start by doing four repetitions every 10 seconds; then increase the number of repetitions by two times every other exercise period until eight, using the same count; then increase the cadence count slightly every other exercise period until approximately nine repetitions are completed every 15 seconds.

Example

First week: four repetitions, 10 seconds
Second week: six repetitions, 15 seconds
Third week: eight repetitions, 20 seconds
Fourth week: eight repetitions, 17 seconds
Fifth week: eight repetitions, 17 seconds
Sixth week: nine repetitions, 15 seconds

Precautions. Be sure that this movement is a trunk-rotating movement and not a side-bending movement. There is no side-to-side movement. The exercise should be done in precise fashion by going through the complete motion on every count. Do not do half motions.

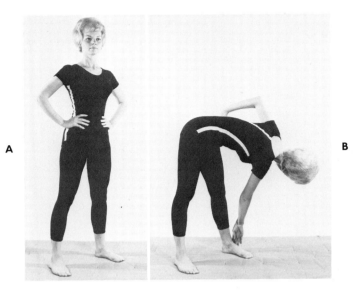

A B

Fig. 79. Exercise 74.

Exercise 75

> *Purpose.* To slenderize the hip and thigh areas.
>
> *Starting position.* Lie on side. Place the right hand on the left shoulder, with the arm perpendicular to the body. Place the left arm in an extended position with the palm on the mat and perpendicular to the body. Keep the head, shoulder, hip, knees, and ankle in straight alignment (Fig. 80, A).
>
> *Movement.* Raise both legs off the floor and kick back and forth alternately in a scissor motion (Fig. 80, B). Repeat the exercise on the left side.
>
> *Progression.* Start by doing ten repetitions to a cadence count of one repetition per second. Increase five repetitions every other exercise period until thirty. Then increase the count to thirty repetitions every 10 seconds. When the exercise can be done to this count, a suggested sequence would be to do fifteen repetitions to this count, rest one-half minute; then do twenty repetitions, rest one-half minute; then do thirty repetitions.
>
> *Precautions.* Good body alignment should be maintained at all times. The abdominal wall should be maintained in good posture and should not be allowed to protrude. Do not allow the pelvis to tilt forward and cause the back to arch. Also, do not bend forward at the hips. Make sure kicking motions pass beyond the midline on both forward and backward motions. Do not bend the knees.

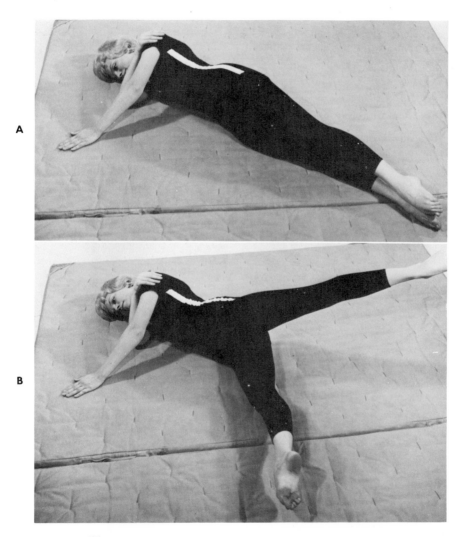

Fig. 80. Exercise 75.

Exercise 76

Purpose. To slenderize the waistline.

Starting position. Stand, with hands on the hips (Fig. 81, *A*).

Movement. Raise the right arm to shoulder level to the front. Raise the right leg with the knee extended (Fig. 81, *B*). Keep the arm at shoulder level, touch the foot to the hand, and return to the starting position.

Progression. Start by doing five to each side to a cadence of one repetition per second. Increase one time every other exercise period until ten. After ten, increase the speed of the exercise to tolerance.

Precautions. Eliminate bending forward from the waist or knee-bending to complete the motion. When increasing the speed of the exercise, be sure that the complete movement is performed.

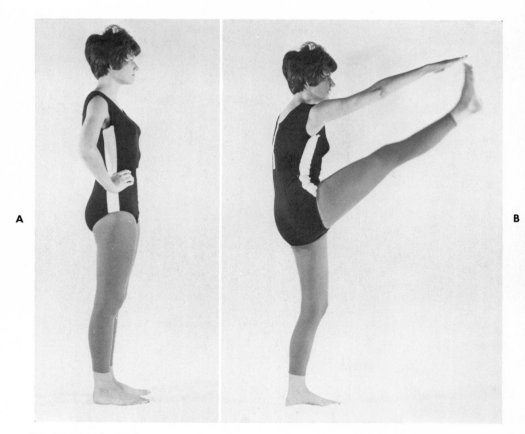

A   B

Fig. 81. Exercise 76.

Exercise 77

Purpose. To slenderize the waistline.

Starting position. Stand, with hands on the hips.

Movement. Raise the right arm to shoulder level and kick with the left leg and touch the right hand by rotating the trunk and pelvis during the movement (Fig. 82).

Progression. Start by doing five to each side to a cadence of one repetition per second. Increase one time every other exercise period until ten. After ten, increase the speed of the exercise to tolerance.

Precautions. Eliminate bending forward from the waist or knee-bending in order to complete the motion. When increasing the speed of the exercise, be sure that the complete movement is performed.

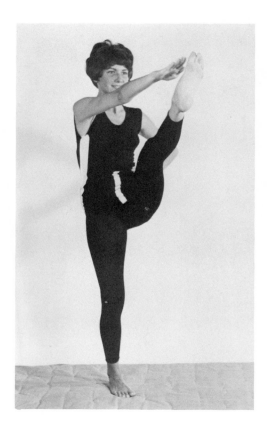

Fig. 82. Exercise 77.

Exercise 78

Purpose. To slenderize the waist and midriff.

Starting position. Sit with the legs spread apart and extended and the hands at the hips (Fig. 83, *A*).

Movement. Rotating and bending the trunk forward, reach to the right foot with the left hand. Derotate and return to the starting position (Fig. 83, *B*). Repeat with the right hand to the left foot.

Progression. Start by doing five to each side to a count of four. On the count of one, reach to the opposite foot; on the count of two return to the starting position; on the count of three reach with the alternate hand to the alternate foot: on the count of four return to the starting position. The cadence of this exercise should be five repetitions every 10 seconds.

Precautions. Keep the arms straight and elevated throughout the movement. Be sure that the knees are straight. Do not allow the hips to rotate or the buttocks to lift from the mat.

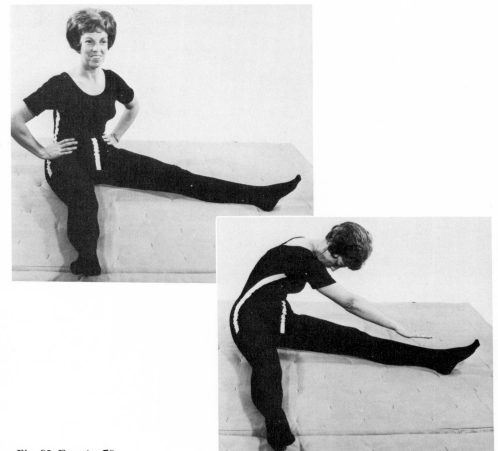

Fig. 83. Exercise 78.

Exercise 79

    Purpose. To slenderize the waistline.

    Starting position. Lie on the back, with the arms outstretched over the head, the palms up, and the legs extended (Fig. 84, *A*).

    Movement. Swing forward to a sitting position by bringing the arms and trunk forward and at the same time bringing the knees to the chest with the feet slightly off the floor (Fig. 84, *B*). Return to the starting position.

    Progression. Start by doing five; then increase one time every other exercise period until ten. This exercise should be done to a cadence count of approximately three repetitions every 5 seconds until ten repetitions; then the count should be one repetition every second.

    Precautions. This movement should be performed in a curling motion even though it is done to a fast count. Be sure that the back does not arch. The pelvis should not be allowed to tilt forward.

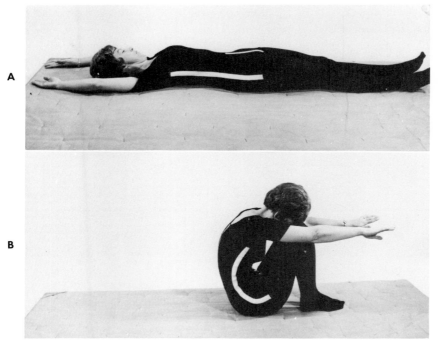

Fig. 84. Exercise 79.

Chapter 6
Exercises to be performed
on apparatus

These exercises, designed to strengthen and to tone muscle groups programmed previously, could have been included in the chapter on strengthening and toning. They should be a part of an exercise program, but since they require the use of apparatus, they should be introduced only after most of the students are in the second progression of the suggested exercises for the abdominal muscles. It is advantageous to have the work with apparatus a part of the regular exercise period.

At this time it should be repeated that in order to increase strength the muscles must be contracted regularly against heavy resistance, and the resistance must be progressively increased as the muscles become stronger. To increase endurance without much increase in strength, the muscles should be contracted regularly against relatively light resistance, and the contractions should be repeated many times in succession. Endurance overload may be applied by either increasing the number of repetitions or the amount of resistance against the muscle contractions.

Exercise 80

Purpose. To increase strength and endurance of the muscles which form the abdominal wall.

Starting position. Hang from the stall bars or horizontal bar (Fig. 85, A).

Movement. Curl the abdominal wall to flatten the back against the stall bars or wall, bringing the knees to the chest as far as possible (Fig. 85, B). Hold the position 5 seconds and return to starting position.

Progression. Begin with three and increase one time every other exercise period.

Precautions. Be sure that the lower abdominal wall maintains the pelvis, as described in the starting movement.

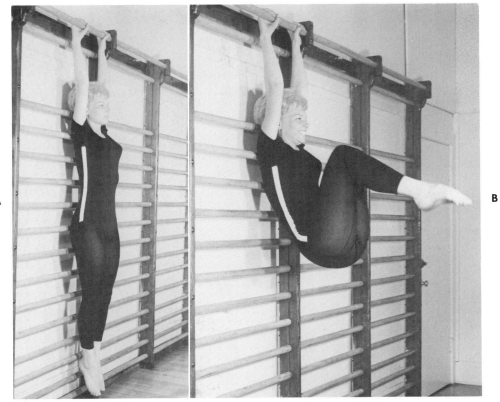

A   B

Fig. 85. Exercise 80.

Exercise 81

Purpose. To increase strength and endurance of muscles which form the abdominal wall.

Starting position. Hang from the stall bars, horizontal bar, or other apparatus.

Movement. Tighten the lower abdominal muscles to flatten the back. Bring the knees to the chest; then raise the pelvis toward the chest in a curling motion (Fig. 86). Hold position 3 seconds. Return slowly to starting position.

Progression. Do exercise three times; increase one every other exercise period.

Precautions. Be sure that the lower abdominal wall maintains the pelvis, as described in the starting movement.

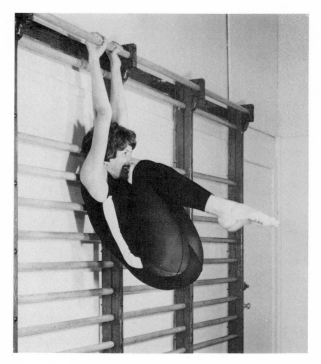

Fig. 86. Exercise 81.

Exercise 82

Purpose. To increase strength and endurance of the adductor muscles of the shoulder and shoulder girdle depressor muscles.

Starting position. Sit on a bench with the feet flat on the floor, the legs 2 to 3 inches apart, and the body in good sitting position.

Movement. Grasp with the palms forward the bar of the pulley weight apparatus, bringing the bar down in front of the body close to the chest to the thigh, in a slow rhythmic motion (Fig. 87, *A*). Return to the starting position and then bring the bar down behind the head and neck, maintaining good posture at all times (Fig. 87, *B*). Return slowly and rhythmically to the starting position.

Progression. Do the exercise five times to the front and five to the back, using a weight of 20 pounds. Increase two times front and back every exercise period until ten. After ten times, add 2½ to 5 pounds resistance and repeat the exercise progressively.

Precautions. Keep the bar motion close to the body at all times. Maintain good sitting posture by eliminating forward tilting of the pelvis and arching of the back (Fig. 87, *C* to *E*). Pull evenly with both arms at all times.

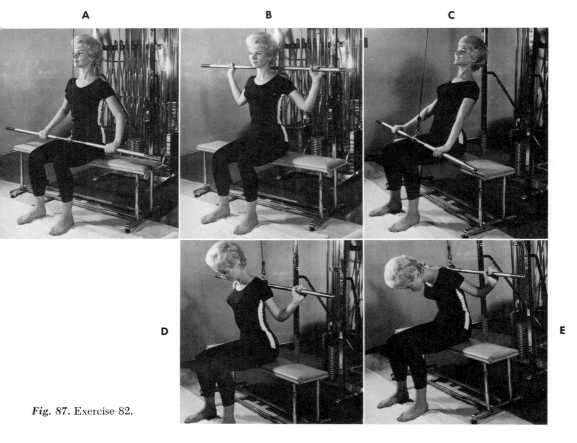

A   **B**   **C**

D   **E**

Fig. 87. Exercise 82.

Exercise 83

Purpose. To increase strength and endurance of the muscles of the calf and upper extremities and the back and hip extensor muscles and to develop the proper body mechanics of lifting.

Starting position. Stand in good posture, one foot advanced slightly ahead of the other and the feet 3 to 4 inches apart.

Movement. Using correct body mechanics, pick up the bar from the floor (Fig. 88, *A*) and return to a standing position (Fig. 88, *B* and *C*). Bring the bar over the head (Fig. 88, *D*) and raise the heels off the floor into a toe-standing position (Fig. 88, *E*). Lower the heels back to the floor; then lower the bar behind the head (Fig. 88, *F*). Place the bar back over the head, arms extended. Raise the heels off the floor to a toe-standing position; then lower the heels again to a standing position. Lower the bar to the front in a normal standing position. Using good body mechanics, return the bar to the floor.

Progression. At the first session of the exercise, use the barbell with the bar and 1¼ pound weights on each side to do three progressions; increase two times every exercise period until ten. After ten repetitions can be accomplished, increase the resistance by 1¼ pounds to each side of the bar, a total of 2½ pounds, and repeat progressively.

Precautions. Be sure that the proper body mechanics of lifting are observed at all times. Keep the barbell close to the center of gravity at all times in order to lessen the strain to muscle areas which are not to be used during the motion. Do not use a jerky, compensatory motion. The exercise should be formed in one smooth, rhythmic motion.

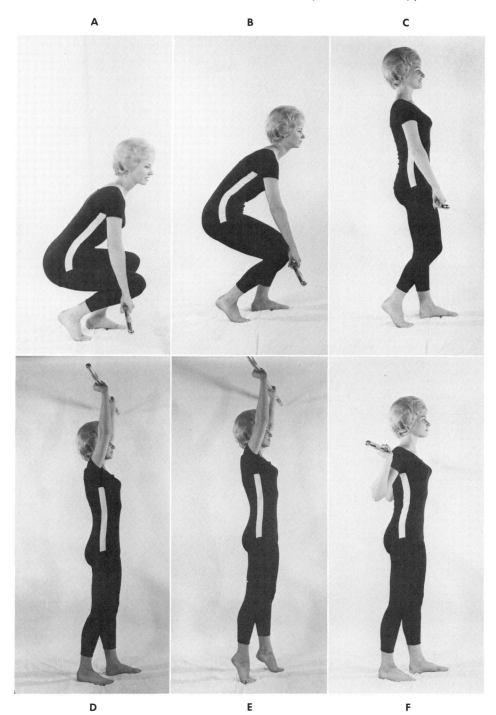

Fig. 88. Exercise 83.

Exercise 84

Purpose. To strengthen the anterior chest and shoulder girdle muscles.

Starting position. Lie on the back on the slant board, with the hands in a functional position and the palms facing the body, with dumbbells in each hand, and with the body in good postural alignment (Fig. 89, *A*).

Movement 1. With the arms extended, elevate the arms forward to a vertical position (Fig. 89, *B*). Lower the arms slowly to the starting position.

Movement 2. In the movement, the arms should be elevated and horizontally adducted at approximately a 30-degree angle (Fig. 89, *C*). Return slowly and rhythmically to the starting position.

Movement 3. Bring the arms to a horizontal position beside the body (Fig. 89, *D*). Return to starting position.

Movement 4. Bring the arms to an overhead position at a 135-degree angle (Fig. 89, *E*). Return to the starting position.

Movement 5. From the horizontal position as in Movement 3, bring the arms straight back to a position of 180 degrees or in line with the head. Let the arms hang freely to stretch, then bring the arms smoothly and rhythmically back to the horizontal position beside the body (Fig. 89, *F*). Then return to the starting position, as described in Movement 1.

Progression. Start by doing three repetitions of the movement using 1-pound dumbbells. Increase one repetition each exercise period until ten repetitions. Then increase the resistance to 2 pounds, starting with five repetitions and working up to ten.

Precautions. Keep the lower back flat on the board. The hands remain in a functional position, except in Movement 3 (Fig. 89, *D*), in which palms are up.

NOTE: These exercises may be done without the slant board and dumbbells by using a bench at home and books or other pieces of equipment to give resistance, or one could do these exercises by having a partner resist the motions.

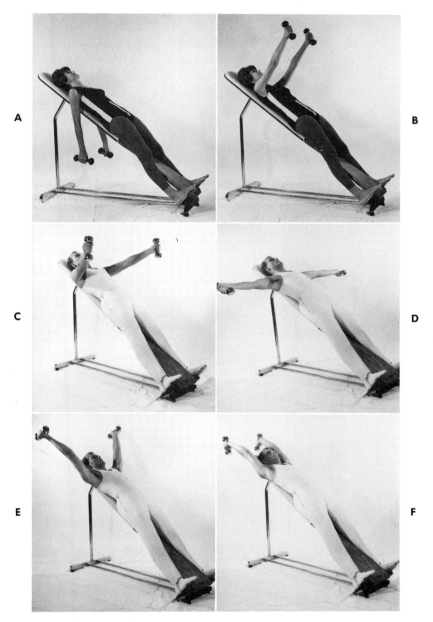

Fig. 89. Exercise 84.

Exercise 85

Purpose. To increase strength and endurance of the abdominal muscles.

Starting position. Lie on the back on an abdominal board, with the arms to the side and the feet placed in the loops on the abdominal board (Fig. 90, *A*).

Movement. Tilt the pelvis to flatten the back to the board. Reach toward the toes and curl to a sitting position as previously described for abdominal exercises (Fig. 90, *B*).

Progression. Progress the same as in the exercises described previously for the abdominal exercises, except that the abdominal board is used to add resistance to the exercise.

Precautions. Observe precautions as prescribed for abdominal exercises previously given.

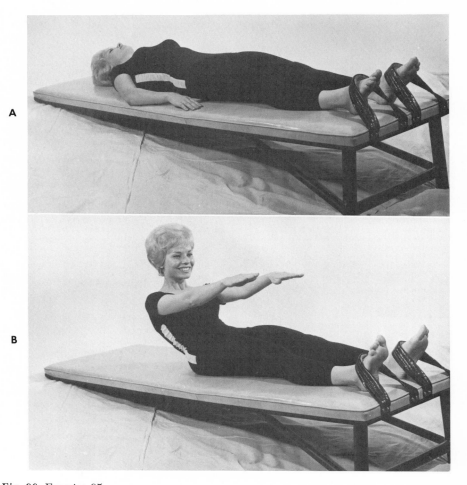

A

B

Fig. 90. Exercise 85.

Exercise 86

> *Purpose.* To increase strength and endurance of the hip flexor muscles.
>
> *Starting position.* Lie on the back on an abdominal board, with the arms outstretched and the hands in the loops.
>
> *Movement.* Bring the right knee toward the chest. Return to the starting position by lowering and extending the leg rhythmically (Fig. 91).
>
> *Progression.* Do the exercise five times with each leg and increase one time with each leg each exercise session.
>
> *Precautions.* Do not allow the pelvis to tilt forward. Keep the extended leg straight.

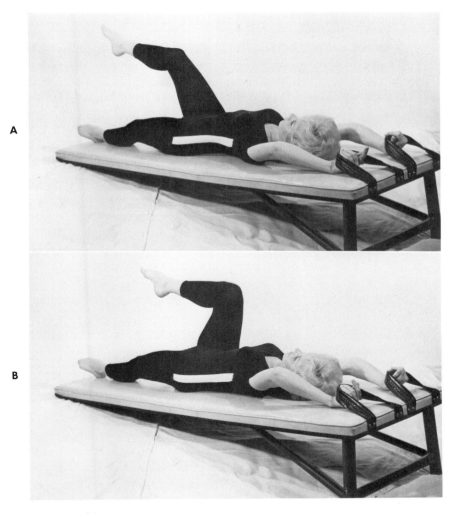

Fig. 91. Exercise 86.

Chapter 7
Relaxation

Stress and strain, either physical or mental, may result in a condition known as neuromuscular hypertension. This is a condition whereby muscles, which are controlled by their motor nerves, have a greater amount of tension than normal. Relaxation, which is opposite to neuromuscular hypertension, is a physical state which may be affected by mental or emotional stress. Relaxation exercises of the type described in this chapter are effective antidotes for neuromuscular hypertension.

Another type of relaxation is that which must occur in antagonistic muscles to allow for movement. Joints in the body are surrounded by paired muscles that are agonistic and antagonistic in their actions. When the agonistic muscle contracts concentrically (muscle shortens), the antagonistic muscle contracts eccentrically (muscle lengthens). This muscle-lengthening is referred to as relaxation. One of the most common examples of this is the flexing or bending of the elbow. One muscle, the biceps, concentrically contracts and the arm bends, but at the same time the biceps eccentrically contracts to allow for the movement. To straighten the bent arm, the actions of the muscles are reversed. If both muscles relax, there is no movement. If both muscles do not contract proportionally as to their antagonistic action, smooth movement will not occur, and there will be tense, jerking, and ungainly movement. Through participation in a controlled exercise program, a person can improve his skill to coordinate these agonistic and antagonistic muscle movements. He then can incorporate the same practice into his daily living.

Today's highly accelerated living pace has caused increased stress to be placed upon man's physical and mental health. The ability to relax one's muscles at will is a desirable and effective skill to be learned by persons desiring to cope with the stresses of modern society.

The following exercises can be practiced in the gymnasium under the direction of the instructor and can then be used during periods of tension outside the exercise classroom.

Exercise 87

The back-lying position on the abdominal board with the head at the lowered end is used. Lace the fingers across the chest and let the total body relax. Assume this position for approximately 15 minutes.

Exercise 88

The back-lying position is used, with the arms at the side and the legs outstretched. Let all of the muscles relax as completely as possible. From this position, contract the muscles in the following manner until tension is felt.

1. Curl the toes down as far as possible until a slight discomfort is felt and slowly and passively just let them relax until complete relaxation is accomplished.
2. Extend the toes and bring them toward the legs. Contract the muscles vigorously until slight discomfort is felt and slowly let them return to the normal position until no tension can be felt at all.
3. Push the heel toward the floor vigorously until tightening of the muscles from the buttocks to the heel is felt. Contract these muscles vigorously until slight discomfort is attained and slowly and progressively let the muscle relax until relaxation is accomplished.
4. Turn the feet away from the body in an attempt to touch the mat with the toes or with the feet. Contract the muscles in this area vigorously until discomfort is felt and slowly and progressively let the muscle relax until no tension is felt at all.
5. Rotate the legs inwardly. Attempt to touch the mat with the big toe. Contract these muscles vigorously until slight discomfort is felt and then progressively relax the legs until no tension can be felt.
6. Pull the legs together as vigorously as possible and then progressively let them relax.
7. Move the legs in abduction as far from each other as possible, maintaining proper alignment with the trunk. Contract these muscles vigorously and, in the manner previously described, let the muscles relax.
8. Squeeze the hands or make a fist, tightening the muscles as vigorously as possible. Relax them as previously described.
9. Push the arms down against the mat, palms down, vigorously and relax as previously described.
10. Push the arms against the mat vigorously with the back of the hands and arm facing the mat. Relax as previously described.
11. Adduct the arms or place them against the sides of the body vigorously. Do as previously described in other exercises.
12. Pull the shoulder blades together, flatten the back on the mat, and

bring the back against the mat vigorously. Relax tension slowly as described previously.

13. Close the eyes vigorously. Relax tension as previously described.
14. Close the jaws together vigorously and progressively and relax tension as previously described.
15. Wrinkle the forehead vigorously and progressively relax the tension as described previously.
16. Push the head against the mat and extend the neck vigorously. Flatten the back against the mat with the heels and arms. Relax the tension slowly and progressively as previously described.

Precautions. This exercise should be done in the manner just prescribed in order that one will gain a feeling of tenseness followed by a feeling of relaxation. If this exercise is done properly, by the completion of the exercise the whole body should be relaxed to the point that a feeling of light sleepiness would occur. Relaxation is definitely a skill which must be learned and practiced.

Exercise 89

1. Stretch the right side of the chest and the right arm upward toward the fingertips. Slowly and with resistance pull the arm downward and place it alongside the body.
2. Repeat to the left side.
3. Stretch downward the lower right side of the body. Use a slow count of five. Do not raise the leg from the mat. Spend the same amount of time in pulling slowly all of the muscles back to the normal position.
4. Repeat to the left.
5. Slowly open the mouth to the full extent. Resist opening it as though the teeth were wired together.
6. Stretch the neck toward the right shoulder, then toward the left shoulder, and pull it back to a normal position. Slowly stretch the neck toward the chest and then toward the back.
7. Breathe in slowly; then exhale fully at a much slower rate, slightly forcing the residual air out of the lungs.

Exercise 90

Starting position. Stand with the arms at the sides.

Movement. Shrug the shoulders. Tighten all of the muscles of the arms and shoulders. Hold five counts and relax.

Exercise 91

Starting position. Stand with the feet apart; let the head, arms, and trunk hang heavily downward.

Movement. Swing the trunk from side to side; let the arms "flap around" as if they were an elephant's trunk.

Exercise 92

    Starting position. Lie on the back with the arms stretched overhead.

    Movement. Raise one hip and try to swing it across the body; let the rest of the body follow heavily until the body is turned over facedown.

Exercise 93

    Starting position. Sit with the head bent forward.

    Movement. Swing the chin toward the right shoulder; slowly raise the head upward and keep the chin pointed toward the right shoulder; let the head fall back as far as possible. Swing the chin across to point behind the left shoulder. Repeat, starting to the left side.

Chapter 8
Body mechanics

Good body mechanics denote the ability to maintain the best possible balance of body parts either at rest or in motion.

Correct body mechanics result in gaining mechanical advantage, which assists in body movement and posture. Whenever the body deviates from a good mechanical position, the resistance upon the antigravity muscles which maintain body balance is increased, and thus extra strain is added to these muscles. This extra strain will cause the muscles to fatigue more readily and may cause poor posture (Fig. 92).

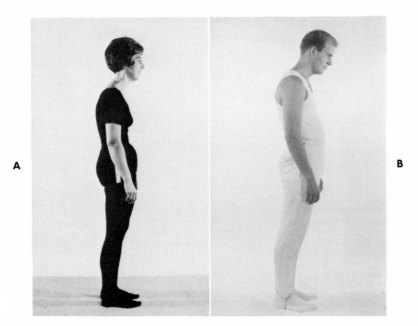

Fig. 92. Poor postural attitudes.

If all segments of the body are balanced directly over their base of support, almost no muscular effort is required to maintain this position. Whenever a body segment is displaced from its base of support, gravity pulls the segment away from the center of alignment, and muscle force is required to overcome this gravitational pull. This displacement increases the muscular work required to maintain a given postural position. In order to acquire a good mechanical position, one must learn to detect awareness of body parts in space. This can be accomplished only by consistent practice.

In order to assume a good balanced position when standing, do the following: (1) stand with the feet 4 to 6 inches apart and parallel to each other, (2) balance the pelvis over the feet by contracting the lower abdominal muscles, and (3) balance the trunk over the pelvis by lifting the chest upward (Fig. 93).

When teaching proper body mechanics in movement, the instructor should observe these same general principles. The pelvis should be balanced over the feet, and the trunk should be balanced over the pelvis. In order to maintain this balance in movement, one must move the body in such a manner as to compensate for the momentary loss of balance required for the movement to occur. For example, when walking, the movement should be initiated from the center of gravity (hips) and not from the distal segments such as the head, trunk, or legs. If this principle is not observed, the body will be moved diagonally or rotated about the center of gravity instead

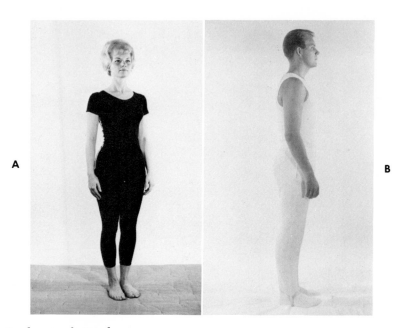

A   B

Fig. 93. Good postural attitudes.

of moved directly forward. This is the reason so many variations of extraneous body movements in walking postures are seen.

Physical educators have found that good body mechanics are learned skills. This means that one must constantly practice.

To develop good body mechanics, the individual must be taught the proper techniques of good standing posture, bending, stooping, reaching, pushing, walking, sitting, and climbing. These techniques must be clearly defined and practiced in order for them to become a part of an individual's daily life.

When lifting a weight or lowering the body to lift an object from the floor, one should observe the same principles (Fig. 94). Unbalanced body segments in lifting posture are illustrated in Fig. 95. If a task requires more stability, then the base of support should be made larger by modifying the stance. If these simple mechanical principles are observed and learned correctly, they can be applied to any task one wishes to perform. The correct

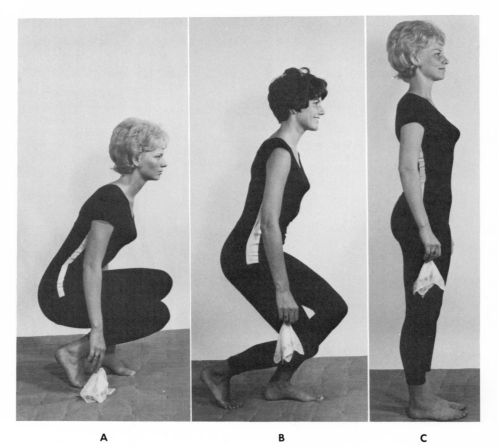

A   B   C

Fig. 94. Good body mechanics of lifting.

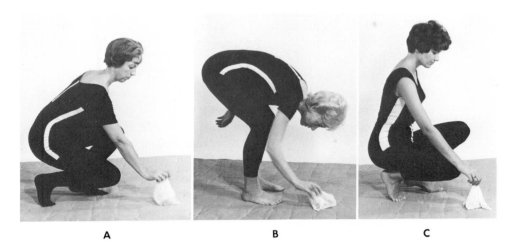

A **B** **C**

Fig. 95. Poor body mechanics of lifting.

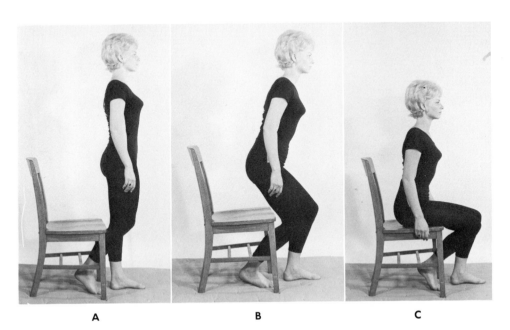

A **B** **C**

Fig. 96. Good sitting attitude.

body mechanics of moving from the standing position to the sitting position are illustrated in Fig. 96.

These principles can be observed during most of our daily living practices. There are some activities, such as lifting a frozen turkey from a chest type of deep freezer, lifting a sleeping child from a playpen, or scouring the bathtub, that do not follow the pattern of good body mechanics. It should be remembered that whenever possible the pelvis should be balanced over the feet, and the trunk should be balanced over the pelvis in order to place the muscular strain where no damage will be done.

Developing and practicing the principles of good body mechanics are satisfying to the learner. When standing correctly with enough muscle tone to maintain the posture, he can feel immediate results. He finds it exciting to walk or run correctly because fatigue does not result as rapidly when the body segments are balanced as when they are unbalanced. The student also responds to a new awareness of muscle action when he lifts, pulls, or pushes heavy objects correctly because he no longer fears injury and soreness.

Chapter 9
Corrective and therapeutic exercises

Exercises may be classified into two general types: (1) those used in programs of education and physical training and (2) those used for the purpose of correcting physical deviations. The principles of exercise remain the same for either type. The differences lie in the objectives of the exercise program.

It is important in any exercise program to keep an accurate record of the progress made by the person performing the exercises. This record can serve as an incentive to improve and as a progress report for diagnosis and evaluation. Also it is important that the exercises be specifically selected to suit the purpose the performer has in mind.

Corrective and therapeutic exercises are those prescribed and supervised by persons specializing in corrective and therapeutic exercises for the cure and prevention of certain physical defects. For many people with poor posture or other physical deformities, corrective exercises are very beneficial.

A prescribed corrective program may call for several types of exercise, some of which are included in this book. For corrective purposes, exercises are generally classified as follows:

1. *Passive* exercise accomplished by a therapist or mechanical device with no active muscle contraction of the involved part by the patient.
2. *Active-assistive* exercise accomplished by active contraction by the patient with the assistance of the therapist or mechanical device.
3. *Active* exercise accomplished by the patient without assistance or resistance.
4. *Resistive-active* exercise accomplished by the patient against resistance, either manual or mechanical.
5. *Stretching* exercise involving forced motion, either passive or active.

The first and second types of exercise are used only in cases of extreme disability and are therefore not included in this text.

EXERCISES FOR THE LOWER BACK

Nonorganic low back pain is one of the most common ailments. It appears that poor muscle tone and strain to the muscles and ligaments involved are important contributors to this condition. The following exercises will improve the condition of the muscles and connective tissues in the lower back. These exercises should be performed as prescribed by the physician recommending the exercises. The progression listed is only suggestive.

Exercise 94

Purpose. To strengthen the hip extensors, primarily the gluteus maximus muscles.

Starting position. Stand with the feet 2 to 3 inches apart and parallel to each other and the arms outstretched to the front, with the weight in the hands (Fig. 97, *A*).

Movement. Move to a semisquatting position and bend the knees and trunk while keeping the back straight (Fig. 97, *B*). Return to the starting position.

Progression. Do five repetitions the first exercise session, seven the second session, and ten the third session.

Precautions. Keep the back straight. Do not allow the weights to lower.

A 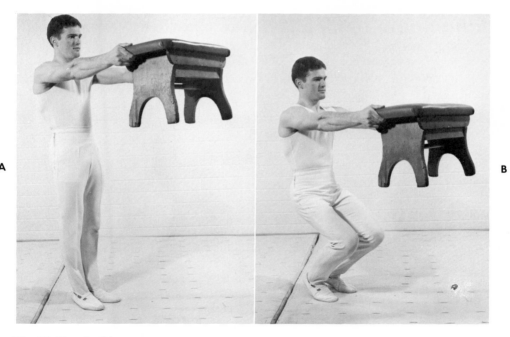 B

Fig. 97. Exercise 94.

EXERCISES FOR THE FEET

Ailments of the feet seem to be very common, and they are often over-looked. For this reason, specific exercises for the feet are included in this chapter.

Most exercises designed for the development of the arch or ankle in-volve the majority of the muscles of the foot. Practically every muscle con-cerned with the foot and ankle acts upon several joints. The anatomic and functional features of the foot and ankle make it almost impossible to devise effective exercises to provide isolated action. Therefore, the following exer-cises for corrective purposes are designed for the development of strength of all the muscles of the foot and ankle.

These exercises are in no way intended to be all-inclusive, but they have proved helpful as corrective measures for painful feet.

EXERCISES FOR ROUNDED SHOULDERS AND FORWARD HEAD TILT

One of the most common and unattractive postural deviations is rounded shoulders and forward head tilt. To correct this condition the muscles in the chest region must be stretched while the muscles in the upper back are increased in strength and tone. The following are exercises designed to cor-rect this condition.

EXERCISES FOR SWAYED BACK AND FORWARD PELVIC TILT

Swayed back and forward pelvic tilt are conditions which result in poor postural alignment and an unattractive profile. This lack of alignment places undue stress on muscles of the lower back and pelvic regions, and this contributes to fatigue of those muscles. The following are exercises which will help correct this condition.

Exercise 18	page 43
Exercise 19	page 44
Exercise 20	page 45
Exercise 39	page 67
Exercise 40	page 68

EXERCISES FOR ABDOMINAL SAG

Many people of middle age and older and some young people suffer from sagging abdominal muscles. This not only detracts greatly from their attractiveness, but it also causes them discomfort and reduces their ability to perform physical tasks. Following are exercises designed to correct abdominal sag. It is important to recognize that this condition usually results from a combination of (1) weak and poorly toned abdominal muscles, and (2) too much bulk within the abdominal cavity pressing outward (overweight).

Exercise 18	page 43
Exercise 19	page 44
Exercise 20	page 45
Exercise 21	page 46
Exercise 22	page 47
Exercise 23	page 48
Exercise 24	page 49
Exercise 28	page 53
Exercise 29	page 54
Exercise 30	page 55
Exercise 31	page 56
Exercise 32	page 58
Exercise 34	page 60
Exercise 35	page 62
Exercise 36	page 64
Exercise 37	page 65
Exercise 38	page 66
Exercise 39	page 67
Exercise 40	page 68
Exercise 80	page 115
Exercise 85	page 122

Index

ERRATUM

Page	Line	Should Read
37	2 (of legend)	. . . *X* chromosomes a recessive mutant . . .
89	4	. . . of two progenies bred after . . .
92	col. 2, line 6	blank
	col. 2, line 7	Albino
		Department of Surgery
	col. 3, entry 17	Albino
96	2 (of legend)	. . . system. Each square . . .
98	Table 5.7 heading	$\overline{H\text{-}2}$ (Haplotype[a])
107	5	. . . a1-positive (a1$^+$) and a1-negative (a1$^-$) . . .
	29	$f_m = f_{a1}^2 \times f_{a1} f_{a2}$
112	8 (of legend)	. . . (molecular weight of 68,000); . . .
132	31	enzyme 1 and the undigested . . . from enzyme 2.
	32	fragment from enzyme 1, . . .
148	col. 2, line 2	V_H; C_H : . . .
166	2 (of legend)	. . . (**$C_{H\mu}$1-$C_{H\mu}$4**), . . .
235	11	. . . the absence of the *Se* allele . . .
252	26	. . . of the P_1^k allele, galactosyl . . .
	35	. . . A P^k
257	17	. . . antigen often produces . . .
271	15	. . . the selected traits . . .
	16	. . . merely reflects the . . .
280	37 (entire line)	not dominant and recessive
320	9	. . . H-2L, H-2M, and H-2R . . .
321	col. 6 ("4*")	delete + for Molecule L2, add for Molecule M
(Table	col. 9 ("[28]")	delete superscript a for Molecule K1
16.5)	col. 10 ("31*")	delete superscript a for Molecule K1 and insert + for **Molecule K2**
	col. 12 ("64")	insert + for Molecule R and delete + for Molecule K1
349	10	. . . by the lymphocytotoxic . . .
362	7	. . . the phenomenon of immune . . .
410	5	. . . Kourilsky, F. M. . . .
418	1	. . . by the (T × A.x^b) F1 . . .
436	28	. . . at which Thy-1.1 has . . .
	29	. . . Thy-1.2 has glutamine.
437	20	. . . β_2m) both by amino . . .
	28	. . . given the designation THY. This . . .
440	col. 3 ("Chromosome Position")	for Gene Ly-6 should read 2(?)
455	footnote	should be on page 453
457	10	23.9 The *Pca* Genes . . .
485	14	. . . in fact differentiation antigen . . .
489	30	. . . the G_{IX}^- antigen . . .
494	28	. . . osteoporosis, the *bg* gene. . . .

IMMUNOGENETICS

Marek B. Zaleski
Department of Microbiology, School of Medicine and
Dentistry, State University of New York, Buffalo

Stanislaw Dubiski
Departments of Medical Genetics, and Clinical Biochemistry,
Institutes of Immunology and Medical Sciences, University of
Toronto

Edward G. Niles
Department of Biochemistry, School of Medicine and
Dentistry, State University of New York, Buffalo

Roger K. Cunningham
The Ernest Witebsky Center for Immunology, State University
of New York, Buffalo

Pitman

Boston · London · Melbourne · Toronto

Pitman Publishing Inc.
1020 Plain Street
Marshfield, Massachusetts 02050

Pitman Books Limited
128 Long Acre
London WC2E 9AN

Associated Companies
Pitman Publishing Pty Ltd., Melbourne
Pitman Publishing New Zealand Ltd., Wellington
Copp Clark Pitman, Toronto

Library of Congress Cataloging in Publication Data
Main entry under title:

Immunogenetics.

Includes bibliographical references and index.
1. Immunogenetics.   I. Zaleski, Marek B.
[DNLM: 1. Immunogenetics.   QW 541 I642]
QR184.I55   1983   616.07′9   82-22486
ISBN 0-273-01925-2

Manufactured in the United States of America

10   9   8   7   6   5   4   3   2   1

To LECH WAŁĘSA

Żeby Polska była Polską
" . . . Non piu schiavo!
Non ti e permesso di essere schiavo! . . . " John Paul II

M. B. Z.

To my teachers

LUDWIK HIRSZFELD and FELIX MILGROM

S. D.

To my wife JOAN
and
my children, AMY and DAVID

E. G. N.

To A. E. C.

R. K. C.

Contents

IV / Major Histocompatibility Systems

Preface

Any author experiences a certain degree of apprehension when his book is about to be released. However, when the book is an attempt to present in a didactic manner a science that is literally *in statu nascendi*, the apprehension becomes true anxiety. It is, therefore, with a great deal of trepidation that we are surrendering this book into the hands of readers. Although we have made the utmost effort to present the topics both comprehensively and comprehensibly, certainly there are areas in which we did not succeed fully in doing so.

One is always tempted to find an easy excuse, but the truth of the matter is that the field we tried to cover is growing so rapidly that even during the months of writing new facts and ideas were constantly added. The tremendous expansion of immunogenetics witnessed in recent years is the result of contemporary research in which classic immunologic and genetic methods are used in conjunction with the most modern biochemical and molecular techniques. This coordinated assault into unexplored areas has resulted in the isolation and purification of a variety of immune system components (immunoglobulins, cell-surface molecules) and in the definition of the structure and expression of the corresponding genes. The rapidity of development always creates problems for those who aspire to describe the field comprehensively. Surely, some of the ideas, findings, and concepts will have been challenged or changed before we have laid our pens to rest and the printers have shut down their presses. Indeed, we are very much like the man, in a story told by J. Klein, who set out to paint a huge bridge by himself but before he finished painting the last span of the bridge, the first span already required repainting.

This book is really more of a snapshot than it is a portrait. It is a glimpse of a rapidly developing subject that has been artificially "frozen" for examination. Such an examination is necessary to gain an appreciation of both the current state and the future directions of the ongoing quest for a full understanding of the workings of the immune system. In this book, we attempted to combine a description of well-established facts with a presentation of current concepts. However, the reader must be aware that life and continuing progress will certainly thaw the frozen picture created by our writing and force the retaking of the snapshot in the foreseeable future. It is with this in mind that the book should be considered as a framework for expansion rather than as a dogmatic treatise. Accordingly, the references are limited to a minimum and include the most current reviews and monographs. They are organized by, and placed at the end of, each section. Although we may have excluded some valuable contributions, such an omission certainly was not intentional. We believe that an interested reader will be able to locate the relevant literature by following the references that are provided.

The book has been written with graduate, medical, and dental students in mind. While presupposing a basic understanding of biology by the reader, the book has been organized as a self-contained entity. It is primarily designed as a textbook for use in various immunogenetics courses, but we hope that many investigators will find it useful as a resource in their daily work. The material presented is organized into the following sections: basic concepts of genetics; methods of genetic research; and the three traditional subjects of immunogenetics—immunoglobulins, blood groups, and cell-surface molecules of nucleated cells.

The amount of material and the complexity of the concepts made our task a trying experience. We would not have been able to carry it out were it not for the moral and practical support and encouragement of our families, colleagues, and friends. We want to say to all of them, from the bottom of our hearts, THANK YOU. There are too many of them to list all by name, but certainly those who found the time and patience to review parts or the entire manuscript deserve to be mentioned: C. David, M. Dorf, E. Gorzynski, K. Kano, M. Klein, H. Köhler, R. Lambert, M. Long, W. Mandy, R. Melvold, J. Minowada, A. Nisonoff, H. Ozer, D. Shreffler, and N. Tanigaki provided us with the invaluable gift of their expertise, and their suggestions and comments certainly improved the rough text they read.

There are two other people to whom we owe a special gratitude. We are grateful to Jonathan S. Reichner for his many nights spend reading and editing the manuscript. Jonathan, himself a student of immunogenetics, was our first and foremost critic; we and future readers are beneficiaries of his input. Rosalind J. Forse deserves a great deal of credit for typing the manuscript and patiently, day after day, struggling with our handwriting, corrections, and innumerable changes and modifications.

We would also like to express our appreciation to the people of Pitman Publishing Inc.: M. Weinstein—Production Manager; S. Badger—copy editor; and M. Erikson—artist for the speed, effectiveness, and quality of their efforts in publishing this book in record time.

Last but not least, we would like to acknowledge the financial support from various sources (for M. B. Zaleski, NIH-NIAID grant AI-13628; for S. Dubiski, Medical Research Council of Canada; for E. G. Niles, NIH-GMS grant GM-23259; for R. K. Cunningham, The Ernest Witebsky Center for Immunology), which permitted us to carry out our research without interruption while writing this book. Without this support, we would not have been able to concentrate fully on the task at hand. In this regard, though indirectly, these agencies contributed immensely to this book and, therefore, should receive credit for any success that the book might achieve.

Buffalo, January 1983

I / *Fundamentals of Genetics*

1 / Introduction to Formal Genetics

HISTORICAL PERSPECTIVES

The phenomenon of the inheritance of various physical and behavioral characteristics has attracted the interest of man since immemorial times. This interest has been prompted not only for fulfillment of natural human curiosity but also for pragmatic reasons. After man began to breed domestic animals, the selection of individuals with the most desirable characteristics and the maintenance of these characteristics in stock animals proved to be pivotal to the success of this new endeavor. Thus, the farmers and shepherds of our earliest recorded civilization unwittingly became the forefathers of modern geneticists. Indeed, from the ruins of the ancient Sumerian city of Ur, a clay tablet, containing the pedigree of horse, has been unearthed that is believed to be the oldest known record of genetic information.

The almost universal restriction against marriages between close members of a family might have resulted from empirical observations of the adverse effects that such marriages have had on the inheritance of certain characteristics. Although amazingly accurate, these observations were too fragmentary to constitute a real basis for a scientific interpretation of all the facts. According to Hippocrates, the characteristics of parents blended in their progeny to form new and unique qualities. Blind acceptance of this quasi-scientific concept of inheritance, proposed as dogma, was a stumbling stone to the consummation of related facts and the birth of genetics as a science.

A scientific approach to genetics finally emerged in the serenity of the courtyard of an Augustinian monastery in the capital of the Czechoslovakian province of Moravia, Brno. Here, a monk named Gregor Mendel painstakingly cultured and observed the varieties of flowers growing in the beds of the monastery garden. These beds have been preserved and continue to provide flowers for the church altar. Unfortunately, Mendel reported his observations in 1866 in a rather obscure journal—Proceedings of the Natural History Society of Brno—where they remained neglected until they were rediscovered by De Vries, Correns, and von Tschermak nearly 34 years later, 16 years after Mendel's death.

At approximately the same time, Weismann proposed that inheritance might be mediated by **idioplasm** (germ plasm), which, according to his theory, was duplicated at the time of each cell division, thus ensuring that each progeny cell (the **soma**) received all the factors that determine its set of characteristics. Considering that Weismann had no knowledge of nucleic acids or even chromosomes, one must acknowledge and admire his ingenuity in predicting the true basis of inheritance.

Shortly thereafter, Sutton and Boveri independently suggested that genetic factors (**genes**) may be transmitted in units located on the recently discovered chromosomes, which would correspond to Weismann's idioplasm. Their concept was expanded by Morgan who proposed that genes are linearly arranged in pairs of chromosomes and that the two genes for each characteristic occupy the corresponding sites, called a **loci** (singular, **locus**), in the chromosomes that form a homologous pair. Putting his concept into practical use, Morgan initiated attempts to assign particular genes to specific points along the chromosome, thus creating the concept of a **genetic map**.

Morgan's concept, still alive today, and his contribution to formal genetics are honored by the term **centimorgan** (cM), which defines a unit of the genetic map.* In 1913, employing Morgan's idea, Sturtevant constructed the first gene map of a chromosome.

The set of all genes present in an individual became known as the **genotype**, or **genome**, whereas the set of characteristics determined by the genotype and expressed in the individual was defined as the phenotype.† Further development of genetics was inseparably connected with progress in the field of cytology and led to the development of a subdiscipline called cytogenetics (Chapter 2), which, together with advances in biochemistry, resulted in the development of molecular genetics (Chapter 3).

Immunogenetics as a branch of formal genetics originated in 1900 when Landsteiner described the ABO blood groups of man, and Ehrlich and Morgenroth made a similar discovery in goats. In each case, immunologic methods were applied to detect a genetically determined trait and define its variants. Soon thereafter, the genetic control of tumor graft rejection was established by Little and Tyzzer (Chapter 14). The scope and emphasis of immunogenetics changed with time and included the genetic determination and mode of inheritance of the blood groups, histocompatibility antigens, immunoglobulins, and allogeneic markers of various immune cells.

In this book, an attempt will be made to summarize the present state of the art in three traditional areas of immunogenetics—immunoglobulins, blood groups, and histocompatibility antigens. Emphasis is placed on well-established facts, but at the same time new frontiers in each field are outlined. A full understanding of each field requires of the reader a fundamental background in formal, cellular, and molecular genetics as well as a familiarity with the principles, of the methodology employed in immunogenetic studies. Having this in mind, the first two sections of the book are written to facilitate the understanding of the complex topics discussed in the other sections. From the vast body of genetics, only those facts and concepts that are directly relevant to immunogenetics are presented.

TRAIT AND THE GENE

A **trait,** or character, represents a detectable feature that is genetically determined and transmitted in a predictable manner from one generation to the next. A trait corresponds to either a specific structure such as a molecule or to a functional property conferred by such a molecule. Most traits have two or more variants; progeny expressing these variants permit a formal genetic analysis. Those traits that are invariant—i.e., traits that have only one form in all individuals of the species—are not amenable to ordinary methods of analysis since it is impossible to demonstrate that the trait in question is indeed inheritable.

---

*1 cM corresponds to the distance between two genes that recombine with a frequency of 0.01, i.e., in 1 percent of the individuals comprising a population.

† Originally, the term genotype indicated individuals with the same genetic makeup, while the term phenotype referred to individuals with the same appearance.

A gene is the unit of genetic material that determines a given trait or its variant. It corresponds to a segment of chromosomal DNA located at a strictly defined position (locus) along the chromosome. Since there are variants of a given trait and a trait is determined by its corresponding gene, it follows that the gene must also have variants. Variants of genes are called **alleles**, and obviously they must occupy the same locus. In this sense, alleles are mutually exclusive since the presence of one allele of a given gene at its locus precludes the simultaneous presence of another allele of the same gene at the same locus in the same chromosome. A gene that has at least two alleles is considered to be **polymorphic**, but from the point of view of formal genetics this statement requires additional qualification. A gene can be considered polymorphic only when at least two of its alleles are present in the population each with a frequency of greater than 1 percent.* A gene with only two alleles of which one is found less frequently than in 1 percent of the individuals in the population is, for all practical purposes, nonpolymorphic.

1.1. Development of the Concept of the Gene

The original concept of the gene assumed that a given characteristic or trait is determined by a single factor that could occur as two or more variants. Systematic analysis of various traits and their inheritance soon revealed, however, that this assumption was an apparent oversimplification. Many traits turned out to be determined by several factors (polyfactorial or polygenic), and it was thus necessary to identify the primary traits, i.e., the traits determined by a single gene only. The discovery of the relationship between genetic material and protein synthesis (Section 3.7) led to a definition of the gene as the unit determining a given protein. Originally formulated in a lapidary form, "**one gene–one enzyme**," the definition was subsequently revised to "**one gene – one protein**" to accommodate the fact that not all proteins are enzymes. The finding that numerous proteins consist of several distinct, independently synthesized polypeptides resulted in a further modification of the definition, which now reads "**one gene – one polypeptide**." According to this definition, a gene determines the primary and hence the secondary and tertiary structure of a particular polypeptide. Such a gene is often referred to as a **structural** as opposed to a **regulatory** gene. The latter class of genes is vested with the capacity to alter quantitatively the expression of certain structural genes. The actual mechanism of such regulatory activity in higher organisms still remains speculative. However, rapid progress is being made in this field. If such regulation is mediated by specific repressor or activator proteins, then, for all practical reasons, regulatory genes are structural genes themselves.

The structural gene that determines the amino acid sequence of a given polypeptide may determine the entire detectable trait. For example, the gene that determines serum albumin determines the whole trait. However, in many instances, a given trait requires the presence of and/or the activity of several different polypeptides. Such a trait is called **polygenic** because it requires the coordinated expression of more than one structural gene. For example, the formation of a single hemoglobin molecule results from the joining of two distinct polypeptides

---

*Some authors arbitrarily accept a larger value, e.g., 5 percent.

(α and β). Hence, production of a hemoglobin molecule requires the expression of two structural genes. In prokaryotes the set of genes that determines certain polygenic traits, especially in the case of metabolic pathways, is given the name **operon**. Contained within this set are several structural genes as well as one or more regulatory genes. Regardless of whether it exists independently or is contained within an operon, a single structural gene is responsible for the synthesis of a specific polypeptide called a **primary product**. In some instances, the primary product, if it is an enzyme, is involved in the synthesis of another molecule, either protein or nonprotein, and this molecule is called a **secondary product**. The allele that may not be able to control the synthesis of a primary product is called **silent**. The allele whose product, even when synthesized, is undetectable by available methods may appear as silent.

The molecular structure of the gene will be discussed later (Sections 3.1 and 3.3). Here it is sufficient to say that genes consist of specific purine and pyrimidine base sequences of DNA that are copied during the premitotic **replication** of DNA, thus supplying the progeny cells with copies of the parental genes. Although the process of DNA replication usually results in the exact copying of each gene, an occasional alteration may occur. An alteration of a given gene is called a **mutation** and results in the formation of a variant of the gene, i.e., an allele. An allele of a structural gene determines a variant of the primary product, which is called an **allelic product**. Since any gene may undergo several independent mutations, a gene may have several alleles, with each determining its corresponding allelic product. It can be envisioned that in each case, through random mutations, a single gene gave rise to a number of alleles determining a number of allelic products and a corresponding number of variants of a given trait. We shall return to the topic of mutation at the end of this chapter. Each somatic cell has two copies of a given gene—one copy contributed by the male and the other by the female parent. Each of the two copies is located on one of the homologous chromosomes. If both copies are identical—i.e., are the same alleles of the gene—the individual (cell) is called a **homozygote** (homozygous) for this gene, whereas if two different alleles are present, the individual or cell is called a **heterozygote** (heterozygous) for this gene. An exception occurs in the case of sex chromosomes (Section 2.6). Male cells have only one female sex chromosome, the X chromosome, and, thus, only one copy of most genes located on this chromosome; a condition called **hemizygosity**.

1.2 Expression of a Gene and Its Alleles

A structural gene on its own, or upon activation by the appropriate regulatory gene, directs the synthesis of its product and thus becomes phenotypically expressed. A homozygote may express either one or both identical copies it carries. On the other hand, a heterozygote may express either allele alone or both alleles simultaneously. An allele that is expressed both in homozygotes and in heterozygotes is commonly referred to as **dominant**, and its corresponding variant of the trait is called the **dominant trait**. An allele, and its corresponding trait variant that is expressed only in homozygotes, are called **recessive**. This simple distinction introduced in early studies now seems to be a gross oversimplification.

In reality, the expression of an allele is affected by two distinct properties called **expressivity** and **penetrance**. Expressivity reflects the degree of expression of a given allele and ranges from **overdominance** through **full dominance, codominance,** and **incomplete**

dominance to **recessiveness**. Overdominance refers to a more pronounced expression of a given allele in heterozygotes than in homozygotes. Full dominance is an expression of an allele to the same extent in heterozygotes and homozygotes. Codominance corresponds to equal expression of both alleles in heterozygotes. Incomplete dominance is the expression of both alleles with one being more pronounced than the other but still less apparent than in the corresponding homozygote. Recessiveness is the very weak expression or total absence of expression of an allele in heterozygotes. The expressivity of any allele is a relative property; variation depends on the other allele of the same gene that is present at the same time in the genome.

Penetrance corresponds to the frequency of expression of a given allele among individuals carrying such an allele. Even an allele with full expressivity may have incomplete penetrance, resulting in some fraction of individuals not expressing the allele. Differences in the expressivity and penetrance of an allele may be caused by environmental or genetic factors. Among the latter, a special role is played by two types of genes called **modifier genes** and **epistatic genes**. A modifier gene quantitatively affects the phenotypic expression of a given allele of another gene, whereas an epistatic gene exerts a qualitative effect preventing the expression of alleles of another gene.

A single trait can be affected by several genes that may determine the trait itself or influence its expression. The reverse situation occurs when a single gene affects several seemingly different traits. A gene with a wide range of effects is called **pleiotropic**. Some genes displaying remarkable pleiotropism will be discussed in the latter part of the book (Chapters 15–17).

Along the development of the concept of the gene, it was assumed that a gene determines a trait that is more or less independent of any other trait. It was found, however, that this is not always the case. The products of certain genes could not be detected unless the products of some other gene(s) were expressed simultaneously. Apparently, some traits are the result of the interaction of two or more genes or their products. In this case, the products of each individual gene when expressed separately do not produce the trait. The phenomenon is called **intergenic complementation**, and the genes involved are referred to as **complementary**. Occasionally, complementation takes place only between particular alleles of two complementary genes but does not occur between other alleles of these genes. In cases where the complementary genes are on the same chromosome the two complementing alleles may be either on the same chromosome (i.e., in the *cis* **position** [coupling]) or on the two homologous chromosomes (i.e., in the *trans* **position** [repulsion]). Accordingly, two types of complementation are distinguished—*cis* **complementation** and *trans* **complementation**. Intergenic complementation plays a significant role in the expression of some histocompatibility antigens (Section 16.8). In other instances, complementation may occur between two distinct alleles of the same gene, and such a phenomenon is called **interallelic** or **intragenic complementation**. This type of complementation occurs provided that the gene determines a product that ordinarily forms a homopolymer composed of two or more identical polypeptides. However, any of the alleles of such a gene may determine a polypeptide that cannot form the bonds required for the formation of the homopolymer. The polypeptide determined by this allele may still be able to form the heteropolymer with the product of the other allele (Fig. 1.1).

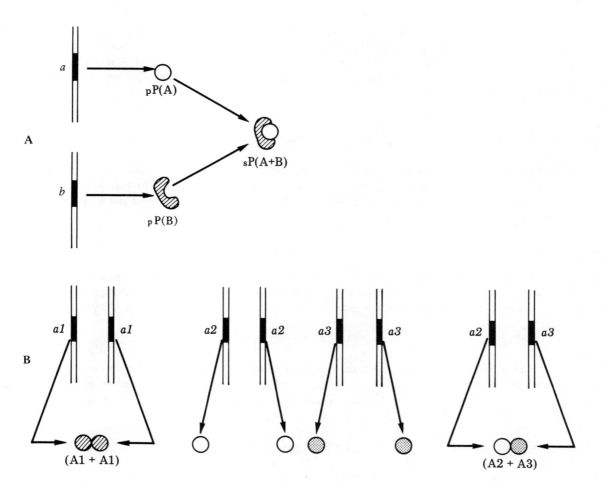

FIG. 1.1. Intergenic (**A**) and intragenic (**B**) complementation. (**A**) Primary products (**pP**) of two genes, **a** and **b**, form a secondary product (**sP**). (**B**) products of **a1** allele form a homopolymer (**A1 + A1**) but the products of **a2** or **a3** alleles cannot form corresponding homopolymers. However, products of **a2** and **a3** form a hetero-polymer (**A2 + A3**).

An unusual case of the expression of codominant alleles is represented by the phenomenon of **allelic exclusion**. In this case, of the two codominant alleles present in the heterozygous cell, only one is expressed while the other is totally suppressed. Allelic exclusion is discussed in greater detail in connection with the genes determining the immunoglobulins (Sections 8.5 and 9.22).

1.3 Relationship between Genotypes and Phenotypes

Both alleles of a single gene make up the genotype of a given individual. Such a genotype consisting of the alleles of a single gene is called the **monogenotype**. The number of distinct monogenotypes (n_g) depends on the number of alleles (n_a) of the gene, and the relationship is expressed by the formula

$$n_g = 0.5 n_a(n_a + 1).$$

When alleles of several discrete genes are considered, they form the **polygenotype**. The number of different polygenotypes (n_G) depends on the number of monogenotypes (n_g) contributing to the particular polygenotype. This relationship can be expressed by the formula

$$n_G = n_{g1} \times n_{g2} \times \ldots \times n_{gn}.$$

Either the monogenotype or the polygenotype determines the corresponding **mono-phenotype** or **polyphenotype**. The number of phenotypes equals the number of genotypes only when all alleles involved are codominant. When some alleles are recessive or silent, the number of phenotypes is lower than the number of genotypes.

Allelic phenotypes may be distinguished from each other qualitatively or quantitatively. Qualitatively, phenotypes are distinguishable on the basis of the presence or absence of a given trait variant (**dichotomy**) or on the basis of several distinct qualitative variants (**polychotomy**). Quantitatively, phenotypes are distinguishable by quantitative variants of the qualitatively same trait.

PRINCIPAL RULES OF GENETIC TERMINOLOGY

Genetic nomenclature, symbols, and abbreviations often cause a great deal of frustration, if not confusion, for an inexperienced reader. It seems that such frustration can be, at least partially, avoided if some basic rules and the exceptions are outlined briefly.

Specific genes are customarily designated by two- or three-letter abbreviations of the name of the trait or the product they determine with the first letter capitalized and the remaining letters lower-case. Since similar products or traits may be determined by more than one gene, different genes may be distinguished by an Arabic number separated from the abbreviation by either a period or preferably a hyphen. Different alleles of a given gene are designated by superscripts consisting of a lowercase letter(s) or an Arabic number(s) or sometimes both. For example, the designation *Igh-1*^{a} means allele *a* of *i*mmuno*g*lobulin *h*eavy chain gene one (*1*).

At one time, it was customary to indicate dominant allele by writing the gene abbreviation in capital letters and the recessive allele by the same abbreviation in lowercase letters. Contemporary nomenclature, which frequently deals with multiple alleles and often their variable expressivity, had to abandon this usage. Finally, the allele most frequently found in a given population is often considered the standard one and is called the **wild-type** allele, whereas alleles less frequently found are considered mutants of the wild type. In this case the wild-type allele is often designated by the plus sign (+) and the mutant alleles by their appropriate superscript symbols. The major exceptions to the rules outlined above are those genes that were arbitrarily given one-letter symbols that have become fixed in the scientific literature. Regardless of the type of symbols and abbreviations, it is a general convention that the specific terms or symbols referring to the genotype (gene, allele, haplotype, mutant gene, etc.) are written in italics, while the phenotypic expressions (trait, product, phenotype, etc.) are written in roman type.

When two or more genes are known to be on the same chromosome, their symbols are written in sequence and separated from each other by either a dash or an ellipsis. Genes known to be on different chromosomes are also written in sequence but are separated by a comma. Two putative genes that seem to be so close to each other that they are indistinguishable or appear as identical are designated by two appropriate symbols with the second symbol written in parentheses. Confusion arises when the parentheses are replaced by the virgule (slash) sign; the virgule sign between two symbols or abbreviations should be reserved for separating two alleles of the same gene.

A product or trait is conventionally designated by the same symbol or abbreviation as its corresponding gene but written in roman type and in capital letters. Allelic products or trait variants are designated by sequential Arabic numbers following the gene symbol and separated from it by a period.

BASIC RULES OF HEREDITY

1.4 Mendel's Laws

The basic rules of heredity in higher organisms are most succinctly stated in the two laws formulated by Mendel and his successors. Using modern terminology, the two laws can be stated as follows:

The Law of Segregation or Purity of Gametes

Each somatic cell has two alleles of a given gene, and these alleles segregate during gametogenesis in such a way that each gamete receives only one of the two alleles, and they are passed in equal frequency to the progeny.

The Law of Independent Assortment

Alleles of two distinct genes segregate during development of gametes independently of each other.

These laws were derived from empirical observations of the frequencies of the expression of two parental variants (P1 and P2) of a given trait in the progeny of the subsequent generations. Such generations include the **first filial** (F1), consisting of the progeny of a cross between two parents—P1 × P2; the **second filial** (F2), produced by the crossing of two F1 individuals—F1 × F1; the **backcross** (BC), resulting from crossing the F1 with one or the other parent—F1 × P1 (or P2); and the **third filial** (F3), which includes the offspring of the cross of two F2 individuals—F2 × F2.

Once the laws were formulated and their validity was proven, it became possible to determine genotypes from the observed phenotypes and vice versa. Such a determination constitutes an essential step in any genetic analysis (Section 5.7). Although generally valid, the laws have certain important exceptions. For example, the somatic cells of a male having only one chromosome X have only one allele of the many genes that are located on this chromosome (Section 2.6). More important, the law of independent assortment applies fully to the genes located on different chromosomes but only partially to the genes located on the same chromosome.

1.5 Recombination and Linkage

The law of independent assortment of alleles of two genes was introduced because of observations of the backcross generation obtained by crossing an F1 individual with a parent who was a recessive homozygote for two genes under study. Among such individuals, 25 percent had the phenotype of the F1 parent and 25 percent had the phenotype of the P1 parent, while the remaining 50 percent had the two phenotypes (R1 and R2), which were the combination of parental traits and were found in the ratio 1:1. This is illustrated in the following table:

Phenotypes of the Progeny of an F1 ×P1 Backcross

	F1 parent		
	Genotype: *a2,b2/a1,b1*		
	Phenotype: a2b2		
	Alleles in gametes:		
	a2b2	*a2b1*	*a1b2*	*a1b1*
P1 parent	a2b2	a2b1	a1b2	a1b1
Genotype: *a1,b1/a1,b1*	25%	25%	25%	25%
Phenotype: a1b1	(F1)	(R1)	(R2)	(P1)
Alleles in gametes: *a1b1*				

From the table and Fig. 1.2, it is obvious that a2b1 and a1b2 phenotypes resulted from a random segregation of F1 chromosomes carrying *a1* or *a2* and *b1* or *b2* alleles. This random segregation produced phenotypes different from those found in the F1 and P1 parental individuals; this phenomenon is called **recombination**, and accordingly the terms

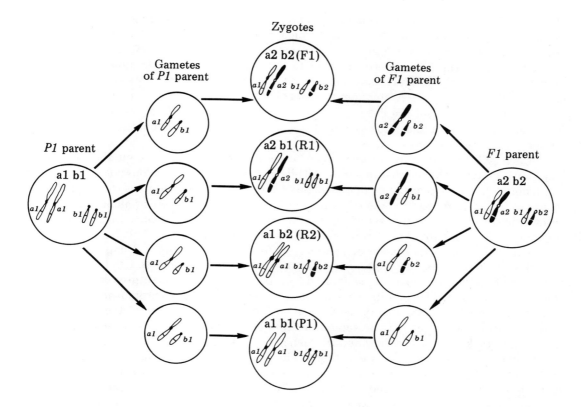

FIG. 1.2. Recombination of alleles of two nonlinked genes, *a* and *b*. Random segregation of chromosomes produces in the heterozygous *F1* parent four types of gametes. These gametes form four types of zygotes with a single type of gamete of the homozygous *P1* parent. Assuming that *a2* and *b2* alleles are dominant, the phenotypes are indicated in circles representing parents and zygotes.

recombinant genotypes and **phenotypes** (R1 and R2) are used. Those individuals carrying and expressing the recombinant genotype are called **recombinants**. The frequency of all recombinants in a given population is called the **recombination frequncy** (f_r), and for two independently segregating genes, it is equal to or close to the value of 0.5 (50 percent).

In many instances, however, recombinant genotypes and the corresponding phenotypes are found with a frequency lower than the predicted 0.5. Since the total frequency of all genotypes and phenotypes (recombinant and nonrecombinant) must be 1.0 (100 percent), a decreased frequency of the recombinants is accompanied by the simultaneous increase in the frequency of parental phenotypes. Therefore, a frequency of parental phenotypes higher than 0.5 indicates that the genes determining these phenotypes are more often transmitted together than separately. This in turn indicates that the two genes are on the same chromosome, and such genes are called **linked**. All genes on a given chromosome form a **linkage group**, and it follows that any cell or organism has as many linkage groups as they have pairs of homologous chromosomes. In fact, before individual chromosomes could be identified and have genes assigned to them, the genes were assigned to linkage groups, each designated by a roman number. Subsequently, when chromosomes were identified, each was designated by an Arabic number. Unfortunately, the Arabic number assigned to a chromosome often did not correlate with the roman number of the corresponding linkage group. Since both a chromosome and a linkage group represent the same group of linked genes, the occasional use of two different numbers often creates confusion.

Each cell has two copies or two alleles of each gene; therefore, the number of copies of alleles must be twice the number of genes. All alleles present in the cell constitute the genotype (polygenotype). The set consisting of one allele of each gene is referred to as the **haplotype**. In recent years, the term haplotype has been used in reference to the set of alleles on any given chromosome or its part, i.e., the set of alleles of linked genes. In concordance with this unwritten convention, the term haplotype in this book will be used to define a set of alleles of any number of genes that are linked—i.e., genes of a major histocompatibility complex (Chapters 15 and 16).

Two linked genes, although present on the same chromosome and thus preferentially transmitted together, may become separated by a process called **crossing-over** (Section 2.2). Crossing-over consists of a simultaneous breaking of two homologous chromosomes at the same point, an exchanging of fragments between them, and a reconnecting of the chromosomes. Alleles of two linked genes may be separated from each other if they are located on opposite sides of the break. The probability and frequency of separation of two linked genes is directly proportional to the distance between them. The f_r of genes located far apart—e.g., on two opposite ends of the chromosome—is often close to 0.5. The closer any two genes are, the lower will be the f_r between them, and when two genes are very close—e.g., side by side—their recombination frequency will approach the value of 0.0. Therefore, the f_r between any two genes is directly proportional to the distance that separates them on the chromosome. Two genes that are close to one another on a given chromosome will be separated by recombination less often and are said to be strongly linked. Genes that are not linked have $f_r = 0.5$, whereas linked genes have an f_r ranging from 0.0 to 0.5, depending on the linkage strength.

It may be difficult to distinguish whether two genes are not linked at all or are very weakly linked, since in both situations the f_r is close to 0.5. Conversely, it is also difficult to demonstrate that two putative genes are very closely linked ($f_r \approx 0.0$) or are actually alleles of the same gene ($f_r = 0.0$). When two genes are very closely linked, the alleles of both genes are almost invariably transmitted together and appear as a single allele referred to as **pseudoallele**. If unopposed, after a certain number of generations the phenomenon of crossing-over should produce all possible combinations of alleles for any pair of linked genes. Such a state is called **linkage equilibrium** and represents a situation in which the frequency (f) of any combination of alleles (haplotype) equals the product of the frequencies of alleles forming the haplotype:

$$f_{ab} = f_a \times f_b.$$

In this formula, *a* and *b* represent alleles, and *ab* is the haplotype composed of these alleles. In cases where the experimentally established value of f_{ab} is either larger or smaller than the product of f_a and f_b, the alleles are said to be in **linkage disequilibrium**. Disequilibrium is measured by the value Δ calculated from the formula

$$\Delta = f_{ab} - (f_a \times f_b).$$

Linkage disequilibrium may be either transient or permanent. Transient disequilibrium occurs when a given allele has recently developed by mutation and the random process of crossing-over has not had enough time to separate it from the allele to which it was linked at the time of its development. In this case, given sufficient time, equilibrium will be reestablished. However, in some instances, linkage disequilibrium is retained even after a long period of time and appears to be permanent. It has been speculated that in such a case either crossing-over between two genes is somehow suppressed or a particular haplotype confers certain advantages to the organism and is retained while the recombinant haplotypes are eliminated from the population.

1.6 Frequencies of Genotypes and Alleles

A familiarity with some basic concepts and formulas of population genetics is necessary for an understanding of many topics discussed in this book. The presentation will be kept as simple as possible because detailed mathematical derivations of the formulas are amply explained in many excellent textbooks of general genetics. Mendel's laws, although derived from observations of populations, define the rules of transmission of a gene and its alleles from one individual to another but not among many individuals or between consecutive generations of a population. To obtain insight into inheritance patterns within the populations and between generations, one must characterize the population with respect to its phenotypic (f_p), genotypic (f_g), and allelic (f_a) frequencies. Determination of f_p is relatively easy, since it can be made by direct observation or testing; f_g and f_a must be either deduced or calculated.

The value of f_p is the ratio of individuals expressing a given trait, variant, or allelic phenotype (n) to all individuals studied (N):

$$f_p = n/N.$$

If the relationship between a given phenotype and genotype is known, f_g can be derived from f_p by using the same formula. In general, $f_p = f_g$ if the alleles involved are codominant. However, in the case of dominance and recessiveness of alleles, the heterozygotes and dominant homozygotes will be phenotypically identical. Therefore, f_p of a dominant phenotype will represent the sum of the f_g for dominant homozygotes and the f_g for heterozygotes. To determine the actual f_g, a special formula must be employed, as discussed below.

It is often preferable to calculate f_a rather than f_g because the number of alleles (n_a) is always smaller than the number of possible genotypes (n_g) according to the formula given earlier (Section 1.3). The value of f_a can be derived from either the number (n) or frequencies (f) of genotypes according to the following formulas:

$$f_a = (2n_{ho} + n_{he})/2N.$$

In this formula, n_{ho} and n_{he} correspond to the number of homozygotes and heterozygotes, respectively, found in a population consisting of N individuals. Alternatively,

$$f_a = f_{ho} + 0.5f_{he},$$

where f_{ho} and f_{he} represent the frequencies of homozygotes and heterozygotes, respectively, in a population studied.

In the case of more than two alleles of a given gene, the calculation of f_a for any allele must include the sum (Σ) of various heterozygotes carrying this allele. Hence, the formula must be modified as follows:

$$f_a = (2n_{ho} + \Sigma n_{he})/2N.$$

1.7 Genetic Equilibrium and the Hardy-Weinberg Law

Under ordinary circumstances, f_a remains relatively constant in any particular population provided that two conditions are fulfilled. First, the population must not be the subject of forces that induce variability (see below). Second, mating in the population must be random. Random mating is mating that occurs between individuals regardless of their genotypes. In such a case, the frequency of mating (f_m) between individuals with two genotypes, *g1* and *g2*, is proportional to the product of the frequencies of these genotypes (f_{g1} and f_{g2}). This can be expressed as

$$f_m = f_{g1} \times f_{g2}.$$

A population with random mating maintains constant f_g and f_a and is said to be in **genetic equilibrium**.

Inasmuch as f_g and f_a in any population determine the pattern of inheritance of a given trait, the process of inheritance by itself does not change these frequencies. This principle, formulated at the beginning of this century, became known as the Hardy-Weinberg law and can be stated as follows:

> In the absence of variability-producing processes, the allelic and genotypic frequencies of a given population are related and achieve a state of equilibrium in a single generation of random mating and remain constant thereafter.

The Hardy-Weinberg law can be expressed mathematically as a square binomial expansion representing the relationship between the frequencies of the alleles (*a1, a2, a3,* etc.) and the frequencies of all possible genotypes:

$$(f_{a1} + f_{a2} + f_{a3})^2 = f_{a1}^2 + f_{a2}^2 + f_{a3}^2 + 2f_{a1}f_{a2} + 2f_{a1}f_{a3} + 2f_{a2}f_{a3}.$$

In this formula, the expressions f_a^2 represent the frequencies of homozygotes, and the expressions $2f_a f_a$ correspond to the frequencies of heterozygotes. If there are two alleles present in the population, then, given random mating, the gametes that form each new individual will combine at a rate proportional to their population frequency. That is, if the frequency of males bearing allele *a1* is f_{a1}, the frequency of females bearing allele *a1* is also f_{a1}. The random chance that a mating will occur between an *a*-bearing male and an *a*-bearing female will be $(f_{a1} \times f_{a1})$ or f_{a1}^2. Similar reasoning applies to individuals bearing *a2* alleles. Since the sum of the allele frequencies or the sum of the genotype frequencies must each equal 1.0, it follows that

$$f_{a1} + f_{a2} + f_{a3} = 1.0.$$

Therefore,

$$(f_{a1} + f_{a2} + f_{a3})^2 = 1.0$$

and

$$f_{a1}^2 + f_{a2}^2 + f_{a3}^2 + 2f_{a1}f_{a2} + 2f_{a1}f_{a3} + 2f_{a2}f_{a3} = 1.0.$$

Obviously, the formula is valid only if the frequencies of all alleles of a given gene are known and considered. Second, it must be emphasized that the law applies only to populations that are in genetic equilibrium—i.e., there are no significant changes in the frequencies elicited by external factors (see below) and the frequencies are the same in males and females.

As mentioned earlier, the calculation of f_g from the corresponding f_p for the combination of dominant and recessive alleles poses a problem since different genotypes (heterozygotes and dominant homozygotes) have the same phenotypes. The problem can be resolved by using the transformed Hardy-Weinberg formula:

$$f_{a1}^2 + f_{a2}^2 + 2f_{a1}f_{a2} = 1.0.$$

If *a1* is a recessive allele and *a2* is a dominant allele and since f_{a1}^2 is the frequency of recessive homozygotes (f_{hor}), the frequency of the recessive allele (f_{a1}) is

$$f_{a1} = \sqrt{f_{hor}}\ .$$

Since by definition $f_{a1} + f_{a2} = 1.0$, the frequency of the dominant allele (f_{a2}) is

$$f_{a2} = 1 - f_{a1}$$

or, by substitution from the previous formula,

$$f_{a2} = 1 - \sqrt{f_{hor}}\ .$$

Since the frequency of recessive homozygotes can be determined by direct observation of the population, it is possible to calculate the frequency of heterozygotes (f_{he}) from the following equations:

$$f_{he} = 2f_{a1}f_{a2}$$

$$f_{he} = 2 \times \sqrt{f_{hor}} \times (1 - \sqrt{f_{hor}})$$

$$f_{he} = 2(\sqrt{f_{hor}} - f_{hor}).$$

FACTORS INDUCING GENETIC VARIABILITY

In all preceding considerations, it was assumed that mating is random and that there are no forces inducing changes in the frequencies of existing alleles. To put it differently, it was assumed that genetic stability is maintained by random mating and that there is neither loss of existing alleles nor appearance of new alleles. Such a situation would maintain the status quo, and there would be no evolution. In fact, such a situation rarely takes place, as genes and alleles are subject to constant changes that can either be random or selective. It is the interplay of the processes causing these changes that constitutes the basis of evolution and is the subject of evolutionary genetics. Since genes that determine immunogenetic traits are by no means immune to the variability-inducing factors, these factors must be briefly discussed.

1.8 Genetic Drift

Drift represents a random variation of allelic frequencies in any two consecutive generations. Such a variation is due to the fact that the actual frequency of gametes carrying a given allele may occasionally deviate from the expected frequency. Such deviation is purely accidental both in size and direction, and it is inversely related to the size of the effective population (N)—i.e., to the number of individuals producing offspring. Genetic drift is governed by the classic laws of probability and in a large population has little, if any, effect upon genetic changes. To produce a permanent change in the allelic frequencies of a population, genetic drift would require 4N generations—i.e., for 100 individuals, as many as 400 generations or 12,000 years would be required for genetic drift to cause a permanent genetic change.

In practice, the conditions under which genetic drift would produce an appreciable change in allelic frequencies may be defined as $4Nx \ll 1.0$, where x represents a specific indicator of other variability-inducing processes such as mutation, migration, or selection (see below). This is precisely the condition that is fulfilled in two situations known as the **founder effect** and the **bottleneck effect**. The founder effect refers to the development of a distinct population from relatively few individuals (founders). Owing to their small number (N), genetic drift can result in allelic frequencies of the new population being significantly different from the frequencies in the population from which the founders originated. The bottleneck effect refers to a similar event in which a population returns to its original size after being reduced to relatively few individuals. Here, again, genetic drift, acting on the small number of survivors, may cause a change in the allelic frequencies such that they become strikingly different from those found before the reduction in population size.

1.9 Mutation

Mutation is the primary source of all variability underlying evolution since only an alteration of existing alleles can lead to new variants of a given trait and to the development of new species. However, mutation alone, unaided by other processes, especially selection, would produce an extremely slow change in the allelic frequencies of a population. This is because the mutation rate (M) of a given gene (i.e., frequency of formation of an altered gene [new allele]) is extremely low—on the average, 10^{-5}/gamete/generation. It can be demonstrated that a change in the frequency of an original allele (Δf_a) in a population would be very slow:

$$\Delta f_a = f_a - f_a(1 - M)^g.$$

In this formula, g corresponds to the number of consecutive generations in which the mutated allele is transmitted by random mating. The above calculation assumes that M is constant, that the mutation is unidirectional, and that there is no selective pressure on the mutant allele. In reality, more often than not, all these assumptions are only partially true. As a result, the change initiated by mutation is affected by a number of factors, with selection being the most important.

It is implicit in the above considerations that to change the population a mutation must occur in germ cells or their precursors. Mutation occurring in non-germ cells, called a **somatic mutation**, although capable of changing the phenotype of an individual, will be eliminated at the time of death of this individual regardless of whether the individual produced progeny. Even a germ cell mutation may be quickly eliminated if it is a **lethal mutation**, i.e., incompatible with survival or reproduction of the carrier. From a morphological point of view, mutations can be divided into two categories: **chromosomal** and **gene mutation**. Chromosomal mutations (Section 2.7) consist of alteration in size, shape, and number of chromosomes and can often be detected by an analysis of the chromosomes (**karyoanalysis** or **karyotyping**). Gene mutation affects a single gene without creating a visible change in the chromosome. The molecular basis of gene mutations will be discussed later (Section 3.8).

1.10 Migration

Migration, or **gene flow**, refers to the phenomenon of influx of a new allele(s) into a given (resident) population from another (migrant) population. Although migration by itself cannot produce a change in the species since no alteration of genes is involved, it influences the allelic frequencies in the two populations involved and may aid in the spreading of mutant genes. The overall effect of migration depends on several factors such as the rate of migration (m), frequencies of a given allele in the two populations, and the number of generations (g). One can calculate m using the formula

$$m = 1 - [(f_F - f_o)/(f_I - f_o)]^{1/g},$$

where f_I and f_F are the initial and final frequencies, respectively, of a given allele in the resident population and f_o is the frequency of the same allele in the migrant population. If neither favored nor opposed, migration will ultimately lead to the establishment of equal frequencies in both populations at which point migration will stop.* However, if the process of selection becomes superimposed upon migration, the latter may result in significant changes of allelic frequencies in one of the populations.

1.11 Selection

The three phenomena described above—genetic drift, mutation, and gene flow—may change the allelic frequencies in a population. For mutation and migration, both the rate and direction of change can be predicted, while only rate can be anticipated for drift. None of the three events, however, is oriented in regard to the adaptation of an individual or a species. To put it differently, all three processes are random with respect to adaptation. Therefore, all three processes alone or in combination, especially mutation, would produce uncontrollable changes and would totally disorganize the genetic makeup of a population. This "destructive" effect is counteracted by the effect of another process called **selection**. Natural selection is a process by which survival and reproduction maintain the desirable and eliminate the undesirable changes brought about by the other processes. It goes without saying that animal husbandry and agriculture mimic natural selection, although trait variants selected for during breeding are often different from those selected in nature.

Natural selection is commonly measured by the relative net fitness (w) and selection coefficient (s). Relative net fitness reflects the reproductive efficiency of a given genotype and depends on various components of which the most important are survival and fertility. Net fitness is a product of survival and fertility and can be determined from the formula

$$w = n2/n1 \times max.$$

In the formula, n1 and n2 are numbers of progeny in two consecutive generations of a given genotype and max corresponds to the largest n2/n1 ratio among the different genotypes studied. Knowing the net fitness, one can calculate the **selection coefficient(s)** from the formula

$$s = 1 - w.$$

---

*In fact, migration as a process may continue, but it will have no visible effect on the frequencies of alleles.

This coefficient measures the reduction of fitness caused by relative net fitness, and the genotype with the highest possible w (i.e., $w = 1$) will have $s = 0$, i.e., no reduction. Fitness allows one to predict the direction of changes; but since it is only a relative measure, it does not permit the prediction of changes in the size of a population.

Selection, operating through fitness, leads to either the elimination of a deleterious allele (with low fitness) or the establishment of a stable equilibrium, according to the Hardy-Weinberg law. Such an equilibrium can be established with polymorphism if selection favors heterozygotes or without polymorphism by selecting and retaining a single allele if selection favors homozygotes. In this case, it is referred to as **fixing** an allele. It is reasoned, therefore, that mutation and migration, by providing new alleles, and drift, by creating a temporary change in allelic frequencies, result in temporary disequilibrium. On the other hand, selection tends to bring the population back to equilibrium. Thus, the effects of mutation and selection are, in a sense, antagonistic; they cancel each other if their quantitative outcomes are the same. However, since mutation is a rather slow process whereas selection may work relatively quickly, the overall outcome is dictated by selection. It should be emphasized that mutation is a random process that constantly produces changes that are subject to selection - for or against. In conclusion, one may say that mutation, being random and disordered, is a primary source of variability that is subsequently subject to the ordering force of selection. The interplay of the two processes results in a slow but constant evolution.

1.12 Evolution

From a genetic point of view, **evolution** may be considered to be the result of random mutations and subsequent selection. However, the direction of selection depends on a variety of factors in addition to genetic ones. The *modus operandi* of evolution depends on the genetic makeup of a population.

Two alternative models of population have been proposed. The **classic model** assumes that the individuals comprising a population are homozygous and carry predominantly wild-type alleles. According to this concept, an occasional mutation creates a mutant allele that, if advantageous, is selected and ultimately replaces the wild-type from which it developed and returns the population to homozygosity. The **balanced model** proposes that most of the genes are polymorphic and that the individuals are predominantly heterozygous. Heterozygosity for one gene influences the genotype of other genes and so on. The selection of an occasional mutant is accompanied by a simultaneous selection of other alleles, thus maintaining the overall predominance of heterozygosity but with the new alleles. Both models agree that too many mutations at the same time would have a deleterious effect on the individual and species and such multiple mutations are promptly eliminated. Neither of the models is entirely acceptable, and it is likely that an intermediate model—with prevalence of homozygosity at some loci and prevalence of heterozygosity at other loci—would best reflect the random population presently in existence.

2 / *Principles of Cytogenetics*

The critical steps of inheritance occur during reproduction of the cell or the organism. The development of an understanding of the processes underlying inheritance at the cellular level is the admitted goal of both cytologists and cytogeneticists. In this chapter, some basic facts about these processes and the consequences of their alterations will be briefly presented.

THE CELL CYCLE

The life story of any cell is divisible into several phases that occur in a repetitive sequence called the **cell cycle**. Although the duration of the cell cycle may vary significantly from one cell to another, the basic phases remain essentially the same. The four phases called **G1** (gap), **S** (synthesis), **G2** (gap), and **M** (mitosis) are shown in Fig. 2.1. The first three phases occur during **interkinesis** or **interphase** during which time the cell performs its normal vital functions, and the last, M phase, corresponds to **cell division**.

From a genetic standpoint, one can view the cell cycle as a process consisting of the decoding (G1 and G2), replication (S), and, finally, the transmission (M) of genetic information from parental to progeny cells. Utilization and replication of the genetic information will be discussed in Chapter 3, which deals with the principles of molecular genetics.

During the S phase, the genetic information contained in the nuclear DNA is replicated; thus, if the amount of DNA in the G1 phase is designated 2n, it becomes 4n after the S phase. Most of the cellular DNA is distributed among the chromosomes, and the result of the S phase is also an increase in the number of interkinetic (interphasic) chromosomes from 2N to 4N. However, the newly produced copies of the chromosomes remain in physical association with the original copies as pairs of **sister chromatids** until they are actually separated during cell division and become new chromosomes. The replication of DNA and chromosomes usually, but not always, leads in a short time to cell division, **mitosis**. Some cells, however, may remain arrested in the G2 phase for prolonged periods of time during which they retain a 4n amount of DNA and a 4N number of chromosomes.

2.1 Mitosis

Morphologically, the M phase consists of two consecutive and partially overlapping periods: division of the nucleus—**karyokinesis**—and division of the cytoplasm—**cytokinesis**. Under ordinary circumstances, the two periods usually follow each other, but in some normal, as well as some pathological, cases there may be no cytokinesis, and the resulting cells will have two nuclei (a **binuclear** cell). If karyokinesis takes place several times in succession without accompanying cytokinesis, a cell will have several nuclei (a **polynuclear** or **polykaryotic** cell). This may happen in some normal cells, but it is most commonly observed in neoplastic cells. Once initiated, the entire process of karyokinesis usually takes about two hours and consists of four phases, which are identified rather arbitrarily (Fig. 2.2).

Prophase is characterized by the condensation of chromsomes, which during interphase are threadlike structures that are indistinguishable from each other and form **nuclear chromatin**. Upon completion of prophase, the chromosomes become easily identifiable. At this

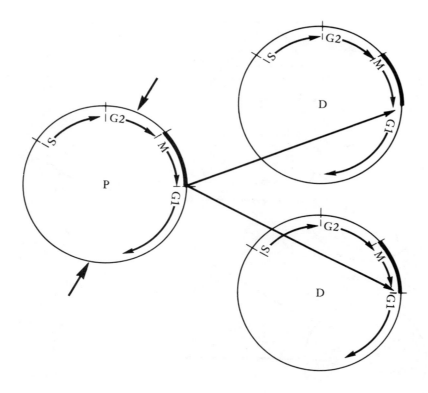

FIG. 2.1. Cell cycles of parental (**P**) and daughter (**D**) cells. Each cell begins the cycle with the
G1 phase and proceeds through **S**, **G2**, and **M** phases. The cell cycle may be arrested
for various periods of time at G1 or G2 phases as indicated by arrows in the P cell.

stage, each chromosome consists of two sister chromatids that initially are tightly connected
along their entire length but at later stages become disconnected except at one point called the
centromere. As mentioned earlier, two sister chromatids are copies of each other formed
during the S phase. The condensation of the chromosomes is accompanied by a gradual
disappearance of the **nucleolus** and the breakdown of the **nuclear membrane**. Simultaneously, the **centrioles** in the cytoplasm duplicate and begin to migrate toward opposite
poles of the cell.

    Metaphase begins when the nuclear membrane has disappeared completely and the
chromosomes are lying free and in disarray in the cytoplasm. Subsequently, they aggregate in
the midpart of the cell in the form of an **equatorial plate** if looked upon from the side or of a
maternal star if looked upon from either cell pole. At this time their centromeres are usually
directed centrally and connected to minute fibers originating from the centrioles. The fibers and
the centrioles comprise a characteristic **spindle apparatus** or **achromatic figure**. It is at this

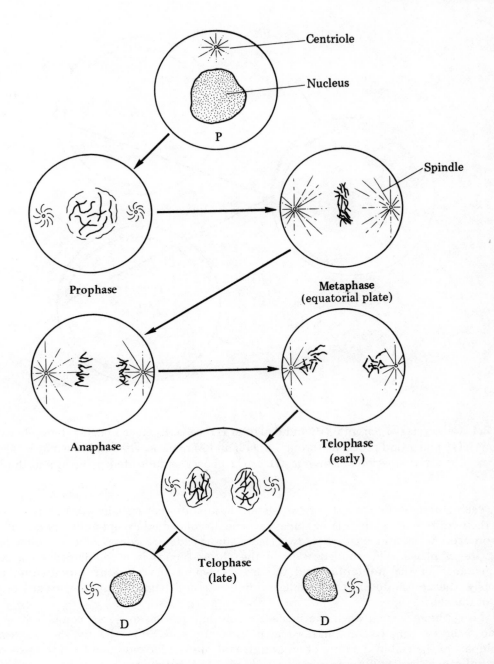

FIG. 2.2. Mitosis. Stages of karyokinesis of the parental (**P**) cell preceding its division into two daughter (**D**) cells. For details, see text.

stage that the two sister chromatids may occasionally break and become reconnected after exchanging fragments between them. This phenomenon is called **sister chromatid exchange** (SCE). Although normally the process by itself does not change the genetic information since the two chromatids are identical, occasionally it may lead to an alteration when the break points in the two chromatids are located at different sites; one chromatid gains and the other loses some genetic material.

Anaphase begins abruptly when the two sister chromatids separate and each begins to move toward the opposite cell poles with a velocity of about 0.2-4 μm/min. The movement is caused by contraction of the spindle fibers, which pull at the centromeres of each chromatid so that each centromere moves first and is followed by the rest of the body of the chromatid. Once separated, chromatids become new chromosomes.

Telophase begins when the chromosomes complete their movement toward their selected cell poles and gather there to form two clusters called **daughter stars**. Subsequently, the clusters become surrounded by a membrane, the chromosomes begin decondensing, and the nucleolus reappears. One may say that telophase is a reverse prophase. After telophase, the cell has two nuclei for a brief period of time.

Since each chromosome consisted of two sister chromatids that separated at the beginning of anaphase, the two nuclei have exactly the same number of chromosomes (2N) and the same amount of DNA (2n) as was present in the cell before S phase. Obviously, since sister chromatids are exact copies of each other, they contain the same genetic information, even in the event that SCE occurs. On occasion, some of the sister chromatids will not separate and both will travel to the same cell pole. This phenomenon, called **nondisjunction**, is responsible for an abnormal and unequal number of chromosomes in two newly formed nuclei and subsequently in two newly formed cells.

Cytokinesis begins during telophase, and its onset is marked by the development of a cell membrane constriction (at the equator) of the cell. This constriction becomes increasingly pronounced and eventually divides the cell into two progeny cells. The mitotic process is the basic mode of division of somatic cells and ensures the quantitative and qualitative transmission of the same genetic information to the progeny cells.

2.2 Meiosis

In contrast to somatic cell division (mitosis), cells that differentiate into gametes (germ cells) must at some point during their development eliminate half of their chromosomes and, therefore, half their DNA. This reduction is necessary since two gametes must eventually join together to form a **zygote** from which a new organism develops. Without such an elimination or reduction in the amount of DNA and in the number of chromosomes, zygotes of each consecutive generation would double both values. Reduction takes place during **gametogenesis** or more specifically during two consecutive cell divisions called **meiosis I** and **meiosis II**. Meiosis I serves to segregate two diploid sets of chromosomes, whereas meiosis II further divides these diploid sets into haploid sets. In both divisions, the four typical phases of mitosis can be distinguished even though they are appreciably modified.

The first division is called meiosis I, or **reductional division** (Fig. 2.3) and is preceded

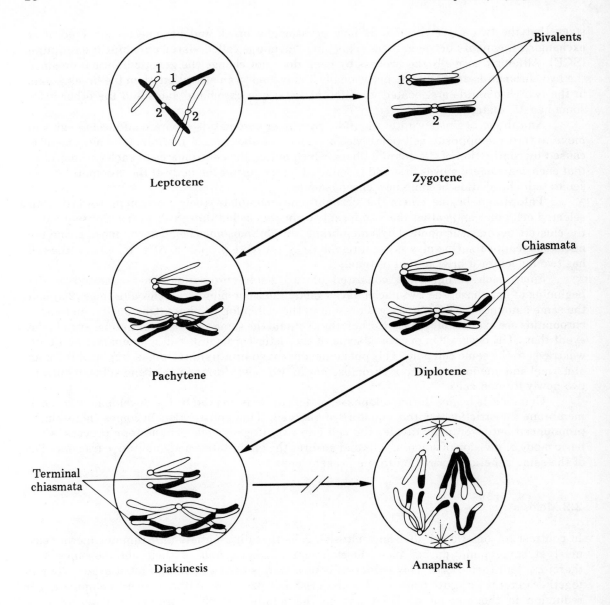

FIG. 2.3. Prophase of meiosis I. For simplicity, only two pairs (**1** and **2**) of chromosomes are represented. Maternal chromosomes of each pair are white, and paternal chromosome are black. At anaphase recombinant chromosomes, each carrying a combination of maternal and paternal alleles, are moving to the opposite poles of the cell.

by the S phase during which time the amount of DNA increases from 2n to 4n and the number of chromosomes increases from 2N to 4N. In the prolonged prophase of meiosis I, the following five substages can be distinguished.

The **leptotene** substage is characterized by a partial condensation of all chromosomes, which now become visible but are still indistinguishable from each other.

The **zygotene** substage consists of a tight, side-by-side joining of the homologous chromosomes into structures called **bivalents**. Since each individual chromosome has two sister chromatids and bivalent is composed of two homologous chromosomes it has a total of four chromatids (tetrad). The four chromatids form two pairs that are morphologically identical, although each pair contains distinctly different genetic information. This is because one chromatid pair comes from the paternal chromosome, while the other comes from the homologous maternal chromosome, and two parental organisms (paternal and maternal) usually have, at least for some genes, different alleles.

The **pachytene** substage is characterized by a further condensation of the chromosome, forming each bivalent.

The **diplotene** substage consists of the beginning of the separation of the bivalents into two chromosomes. The separation begins at the centromere and proceeds toward both ends of the chromosomes. As the process progresses, the two chromosomes become almost entirely separated except for two to three sites at which the chromatid of one chromosome is connected to a chromatid of the other chromosome. These sites are often easily discernible under the light microscope and are called **chiasmata** (singular, **chiasma**). Each chiasma represents a break and rejoining of two chromatids. In meiosis the break and subsequent exchange occurs not between sister chromatids but between chromatids of homologous chromosomes. Exchange or crossing-over that occurs between non-sister chromatids results in a recombination of alleles present in the homologous chromosomes. Thus, crossing-over is the phenomenon responsible for the recombination of linked genes (Section 1.5). Morphologic proof for fragment exchange between homologous chromosomes has been obtained by correlation of genetic recombination with the exchange of microscopically detectable markers of the homologous chromosomes. The two sister chromatids remain connected with each other at the centromere during the entire process.

Diakinesis, the last substage of meiosis I prophase, is characterized by the separation of the bivalents over their entire length except at the ends where the two chromosomes remain connected by **terminal chiasmata**. Toward the completion of diakinesis, the nuclear membrane disappears, signaling an end to prophase and the beginning of metaphase.

In metaphase the bivalents, connected by terminal chiasmata, are arranged at the equatorial plate. The centromere of each chromosome is attached to a spindle fiber originating at one of the two poles of the cell. At the onset of anaphase, each bivalent finally separates into two chromatid pairs that move toward opposite poles. It should be noted that, in contrast to mitosis in which spindle fibers pull individual chromatids, in meiosis I spindle fibers pull a chromosome that consists of a pair of connected chromatids. As a result, the new nuclei formed at the end of telophase will have an amount of DNA reduced from 4n to 2n and a reduced number of chromosomes; however, each chromosome consists of a pair of chromatids. Because during meiosis I the chromatids undergo crossing-over, they may differ with respect to the genetic information they carry and should not be called sister chromatids. Meiosis I (reductional division is almost immediately followed by the next division called meiosis II (equational division).

Meiosis II is not preceded by the S phase since each chromosome already consists of two chromatids. The prophase of meiosis II is very brief, and the remainder of the meiotic process is identical to mitosis. During metaphase, the two chromatids of each chromosome are attached to new spindle fibers and migrate to opposite poles of the cell at anaphase. The two new nuclei will now have half of the original (2N) number of chromosomes, i.e., N, and are termed **haploid** as opposed to somatic cells, which, after completion of mitosis, have a **diploid** number of chromosomes (2N).

2.3 Gametogenesis

The two meiotic divisions are essential steps in the process of germ cell (gamete) formation. The first division allows a random distribution (recombination) of homologous chromosomes with the possible number of recombinants of nonlinked genes equal to 2^x where x represents the number of homologous pairs. In man the number of somatic homologous pairs is 22, 23 including the X and Y chromosomes. Therefore, the first meiotic division can produce 2^{23} recombinants, i.e., 8,388,608. In the second meiotic division, a random distribution of the recombinant chromatids formed by crossing-over further increases the number of recombinant haploid cells. At this step, the number of recombinants for each chromosome may be expressed by 2^y where y is the number of chiasmata (an average of 2/bivalent). As can be seen, meiosis not only reduces the amount of genetic information to be transmitted, but it also generates enormous variation in the combination of alleles, linked and nonlinked, that are transmitted to haploid germ cells. Gametogenesis in the male and the female is schematically presented in Fig. 2.4.

In the male, gametogenesis is called **spermatogenesis**. The first meiotic division occurs between **spermatocyte I** and **spermatocyte II**, and the second division occurs between spermatocyte II and **spermatid**. Each spermatid is transformed into a mature male germ cell, a **spermatozoon** (plural, **spermatozoa**), by the process of differentiation (**spermiogenesis**). In the female, gametogenesis is called **oogenesis**. The first division occurs between **oocyte I** and **oocyte II** and results in the formation of oocyte II and the **first polar body** (**polocyte I**). Oocyte II then enters the second division, which becomes arrested at metaphase. Division becomes reactivated by **fertilization**, i.e., the penetration by a spermatozoon, and results in the formation of an **ovum** and the **second polar body** (**polocyte II**). The spermatozoon and the ovum each has the haploid number of chromosomes (N); hence the zygote, a cell formed by their union, will have double that number and will be diploid (2N). One half of the diploid set of chromosomes is contributed to the zygote by the spermatozoon and carries paternal alleles, and the other half consists of ovum chromosomes and carries maternal alleles.

When the zygote develops into an adult organism capable of producing germ cells, each germ cell will have half of all the organism's alleles. Among them, 50 percent will be paternal and 50 percent will be maternal. It is quite easy to demonstrate that as a result of recombination of nonlinked and linked genes and the reduction during gametogenesis each generation has a certain fraction of alleles from each preceding generation. It can be calculated that such a fraction is equal to 2^x where x is the number of the generation in question. Assuming that an

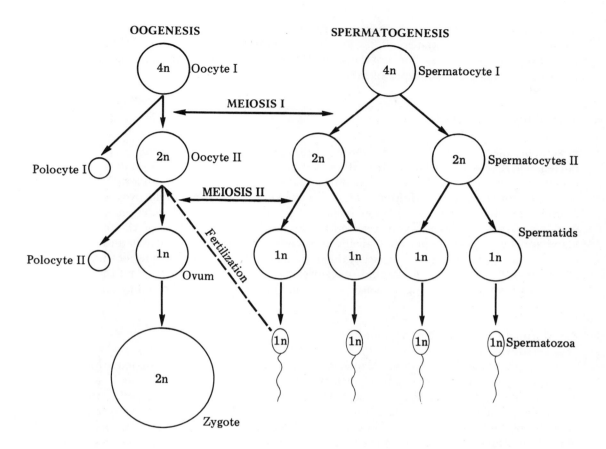

FIG. 2.4. Gametogenesis in the female (**oogenesis**) and in the male (**spermatogenesis**). From original diploid cells, the haploid gametes—one ovum and four spermatozoa—are formed. Fusion of two haploid gametes forms a diploid zygote. The value **n** indicates the amount of DNA.

individual is generation 0, his parents are generation −1, and the alleles of each parent constitute $(2)^{-1}$ or ½ of the genotype; grandparents are generation −2, and the alleles of each grandparent constitute $(2)^{-2}$ or ¼ of the individual's genotype, etc. This important fact forms the basis of producing certain types of inbred animals (Section 5.4).

THE CHROMOSOME

Essentially all the genetic information in a cell, and thus in an individual, is contained in the nuclear DNA (Section 3.1). Nuclear DNA is organized into distinct morphological structures called chromosomes. Each species has its characteristic and constant number of chromosomes, or its **chromosomal complement**. The set consists of **autosomes** and two **heterochromosomes** (sex chromosomes). Autosomes can be arranged into homologous pairs in which one member of the pair has been contributed by the mother and the other by the father. The two members of each pair are morphologically very similar, if not identical. The heterochromosomes form the pair that determines the sex of the individual, and the chromosomes of this pair may be strikingly different. Although chromosomes preserve their integrity throughout the life of a cell, their morphology changes significantly, depending on the phase of the cell cycle.

2.4 Morphology of the Chromosome

The interphase, or interkinetic, chromosome is sometimes called the **prochromosome** and constitutes the major component of nuclear chromatin. Its fine structure has been elucidated with the aid of the electron microscope. The basic component of the interphasic chromosome is a double-stranded DNA forming the smallest nuclear fibril—**protochromonema**—with a diameter of 20–50Å. When the protochromonema coils around the nuclear proteins, histones, a thicker fibril (about 100 Å) called the **subchromonema** is formed. Further condensation of the subchromonema results in a still thicker fibril (250–300 Å) called a **chromonema**. Some segments of the chromonema are still more condensed and stain readily with basic dyes. Such condensed segments are known as **heterochromatin**. It is the chromonema that becomes replicated during the S phase of the cell cycle and subsequently forms the chromatid. The early chromatid represents a coiled chromonema that is folded lengthwise five to seven times. Both chromatids are very closely packed at a common point and are joined by a structure called a centromere.

The basic structure of the mitotic chromosome has been known since the discovery of mitosis at the end of the past century. However, a more detailed description became possible only when metaphase chromosomes could be separated and studied in greater detail. Fig. 2.5 shows typical metaphase chromosomes. Each chromosome has two major components: a centromere, or **primary constriction**, and either one or two **arms**. During late prophase, the arm(s) consists of two closely connected sister chromatids. At a later stage, the chromatids separate along their entire length except at the centromere. Each arm stains unevenly with various histologic stains and shows lighter and darker zones or **bands**. Depending on the stain and procedure employed, the bands are referred to as Q after staining with quinacrine, G after

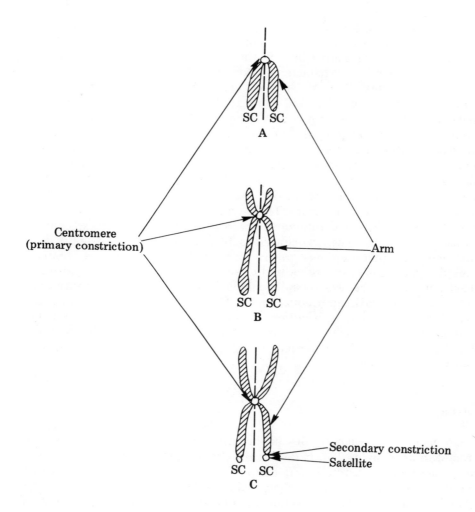

FIG. 2.5. Three types of late metaphasic chromosomes. (**A**) Telocentric with only one arm and a centromeric index equal to 0.0. (**B**) Acrocentric with one arm shorter than the other and a centromeric index of about 0.25. (**C**) Metacentric with equal arms and a centromeric index equal to 0.5. Each chromosome consists of two sister chromatids (**SC**) connected at the centromere.

staining with Giemsa reagent, or C after staining with Giemsa reagent following treatment with alkali. It is believed that bright Q bands and dark G bands represent **nontranscribable spacers**, whereas active genes are located in the dull Q bands and light G bands. The number and position of these bands are characteristic for each chromosome and are similar in the two homologous chromosomes. The staining of chromosomes to demonstrate these bands (**banding**) permits the identification and pairing of homologous chromosomes. Occasionally, a **secondary constriction** of the chromosome occurs close to one end, separating the main body of the chromosome from a small fragment called a **satellite**. At the tip(s) of the arm(s), there is an ill-defined structure called a **telomere**, which purportedly prevents the connection of the two chromosomes end to end. Such a connection would interfere with separation of chromosomes during mitosis.

The position of the centromere along the chromosome is an important feature in the identification of particular chromosomes. Three types of chromosomes are distinguished on the basis of centromere position. The **telocentric** chromosome has its centromere at the very end, and thus it has only one arm. The **acrocentric** (subtelocentric) chromosome has its centromere close to the end, and, therefore, one arm is significantly longer than the other. Finally, the chromosome that has its centromere located close to the midpoint is called **submetacentric**, and that having its centromere exactly in the middle is referred to as **metacentric**. The arms in both instances are of approximately equal length. Morphologically, chromosomes are classified on the basis of their **relative length** and/or their **centromeric index**. The relative length of the chromosome is expressed in arbitrary units corresponding to 0.001 of the total length of the entire set of chromosomes. The centromeric index is the ratio of the shorter arm to the total length of a given chromosome.

2.5 Karyotype

As previously mentioned, each species has a characteristic set of chromosomes varying in number from 2 to as many as 254. However, the average number is between 30 and 50. The chromosomes can be arranged into pairs that are numbered in sequence (Fig. 2.6) by Arabic numbers and further assigned to groups* according to their relative length and/or centromeric index. Isolated chromosomes can be photographed and arranged in pairs and in groups. After arrangement, the complement of chromosomes is called a **karyotype**, or **ideogram**. Preparation of the karyotype is an important step in a chromosomal analysis when searching for possible abnormalities. In the early days of karyoanalysis, only morphological features were used to prepare a karyotype, but the subsequent development of banding techniques has made karyotyping much more accurate. Karyoanalysis performed on artificially formed interspecies **cell hybrids** permitted, in several instances, the assignment of a specific gene to a specific chromosome. Since hybrids are formed by the fusion of two different cells, they carry two distinct sets of chromosomes. However, in most instances the hybrid cells gradually lose chromosomes of one species, and such a loss is often correlated with the loss of certain

---

*With respect to human chromosomes, this classification is commonly known as the Denver classification.

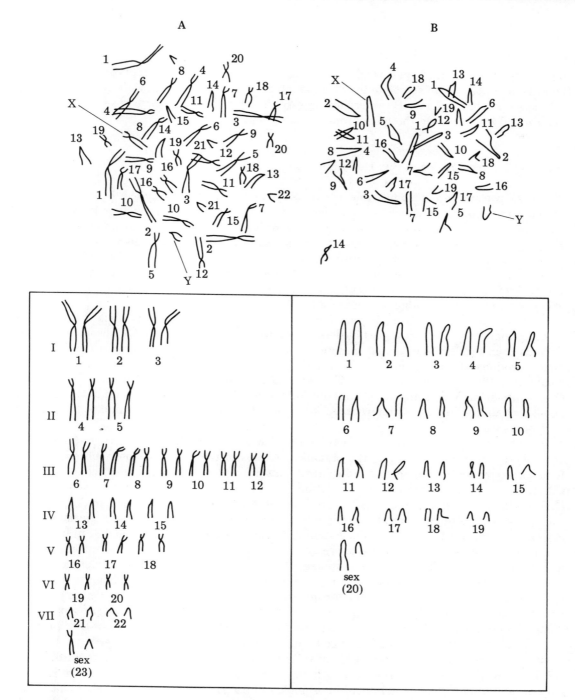

FIG. 2.6 Karyotypes (ideograms) of the man (**A**) and laboratory mouse (**B**). The karyotypes were prepared from a preparation of metaphase chromosomes by arranging them into homologous pairs; in the case of man, into seven groups (Denver classification).

phenotypic traits of that species. By analyzing the karyotypes and phenotypes of various cell hybrids, it is possible to correlate the disappearance of a particular trait with the disappearance of a specific chromosome. By inference, one could draw the conclusion that the lost trait is determined by a gene on the lost chromosome.

2.6 Sex Chromosomes and Sex Determination

There are two sex chromosomes, one designated X, for the female, and the other Y, for the male chromosome. For essentially all mammalian species discussed in this book, females are X/X and males are X/Y. This type of sex determination in which the males are heterogametic is called the **Drosophila** or **Tenebrio** type. Other types of sex determination are also known to exist in various species and are called **Protenor** (females are X/X and males are X/O), **Abraxas** (females are X/Y and males are X/X) and **haploidy-diploidy** (males are haploid and sterile, whereas females are diploid and fertile). The names are derived from the names of the insect in which a given type was originally observed.

The male Y chromosome is smaller than its female X counterpart since the Y chromosome probably evolved by a partial deletion of what was originally an X chromosome. It is obvious from Fig. 2.7 that females produce ova that carry one of the X chromosomes, whereas males produce spermatozoa that carry either the X or the Y chromosome. Under normal conditions, the ratio of the X and Y spermatozoa produced is close to 1:1. The random fertilization of an X-carrying ova should produce either X/X (female) or X/Y (male) zygotes with equal probability. Indeed, with few exceptions, the ratio of females to males in most populations is close to 1.0.

The X chromosome carries a set of genes that determines a wide variety of traits that do not necessarily affect the sex of the organism. Alleles of the genes on the X chromosome in females segregate according to simple Mendelian principles (Section 1.4). In contrast, the Y chromosome, being the product of a deletion, lacks many, but not all, genes present on the X chromosome. Therefore, Y/O zygotes are incapable of survival as opposed to X/O zygotes, which, although often abnormal, are capable of surviving. Nevertheless, the Y chromosome is not entirely deprived of genetic information. The sex-related genes of the male can be divided into two categories. Genes that are expressed in males and not in females are transmitted only from fathers to sons. This type of inheritance is called **holandric**, and the best example of this is the inheritance of maleness and fertility. Another example of holandric inheritance occurs during transmission of a particular histocompatibility antigen (H-Y) that is present in males but not in females (Section 21.8). Another group of genes consists of those that are present on both Y and X chromosomes and, thus, are transmitted from fathers to both sexes of ther progeny.

The difference in the number of genes on the X and Y chromosomes is responsible for the phenomenon of sex-linked transmission of various traits. This transmission is illustrated in Fig. 2.7. It can be seen that the female, being heterozygous and carrying a wild-type (normal) and a mutant (abnormal) allele on her X chromosomes, will transmit the abnormal allele to half of her sons and daughters. If the abnormal allele is recessive, none of her daughters will express the abnormal phenotype since they will have a dominant normal allele obtained with the father's X chromosome. However, all of her sons who receive the abnormal allele will express the abnormal

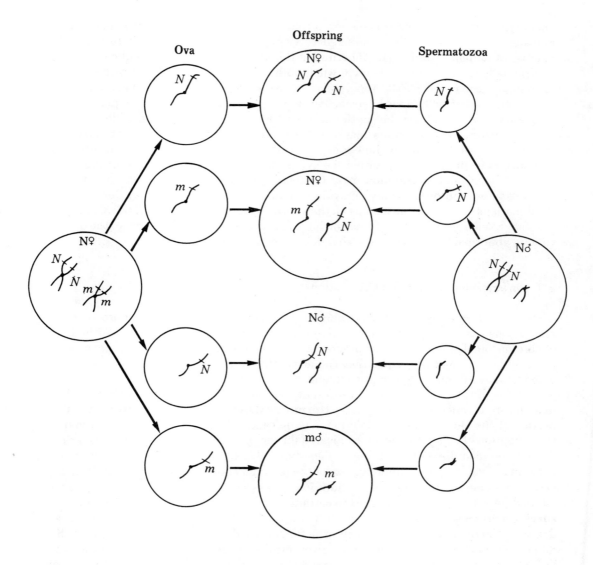

FIG. 2.7. Drosophila (Tenebrio) type of sex determination and transmission of sex-linked genes. Female (**N♀**) that carries on one of her *X* chromosomes to a recessive mutant allele (***m***) transmits it to half of her ova. The *m* allele is expressed only in a male zygote (**m♂**) formed with a *Y* chromosome of a normal male (**N♂**).

phenotype if their *Y* chromosome does not have a dominant counterpart of the abnormal allele. Females are carriers of the sex-linked recessive allele and transmit it to their offspring. A number of human disorders are inherited in this way, e.g., hemophilia and color blindness. It is easy to deduce that in rare instances when both the female and male carry the abnormal allele, the daughters may receive the abnormal recessive allele from both parents and will express it. In man, such a situation happens extremely rarely, since abnormal alleles are present in a very low frequency and the chance that both parents carry them is usually negligible.

A distinct group of abnormalities that are associated with the sex chromosomes consists of cases caused by a nondisjunction occurring during gametogenesis and affecting the sex chromosomes. In these cases, either the ovum carries two *X* chromosomes or the spermatozoon carries both *X* and *Y* chromosomes. Correspondingly, some spermatozoa will carry no sex chromosomes, and occasionally an ovum lacking a sex chromosome may develop. A variety of combinations of sex chromosomes can then occur resulting in *XX/Y, XX/X, X/XY, X/O,* or *Y/O* zygotes. Except for the last case in which the individual is unable to survive, the others produce various abnormalities mostly of sexual development and function.

2.7 Chromosomal Mutations (Aberrations)

The sex abnormalities mentioned above are examples of one large group of chromosomal aberrations that can be classified into several types as shown in Table 2.1. Although the study of chromosomal aberrations falls predominantly into the realm of traditional genetics, they must be briefly mentioned here since they can affect the expression and function of genes connected with virtually all immunologic phenomena.

A **deletion**, or deficiency, represents the loss of a segment of a chromosome. Such a deletion may concern the peripheral (**terminal deletion**) or middle (**interstitial deletion**) portion of the chromosome. A deletion may be caused by the breaking of a chromosome or by the formation of a loop that is not replicated during the S phase and, therefore, is ultimately lost. A deletion can be detected both phenotypically, by the absence of certain traits, and karyoanalytically, by the abnormal size of the affected chromosome. Observation of phenotypes and karyotypes with deletions, in addition to assessment of interspecies cell hybrids, is a method for the assignment of genes to certain chromosomes when a karyotypic abnormality of a specific chromosome is correlated with a specific alteration of the phenotype. A physical deletion should not be confused with a functional deletion. In the first case, changes are detectable both phenotypically and karyotypically, whereas in the second case, no morphological changes in the chromosome can be seen. Functional deletion is due to either the suppression of certain genes or the presence of silent alleles, i.e., alleles that do not encode a product.

A **duplication** is the presence of a repeated segment of a given chromosome. The repeated segment may be located terminally or interstitially and often occurs in tandem—i.e., the repeated segments are side by side. A duplication, if large enough, is detectable in karyotypes as a change in the size of the chromosome. Phenotypically, the duplication may remain undetectable since it encodes the same traits, although repeatedly. However, the two originally identical segments may mutate independently, and a mutation limited to one of the

TABLE 2.1. Classification, Definitions, and Characteristics of Major Chromosomal Aberrations

Type of Aberration	Definition	Phenotypic Changes	Karyotypic Changes	Subtypes
Deletion	Loss of segment of chromosome	Absence of trait(s)	Decrease in size of chromosome	Terminal Interstitial
Duplication	Presence of extra segment of chromosome	New trait(s) after mutation of duplicated segment	Increase in size of chromosome	Terminal Interstitial
Inversion	Change in orientation of a fragment within chromosome	Change in linkage strength and suppression of recombination	Change in position of centromere*	Pericentric Paracentric
Translocation	Change of the position of a fragment within chromosome or transfer to different chromosome	Change in linkage strength	Change in size of chromosome	Simple Reciprocal a. Homozygous b. Heterozygous
Robertsonian changes	Joining of two chromosomes or break of single chromosome at centromere	Change in linkage strength	Change in the number and size of chromosomes	Fusion Fission

*Changes are detectable only in some pericentric inversions.

repeated fragments may become phenotypically detectable. A duplication may develop as the result of the breaking of a chromosome during S phase or by unequal crossing-over in meiosis. In the latter case, the two chromatids break at different sites, and after rejoining one chromatid has an extra segment (duplication) and the other lacks a segment (deletion). It is believed that duplication might play an instrumental role in the development of clusters of genes that, by independent mutations, acquire new functions but still preserve a certain similarity owing to their common origin. This is one of several concepts proposed for the development of the major histocompatibility complex (Chapters 15–17) and immunoglobulin genes (Chapter 8).

An **inversion** refers to the breakage of a chromosomal fragment and its return to its original place in the chromosome, but in a reversed position. If the change includes the centromere, the inversion is called **pericentric**, and if it concerns only one arm, it is called **paracentric**. Inversion, by definition, changes the linkage strength between genes in the affected chromosome. Paracentric inversion is undetectable in a karyotype. Pericentric inversion may change the morphology of the chromosome if it involves the repositioning of unequal fragments on both sides of the centromere. Inversion will cause an atypical pairing of

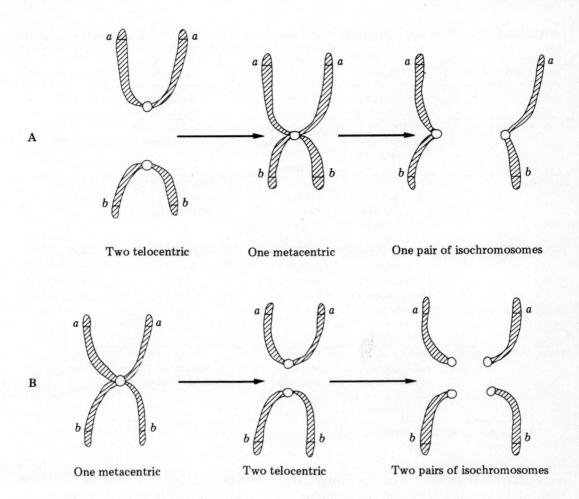

FIG. 2.8. Robertsonian changes. (**A**) Fusion of two telocentric chromosomes results in formation of a single metacentric chromosome, which during anaphase forms a pair of
isochromosomes. (**B**). Fission of a single metacentric chromosome produces two
telocentric chromosomes. From each chromsome a pair of isochromosomes is formed
during anaphase.

chromosomes during meiosis. Phenotypically, the most common effect of an inversion is a significant reduction in recombination (crossing-over) between genes within and outside of the inverted segment.

A **translocation** is an event in which a fragment of a chromosome changes its position. Two types of translocation can be distinguished. **Transposition**, or simple translocation, refers to the unidirectional transfer of a chromosomal fragment, either to a different location within the same chromosome or to a different, nonhomologous chromosome. Transposition from one arm to another of the same chromosome, or from one chromosome to another, is usually detectable in the karyotype. A **reciprocal translocation**, on the other hand, consists of an exchange of fragments between two nonhomologous chromosomes. Such an exchange can affect both members of the two involved pairs (homozygous) or only one member of each pair (heterozygous). In either case, the resulting chromosomes are grossly altered and easily detectable, especially during meiosis, since they form complexes, called **quadrivalents**, that consist of four rather than two chromosomes with the characteristic shape of a cross or circle. Apparent changes in the linkage between genes involved in translocation are easily detected phenotypically.

Robertsonian changes can be of two kinds—the **fusion** of two nonhomologous chromosomes through their centromeres or the **fission** of a single chromosome at the centromere (Fig. 2.8). In the first case, two chromosomes coalesce, and this results in a reduction in the number of chromosomes. In the second case, a single chromosome is converted into two **isochromosomes**; this results in an increase in the number of chromosomes. These changes alter neither the total amount of DNA nor the genetic information, but both result in a morphologically detectable aberration of the karyotype. By definition, fusion usually generates metacentric or submetacentric chromosomes, whereas fission forms telocentric chromosomes. Interestingly, the normal karyotype of the laboratory mouse consists of only telomeric chromosomes, strongly suggesting that multiple Robertsonian changes have occurred in this species. Also, exceptional cases in which chromosome complements are composed of a few or very many chromosomes suggest that such karyotypes developed by means of multiple Robertsonian changes. This concept is supported by the finding that all apes have 24 chromosome pairs, whereas man has only 23; a Robertsonian fusion may have occurred in man, reducing the number of chromosomes.

It was mentioned earlier that each species has a constant and characteristic diploid number of chromosomes in its somatic cells and a haploid number in its germ cells. These numbers, when present in the respective cells, are defined as **euploidy**. A lack or an excess of one or more chromosomes is called **aneuploidy**. Aneuploidy can originate from an abnormal segregation of chromosomes during meiosis or at early stages of embryogenesis. In the case of abnormal segregation during meiosis, all cells may lack a given chromosome pair (**nullisomy**), lack one member of the pair (**monosomy**), or have an excess of some chromosomes (**trisomy**, **tetrasomy**, **polysomy**). Generally, nullisomy is lethal as is monosomy, though less often. Polysomy often, but not always, has deleterious and even lethal effects. A deviation that occurs at a very early stage of embryogenesis results in aneuploidy that affects only a certain fraction of the cells, and such an individual is referred to as a **chromosomal mosaic**. In some instances, an entire haploid set of chromosomes can be missing (**monoploidy**), or an entire extra set may be present (**polyploidy**). While these types of abnormalities are extremely rare in the whole organism, they often affect certain cells, especially those undergoing neoplastic transformation.

3 / *Molecular Genetics*

A brief review of gene structure and expression in eukaryotes is in order before discussing the expression of various specific genes that determine immunogenetic traits.

GENETIC MATERIAL

Fig. 3.1 depicts a general outline of the processes underlying gene expression in higher organisms. Genes, composed of double-stranded *deoxyribonucleic acid* (DNA), are complex structures in themselves, often separated into coding and noncoding portions called **exons** and **introns**, respectively. In many genes, each exon encodes a distinct functional domain in the protein product. A gene is transcribed by **RNA polymerase**, and, initially, a **precursor** ribonucleic acid (preRNA) molecule is synthesized as a complementary copy of both the exon and intron components of the gene. The preRNA molecule is subsequently modified by a series of specific enzymatic events that generate a mature RNA molecule. These modification steps are collectively referred to as **RNA processing**. The mature RNA molecule proceeds to carry out its specific function. There are three classes of RNA. The **ribosomal RNA** (rRNA) consists of four types—28S, 18S, 5.8S, and 5S—which are found as structural components of **ribosomes**. **Messenger RNA** (mRNA) encodes the information needed to form a polypeptide chain. **Transfer RNA** (tRNA) or **soluble RNA** recognizes the triplet code in the mRNA and converts the code into an amino acid sequence.

3.1 Molecular Structure of Chromosomes

In higher organisms most DNA is found in the nucleus as a nucleoprotein complex forming a structure called a chromosome (Section 2.4). Protein components of chromosomes can be divided into two groups: the basic **histones** and a multitude of nonhistone chromosomal proteins.

The histones form stable octamers, each containing two molecules of histones H2A, H2B, H3, and H4. A double-stranded DNA chain (DNA duplex) 146 base pairs in length is wrapped 1¾ times around the histone octamer in a structure called the **nucleosome core** (Fig. 3.2**A**). The DNA-protein complex forms a structure resembling a string of beads in which each bead corresponds to a nucleosome core. Between adjacent nucleosome cores lies a **spacer DNA** segment, which serves as the binding site for histone H1 (Fig. 3.2**B**). The nucleosome can form a supramolecular structure in which each string of nucleosomes is coiled and placed one on top of the other (Fig. 3.2**C**). It is believed that the enormous contraction of DNA into chromatids during the prophase stage in mitosis is accomplished by the formation of this supramolecular structure.

The nonhistone proteins form a very heterogeneous group. There is evidence that some of these proteins can affect the nucleosome structure and, thus, promote gene expression by exposing a segment of the DNA to RNA polymerase. The sensitivity of an active gene to digestion with nuclease (Section 6.1) is directly correlated to the level of its expression in a cell. Genes that are being expressed, or have been expressed, are more exposed and more readily digested, whereas genes that are not being expressed, or have not been expressed, are less

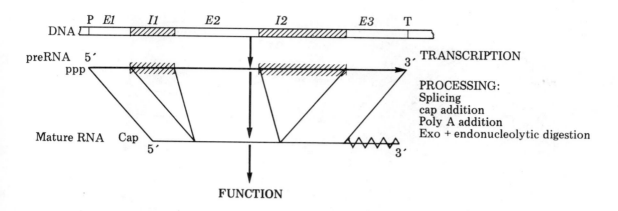

FIG. 3.1. Enzymatic steps involved in the expression of a complex eukaryotic gene: **P** = promoter or transcription initiation site; **I1** and **I2** = introns; **E1**, **E2**, and **E3** = exons; **T** = terminator or transcription termination site.

exposed and relatively resistant to nuclease digestion. This fact suggests that the level of condensation of the gene is altered prior to and during its expression, implying that a change in the nucleosomal structure of the gene must have occurred.

3.2 DNA Replication

During S phase of the cell cycle (Chapter 2), the DNA content and the number of chromosomes double owing to the replication of the nuclear DNA. During this period, in addition to a doubling of the DNA content, there is a twofold increase in the content of histone and nonhistone chromosomal proteins. The precise mechanism of nuclear DNA and chromosomal protein synthesis is largely unknown, but borrowing heavily from studies of prokaryotic DNA replication, in addition to utilizing information from recent research on eukaryotic DNA synthesis, one can arrive at a very general working model.

Replication is semiconservative—i.e., each new DNA duplex has one new and one old strand—and bidirectional—i.e., it proceeds from the point of origin in both directions. However, while one strand is continuously elongated in the 5′ to 3′ direction, the other strand replicates discontinuously and requires multiple initiation events. On each chromosome there are many

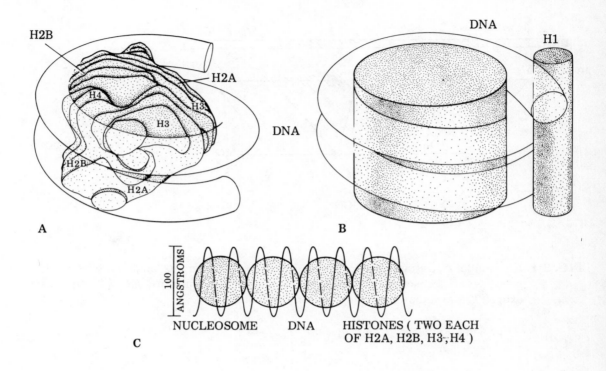

FIG. 3.2. Structure of nuclear DNA. (**A**) Model of a nucleosome core consisting of pairs of H2A, H2B, H3, and H4 histones surrounded by a stretch of double-stranded DNA 146 base pairs in length. (**B**) Model of a nucleosome core with position of H1 histone indicated. (**C**) Model of multiple histone cores wrapped by double-stranded DNA that consists of loops surrounding individual cores and spacer segments between cores. (Reprinted from: Kornberg, R. D., Klug, A., The nucleosome. Sci. Amer. **244**: 52–64, 1981. Used with permission.)

sites where replication may be initiated, and these sites are spaced at an average distance of 10,000 to 50,000 base pairs. Multiple initiation events require the synthesis of short RNA primers, which are removed after DNA synthesis proceeds, leaving a short gap in the DNA sequence. This gap is filled by a **DNA polymerase**, and the DNA segments are ligated together by a **DNA ligase**. This activity takes place at the **replication fork** (Fig. 3.3) and requires a great many enzymes—e.g., DNA polymerase, DNA ligase, and RNA polymerase or primase—and protein factors such as **DNA unwinding proteins** and other DNA binding proteins. As replication proceeds along the DNA molecule, one of the daughter duplexes associates with the original histone octamer. The other DNA duplex associates with a newly synthesized histone octamer, and thus the nucleosomal structure of the chromosome is maintained.

Genetic recombination (Chapters 1 and 2) requires specific cleavage and religation of the

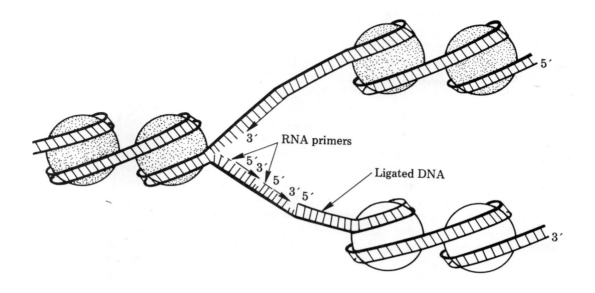

FIG. 3.3. DNA synthesis at the replication fork. The "old" nucleosome cores are dotted and the "new" cores are white. The "old" DNA strands are represented by a thick line, and the "new" DNA strands are marked by a thin line.

duplex DNA in the two homologous chromosomes. The mechanisms responsible for DNA recombination are unknown. It is likely, however, that DNA recombination utilizes many of the enzymes and factors employed in DNA replication in addition to specific proteins that are needed for DNA repair reactions.

GENE EXPRESSION

3.3 Transcription

In eukaryotes there are three forms of RNA polymerase, polymerase I, II, and III, which are responsible for the synthesis of precursors of the three classes of RNA; rRNA, mRNA, and tRNA and 5S rRNA, respectively. Each enzyme is a complex of several subunits, some of which are shared among the three forms of RNA polymerase, whereas others are unique to a given form of the enzyme.

Transcription is a highly specific process consisting of the following steps that take place after binding of RNA polymerase to DNA: **initiation**, **elongation**, and **termination** (Fig. 3.4). RNA polymerase must first recognize a particular DNA sequence called a **promoter**, bind to the DNA, and separate the strands of DNA duplex in the promoter region. This recognition requires a very specific interaction between the RNA polymerase and the promoter DNA sequence. Transcription is initiated by the formation of a phosphodiester bond between the first two nucleoside monophosphates.* Elongation, the sequence-directed addition of nucleoside monophosphates, continues until termination occurs. Termination, an event triggered by a particular DNA sequence called a **terminator**, results in RNA polymerase ceasing elongation of the transcript, release of a preRNA molecule from the transcription complex, and dissociation of the enzyme from the DNA.

In eukaryotes the level of expression of many genes is controlled by the modulation of the rate of preRNA synthesis. For example, the level of transcription of the 5S rRNA gene is controlled, in part, by the binding of a positive regulatory protein to the gene itself. In addition, steroid hormones, which can increase the expression of specific genes by several orders of magnitude, appear to work by binding to a specific activator protein that interacts with the activated gene and increases the level of preRNA synthesis. Since these activator proteins are gene products themselves, their structure must be determined by modifier genes (Section 1.2).

3.4 RNA Processing

Before being released from the nucleus to the cytoplasm, the preRNA is chemically modified during one or more enzymatic steps required for the production of a mature RNA species.

PreRNA may be shortened by endonucleolytic cleavage, in which an internal portion of the molecule is excised, and/or by exonucleolytic cleavage, which removes either the 3' or 5' tail of the precursor molecule. These processing reactions are especially important in rRNA maturation (Fig. 3.5). As mentioned above, many genes are mosaic structures in which coding portions, exons, are interrupted by noncoding intervening sequences, introns. Both exons and introns are transcribed into the preRNA molecule (Fig. 3.1). During RNA processing, a complex series of RNA **splicing** reactions take place in which the intron regions of transcript are excised and the exon-derived sequences are spliced together to form the active and mature RNA. A high degree of sequence conservation was found when several RNA sequences at the splice points of intron-exon junctions were compared. On the basis of these observations, a consensus **splice junction RNA sequence** was deduced. This led to the development of a model for RNA splicing that requires the use of a nuclear ribonucleoprotein that contains **U1 RNA**, a molecule that is complementary to the RNA splice junction sequence. It has been proposed that U1 RNA holds the splice points together by base pairing with the RNA in the region of the intron-exon

---

*Nucleosides are abbreviated A (adenosine), T (thymidine), U (uridine), C (cytosine), and G (guanosine).

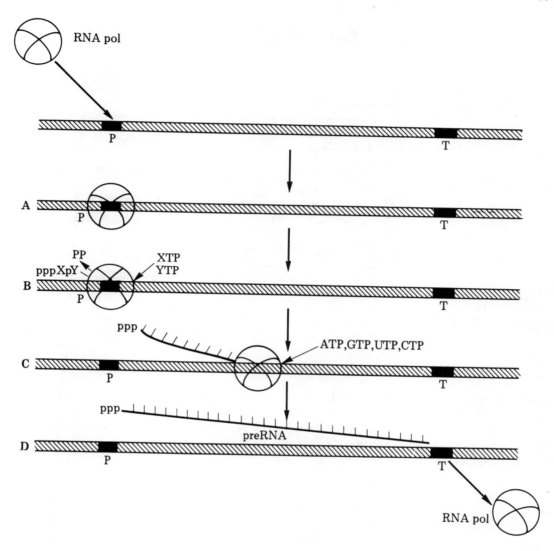

FIG. 3.4. Consecutive steps of transcription. (**A**) Binding of RNA polymerase (**RNA pol**) to the promoter (**P**). (**B**) Initiation of transcription by linking two nucleoside triphosphates (**XTP** and **YTP**) via phosphodiester bond and release of pyrophosphate (**PP**). (**C**) Elongation of mRNA chain by incorporation of nucleoside triphosphates (**ATP, GTP, UTP,** and **CTP**) according to base sequence of the DNA template. (**D**) Termination of transcription by dissociation of mRNA and RNA pol at terminator (**T**).

rRNA GENE

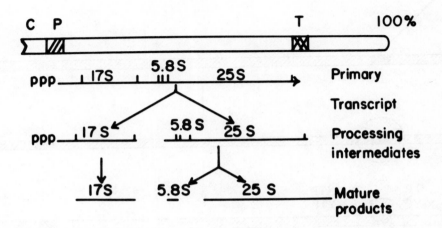

FIG. 3.5. The *rRNA* gene of *Tetrahymena pyriformis* and major synthetic and processing steps leading to the production of three kinds of rRNA: 17S, 5.8S, and 25S.

junctions. Splicing is a highly specific process, and a single base mistake will make most RNA molecules inoperative.

The 5′ ends of most mRNA molecules are joined by a 5′-5′ triphosphate linkage to 7-methyl-guanosine in a form called **cap structure** shown below.

Since this capping reaction is carried out in the nucleus at the level of the unprocessed RNA molecule, the cap site of an mRNA defines the promotor sequence or the site of transcription initiation. The cap structure plays a role in the binding of the mature mRNA to the ribosome during initiation of translation.

At the 3′ end of most mRNA molecules, an enzyme, **poly A polymerase**, catalyzes the addition of 200–250 adenosine monophosphate (AMP) residues. According to the following reaction,

$$\underrule{\hspace{1cm}}\text{AAUAAA}\underrule{\hspace{1cm}} \quad \xrightarrow[\text{poly A polymerase}]{\overset{\displaystyle (\text{ATP})_n \quad\quad P \sim P \to (2P)_n}{}} \quad \underrule{\hspace{1cm}}\text{AAUAAA}\underrule{\hspace{1cm}} (\text{A})_n$$

poly A polymerase recognizes the sequence AAUAAA near the 3′ end of the pre-mRNA. The addition of the poly A sequence is believed to play an essential role in ribonucleoprotein formation and in stabilizing the mRNA against nuclease digestion, thus slowing down the rate of mRNA turnover.

Different classes of RNA undergo a variety of chemical modifications of their bases and sugar backbone. For example, modification of tRNA plays an essential role in the folding of the rRNA and about 50 proteins and a small subunit containing the 16S—18S rRNA, and about 30 modified, and modified bases may play a role in ribosome formation. Finally, mRNA possesses a few specific modifications that include the cap and internal base methylation, but the significance of the latter remains unknown.

During or subsequent to the processing events, RNA molecules are complexed with proteins to form ribonucleoprotein complexes. For example, rRNA serves as a structural unit in the formation of ribosomes. Secondary structures in the rRNA serve as specific binding sites for ribosomal proteins and, thus, allow the construction of this complex protein-synthesizing machine, which consists of a large subunit containing the 23S-28S rRNA, the 5.8S and 5S rRNA, about 50 proteins and a small subunit containing the 16S–18S rRNA, and about 30 different proteins. The mRNA also binds specific proteins that may play a role in its transport from the nucleus to the cytoplasm and in maintaining stability of mRNA.

DECODING GENETIC INFORMATION

3.5 Translation

A functional mRNA can be thought of as possessing four regions essential for its decoding into protein sequences (Fig. 3.6). The four regions are (1) a **ribosome binding site**, (2) an **initiation triplet** (AUG or GUG), (3) **a sequence of coding triplets**, and (4) **termination triplet** (UAG, UAA, or UGA). The ribosome binding site is near the cap structure on the 5′ end of the mRNA. This sequence interacts with the 18S rRNA (i.e., 40S ribosome subunit) and permits the precise alignment of the mRNA on the ribosome as required for initiation of translation. AUG, the triplet sequence at the ribosome binding site, directs the binding of initiator tRNA-methionine (tRNA^{fmet}) and permits specific initiation of protein synthesis. The main

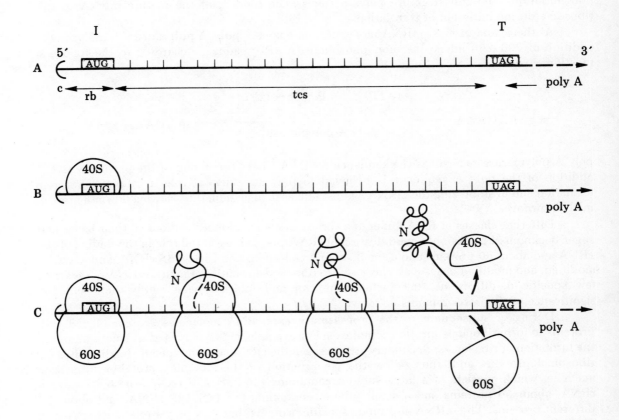

FIG. 3.6. Protein synthesis (translation). **(A)** Structure of mRNA with cap **(c)**, ribosome binding site **(rb)** that contains initiation **(I)** codon **AUG**, triplet-coding sequence **(tcs)**, terminator **(T)** codon **UAG**, and **poly A** sequence. **(B)** Initiation complex consisting of 40S subunit of ribosome bound to rb site. **(C)** Polysome consisting of three ribosomes and composed of 40S and 60S subunits and involved in synthesis of a polypeptide **(N)**. The fourth ribosome is being released at the T codon.

body of the mRNA is a collection of **codons**, each codon consisting of three bases (triplet), which permit the binding of a specific tRNA and allow the proper amino acids to be joined with each other in the growing polypeptide chain. Finally, a specific subset of triplets—UAG, UAA, or UGA—signals termination of translation and the binding of release factors, which, upon completion of translation, dissociate the mRNA from the ribosome. Synthesis of a protein begins at the amino terminal end and proceeds in the direction of the carboxy terminal end.

During translation, more than one ribosome binds to a single mRNA at any one time (Fig. 3.6 C). The structures, which are called **polysomes**, have from 5 to more than 20 ribosomes per single molecule of mRNA, depending on the size of the mRNA. Polysomes involved in the synthesis of soluble cytoplasmic proteins are randomly dispersed in the cytoplasm. However, polysomes participating in the synthesis of membrane-bound proteins or proteins that ultimately will be secreted are associated with the membranes of the endoplasmic reticulum. This binding of the ribosome to the endoplasmic reticulum is mediated by a 15–25 amino acid long **hydrophobic tail** on the nascent protein that becomes embedded in the membrane of the endoplasmic reticulum. In the case of membrane-bound protein, the tails anchor the protein in

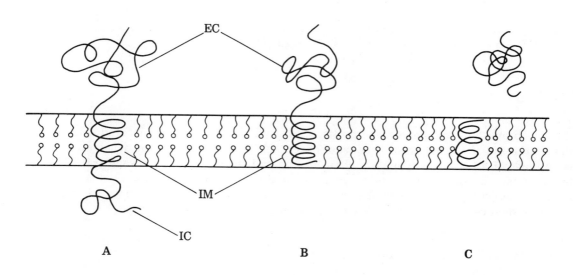

FIG. 3.7. Three types of relationships between protein and membrane. (**A**) Transmembrane protein is anchored into the membrane by a hydrophobic intramembrane portion (**IM**) inserted between hydrophilic extracellular (**EC**) and intracellular (**IC**) portions. (**B**) External protein is attached to the membrane by a hydrophobic tail (**IM**). (**C**) Secreted protein is released after clipping off an N terminal hydrophobic tail.

TABLE 3.1. Genetic Code as Base Triplets (codons) in mRNA

First Position (toward 5′ end of strand)	Second Position				Third Position (toward 3′ end of strand)
	U	C	A	G	
U	Phe	Ser	Tyr	Cys	U
	Phe	Ser	Tyr	Cys	C
	Leu	Ser	Stop	Stop	A
	Leu	Ser	Stop	Trp	G
C	Leu	Pro	His	Arg	U
	Leu	Pro	His	Arg	C
	Leu	Pro	Gln	Arg	A
	Leu	Pro	Gln	Arg	G
A	Ile	Thr	Asn	Ser	U
	Ile	Thr	Asn	Ser	C
	Ile	Thr	Lys	Arg	A
	Met*	Thr	Lys	Arg	G
G	Val	Ala	Asp	Gly	U
	Val	Ala	Asp	Gly	C
	Val	Ala	Glu	Gly	A
	Val	Ala	Glu	Gly	G

*AUG is a codon that also signals "start," though not in all cases.

the membrane. For transmembrane proteins, the hydrophobic region is located within, rather than at the end of, the amino acid sequence of protein. The hydrophobic tail of secreted proteins is clipped off after the polypeptide chain has passed through the membrane (Fig. 3.7). The hydrophobic tails play an important role in the production and secretion of all immunoglobulin chains. Interestingly, the former are encoded in discrete exons that are separated by an intervening sequence from the main body of the coding region of the genes.

3.6 Chemical Basis of Mutation

As mentioned above, the amino acid sequence of a polypeptide chain is determined by the triplet code of the mRNA. Any alteration in the mRNA sequence may cause a change in the amino acid sequence or even result in the inability of an mRNA to be translated. The genetic code is degenerate (see Table 3.1), i.e., more than one triplet encodes a given amino acid. Thus, not every DNA base change will produce an alteration in the protein sequence. The chemical basis of genetic mutation lies in the DNA sequence changes, and these changes can be easily categorized. In **initiation mutants**, an alteration in the initiation tRNA-methionine binding sequence AUG at the ribosome-binding site will prevent the proper initiation of protein synthesis and, thus, will result in the lack of synthesis of a particular protein. **Nonsense mutants** are caused by a change in the DNA sequence and result in the generation of termination triplet UAG, UAA, or UGA within mRNA. Synthesis is interrupted at the site of this termination triplet. Therefore, instead of a peptide of normal length, a shortened polypeptide chain will be produced. In **frameshift mutants**, the deletion of a coding region of the DNA, or the insertion of one or more bases (except multiples of three) into the coding region of the DNA, will result in the reading of all following triplet codons out of frame. However, the deletion or insertion of bases in multiples of three will cause a deletion or insertion or one or more amino acids but will not produce frame shift. **Readthrough mutants** are the result of the removal of the termination triplet, which causes the production of an elongated polypeptide chain. **Missense mutations**, alterations in the triplet sequence that changes the code from one amino acid to another, will result in polypeptide chains with altered amino acid sequences. Finally, **structural mutations** result from any alteration—base change, insertion, or deletion variety—that affects the secondary or tertiary structure of an mRNA. These changes in structure may affect the translation of an mRNA by modifying one or more of its processing steps, i.e., cap or poly A formation, or a splicing reaction.

I / *Suggested Supplementary Reading*

The following list of publications has been compiled to provide the reader with a source of specific references. It consists predominantly of the most recent textbooks, monographs, reviews and some selected original papers. Each publication listed has an extensive list of references that may be useful for the reader who desires to pursue in depth some topics discussed in the preceding section.

Abelson, J., RNA processing and the intervening sequence problem. Ann. Rev. Biochem. **48**: 1035–1049, 1979.

Ayala, F. J., Kiger, J. A., *Modern Genetics*. The Benjamin/Cummings Publishing Co., Menlo Park, London, Amsterdam, Sydney, 1980.

Breathnach, R., Chambon, P., Organization and expression of eukaryotic split genes coding for proteins. Ann. Rev. Biochem. **50**: 349–383, 1981.

Cavalli-Sforza, L. L., Bodmer, W. F., *The Genetics of Human Populations*. W. H. Freeman and Co., San Francisco, 1971.

De Robertis, E. D. P., Nowinski, W. W., Saez, F. A., *Cell Biology*. W. B. Saunders Co., Philadelphia, London, Toronto, 1970.

Dun, O. J., *Basic Statistics: A Primer for Biomedical Sciences*. J. Wiley & Sons, New York, London, Sydney, 1964.

Dyson, R. D., *Cell Biology. A Molecular Approach*. Allyn and Bacon, Boston, 1974.

Fraser, F. C., Nora, J. J., *Medical Genetics, Principles and Practice*. Lea and Fibiger, Philadelphia, 1981.

Fudenberg, H. H., Pink, J. R. L., Wang, An-C., Douglas, S. D., *Basic Immunogenetics*. Oxford University Press, New York, 1978.

Goodenough, U. *Genetics*. Holt, Rinehart and Winston, New York, 1978.

Green, F. L., *Genetics and Probability in Animal Breeding Experiments*. Oxford University Press, New York, 1981.

Greep, R. O., Weiss, L., *Histology*. McGraw-Hill, New York, 1973.

Hildeman, W. H., Clark, E. A., Raison, R. L., *Comprehensive Immunogenetics*. Elsevier, New York, 1981.

Klein, J., *Biology of the Mouse Histocompatibility-2 Complex*. Springer-Verlag, New York, Heidelberg, Berlin, 1975.

Kornberg, R. D., Klug, A., The nucleosome. Sci. Amer. **244**: 52–64, 1981.

Latt, S. A., Schreck, R. R., Sister chromatid exchange analysis. Am. J. Hum. Genet. **32**: 297–313, 1980.

Levitan, M., Montagu, A. *Textbook of Human Genetics*. Oxford University Press, New York, 1977.

Little, M., Paweletz, N., Petzelt, C., Ponstingl, H., Schroeter, D., Zimmermann, H-P. (eds.), *Mitosis Facts and Questions*. Springer-Verlag, Berlin, Heidelberg, New York, 1977.

Maltus, D., Oudet, P., Chambon, P., Structure of transcribing chromatin. Prog. Nucleic Acid Res. **24**: 1–55, 1980.

de Pamphilis, M. L., Wasserman, P., Replication of eukaryotic chromosomes. A close up of the replication fork. Ann. Rev. Biochem. **49**: 627–666, 1980.

Strickberger, M. W., *Genetics*. Macmillan, New York, 1976.

Sturtevant, A. H., *A History of Genetics*. Harper & Row, New York, 1965.

Sutton, H. E., *An Introduction to Human Genetics*. Holt, Rinehart and Winston, New York, 1965.

Watson, J. D., *Molecular Biology of the Gene*. W. A. Benjamin, Menlo Park, 1976.

II / Basic Methods of Immunogenetics

4 / *Basic Immunologic Methods*

4.1. Overview of Immunogenetics

During the course of its history, the science of genetics has evolved into several distinct branches. Immunogenetics can be defined as that branch of genetics that is concerned with traits detectable by immunologic methods. Specifically, immunogenetics studies the determination and inheritance of moieties that elicit an immune response, i.e., **antigens**, and the determination and inheritance of the capability to respond (**responsiveness**) to a variety of antigens.

Although genes that determine antigens are found in all living organisms, the antigens of higher animals have always been in the center of interest for immunogeneticists. From the repertoire of an animal's antigens, **alloantigens**, which distinguish individuals within a given species, have attracted special interest. Alloantigens can be subdivided into three distinct, but overlapping, categories. Alloantigens present predominantly as blood group antigens on erythrocytes constitute one category, while antigens present mainly on nucleated cells and antigens present in a cell-free form in body fluids make up the second and third categories, respectively. This division is far from precise because many blood group antigens may also be found on nucleated cells, and antigens of nucleated cells occasionally are detectable on erythrocytes. Furthermore, cell-bound antigens may be released into body fluids, whereas cell-free antigens can be passively adsorbed onto cells.

The ability to respond to a given antigen, i.e., immunologic responsiveness, is a feature of vertebrate animals since these animals have a more fully developed immune system than their primordial ancestors. Responsiveness is determined and influenced by a wide variety of elements that are either specific or nonspecific. Specific elements include antibodies (Chapter 7), antigen-specific *Ir* genes (Section 19.3), and antigen-specific receptors (Section 19.13). These elements selectively influence the response to a particular antigen and may permit only minimal response to one antigen while allowing maximal response to other antigens. Nonspecific elements affect virtually all responses regardless of the antigen. This category includes, but is not limited to, the effects exerted by molecules expressed on the cell surface of functionally distinct subsets of lymphoid cells, the capacity to synthesize protein and the ability of lymphoid cells to proliferate.

The ability to understand the data generated by immunogenetic studies, to interpret such data, and to formulate various working concepts and hypotheses is contingent on a sound knowledge of the principles and limitations of the methods used to generate the data. An **immunogenetic analysis** ordinarily consists of three steps: the immunologic identification of the trait, genetic analysis of the trait, and biochemical isolation and characterization of the corresponding gene product. Each consecutive step of the analysis employs a specific set of methods; therefore, it seems appropriate to discuss the principles of the most fundamental methods.

4.2 The Principal Rules of Immunogenetics

The first step of an immunogenetic analysis consists of the identification of a trait by a single or several different immunologic methods. These methods are used to elicit or examine a specific immune response and determine its nature, character, and magnitude. The use of these methods hinges on two primary assumptions of immunogenetics that concern the genetic determination of an antigen and the ability of an individual to respond to that antigen. The two rules can be formulated as follows:

> Each antigen is determined by one or more structural genes; the alleles of each gene, which determine variants of the antigen, are either dominant or codominant.

> An individual is able to respond to an antigen that is not expressed in this individual but cannot normally respond to an antigen that is expressed in this individual.

According to the first rule, a homozygous individual carrying an allele for a given variant of an antigen will express this variant, while the heterozygous individual, carrying two different alleles, will express both corresponding variants of the antigen. The expression of an antigen may be influenced by regulatory genes that may temporarily or even permanently prevent the expression of the antigen. Moreover, some antigens may be expressed in some but not all cells of a given individual. Finally, some antigens may be the result of interaction between complementary genes, and thus their expression requires the simultaneous presence of the appropriate alleles of two discrete structural genes (Section 1.2).

According to the second rule, an immune response can be elicited only by an antigen that normally is foreign to an individual's immune system. The response is influenced qualitatively and quantitatively by a variety of elements. Among these elements are the dose of antigen, its physicochemical form, the route of administration, and the age, sex, and physiologic status of the responder. From the immunogenetic point of view, perhaps the most important effect is exerted by the antigen-specific *Ir* genes (Section 19.3). These genes control the recognition of an antigen and can cause an otherwise permissible response to be very low or even undetectable. Finally, it should be pointed out that under abnormal conditions an immune response to antigen(s) normally present in an individual may develop. Such a situation, called **autoimmunity**, is the subject of general immunology and will not be discussed here.

Despite some limitations of and exceptions to the two cardinal rules, they constitute a sound basis for the use of various immunologic methods in the identification of a trait. The methods fall into two broad classes corresponding to the two basic types of immunity: **antibody-mediated** (humoral) and **cell-mediated** (cellular).

HUMORAL IMMUNITY AND ITS CONSEQUENCES

4.3 Principal Mechanism of the Humoral Response

Although a description of an immune response and its mechanism is within the domain of immunology, a brief schematic presentation of the topic should be helpful for subsequent discussions. Inasmuch as any immune response may be considered a continuous process, one can still distinguish three consecutive and interrelated phases.

The first phase is composed of several successive events—introduction, processing, presentation, and recognition of the antigen. The processing of the antigen is attributed to **macrophages** (mϕ) and results in the disassembly of the native molecule into small fragments that carry specific antigenic determinants. A **determinant** corresponds to a unique sequence and/or spatial arrangement of a few (two to six) amino acids, monosaccharides, or simple organic compounds. It is the determinant per se that is presented and recognized and against which the ensuing response is directed. Since a single macromolecule of an antigen may contain one or several different determinants, the response elicited by such a macromolecule represents a sum of responses against the individual determinants. The **antigen-processing** cells or mϕ are believed to select unspecifically the determinants that are to be subsequently presented. The successful presentation of determinants requires an association of those determinants with certain molecules in the cell membrane of the macrophage. This requirement constitutes the basis of **associative recognition**—a phenomenon believed to be the basis of both the **Ir phenomenon** and **genetic restriction** (Chapter 19). Purportedly, after the association takes place, a determinant is presented to lymphoid cells that are capable of recognizing the associated determinant and initiating the second phase.

The second phase consists of the activation of specific lymphoid cells. This results in the morphological transformation, proliferation, and differentiation of the activated cells. Functional differentiation requires the interaction of distinct types of lymphoid cells and/or their subsets. At least two types of cells are involved in this phase. One type is referred to as **thymus-derived lymphocytes**, or **T cells**, and the other type is called **bone marrow-derived lymphocytes**, or **B cells**. Although both types initially originate in the bone marrow, the T cells require a subsequent period of maturation in the thymus, whereas B cells subsequently mature in peripheral lymphoid organs such as the spleen, lymph nodes, or solitary lymphatic nodules. The T cells can be further subdivided into several subsets that differ from each other by function and by particular combinations of cell-surface molecules (markers) (Chapters 22 and 23). During a humoral response, two of the major subsets of T cells may be activated to various extents. One of these subsets, the **helper T cells** (T$_h$), interacts with B cells, prompting their activation and differentiation. It should be noted that the interaction of T$_h$ and B cells may be negligible during the first encounter with the antigen (**primary response**), but it becomes more pronounced following a subsequent challenge (**secondary response**). The second subset, called **suppressor T cells** (T$_s$), interacts predominantly, if not exclusively, with T$_h$ cells, preventing the latter from effectively interacting with B cells; therefore, the response is suppressed. The antigens that require T$_h$ cells are called **thymus-dependent antigens**, in contrast to some other antigens that do not require T$_h$ cell activity and are called **thymus-independent antigens**. The degree of involvement of T$_h$ and T$_s$ cells determines the magnitude of the ensuing response. The efficacy and the specificity of the interaction between various lymphoid cells are influenced by cell-surface molecules that restrict the interaction (Section 19.8).

The third and last phase of the humoral response consists of the activation of specific B cells that begin the synthesis and secretion of specific immunoglobulins, or antibodies (Chapter 7). The antibodies produced are specific for the determinants that elicited them and can bind to these determinants alone or to the macromolecule carrying these determinants. The binding between antigen and antibody produces a complex that has several physicochemical characteristics different from those of either of its components. The formation of the **antigen-antibody complex** is a basis for the eventual physiologic and pathologic consequences of a humoral response.

4.4 Precipitation Reaction and the Methods Based on It

When soluble antigen is mixed with specific antibodies, the two react rapidly, forming large aggregates that are no longer soluble and, thus, precipitate or flocculate out of solution (Fig. 4.1). The precipitation is influenced by several factors other than the specificity of antigen and antibody. Among these factors are temperature, viscosity of the solvent, agitation, ionic strength, and pH. However, the most important factor is the proportion of antibody and antigen in the mixture. Usually, the optimal proportion corresponds to equivalent amounts of the two reactants, and an excess of either may slow down or entirely inhibit the precipitation. It should be remembered that the precipitation reaction requires that both components be polyvalent, i.e., each can bind at least two molecules of the other. The capacity to form two "bonds" results in a three-dimensional expansion of aggregates (lattices), while the formation of a single "bond" alone would result in separate and still soluble dimers.

There are many specific methods that utilize the precipitation reaction, but only the most basic will be briefly discussed. The simplest method is the **test-tube precipitation** in which antigen and antibody are mixed and the mixture is examined for the presence or absence of a visible precipitate. This method can be used for the relative or absolute quantitation of either antibody or antigen by using serial dilutions of one reactant and keeping a constant concentration of the other. An important limitation of the test-tube precipitation is that to identify particular components involved in the reaction at least one reactant must be monospecific, since precipitates containing different antigens or caused by different antibodies are indistinguishable from each other. This limitation is circumvented by a method called the **immunodiffusion assay** in which either one or both reactants are permitted to diffuse in a semisolid and translucent medium, e.g., agar. The diffusion establishes a concentration gradient of the reactant(s), and the precipitation of an antigen and its corresponding antibody occurs at the point where the concentrations of both are optimal. Since the velocity and the range of diffusion vary depending on the physicochemical properties of the reactants, the precipitation between different antigens and antibodies occurs at different locations.

Basically, there are two variants of the immunodiffusion assay: single and double (Fig. 4.2). In a **single diffusion** (Fig. 4.2**A**), only one reactant is permitted to diffuse, while the other is incorporated in the gel. As the diffusing reactant travels through the gel, it binds to the one that is incorporated, forming an ill-defined zone of precipitation. The precipitate may be directly visible, but if it is formed in very small quantities, it may be necessary to employ special methods to demonstrate its presence. In one of these methods, **radioimmunoassay** (Fig. 4.2**B**), the antibodies are labeled with isotope and incorporated into the agar. After the diffusion has equilibrated, the unbound labeled antibodies are washed out and the antibodies forming the precipitate are detected by autoradiography. Simple diffusion can be combined with electrophoresis (Section 6.2) to yield a better separation of different precipitates that are formed simultaneously.

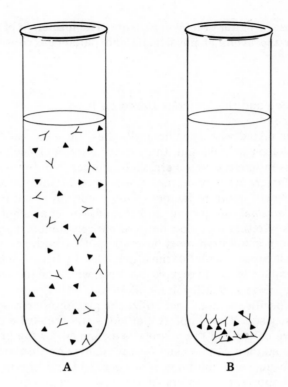

A   B

FIG. 4.1. Test-tube precipitation. (A) Mixture of antigen (▲) and antibody (≻−) in solution.
(B) Precipitation of antigen-antibody complexes.

In **double diffusion** (Fig. 4.2 **C**), both reactants diffuse toward each other and form two concentration gradients. A sharp zone (line) of precipitation develops where the concentrations of both reactants are optimal. An important modification of the double diffusion method is **comparative diffusion** (Fig. 4.2 **D**) in which two or more samples of tested material diffuse against a simple sample of antibodies. Comparing the relationship between the precipitation lines, one can ascertain whether the two samples tested contain the same or different antigens.

4.5 Antigen Redistribution and the Methods Based on It

When the antigen, rather than being in solution, is an integral component of a cell membrane (a cell-surface antigen), linking the antigen molecules by antibodies causes a redistribution of the antigen (Fig. 4.3). Under normal circumstances, most cell-surface antigens are randomly, and

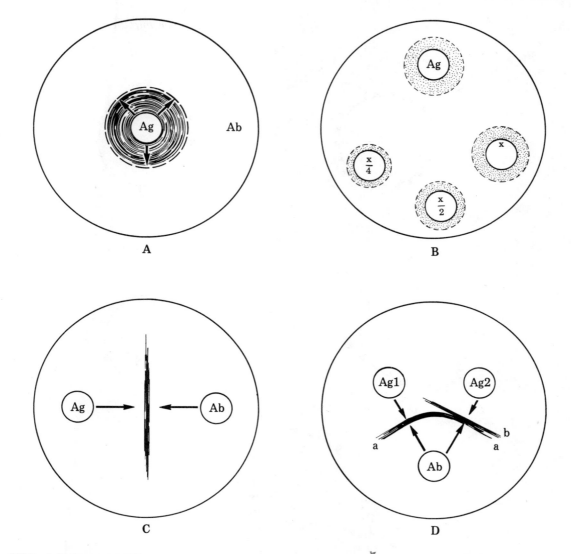

FIG. 4.2. Immunodiffusion methods. (**A**) Simple radial diffusion of the antigen (**Ag**) in the gel that contains antibody (**Ab**). Precipitation forms a ring around the antigen well. (**B**) Radioimmunodiffusion. The antigen (**Ag**) diffuses into the gel that contains radiolabeled antibody. The insoluble precipitate is detected by autoradiography, and the quantity of antigen is determined by comparison of the diameter of the precipitation zone with standards obtained after diffusion of twofold (**x, x/2, x/4**) dilutions of standard. (**C**) Double diffusion. Antigen (**Ag**) and antibody (**Ab**) diffuse toward each other and form a line of precipitation at the site of equivalent concentrations. (**D**) Comparative diffusion. Two antigenic preparations (**Ag1** and **Ag2**) diffuse toward an antibody (**Ab**). A continuous **line** (**a**) indicates that **Ag1** and **Ag2** contain the same molecules. The **line** (**b**) between **Ab2** and **Ab** indicates that **Ag2** contains an additional molecule that is absent from **Ag1**.

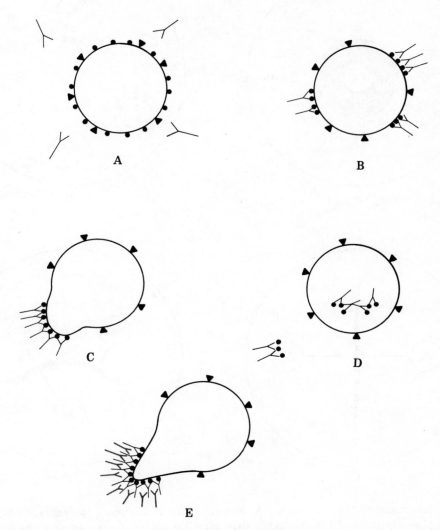

FIG. 4.3. Redistribution of cell surface antigen. (**A**) Normal cell with two uniformly distributed antigens (● and ▲) treated with antibodies (⤙). (**B**) Patching. Antibody binds to one of the antigens, and patches are formed. (**C**) Capping. Patches aggregate at one point forming a cap. (**D**) Lysostrip (modulation). Cap is either phagocytized or shed, depriving the cell of one of the antigens. (**E**) Capping with anti-immunoglobulin—after formation of patches. Anti-immunoglobulin is added to form a cap. Note that a given antibody redistributes only one antigen (●), while the other antigen (▲) remains undisturbed.

more or less evenly, distributed on the surface of the cell (Fig. 4.3**A**), which is not functionally and anatomically polarized. When bound by bivalent antibody, the cell-surface antigen molecules become aggregated into dense patches (Fig. 4.3**B**). **Patching** is temperature dependent but requires little, if any, metabolic energy and can be observed even in the presence of metabolic poisons. Prolonged incubation leads to the formation of a single patch, or **cap**, which is invariably located on the cell surface in the vicinity of the Golgi appratus (Fig. 4.3**C**). In contrast to patching, **capping** seems to require metabolic energy since it is totally inhibited by metabolic poisons. It is speculated that capping results from the accumulation of multiple patches at a single point owing to the active movements of the cell. Further incubation leads to the removal of the cap owing to pinocytosis and/or shedding (Fig. 4.3**D**). The removal of the cap deprives the cell surface, at least temporarily, of the involved antigen and makes the cell resistant to the action of any antibody specific for this particular antigen. The phenomenon is called **antigenic modulation**. In regard to antigen redistribution, it should be mentioned that in some instances redistribution may require the addition of a second antibody. The second antibody is directed against the original antibody that is bound directly to the cell-surface molecules. The actual redistribution is caused by binding of the second antibody with the complex of the antigen and the first antibody (Fig. 4.3**E**). The redistribution is exquisitely specific in that it affects only those molecules to which antibody is directed, while all other cell-surface molecules remain undisturbed.

The redistribution and its consecutive steps can be visualized by labeling the antibody with either fluorochrome or a moiety detectable under the electron microscope. Observation of the redistribution allows one to determine the presence of the antigen on the cell surface and, more important, to study the relationship between two antigenic determinants. If two different antibodies directed to two different determinants are labeled with two distinct fluorochromes, one can distinguish the redistribution caused by each of the antibodies. If patches and caps contain both antibodies, it indicates that the two determinants were coredistributed (cocapped) and, thus, are on the same molecule. Conversely, if two kinds of patches and two caps are formed, it means that the two determinants redistributed independently and thereby are on two distinct molecules. Using antibody against one such antigen, it is possible to remove this antigen from the cell membrane, rendering the cell resistant to the subsequent treatment with antibodies to this particular antigen (**lysostrip**).

4.6 Agglutination Reaction and the Methods Based on It

The **agglutination reaction** consists of the binding of antibody with cell-surface antigens of cells that are in suspension. Such binding results in the formation of multicellular aggregates that cannot remain in suspension and rather rapidly settle out on the bottom of the container in which the reaction takes place. Agglutination is, in principle, identical with precipitation except that the aggregates are composed of cells carrying the antigen molecules and not soluble antigen molecules alone. Perhaps the most important factors that influence agglutination are the density of the antigen molecules on the cell surface and the class of antibodies (Section 7.2). Generally, antibodies of the IgM class cause relatively strong agglutination, whereas antibodies of the IgG class often produce only a weak reaction or no reaction at all. Such a weak reaction can be facilitated by the addition of high molecular weight compounds to the reacting mixture of cells and antibodies.

There are many methods based on the agglutination phenomenon. The major categories are called active and passive (Fig. 4.4). **Active agglutination** involves the binding of antibodies with an antigen that is an integral and natural component of the cell membrane. Many different cell-surface antigens, including blood group substances and transplantation antigens, can be detected by the active agglutination of appropriate cells. **Passive agglutination** consists of the binding of antibodies to an antigen that has been artificially attached to certain cells or particles, usually erythrocytes. The cells or particles, in this case, are only indicators of the reaction between antibodies and the attached antigen. The attachment of the antigen to the indicator cells can be accomplished in two different ways. In some instances, the antigen is chemically conjugated with the cell membrane. Conjugation is often facilitated by special pretreatment of the cells with reagents that alter the cell membrane. In other instances, antibody directed to the native antigens of the cell plays the role of an antigen. The presence of such an antibody bound to the cell membrane can be detected by an agglutination reaction elicited by another antibody that is directed to the antigenic determinants of the antibody bound to the cell membrane. The method, known as the **Coombs test** or the **antiglobulin reaction**, has found multiple applications in studies of blood groups (Section 11.3) and other cell-surface antigens.

4.7 Lysis and Lytic Assays

Ordinarily, the binding of antibody alone to either native or exogenous antigen associated with the cell membrane does not injure the cell. However, the addition of **complement** usually results in severe damage of the cell (**cytotoxicity**), which if extensive enough leads to cell death (**cytocidal effect**) and subsequently to physical dissolution of the cell (**cytolysis**). It is beyond the scope of this book to describe complement and the mechanism of its action. Complement consists of several components present in normal serum and acting in sequence. Upon being activated by an antigen-antibody complex on the cell surface, complement causes damage to the cell membrane and the subsequent death of the cell. While the lysis of erythrocytes is easily detectable by direct examination of the reacting mixture, the detection of lysis of nucleated cells requires application of special procedures. The two most commonly used procedures are based on the detection of primary consequence of immune injury of the cell, i.e., increased permeability of the cell membrane.

In the **dye exclusion assay**, advantage is taken of the fact that under normal conditions the cell membrane prevents the passage of certain supravital dyes (trypan blue, nigrosin, eosin) from the surrounding medium to the interior of the cell. Thus, normal viable cells exclude the dye and remain unstained, while upon antibody- and complement-inflicted damage, the cell membrane is no longer able to exclude the dye and the cell becomes stained. In the one-stage assay, antibodies and complement are added simultaneously, while in the two-stage assay complement is added after a prior incubation of cells with antibodies. The results of the assay can be evaluated qualitatively or quantitatively. In the first case, the presence of stained (damaged) cells as seen under the microscope is indicated by a plus sign (+) or occasionally by using an arbitrary scale of 0–8, depending on the estimated proportion of damaged cells. In the

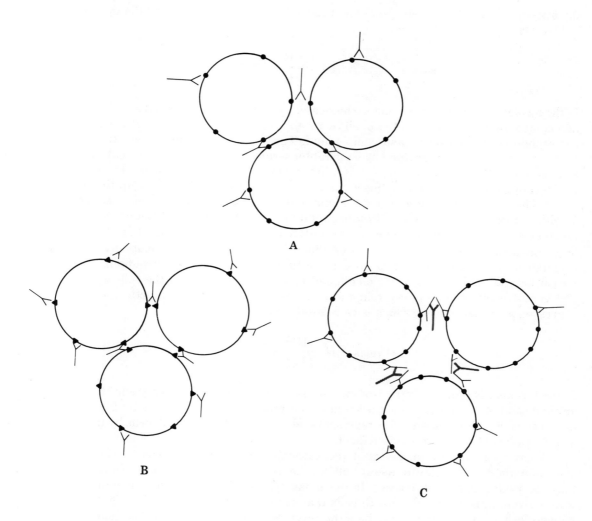

FIG. 4.4. Agglutination. (**A**) Active agglutination due to binding of antibody (⊱) to native antigen (●) of cell membrane. (**B**) Passive agglutination due to binding of antibody to an antigen (▲) artificially attached to the cell membrane. (**C**) Coombs test. Agglutination of cells coated with antibodies and binding anti-immunoglobulin.

quantitative assay, the percentage of the damaged cells is determined and the **cytotoxic index** (CI) is calculated from the formula

$$CI = \frac{E}{C}.$$

In the formula, E and C correspond to the relative numbers of stained dead cells in experimental and control samples, respectively. In all cases, the control should consist of cells treated with a corresponding normal serum and complement. This control is required since the complement for the cytotoxic assay is provided by fresh rabbit serum, which often contains natural cytotoxins against nucleated cells of various species. In fact, the selection of rabbit serum with the lowest possible cytotoxicity is often the most cumbersome undertaking in setting up the test.

The second procedure, called the **chromium release assay**, utilizes the fact that cells labeled supravitally with various isotopes retain most of the internal label as long as they are undamaged. Although at one time several different isotopes (^{51}Cr, ^{42}K, ^{32}P, ^{35}S, or ^{99}Tc) were used, presently ^{51}Cr is by far the most frequently employed. Upon damage by antibody and complement, the supravitally labeled cells release isotope into the surrounding medium. By measuring the radioactivity of the medium after proper incubation of the cells with antibodies and complement, one can ascertain the extent of cell damage. In practice, cell damage is expressed as % net release, which is calculated from the formula

$$\% \text{ net release} = \frac{E - SR}{Max - SR} \times 100.$$

In the formula, E represents the isotope release in the experimental sample in the presence of antibody and complement, SR is the spontaneous release in the absence of antibodies but in the presence of complement, and Max represents release after damage of all cells by treatment with a chemical agent, e.g., hydrochloric acid.

The methods described so far detect cytolytic or cytotoxic antibodies present in serum. A special method called **plaque assay*** allows the detection and enumeration of individual cells that are producing lytic antibodies. In this assay, lymphoid cells from an individual immunized with a given antigen are mixed with cells that carry this antigen (Fig. 4.5). The cells carrying antigen, called **target cells**, may be either erythrocytes or nucleated cells, depending on the particular experimental design. The antigen may be either native or attached artifically to the cells in a similar fashion as described for passive agglutination. The mixture of the immune and target cells is suspended in liquid agar and spread on a microscope slide to form a thin homogeneous layer. Solidification of the agar immobilizes the immune and target cells in such a way that each single cell that produces antibody is surrounded by numerous target cells. During the course of incubation, the antibody-producing cells release antibodies, which diffuse through agar and bind to antigen on the target cells sensitizing them. The addition of complement causes lysis of the sensitized target cells in the vicinity of antibody-producing cells. Lysis is

---

*The ingenious method developed by Jerne and Nordin is often referred to as the **Jerne assay**.

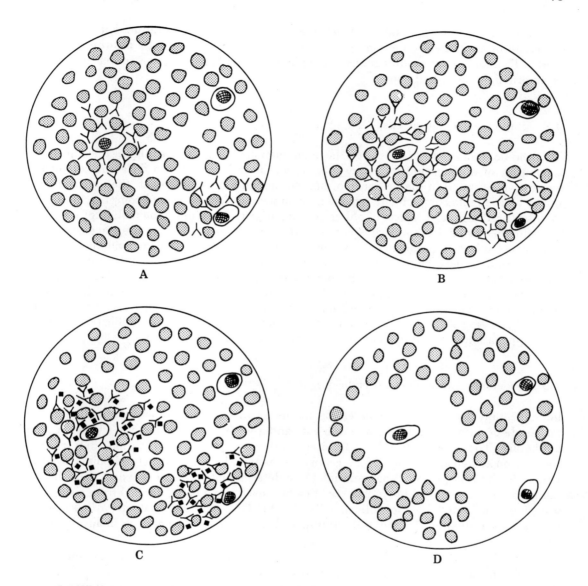

FIG. 4.5. Plaque assay. (**A**) Antibodies (>—) are secreted by immune cells. (**B**) Antibodies bind to target cells in the vicinity of antibody-secreting cells. (**C**) Complement (■) is bound to antibodies. (**D**) Lysis of target cells and formation of the plaques.

visible as a small clear area (about 0.5–1 mm in diameter) called a **plaque**, and since plaque is the result of antibody production by a single cell, such a cell is called a **plaque-forming cell** (PFC). There are many modifications of the plaque assay, but all of them are based on the same basic principle described above.

4.8 Complement Fixation Test

This classic serologic test is based on the phenomenon of quantitative binding of complement by a complex of antigen and its corresponding antibody. Thus, if two different complexes are successively formed in the presence of limited amounts of complement, the first complex will utilize all available complement, leaving no complement for the second complex. In the routine test, the first complex consists of either known antigen and serum to be tested for the presence of antibodies or known antibodies and a material to be tested for the presence of antigen. In either case, if both components are present, they will form a complex that will bind all available complement. Subsequently, when a second complex consisting of erythrocytes coated with specific antibodies is added, there is no complement left to cause cell lysis (Fig. 4.6**B**). On the other hand, if the first complex was not formed because of the absence of either antibody or its corresponding antigen, the complement is still available to produce lysis of the sensitized erythrocytes (Fig. 4.6**A**). The complement fixation test and its various modifications have found wide application in the studies of many antigens or responses to them.

4.9 Monoclonal Antibodies and Hybridomas

Immunization with a native antigen ordinarily results in simultaneous stimulation with a multitude of different antigenic determinants and, thus, the production of a whole spectrum of antibodies. These antibodies differ from each other by specificity for various determinants of the antigen as well as by affinity for a given determinant. From the structural point of view, they may differ by isotypic, allotypic, and idiotypic determinants (Chapters 9 and 10). These antibodies are produced by numerous distinct clones, each clone being derived from a single B cell originally stimulated by the antigen (Chapter 8). One may say that an ordinary antibody response is **polyspecific** and **polyclonal**, owing to the involvement of many clones of B cells.

A clone derived from a single B cell will produce **monoclonal antibody** with all molecules having the same primary structure, binding specificity, and affinity. B cells can be stimulated to produce antibody of desired specificity by immunizing an animal with an antigen of interest. However, these cells cannot multiply indefinitely and have a limited life-span; thus, they cannot be maintained in culture for any significant length of time. On the other hand, a neoplastic B cell (**myeloma cell**) produces antibody of unknown specificity (**myeloma proteins**, Chapter 7), and multiplies without restriction, and can be maintained indefinitely either in vivo or in vitro. By application of a **cell fusion** technique, these two cell types can be used to form a **hybrid cell**, or **hybridoma**, which will produce antibody to an antigen of choice and proliferate continuously.

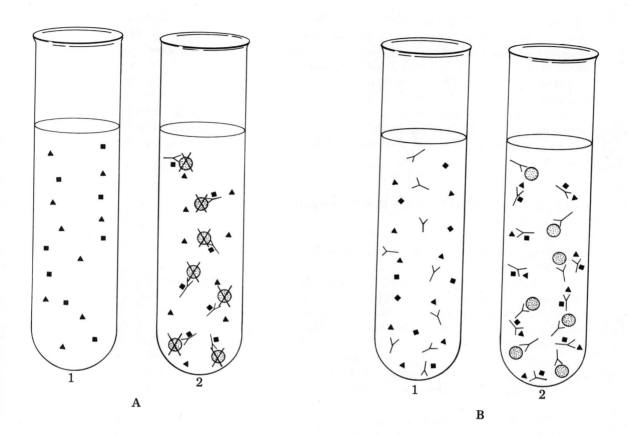

FIG. 4.6. Complement fixation test. (**A**) Antigen (▲) in absence of antibodies (⊱) does not form complexes and leaves complement (■) free (Tube **1**) to react with sensitized erythrocytes (●) and antibodies. The reaction results in lysis (**X**) of erythrocytes (Tube **2**), which indicates a negative result of the test. (**B**) Antigen (▲) and antibodies (⊱) (Tube **1**) form complexes that bind complement (■) (Tube **2**). Binding of complement prevents the lysis of erythrocytes by antierythrocyte antibodies, indicating a positive test.

In principle, a hybridoma is produced by immunizing an animal and mixing its spleen cells with myeloma cells in the presence of a fusing agent, e.g., Sendai virus or polyethylene glycol. The myeloma cells used are variants that cannot produce their original immunoglobulin; additionally the cells cannot produce the enzyme hypoxanthine phosphoribosyltransferase, which is involved in nucleic acid metabolism. Because of this enzyme deficiency, nonfused myeloma cells or myeloma-myeloma hybrids cannot grow in a **selective medium** called HAT (*h*ypoxanthine, *a*minopterin, *t*hymidine), but since B cells provide the missing enzyme, B cell-myeloma hybrids will proliferate. Growing in HAT medium, therefore, selects populations of B cell-myeloma hybrids, each of which produces a different antibody. A single hybrid that produces a single antibody is then selected from this population by a procedure called **limiting dilution** in which each culture has been initiated by a single hybrid cell. This cell is allowed to proliferate; when a sufficient number of progeny cells are generated, the specificity of the antibody produced is defined. This resulting hybridoma can be maintained and perpetuated either in vitro or in vivo or preserved frozen in liquid nitrogen for future culturing. The significance of monoclonal antibodies cannot be overestimated, and at this time they are probably a more precise and powerful tool than any other in serologic and immunogenetic analysis.

CELLULAR IMMUNITY AND ITS CONSEQUENCES

4.10 Basic Mechanism of the Cellular Response

As in the case of humoral immunity, only a very fundamental description of the events leading to a cellular response will be given. The response consists of three main phases.

The first phase consists of the introduction, presentation, and recognition of an antigen. Antigens that elicit cellular responses are either located on the cell surface at the time of their introduction or become associated with cell surface soon after. In each case, the cells with which the antigen is associated function as **antigen-presenting cells**. The effective presentation and/or recognition of many antigens requires that the antigen be associated with specific cell membrane molecules. These molecules restrict both the specificity and magnitude of the ensuing response (Section 19.8).

The recognition of the antigen initiates the second phase of the response. This phase usually involves three different subsets of the T cells since cellular responses are always thymus dependent. They are helper (T_h), suppressor (T_s), and **effector** (T_{ef}) subsets, and their activation, proliferation, and interaction determine the efficacy and magnitude of the third and last phase of the cell-mediated responses.

Among the T_{ef} cells, at least two distinct subpopulations can be defined. One subpopulation consists of T cells, which upon contact with a specific antigen produce **soluble mediators** or **lymphokines.** The lymphokines act on various cells, either activating or damaging them. Since the cells belonging to this subpopulation are responsible for **delayed-type hypersensitivity**, they are commonly referred to as T_{DTH} cells. In addition, there are indications that T_{DTH} cells may be involved in the rejection of allogeneic grafts (see below). The second subpopulation of T_{ef} cells contains T cells that upon direct contact with the target cells inflict injury and cause destruction of the target cells bearing the specific antigen. These cells are commonly called **cytotoxic** T cells (T_c) or **cytotoxic T lymphocytes** (CTL); most likely, CTL are involved in the rejection of some grafts.

The magnitude and specificity of the two essential events in any cellular response—cell proliferation and effectoral activity—can be determined by means of various in vivo and in vitro assays.

4.11 In Vivo Assays of T Cell Proliferation

When the antigen is presented as an allogeneic or xenogeneic graft (Section 20.1), the most pronounced cellular changes occur in the regional lymph node draining the area in which the graft has been placed. The changes consist of blast transformation and proliferation of T cells and result in a significant enlargement of the lymph node. Histologic examination reveals that the **paracortical zones**, normally populated by T cells, are hypercellular and contain an increased number of blast cells. The relative and/or absolute numbers of these blast cells can be determined using standard cytologic methods.

Similar changes take place in the spleen when allogeneic lymphoid cells are grafted systemically (intravenously or intraperitoneally) into a compromised recipient, a host made immunologically incompetent, or an individual genetically incapable of mounting a response to the antigen(s) of the grafted cells. Since the recipient does not reject the grafted cells such a situation results in the cellular response of the grafted lymphoid cells against the antigens of the host and is called a **graft versus host reaction** (GVHR). The intensity of a GVHR can be measured by a variety of semiquantitative methods but the spleen weight assay (**splenomegaly test**) is most commonly used. The assay takes advantage of the fact that during a GVHR the spleen of the host becomes enlarged and the enlargement, within certain limits, is directly proportional to the intensity of the GVHR. The enlargement is expressed as the **spleen index** (SI), which is determined from the formula

$$SI = \frac{E_{sw}/E_{bw}}{C_{sw}/C_{bw}} \,,$$

in which E_{sw} and E_{bw} represent spleen weight and body weight, respectively, of the experimental individuals, whereas C_{sw} and C_{bw} correspond to the same parameters in control individuals. Controls usually consist of animals receiving cells that are incapable of eliciting a GVHR. An SI of 1.3 or higher is conventionally considered as indicative of a GVHR, and it reflects the proliferation of cells within the spleen. However, it should be remembered that overall splenomegaly is caused by the proliferation of grafted as well as host cells, especially at later stages of the reaction. The SI depends on the number of grafted cells—or, to be specific, the number of T cells in the graft—and on the antigenic disparity between the donor and host. Splenomegaly is associated with a GVHR elicited by systemic introduction of the allogeneic cells, whereas local (subcutaneous) grafting of immunocompetent cells results in the enlargement of the regional lymph node. The systemic GVHR can be also assessed on the basis of the perivascular infiltrates in the portal spaces of the liver. The number of such infiltrates correlates well with the intensity of the GVHR.

4.12 In Vitro Assays of T Cell Proliferation

Proliferation of lymphocytes can be elicited in vitro by a large spectrum of agents called **mitogens**, or, more properly, **stimulators**, which may be nonspecific or specific. The nonspecific stimulators* usually induce blast transformation and proliferation in a matter of hours, and such proliferation involves a large proportion of the lymphocytes. On the contrary, specific stimulators, or antigens, require three to four days to induce similar changes in a relatively small fraction of the lymphocytes. In addition, most, but not all, specific stimulators (antigens) are effective only for lymphocytes that were previously exposed to the same stimulator—i.e., the lymphocytes must be primed either in vivo or in vitro by the stimulator. Regardless of the type of stimulator, the changes induced in vitro have several characteristics in common. They are initiated during the first few hours of reaction by a series of biochemical events that are by no means unique to lymphocytes and which can be observed in various cells undergoing activation. Subsequently, small lymphocytes become transformed into blast cells that actively synthesize proteins and at some point enter the S phase and replicate DNA. In the last step, the cells begin to proliferate.

Although the biochemical events of the initial step cannot, as yet, be reliably detected and measured, the morphologic and synthetic processes of the other steps are readily assayed. A morphologic evaluation employs standard cytologic methods by which a percentage of transformed and/or dividing cells is determined. In the latter case, a few hours prior to examination all mitoses are arrested at metaphase by treatment with an antimitotic agent such as colchicine. The synthetic events can be detected and quantitated by adding isotope-labeled precursors of proteins (amino acids) or DNA (thymidine) to the culture and measuring their incorporation (Section 6.3). The incorporation of a radioactive precursor is determined in cells that are killed, separated from the medium, washed, and disrupted before being counted in a scintillation counter. Incorporation is expressed either as a direct count or as a stimulation index calculated from the formula

$$I = E/C,$$

in which direct counts of experimental (E) and control (C) cultures are compared.

Some cell-surface alloantigens (Chapters 15–17) occupy a special position among the specific stimulators in vitro. They are capable of stimulating the proliferation of primed and nonprimed lymphocytes. Since the responses to cell-surface alloantigens are usually studied using lymphocytes as both stimulators and responders, the method is known as **mixed lymphocyte culture** (MLC) and the resulting reaction is termed **mixed lymphocyte reaction** (MLR). Although the degree of MLR can be ascertained by either cytologic or isotopic methods, measurement of DNA synthesis by incorporation of ^{3}H-labeled thymidine is usually used. When lymphocytes of two unrelated individuals are cocultured, the lymphocytes often react against each other, resulting in a so-called **two-way MLR**. However, the relative contribution of the lymphocytes of each individual to the overall MLR cannot be determined. To study the reaction

---

*In mice the most common T cell mitogens are phytohemagglutinin (PHA) and concanavalin A (Con A), whereas bacterial lipopolysaccharide (LPS) is a potent stimulator of B cells.

of the lymphocytes of only one individual, the lymphocytes of the other individual must be prevented from proliferation. This is accomplished by either heavy irradiation or pretreatment of the cells of one individual with actinomycin D or mitomycin C. Such pretreated lymphocytes can act only as stimulators, whereas the untreated lymphocytes are able to respond and will be responsible for the entire MLR. Naturally, when such a **one-way MLR** is employed, appropriate controls must be used. These controls are required to ascertain the effectiveness of the inhibition of the stimulator cells as well as the ability of the responder to respond. The MLR assay has become an invaluable tool in the study of certain cell-surface antigens; some current modifications of the MLR will be discussed later (Section 15.5).

4.13 In Vivo and In Vitro Assays of T Effector Cell Activity

The effector phase of cellular responses in vivo can be determined by various qualitative and semiquantitative methods. One of the methods assesses the active rejection of the allogeneic graft by the recipient, i.e., the HVGR (Section 20.2). The intensity of the HVGR is reflected by the length of time between grafting and rejection, which is expressed as the **median survival time** (MST). Apparently, the shorter the MST, the stronger the HVGR. Because evaluation of rejection is subjective, it is very difficult to decide on its end point, especially in protracted rejection. All attempts to make the determination of the MST more objective have met with failure or, at best, are impractical. The second method detects the ultimate effect (effectoral phase) of the previously described GVHR. This phase is represented by the incidence and the time of the death of the host suffering from GVHR. The two parameters are combined into the **cumulative mortality** in which the number or percentage of individuals that succumbed is determined at various times after the onset of GVHR.

The presence and activity of T_{DTH} cells are assessed by the delayed-type hypersensitivity test. In this test a specific antigen is introduced locally (intracutaneously) into a previously immunized individual. The inflammatory reaction developing at the site of antigen administration reflects the production of lymphokines by the specific T_{DTH} that encountered the antigen. Since the most pronounced signs of inflammation are observed 24–28 hours after introduction of an antigen, this type of reaction is referred to as delayed-type hypersensitivity.

The effectoral phase of some cellular responses is mediated by T_c cells (CTL) that are capable of inflicting damage upon appropriate target cells by direct contact. This damage can be evaluated quantitatively by means of the **cell-mediated lymphocytotoxicity** (CML) assay. This assay, in principle, is analogous to the antibody-mediated cytotoxic or cytolytic chromium release test described earlier. It measures the extent of damage to target cells based on the release of an isotope (usually ^{51}Cr) with which such targets have been labeled. The damage measured in a CML assay is inflicted by T_c cells and not by antibodies and complement. After incubation for 4–16 hours, the amount of radioactivity released into the medium is determined and the net release calculated. The results of CML tests depend on a proper ratio of the target to effector cells, which usually ranges from 1:10 to 1:100 but varies with each system. The specificity of the CML can be demonstrated in one of two ways. Replacing the target cells with labeled target cells not carrying the antigen in question results in only minimal isotope release if the T_c cells are indeed antigen specific. Alternatively, the effector cells may be preincubated with nonlabled ("cold") targets that compete with subsequently added labeled cells and significantly reduce or totally preclude the release. Occasionally, this **competitive inhibition** by cold target cells turns out to be a more sensitive assay than the direct testing procedure.

APPLICATION OF IMMUNOLOGIC METHODS IN IMMUNOGENETIC ANALYSIS

The primary objectives of an immunogenetic analysis are the demonstration of an antigen, the determination of its distribution among individuals of a given species or among different tissues and cells within an individual, and the isolation and characterization of such an antigen. To attain these objectives, certain methods can be successfully employed, depending on the antigen studied.

4.14 Demonstration of an Antigen

Demonstration of an antigen that elicits a humoral response requires the availability of specific antibodies. Such antibodies, or antiserum, once produced can be used in various tests. In the case of soluble antigens, precipitation or immunodiffusion assays are most commonly used. For cell-surface antigens, a wide variety of methods can be employed. Immunofluorescence testing will demonstrate an antigen by its capability of binding with fluorochrome-labeled antibodies. Redistribution, agglutination (either active or passive), lysis, or cytotoxicity also will reveal the presence of an antigen through the changes a target cell undergoes when subjected to the action of specific antibody. A cell-surface antigen that induces a cellular immune response can be demonstrated by its ability to induce delayed-type hypersensitivity, to generate specific T_c cells, or to stimulate the in vitro proliferation of lymphocytes, e.g., MLR. The in vitro response to a soluble antigen can be studied by measuring the proliferation of primed T_h cells upon in vitro challenge with the antigen.

 One must remember that the direct demonstration of an antigen may pose difficulties and necessitate the use of indirect approaches. For example, an antigen may be detected by its ability to absorb specific antisera, to inhibit agglutination, or to compete with labeled targets attacked by T_c cells in a CML assay.

4.15 Testing for Distribution of an Antigen

Any method sensitive enough to detect an antigen can be used to determine the distribution of this antigen in a population or in different tissues or cells of a given individual. When serologic methods are adopted for these studies, a positive reaction indicates the presence of the antigen; however, a negative reaction does not rule out its presence. Certain cells that express an antigen and bind antibodies may not agglutinate or may not be susceptible to lysis, e.g., because of a low concentration of antigen or low affinity of antibodies. In such cases, the method of choice is a quantitative absorption of the antiserum with the cells under study. If after absorption the antiserum no longer reacts with other cells bearing the antigen in question, it is reasoned that absorption removed the antibodies and that the cells used for absorption have the antigen. Conversely, if absorption does not remove or reduce activity of the antiserum, one must conclude that the cells do not possess the corresponding antigen.

4.16 Characterization and Isolation of an Antigen

This objective is usually approached after the antigen has been demonstrated and its distribution determined.

Characterization of an antigen includes the determination of its relationship to other known antigens or determinants expressed by a given cell. At the cellular level, the method most commonly employed is cocapping of the two antigens with two corresponding antibodies labeled with different fluorochromes (Section 4.5). In the case of a soluble antigen, **sequential precipitation** can be used with two antibodies, each directed to one of the two determinants under investigation. If the first antibody abrogates precipitation by the second antibody, it indicates that two determinants are associated with a single molecule, which apparently has been precipitated by the first antibody.

The isolation of an antigen from a crude cell homogenate is an essential step for a subsequent biochemical analysis or characterization. Cells are homogenized and their membrane-bound molecules solubilized either by enzymatic digestion or by the action of detergents. The specific molecules are then separated from the mixture by precipitation with specific antibodies. The precipitate, composed of antibody and corresponding antigen, is isolated from the mixture and dissociated to yield the antigen alone. Once the antigen is isolated in its purified form, it can be subjected to a proper molecular and biochemical analysis (Section 6.5).

5 / Tools and Methods of Genetic Analysis

Because an understanding of the inheritance of immunologically detectable traits is its primary goal, immunogenetics usually employs multicellular higher animals with defined organ systems, since only these animals are fully capable of recognizing and responding to antigens. Because of this, contemporary immunogenetics is limited almost exclusively to studies of higher animals. Although important studies have been done on other organisms such as viruses, bacteria, or plants, this chapter, however, will be restricted to certain animal models and the basic genetic approaches used for genetic analysis of these models.

ANIMALS AS THE SUBJECT OF IMMUNOGENETIC STUDIES

5.1 Outbred Animals

Randomly bred (outbred) animals of some species are often the only material available to the immunogeneticist. These animals, whether derived from a natural environment or from a randomly bred laboratory colony, are genetically heterogeneous. Randomly bred animal populations contain both homozygotes and heterozygotes with frequencies predictable according to the Hardy-Weinberg law (Section 1.7). Inasmuch as studying such animals can provide relevant information about the inheritance of immunologically related traits, this approach often poses a great number of practical difficulties. These difficulties are caused by the simultaneous and independent segregation of alleles of many genes, which may affect the trait under study. The difficulties are further compounded by the need for large numbers of individuals from consecutive generations to carry out a definitive analysis. Unfortunately, many animals, especially large ones, produce only small numbers of progeny and, in addition, may be difficult to breed in captivity. These difficulties can be circumvented if genetically uniform animals that produce a relatively large number of progeny are available for study. Because mice have a relatively short gestation period and produce sizable litters, and because mice can be maintained by sister-brother mating for multiple generations, many strains of mice have been produced and maintained and are readily available. These strains ideally satisfy the requirements for a genetically uniform population, as indicated above.

5.2 Inbred Strains

Although random breeding does not change the allelic and genotypic frequencies of a population, **assortative breeding**—e.g., inbreeding—does. In general, if the probability of matings between similar genotypes is increased over that found in random matings, the frequency of homozygotes will increase. Conversely, a decreased probability of matings between similar genotypes will result in a decreased frequency of homozygotes. Accordingly, breeding of close relatives should increase the frequency of homozygotes for each individual gene and, therefore, for the entire genome, eventually leading to an overall homozygosity. This is precisely the primary goal of **inbreeding**—to produce an increasingly homogeneous population with each successive generation. Inbreeding can be achieved by mating related individuals for a sufficient number of generations. As a result, a single allele for each gene tends to become fixed. Naturally, once a given allele is fixed, all subsequent generations will be homozygous for this allele, provided no mutation arises. Even a sporadic mutation, when it occurs, is eliminated quickly provided there is no selective pressure to maintain it and the population is large enough.

Selective breeding for a single or a few genes was practiced in animal husbandry and in horticulture long before the theoretical basis of heredity was fully comprehended. The breeding strategy in these cases consisted of selecting for successive matings individuals expressing a desired trait variant. After a sufficient number of generations of selection, the allele responsible for the particular variant becomes fixed, and all individuals will be **true-breedings**, i.e., homozygotes for this allele. However, since the selection of mating partners is made on the basis of phenotype and does not necessarily involve related individuals, alleles of other genes do not become fixed and the produced strain will remain heterozygous for most genes other than the desired one.

Selective breeding to achieve more extensive genotypic homozygosity was also attempted before the formulation of genetic principles. It was practiced for ages by dealers raising animals as pets, especially mice, a custom that was common in the Far East and was brought to Europe and the Americas in the nineteenth century. Inbreeding in its rudimentary form was used by many dealers to produce and maintain a stock that expressed a particular combination of traits. The most renowned among the pet mice dealers in this country was Mrs. Abby Lathrop of Brandby, Massachusetts, whose mouse colony was the forerunner of many of the presently maintained inbred strains. The dealers began supplying mice for laboratory purposes and when a high degree of genetic homogeneity was noted, the deliberate production of inbred strains was initiated, resulting in the first truly inbred strains. Although overall inbreeding can be achieved by repeated matings of individuals related to each other in various degrees, **full sister and brother (sib) mating** in each generation is the most effective way to achieve relatively quick fixation of alleles. Sib mating is, therefore, the most commonly used method to produce highly inbred strains of mice and other animals.

If the two individuals used in an initial mating are both heterozygotes, e.g., $a1/a2$, for a given gene, in accordance with Mendel's law, their offspring will have three genotypes: $a1/a1$, $a1/a2$, and $a2/a2$ with frequencies of 0.25, 0.5, and 0.25, respectively. The random selection of mating pairs from these offspring will create four types of matings called **incross** (inx), **cross** (x), **backcross** (bx), and **intercross** (itx). These four types correspond to the mating of two identical homozygotes (inx), two different homozygotes (x), homozygotes with heterozygotes (bx), or two heterozygotes (itx). The expected or probable (p) frequency of occurrence of each mating type can be calculated from the frequencies with which each corresponding genotype is found in the population that serves as the initial source of random breeding pairs. Such calculations must take into account the fact that there are two distinctly different incrosses and backcrosses; hence, the probability derived from the frequencies must be doubled. Furthermore, because the probability of reciprocal matings must be considered for crosses and backcrosses, it is necessary to double the data obtained from the simple multiplication of frequencies. With this in mind, the probabilities of the four mating types in the first generation of full-sib breeding are

$$p_{inx} = 2 \times 0.25 \times 0.25 = 0.125,$$

$$p_x = 2 \times 0.25 \times 0.25 = 0.125,$$

$$p_{bx} = 4 \times 0.5 \times 0.25 = 0.5,$$

and

$$p_{itx} = 0.5 \times 0.5 = 0.25.$$

Noticeably, while in the initial mating (F0) only an intercross was involved ($p_{itx} = 1.0$), in the first (F1) sib mating p_{itx} decreased to 0.25, while p_{inx}, p_x, and p_{bx} increased. In the subsequent generations of sib mating (F2, F3, . . . , Fn), p_{inx} continuously increases, whereas p_x, p_{bx}, and p_{itx} continuously decrease according to formulas

$$p_{inx} = p^*_{inx} + 0.25p^*_{bx} + 0.125p^*_{itx}$$

$$p_x = 0.125p^*_{itx}$$

$$p_{bx} = 0.5p^*_{bx} + 0.5p^*_{itx}$$

$$p_{itx} = p^*_x + 0.25p^*_{bx} + 0.25p^*_{itx}.$$

In these formulas, p^* corresponds to probabilities in the generation immediately preceding the one for which p is calculated. These changes in probabilities of mating are reflected in the increasing probability of homozygosity for any particular gene as well as an increasing degree of homozygosity of the entire genome. Both the particular gene and the genome homozygosity are reflected by the **inbreeding coefficient** (Ic), which can be calculated from the formula

$$Ic = 1 - (1 - Ir)^g.$$

In this formula, Ir represents a constant **inbreeding rate**, which for sib mating is 0.191, and g represents the number of consecutive generations undergoing inbreeding. Using the formula, it is easy to calculate that $Ic = 0.985$ for $g = 20$, which means that in a given individual and in a population any gene has a 98.5 percent probability of being homozygous and that 98.5 percent of all genes are actually homozygous. Ic is also defined as the probability that an individual homozygous for any gene carries both alleles identical by descent, i.e., both alleles are derived from the same allele of an ancestor.

Continuous inbreeding by sib mating results in a progressively increased probability of homozygosity (Fig. 5.1) for all genes and a simultaneous decrease in the probability of heterozygosity. The corresponding probabilities approach the values 1.0 and 0.0, respectively, as the number of generations increases. However, at least theoretically, neither of the above values can actually be achieved since Ic would equal 1.0 only if Ir = 0.0. Thus, even strains bred

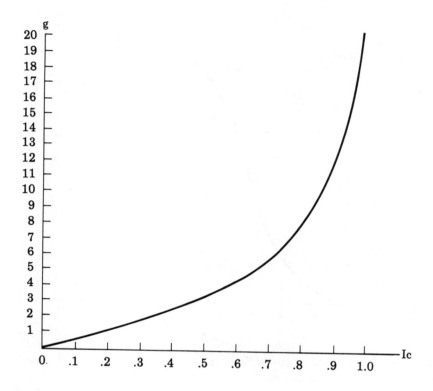

FIG. 5.1. Relationship between the number of generations (**g**) of sib mating and the inbreeding coefficient (**Ic**). The relationship is expressed by the equation $Ic = 1 - (1 - Ir)^g$ and represents the probability of homozygosity at a given locus.

for 200 or more generations may still have **residual heterozygosity**. In fact, **genome purity**—i.e., a situation in which the probability of heterozygous segments (tracts) in the entire genome is in the range of 0.01—is attained only after 60 consecutive sib generations (Fig. 5.2). To eliminate such residual heterozygosity, an intentional selection procedure against particular heterozygotes would have to be used rather than sib mating without specific selection. Furthermore, a perennial problem that cannot be controlled is that an existing homozygosity may be temporarily converted into heterozygosity by random mutation (see below). Having this in mind, an established inbred strain (by convention after 20 sib generations) should be periodically tested for homozygosity. However, such testing usually is very tedious, and it is impractical to monitor all genes.

Separation from the original stock before the F8 generation of full-sib breeding results in production of two distinct **strains** if sib mating is continued for both the original stock (one strain) and the separated animals (second strain). Any strain separated from the original stock

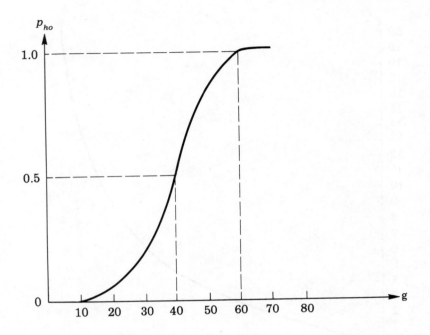

FIG. 5.2. Relationship between probability (p_{ho}) of full homozygosity and number of generations (**g**) of sib mating.

between the F8 and the F19 generations is considered a **substrain** if sib mating has been continued for 12 or more generations afterward.

Differences between strains or substrains are due to three factors: accidental outcrossing, which may introduce new (contaminant) alleles; incomplete inbreeding or residual heterozygosity; and new mutations. The residual heterozygosity due to incomplete inbreeding and new heterozygosity due to mutation tend to equal each other at about the F20 generation. When the animals are separated at this stage, upon further sib breeding as many as 117 substrains may evolve owing to residual heterozygosity. This number approaches the value of 0 at about the F50 generation (Table 5.1).

Since many currently available inbred strains of mice were originally derived from a common ancestral stock and separated at various times, they differ from each other by alleles of different numbers of genes. It can be said that the nearer in time to the ancestral stock such a separation occurred, the greater is the number of the loci carrying different alleles. Owing to the new mutations, the progeny of any strain maintained by sib mating at different locations may

TABLE 5.1. Relationship between the Number of Generations of Sib Breeding and the Extent of Residual Heterozygosity

Generation of Sib Breeding	Contribution by Segments (tracts) of Genome Being Heterozygous (percent)[a]	Number of Heterozygous Loci	Possible Number of Substrains[b]
10	21.5	6,500	975
20	2.6	780	117
30	0.3	93	14
40	~0.0	11	2
50	~0.0	1	0

[a]The total genome is assumed to be 1,500 cM and to contain about 30,000 structural genes.
[b]If animals are separated at this generation and sib breeding is continued.

differ from each other by distinct alleles fixed at a certain number (n) of loci. This number increases with time and can be estimated from the formula

$$n = (g1 + g2 - 7)\mu.$$

In this formula, g1 and g2 represent the numbers of generations of two progenesis bred after separation, and the constant $\mu = 0.3$ is the product of the estimated mutation rate ($\sim 10^{-5}$) and the estimated total number of mutable genes (3×10^4). On the basis of this equation, there is consensus that any established inbred strain separated from its original strain for more than five generations of sib mating should be considered a **subline**.

Occasionally, inbreeding efforts may be complicated by a phenomenon known as **inbreeding depression**. This is not unexpected because inbreeding by definition increases homozygosity for all alleles, both beneficial and deleterious. Fortunately, deleterious alleles usually are relatively infrequent recessive mutants and, therefore, are not expressed in a random population owing to the much more frequent presence of dominant nondeleterious alleles. However, inbreeding does increase the chances that an individual will become homozygosity for all alleles, both beneficial and deleterious. Fortunately, deleterious alleles further by a concomitant homozygosity for the deleterious alleles of several different genes. Phenotypically, the depression results in decreased fertility, lowered resistance to some diseases, and an increased occurrence of degenerative disorders. All of these traits slow down the breeding until the affected animals are self-eliminated. However, in extreme cases, depression may result in the eventual extinction of the particular strain before it is established. This has been a common experience in agricultural attempts at inbreeding.

Presently, there are several hundred distinct inbred strains of mice. Table 5.2 lists the most common. Unfortunately, the nomenclature of inbred strains is quite confusing since the designations were given rather arbitrarily. In general, the symbols consist of capital letters and numbers followed by a virgule and an abbreviation indicating the producer of the strain, substrain, and/or subline. Since the original strains have been exchanged by dealers and

TABLE 5.2. Some Common Inbred Strains of Mice

Strain (Common Abbreviation)	Derivation of Name	Coat Color	*H-2* Haplotype*	Strains Partially Related by Origin
A/Jax (A)	Albino, *Jacks*on Laboratory	White	*a*	BALB
C57BL/6 (B6)	Female #*57*, *bl*ack	Black	*b*	C57BR, C57L, C57BL/10J
DBA/2 (D2)	*D*ilute *B*rown, non*a*gouti, subline *2*12	Dilute brown	*d*	DBA/1J, BDP, STOLI
BALB/c (C)	*B*agg's *alb*ino, *c* gene	White	*d*	A
NZB	*N*ew *Z*ealand *b*lack	Black	*d*	NZW
C3H (C3)	*C3H* stock, Heston	Agouti	*k*	CHI, C/St, CBA, DBA/1, DBA/2
CBA (CB)	*CB* stock *a*gouti	Agouti	*k*	C3H, DBA/1, DBA/2
C57BR/cd (BR)	Female #*57*, *br*own, sublines *c* and *d*	Brown	*k*	C57BL
RF	*R*ockefeller Institute, *F*urth	White	*k*	BRVR
BRVR (RR)	*B*acteria-*r*esistant-*v*irus-*r*esistant	White	*k*	RF
BDP	*B*rown, *d*ilute, *p*ink-eyed	Dilute brown	*p*	P, DBA/1, DBA/2
DBA/1 (D1)	*D*ilute *b*rown, non*a*gouti, subline *1*2	Dilute brown	*q*	DBA/2, BDP, P, STOLI
BUB	*B*rown *U*niversity, stock *B*	White	*q*	BUA
SJL	*S*wiss, *J*ackson Laboratory	White	*s*	DA
PL	*P*neumonia*l*ike or *P*rinceton *L*eukemia	White	*u*	None
SM	*Sm*all line	Gray	*v*	DBA (?)
NZW	*N*ew *Z*ealand *w*hite	White	*z*	NZB

*The *H-2* haplotype determines the murine major histocompatibility complex (Chapter 16).

NOTE: For a more complete list of inbred strains of mice, see: Festig, M. F. V. (ed.), *International Index of Laboratory Animals*. Fourth Edition. Medical Research Council, Laboratory Animal Centre, United Kingdom, 1980.

investigators many times, there may be several abbreviations indicating consecutive holders. To avoid excessive complexity, a convention has been proposed that only the two most recent holders be indicated.

Production of inbred strains has also been undertaken with several other species of laboratory animals. Fully inbred strains of rats (Table 5.3), guinea pigs (Table 5.4), and Syrian hamsters (Table 5.5) are presently available. For other species, such as chickens, rabbits, dogs, or miniature swine, only partially inbred strains are currently available. In some instances, e.g., rabbits, the progress of inbreeding is greatly impeded by an especially pronounced inbreeding depression. The value of inbred strains to genetic and other biologic endeavors can hardly be overestimated. These animals allow studies to be carried out on genetically homogeneous and defined populations, thus eliminating, to a great extent, a primary source of uncontrolled experimental variability.

5.3 Recombinant Inbred (RI) Strains

The number of distinct inbred strains can be increased almost indefinitely by crossing two already established inbred **progenitor** strains and then producing the F2 hybrids and sib mating their progeny for 20 consecutive generations. The F2 hybrids represent recombinants of the alleles by which the two parental inbred strains differed. If sib mating is used for 20 generations, various random combinations of these alleles become fixed, giving rise to new inbred strains. Although such strains are related to each other, as well as to the original parental strains, each has a unique combination of alleles. All RI strains derived from a given cross form a set that may be considered as a stable segregating population of such a cross. The set consists of various recombinant genotypes in which alleles of some, but not all, linked genes are present in those combinations found in the parental strains.

There are presently six sets of RI strains (Table 5.6) in which the distribution of parental alleles at 50–60 loci have been determined. Poor reproduction of the animals belonging to some RI strains of a given set is a major drawback of RI strains. RI strains have several specific applications in immunogenetic studies—e.g., identification of minor histocompatibility genes (Section 21.2) and the study of linkage between genes. Linkage is determined by making a comparison of the **strain distribution pattern** (SDP) for various traits of the original parents. The traits with identical or a similar SDP in the different RI strains must be determined by genes that have been transmitted together for the 20 consecutive generations. By implication, most likely these genes are linked. The probability of detecting linkage depends on the number of genes tested in a given set. For example, there is a 95 percent probability of detecting a linkage when 200 genes in 25 RI strains are identified. However, linkage data obtained in different studies are cumulative and need not be reestablished in each particular experiment.

5.4 Congenic Strains

The availability of inbred strains created an opportunity to produce strains that differ from each other only by a small fragment of a single chromosome. Such strains are called **congenic** since,

TABLE 5.3. Some Common Inbred Strains of Rats

Strain	Derivation of Name	Coat Color	*RT1* Haplotype[a]	Number of Strains[b]	F Generation	Related Strains
ACI	Stock *A*, Cancer *I*nstitute	Black, white belly and feet	*a*	7	>100	ACH
ALB	*Alb*any	Dilute brown	*b* ⎫	7	>40	—
BUF	*Buf*falo	Albino	*b* ⎭		>70	—
AUG	*Aug*ust	Dilute brown, hooded	*c*	11	>40	Several sublines
BDI	*B*erlin, *D*ruckrey	Yellow, pink-eyed	*d*	8	>50	BDIII-BDX
BDVII	*Albino, Department of Surgery*	Sandy, pink-eyed	*e*	—	>50	BDI-BDX
		Albino	*f*	1	>60	—
AS2						
KGH	*K*unz-*G*ill, *H*arvard	Albino	*g*	—	>60	—
HW	*H*omburg	Yellow, hooded	*h*	1	>20	—
WKA	*W*istar, *K*ing *A*	Albino	*k*	2	>200	—
LEW	*Lew*is	Albino	*l* ⎫		>90	Numerous congenic lines
F344	*F*ischer	Albino	*l* ⎭ 14		>100	Several sublines
MNR	*M*audsley, *n*onreactive	Albino	*m*	—	>50	MR, Several sublines
BN	*B*rown, *N*orway	Brown	*n* ⎫	2	>60 .	MAXX
MAXX	*M*icrobio-logical *A*ssociates	Black, hooded	*n* ⎭		>30	BN, LEW
MR	*M*audsley, *r*eactive	Albino	*o*	—	>40	MNR
RP	*R*ecombinant *p*		*p*	—		—
TO	*T*okyo	Albino	*t*	—	>25	—
WF	*W*istar, *F*urth	Albino	*u*	—	>20	—

[a]Determines rat major histocompatibility complex (Section 17.1).
[b]With same *RT1* haplotype.
SOURCE: Based on Altman, P. L., Katz, D. D. (ed.), *Inbred and Genetically Defined Strains of Laboratory Animals*, Federation of American Societies for Experimental Biology. Bethesda, 1979. For a more complete list, see footnote to Table 5.2.

TABLE 5.4. Some Common Inbred Strains of Guinea Pigs

Strain	Derivation of Name	Coat Color	GPLA* (B allele)	F Generation	Related Strains
2	USDA family #2	Spotted (tricolor)	1	>30	—
13	USDA family #13	Spotted (tricolor)	1	>30	—
BIOB	*Bio*logical Institute, genotype *B*	White	1	~20	From a single colony in the Biological Institute, Füllinsdorf, Switzerland
BIOAC	*Bio*logical Institute, genotype *AC*	White	2	~20	
BIOC	*Bio*logical Institute, genotype *C*	White	2	~20	
BIOAD	*Bio*logical Institute, genotype *AD*	White	3	~20	
B(BE)	—	Albino	3	>20	IMM/R —
IMM/R	*I*nstitute *M*edical *M*icrobiology, *r*esistant	Albino	3	>30	IMM/S
PCA (DHCBA)	*P*assive *c*utaneous *a*naphylaxis (*D. H. C*ampbell)	Albino	3	>20	—
R9	*R*ogers	Brown and white	3	>20	—
JY-1	*J*4 fibrosarcoma	Albino	3	>40	—

*Determines guinea pig major histocompatibility complex (Section 17.3). The *B* alleles *1, 2,* and *3* were formerly designated *B, C,* and *D*, respectively.

presumably, they share alleles of all genes except those located in a small fragment of one chromosome. Although congenic strains may differ for any number of alleles in a chromosomal fragment (**passenger alleles**), they are initially selected for an allele of a single gene called the **differential gene**. The production of congenic strains is achieved by various systems of selective breeding, but the most frequently used system involves repeated backcrossing (Fig. 5.3). This system, called NX, consists of an initial cross followed by 12 consecutive backcrosses and a final intercross. The initial cross is made between an animal carrying the differential allele ($a1$) and an inbred animal carrying the other allele ($a2$) of the differential gene. The first parent is a representative of the **donor strain** and may be, but does not have to be, inbred. The second animal is the **background or partner strain** and must be inbred—and thereby an $a2/a2$ homozygote. Assuming that the donor strain is a heterozygote, $a1/x$, for the differential gene, the first cross yields $a1/a2$ and $x/a2$ heterozygotes in the ratio of 1:1. The $a1/a2$ heterozygotes are then selected for backcrossing to the background strain, which, of course, is $a2/a2$ homozygote. The progeny of the backcross will consist of 50 percent $a1/a2$ heterozygotes and 50 percent $a2/a2$ homozygotes. The $a1/a2$ heterozygotes are again selected to be used in a second backcross to produce 50 percent $a1/a2$ and 50 percent $a2/a2$ individuals. The procedure should be repeated for at least 12 consecutive generations, each time selecting the $a1/a2$ heterozygotes for mating to the background strain and rejecting the $a2/a2$ homozygotes. By

TABLE 5.5. Common Inbred Strains of Hamsters

Strain	Derivation of Name	Coat Color	F Generation
ALAC	*Ac*romelanic, *L*aboratory *A*nimal *C*enter	Acromelanic albino	>50
BF	—	—	20
CB	*C*hester *B*eatty Institute	Golden	>60
CD	—	—	20
CLAC	*C*ream, *L*aboratory *A*nimal *C*enter	Cream	>50
LVG	*L*ake *V*iew *G*olden Syrian	Golden	>50
LSH(2.4)	*L*ondon *S*chool of *H*ygiene	Agouti-golden	>70
LHC	*L*ake *V*iew *H*amster *C*olony	Cream	>60
MHA	*M*ill *H*ill *A*lbino	Albino	>60
PD4	*P*ee *D*ee Farm	Acromelanic albino	>80
RL	*R*usty, *L*emonde	Rusty	>40
RY	*R*ijsvijk	—	>20
W/MGH (extinct)	*W*hite *M*agalhaes, *H*arwell	Agouti	>60
XX.B	—	Agouti	>60
X.3	—	Acromelanic albino	>60
X.68	—	Acromelanic albino	>60
BIO[a]	—	Various	>60
MIT[b]	—	Agouti	20

[a]21 strains developed and maintained at the *BIO*-Research Institute, Cambridge, MA. They are designated by a number indicating pedigree and vary in color.

[b]Seven strains developed and maintained at the *M*assachusetts *I*nstitute of *T*echnology from newly captured wild Syrian hamsters.

Source: Based on Altman, P. L., Katz, D. D. (ed.), *Inbred and Genetically Defined Strains of Laboratory Animals.* Federation of American Societies for Experimental Biology, Bethesda, 1979. Personal communications, Charles River Breeding Laboratory, Wilmington, MA.

convention, each backcross generation is designated by a consecutive number preceded by the capital letter N. From the progeny of the N12 generation, the *a1/a2* heterozygotes are selected and intercrossed. Their offspring consist of 25 percent *a1/a1* homozygotes, 50 percent *a1/a2* heterozygotes, and 25 percent *a2/a2* homozygotes. The *a1/a1* homozygotes are selected for further breeding by the full sib system, thus initiating the new congenic strain.

As backcrossing continues, the alleles of genes, other than the differential gene contributed in the original cross by the donor strain, are gradually (via recombination) replaced by the alleles of the background strain. The contribution of donor alleles (d) decreases with each generation removed from the original cross according to the formula

$$d = (1/2)^g.$$

TABLE 5.6. Summary of Available RI Strains of Mice

RI Set	Original F1 Hybrid	Number of Strains in the Set	Number of F Generations*
CXBD	C × B6	7	>20
BXD	B6 × D2	24	25–39
BXH	B6 × C3	14	28–34
SWXL	SWR × C57L	8	13–34
AKXL	AKR × C57L	21	12–35
NB	NZB × BALB	22	15–23

*Different for different lines in a given set.
NOTE: For strain designation, see Table 5.2.

In this formula, g is the number of backcross generations since the original cross with the donor strain. In the N12 generation, d will be $(1/2)^{12} = 0.00024$ or about 0.02 percent. This means that about 0.02 percent of the alleles may be contributed by the donor strain and 99.98 percent of the alleles by the background strain. The intentional selection for the donor differential allele a in each generation ensures that this particular allele is retained and not replaced along with other alleles.

The above calculation applies to the alleles of genes that are not linked to the differential gene (**contaminant alleles**). The replacement of donor alleles linked to the differential gene (passenger alleles) depends on the linkage strength. The probability (p_d) that the donor allele of a linked gene has not yet been replaced at generation g can be calculated from the formula

$$p_d = (1 - f_r)^{g-1},$$

where f_r is the recombination frequency between the differential gene and the gene in question. According to the formula, the probability of the presence of the donor allele of a gene with an $f_r = 0.4$ (40 cM away from the differential gene) is 0.0036 (0.36 percent) at generation N12, but for the gene with an $f_r = 0.1$ (10 cM away from the differential gene), the corresponding value is 0.31 (31 percent) (Fig. 5.4). Obviously, further backcrossing would progressively decrease this probability, even for alleles of genes very closely linked to the differential gene. However, since the decrease is asymptotic even after, e.g., generation N24, the probability for an allele with an $f_r = 0.1$ would still be about 0.09 (9 percent). Prolonged backcrossing, in some instances, can be avoided if, at any stage of breeding, a linked donor allele can be identified and animals that do not carry it are selected for backcrossing. The identification of and selection for either contaminant or passenger alleles permits production of either **derivative congenic strains** or **double congenic strains**. In the first case, two strains are raised to differ exclusively by the contaminant or passenger allele, whereas in the second case two strains differ by alleles of two genes that may be either linked or totally independent.

Congenic strains that differ for alleles determining various traits have been produced (Table 5.7). By convention, congenic strains are designated by the abbreviations of the background strain and donor strain separated by a period. Preferably, the two basic abbrevia-

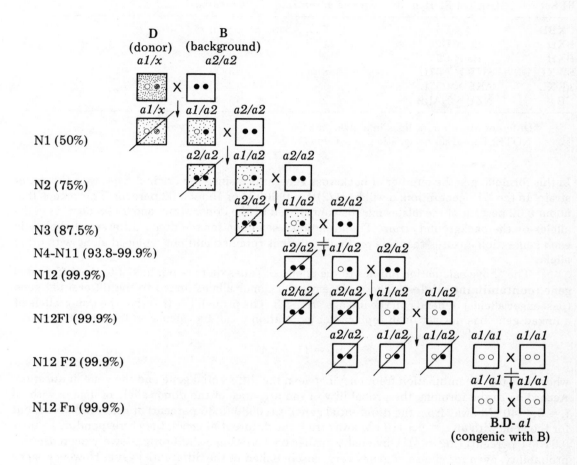

FIG. 5.3. Production of a hypothetical congenic strain **B.D** by a multiple backcross (NX) system). Each **square** represents the entire genome, and each small **circle** represents a differential gene. The donor animal alleles are **open** or **shaded circles**, and the background animal allele is a **black circle**. At each generation, part of the donor genome (**dotted**) is eliminated and replaced by the background genome (**white**). The contribution of the background genome is indicated in parentheses. Homozygotes carrying the background allele of the differential gene are eliminated from breeding (crossed). (Based on: Klein, J., *Biology of the Mouse Histocompatibility-2 Complex.* Springer-Verlag, New York, Heidelberg, Berlin, 1975.)

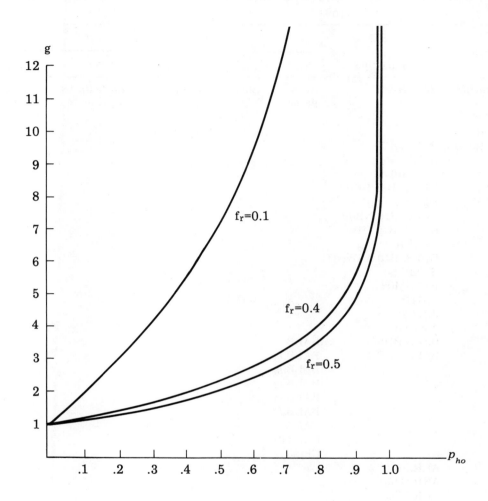

FIG. 5.4. Relationship between number of generations (**g**) of backcrossing and probability of homozygosity (**p_{ho}**) during production of a congenic strain by the NX method. Separate curves for genes linked with different strengths to the differential gene were derived from the equation $p_{ho} = 1 - (1 - f_r)^{g-1}$.

TABLE 5.7. Some Congenic Strains of Mice with Various Alleles of Genes Determining Immunogenetic Traits*

Background Strain	*H-2* (Haplotype[a])	Differential Gene(s)				
		Igh	*Tla*	*Thy-1*	*Lyt-1*	*Lyt-2,3*
C57BL/6(B6)[b]	B6.C-*H-2^d*	BC-8	B6-*Tla^a*	B6.PL(74NS)	B6-*Lyt-1^a*	B6-*Lyt-2^a*
	B6-*H-2^k*	B6.*Ig^e*				B6-*Lyt-2^a,3^a*
B6.C-*H-2^d*				B6.C-*Thy-1^a*		
B10.S(7R)				B10(7R)-*Thy-1^a*		
C57BL/10(B10)	B10.A(*a*)					
	B10.D2(*d*)					
	B10.M(*f*)					
	B10.K, B10.BR(*k*)					
	B10.AKM(*m*)					
	B10.P, B10.NB(*p*)					
	B10.Q, B10.D1(*q*)					
	B10.RIII(*r*)					
	B10.S, B10.ASW(*s*)					
	B10.PL(*u*)					
	B10.SM(*v*)					
A	A.BY(*b*)		A-*Tla^b*	A-*Thy-1^a*		
	A.CA(*f*)					
	A.SW(*s*)					
BALB	BALB.B10(*b*)	BALB-14				
	BALB.AKR(*k*)	BALB.*Ig^b*				
		BALB.*Ig^c*				
		BALB.*Ig^d*				
		BALB.*Ig^f*				
		BALB.*Ig^g*				
		CAL-9				
		CAL-20				
		CB-20				
AKR	AKR.B6(*b*)			AKR/Cum(?)		
	AKR.D2(*d*)					
	AKR.M(*m*)					
C3H	C3H.A(*a*)				C3H.CE-*Lyt-1^b*	
	C3H.B10, C3H.SW(*b*)					
	C3H.D(*d*)					
	C3H.LG/c(*ar1*)					
	C3H.JK(*j*)					
	C3H.NB(*p*)					
	C3H.Q(*q*)					
	C3H.RIII(*r*)					

[a]Only congenic for unrelated and spontaneous recombinant haplotypes are listed.
[b]Several different sublines are included.
NOTE: For other congenic lines, see Tables.
NOTE: For other congenic lines, see Tables 16.1 and 16.3.

tions should be followed by a hyphen and the symbol of the differential allele of the donor. In addition, the subsidiary symbol may include the method of production, the individual designation, the subline designation, and the initial(s) of the producer(s). The common abbreviations for method of production are M for cross-intercross breeding, N for backcross, NS for backcrossing in which the serologic method was used to select breeders in each generation, and R for use of recombinant animals. An individual designation usually consists of an Arabic number. The subline designation consists of a number or a lowercase letter. There is an unwritten convention governing the designation of producer(s) or holders(s).* In principle, if two individuals produced a strain, the one who made the larger contribution or actually keeps the strain is indicated. Among the congenic strains, a special place is occupied by strains that differ for alleles of the histocompatibility genes (Chapters 16 and 21). Since such strains do not accept (resist) allografts exchanged between them, they are commonly referred to as **congenic resistant** (CR) strains.

A special case of congenic strains includes those that carry a specific recombinant haplotype of a gene complex, e.g., the major histocompatibility complex (Chapter 16). Most commonly, recombinants are detected in the F2 progeny of two congenic inbred strains that differ only for the MHC haplotype. Once the recombinant (r) is identified, it is backcrossed to either parent (p), and the resulting heterozygotes, r/p, are intercrossed to obtain 25 percent of offspring that are the recombinant homozygotes (r/r). Since both parental strains were already congenic and shared all background alleles, there is no need for prolonged backcrossing in these cases, and r/r homozygotes can be maintained by standard sib mating.

5.5 Coisogenic Strains and Mutant Strains

The major drawback of congenic strains is that they may and often do differ by alleles of other genes, in addition to the differential allele, especially those closely linked to the differential gene (passenger). Strains differing only by the allele of a single gene are called **coisogenic**. Such strains can be derived by selective breeding of inbred animals in which a point mutation has been identified. Obviously, before any such breeding can be attempted, the specific mutation must be detected using an appropriate procedure. The actual procedure depends on the nature of the mutated gene and its phenotypic expression. In any case, considering that the mutation rate for murine genes varies from 10^{-5}–10^{-7}/gamete/generation, the procedure must involve the screening of a large number of individuals.

Several methods can be used to screen for mutated genes that determine histocompatibility antigens (Chapters 16 and 21), but most frequently a technique called the **reciprocal circle** (Fig. 5.5) is employed. In this method, groups of animals are arranged in such a way that each member of the group donates a graft to two other animals and receives a graft from two animals. Since the animals used are presumed to be genetically identical, all grafts should be accepted unless there is mutation of a histocompatibility gene.

---

*For designation, consult: Festig, M. F. V. (ed.), *International Index of Laboratory Animals*. Fourth Edition. Medical Research Council, Laboratory Animal Centre, United Kingdom, 1980.

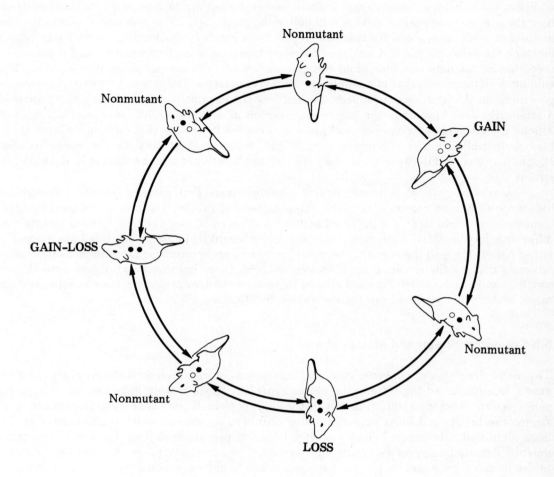

FIG. 5.5. Detection of mutants of *H* genes in F1 hybrids by reciprocal circles method. Each mouse donates grafts to two other mice and receives one graft from each of those two mice in return. Direction of grafting is indicated by the **arrows**. The pattern of rejection (**black circles**) and acceptance (**white circles**) depends on the type of mutation. For details, see text.

The pattern of rejection permits the classification of the mutation as either a **gain** (acquisition of a new determinant) or **loss** (deletion of an original determinant) or **gain-loss** type. A gain mutation will cause the rejection of grafts derived from the mutant, but the mutant itself will accept grafts from other animals. A loss mutation results in the rejection of grafts by the mutant, but its grafts are accepted by other animals. Finally, a gain-loss mutation will lead to the reciprocal rejection of grafts between the mutant and normal animal. In screening for histocompatibility mutations, either F1 hybrids of the inbred strains or the inbred strains themselves can be used. The F1 hybrids permit the detection of all three types of mutations. However, to produce a congenic inbred strain carrying the mutant allele as a differential gene, 12 generations of the backcrossing are required. When inbred mice are used, only a gain or a gain-loss mutation can be detected, since a loss mutation that affects only one allele while the other allele remains normal will permit the acceptance of the graft by the mutant. However, the use of inbred strains facilitates the quick production of a truly coisogenic strain by crossing the detected mutant (m) with a normal (n) individual and subsequently selecting m/n heterozygotes from the progeny. Intercrossing of m/n heterozygotes will produce 25 percent of offspring that are m/m homozygotes for the mutant allele. Once the mutation is detected and appropriate congenic or coisogenic strains are produced, it is necessary to determine which of the many histocompatibility genes has mutated. This is accomplished by a variety of methods that will be discussed later (Section 16.7). The availability of mutant congenic and coisogenic strains has contributed greatly to the detailed analysis of various gene products from both the structural and functional points of view. Mutants of the major histocompatibility complex will be discussed further in Chapter 16.

GENETIC ANALYSIS

5.6 Objectives and Steps

The identification of a trait calls for a series of experiments known collectively as a **genetic analysis**. The two primary objectives of such an analysis are, on the one hand, the determination of the mode of inheritance and, on the other hand, the assignment of the gene or the genes responsible for the trait to a particular chromosomal site. The analysis consists of three consecutive steps. In the first step, experimental data are collected from controlled breeding experiments, random populations, or family studies. The second step involves the selection of a theoretical model, based on genetic principles, that seems compatible with the experimental data. The third and final step consists of the application of an appropriate statistical test or tests to determine the concordance of the experimental findings with those expected on the basis of the adopted model. The extent and complexity of the genetic analysis vary, depending on the trait under study and the available population. However, in virtually all instances the two primary objectives of a genetic analysis are initially approached by the analytical methods that consists of segregation, linkage, and complementation tests (see also Section 21.1).

5.7 Segregation Analysis

By definition, only a trait with at least two allelic variants is amenable to a **segregation analysis**. A segregation analysis is based on a determination of the phenotypes, and subsequently the genotypes, of related individuals that belong to several consecutive generations. Specifically, a segregation analysis is designed to determine the genetic nature of a trait, the expressivity and penetrance of different alleles, and the extent of its polymorphism. The analysis is greatly facilitated when it can be carried out with individuals that are true-breedings or, even more so, with individuals of inbred strains. Regardless of the origin of the individuals studied, the analysis consists of two consecutive matings and the defining of the phenotypes and their frequencies in each generation.

Assuming that the two original parental individuals are homozygotes, *a1/a1* and *a2/a2* for the two variants, a1 and a2, of the trait in question, all their offspring are expected to be phenotypically identical if the inheritance of the trait is consistent with Mendelian principles. The phenotypes of the F1 hybrids will be determined by the heterozygous combination, *a1/a2*, of the parental alleles. The comparison of the F1 phenotypes with those of the parents permits the determination as to whether the two alleles are codominant when F1 has phenotype a1a2 or recessive and dominant when the F1 phenotype is either a1 or a2. It also allows the determination of the penetrance of each allele. In some instances, the F1 hybrids of two homozygous parents may display a phenotype that is absent in either of the two parents. In such cases, one must consider that intergenic or intragenic complementation is involved (Section 1.2). If the entire population of F1 hybrids has a phenotype that is totally different from those of the parents, it must be concluded that one is dealing with a polyphenotype determined by a polygenotype consisting of several genes (monogenotypes), each being homozygous in the parents.

The second mating in a basic segregation analysis consists of backcrossing the F1 individuals to one of the original parents. In the case of codominant alleles, either parent can be used, but in the case of dominant and recessive alleles, the parent carrying the latter should be used. Mating to the parent carrying the dominant allele would make the segregation of the F1 alleles phenotypically undetectable since all progeny would carry and express a dominant allele. Again, assuming that the original parents were homozygotes (*a1/a1* and *a2/a2*) and that all F1 individuals were heterozygotes (*a1/a2*), the alleles of the F1 cross should segregate in the backcross generation, and generate backcross individuals displaying two parental phenotypes: a1, if backcrossed to an *a1/a1* parent, and a1a2 of the F1 parent. In instances where there is a direct relationship between the genotype and phenotype, the two phenotypes, a1 and a1a2, are expected to be found in a ratio of 1:1. The concordance of the actual findings or "goodness of fit" with those expected can be evaluated using the χ^2 (chi-square) test. The simplest formula applicable to the backcross generation displaying only two phenotypes is

$$\chi^2 = \Delta^2/N,$$

where Δ is the difference between the numbers of animals expressing each phenotype, and N is the total number of individuals studied. The value of χ^2 is subsequently converted into a probability (p) value, which is found in appropriate tables. In principle, the lower the χ^2, the higher the probability that the observed and expected numbers do not differ significantly and that the segregation does not deviate from that postulated by a sampling error in the accepted model. Naturally, a significant deviation from the expected numbers calls for a reconsideration of the model and a search for alternative models.

Perhaps the most frequently encountered deviation from the expected phenotypic ratio of 1:1 is the finding that a backcross generation displays more than the two expected variants of the phenotype. This suggests that the phenotypes studied are determined by more than one gene and that these different genes, which also contribute to the polyphenotype, are segregating more or less independently. The relationship between the number of segregating genes (sg) and the number of discrete polyphenotypic variants (pv) observed in the backcross generation is represented by the formula

$$\mathrm{pv} = 2^{\mathrm{sg}}.$$

The frequencies of the various polyphenotypic variants found among the backcross individuals depend on the linkage of the genes and the dominance or codominance of the segregating alleles. Generally, if all the genes in question are not linked, their alleles will segregate independently, and, thus, each phenotypic variant in a backcross generation will have a similar frequency—$(1/2)^{\mathrm{sg}}$. On the other hand, if some of the genes are linked, the recombinant phenotypes determined by these genes will be less frequent than either of the parental phenotypes. In the case of a very strong linkage, the recombinant phenotypes may only be detected rarely. Occasionally, the extremely low frequency of certain phenotypes may cause doubts as to whether such phenotypes are indeed genetically determined. To dispel these doubts, a **progeny test** is carried out using individuals with the putative recombinant phenotype. The test consists of mating the alleged recombinant individual with the original parent(s) and determining the frequency of the recombinant phenotype. Finding that the progeny of recombinant and homozygous parents display the two phenotypes in the ratio of 1:1 constitutes strong evidence in favor of a genetic basis for a rare phenotype.

5.8 Linkage Analysis

Once the mode of inheritance, the number of genes involved and their expressivity, and polymorphism are established, the determination of the position of the gene(s) within the genome must be attempted. This is done by means of a linkage analysis comprised of three steps. In the first step, two genes linked to the gene in question are identified. In the second step, the linkage strength between the gene in question and the two other linked genes is determined. Finally, in the third step the linear order of the three genes is established.

The second step is carried out in a manner similar to the first step of segregation analysis. Assuming that inbred strains (homozygotes) are available, the F1 hybrids and the backcross generation are raised using strains that differ by alleles of the three genes that determine the polyphenotype (a,x,y) where a is the trait under study and x and y are other traits associated with it. The traits are presumed to be determined by the corresponding alleles *a1* or *a2*, *x1* or *x2*, and *y1* or *y2*. The backcross individuals will consist of the offspring that display either the parental polyphenotype (a1, x1, y1) or the F1 polyphenotype (a1a2, x1x2, y1y2). However, some individuals will express recombinant polyphenotypes resulting from recombinations between the three genes a, x, and y during meiosis in the F1 hybrid parent. The frequency of recombination (f_r) between any two genes depends on the strength of their linkage, which can be calculated as follows:

$$f_r = R/N,$$

where R is the number of particular recombinants and N is the total number of backcross animals studied. The standard error (SE) for f_r can be calculated from the formula

$$SE = \pm [f_r(1 - f_r)/N]^{1/2}.$$

It should be remembered that since f_r in females and males may differ, depending on the species, the determination of f_r should be made on an equal number of progeny of F1 females and F1 males to avoid overestimation or underestimation of the f_r value. According to Mendel's second law, the f_r for any two nonlinked genes should be equal to 0.5, while a frequency lower than 0.5 indicates linkage. The principle can be extended to include a polyphenotype determined by several nonlinked genes. In this case, the frequencies of the parental type and of each recombinant variant should be similar, $(\frac{1}{2})^{sg}$, where sg is the number of segregating genes contributing to the polygenotype. The frequency of parental variants (f_P) if higher than the frequencies of the recombinant variants (f_R) indicates that the genes determining the polyphenotype are linked. The significance of such a preponderance of parental polyphenotypes is established by using the χ^2 test according to the formula

$$\chi^2 = \mathbf{\Sigma}(O^2/E) - N,$$

where O and E are the observed and expected number, respectively, of each polyphenotype, assuming that the genes are not linked, and N is the total number of individuals tested. If the calculated χ^2 converts into $p < 0.05$, it is accepted that there is significant deviation from the expected equal frequencies of recombinant and parental phenotypes and that the phenotypes must be determined by linked genes. This conclusion should always be supported further by showing that the segregation of alleles of each individual gene is not disturbed and produces a ratio of 1:1 of monophenotypes determined by the alleles of such a gene. This is again accomplished by using the formula

$$\chi^2 = \Delta^2/N.$$

The conversion of the calculated χ^2 into $p > 0.05$ indicates that the segregation is indeed undisturbed.

In the final step of linkage analysis, the linear order of the three genes is determined by comparing the f_r values for three pairs of linked genes. Such a comparison always reveals that the f_r for one of the pairs is apparently higher than the f_r values for the other two pairs. The relationship between three f_r values can be written as follows:

$$f_{r1} \approx f_{r2} + f_{r3},$$

where 1, 2, and 3 represent three possible pairs of the genes investigated. Since the f_r between any pair of linked genes is directly related to the distance between the two genes (Section 1.5), the two genes with the highest f_r must be farthest apart, and, accordingly, the third gene must be located between them (Fig. 5.6). The fact that in many instances the highest f_r is smaller than the sum of the two f_r is due to double recombination, which simultaneously separates the centrally located gene from both peripheral genes while the latter are not separated from each other. Because double recombination is a relatively rare event, it produces the two least frequent recombinant phenotypes, which can be eliminated from the calculations. The procedure described above is called genetic mapping, and since it is accomplished by observing the segregation of three distinct genes, it is also referred to as **three-point mapping** or a **trihybrid cross**.

GENETIC ANALYSIS OF AN OUTBRED POPULATION

One is not always so fortunate as to have the inbred animals to carry out a genetic analysis as described above. This is especially true of human beings, which understandably form an outbred population. The genetic analysis in this case is a lengthy and complex undertaking that consists of several steps. In each step a specific assumption must be made, and the search is carried out to prove or disprove this assumption. Perhaps the most common case is the finding of an unexpected antibody in the serum of an individual who has received a blood transfusion. This antibody—e.g., anti-a1—reacts with cells (erythrocytes or nucleated cells) of only some individuals comprising the population.

5.9 Defining a New Alloantigen System

In the first step of the analysis, one makes the assumption that anti-a1 reacts with an alloantigen belonging to a presently known and defined alloantigen system. This assumption is tested by comparing the reactivity of anti-a1 with the reactivities of a battery of standard antibodies to all known antigens. These antigens are expressed in various combinations on the panel of cells that are tested with anti-a1 and with appropriate standard antibodies. It is important to include in the panel the cells of the individual that produced anti-a1 to check the possibility that anti-a1 may be an autoantibody. If the pattern of reactivity of anti-a1 is not consistent or antithetical with the pattern of any known standard antibody, it must be concluded that anti-a1 detects a new alloantigen that does not belong to any known antigenic system.

5.10 Genetic Characterization of the Population

Once the conclusion is made that anti-a1 detects a new alloantigen, it is followed by the assumption that antigen a1 is an allelic product of a gene at a single locus *a* that has two alleles,

Polypheno type	Percentage of Individuals with Given Phenotype	Recombination Frequency (f_r) between Genes		
		$\triangle$ ($\blacktriangle$) – $\bigcirc$ ($\bullet$)	$\triangle$ ($\blacktriangle$) – $\square$ ($\blacksquare$)	$\bigcirc$ ($\bullet$) – $\square$ ($\blacksquare$)
$\triangle\,\bigcirc\,\square$	43.4	———	———	———
$\blacktriangle\,\bullet\,\blacksquare$	44.2	———	———	———
$\triangle\,\bullet\,\blacksquare$	3.2	.032	.032	
$\blacktriangle\,\bigcirc\,\square$	3.1	.031	.031	
$\triangle\,\bigcirc\,\blacksquare$	2.7		.027	.027
$\blacktriangle\,\bullet\,\square$	2.5		.025	.025
$\triangle\,\bullet\,\square$	0.4	.004		.004
$\blacktriangle\,\bigcirc\,\blacksquare$	0.5	.005		.005
		$\overline{.072}\,(f_{r1})$	$\overline{0.115}\,(f_{r2})$	$\overline{.061}\,(f_{r3})$

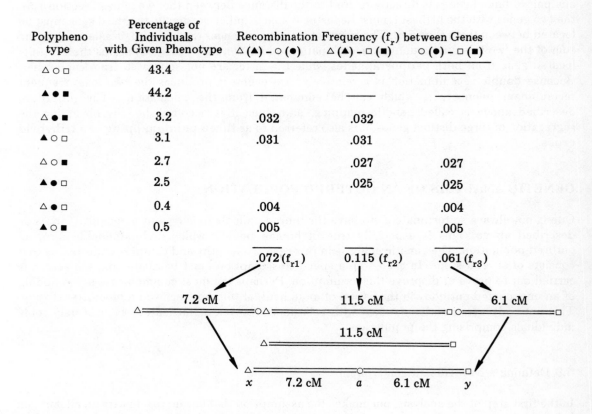

FIG. 5.6. Three-point mapping. Genes *x*, *a*, and *y* have two alleles, each represented by white and black symbols $\triangle$ ($\blacktriangle$), $\bigcirc$ ($\bullet$), and $\square$ ($\blacksquare$), respectively. From the frequency of various phenotypes, the distances between genes and the linear order of genes are determined. For details, see text.

a1 and *a2*. In the next step of the analysis, it is imperative to characterize the population in respect to phenotypic, allelic, and genotypic frequencies. The task would be relatively easy if antibodies to both putative antigens—a1 and a2—were available. This is, however, a rare situation, and usually only one antibody (anti-a1) can be used. Using this antibody, one tests a population to determine the frequencies of a1-positive (a1$^+$) and a1-negative (a1$^-$) individuals. In the subsequent interpretation of the acquired phenotypic data, it is assumed that the population tested is in genetic equilibrium. Therefore, the allelic and genotypic frequencies should be consistent with the Hardy-Weinberg equation. Accordingly, if *a1* and *a2* alleles are dominant and recessive, respectively, the individuals found to be a1$^+$ consist of *a1/a1* homozygotes and *a1/a2* heterozyotes. On the other hand, the a1$^-$ individuals are *a2/a2* homozygotes.

According to the Hardy-Weinberg law, the frequency of homozygotes equals the square of the frequency of a given allele. Thus, if the frequency of a1$^-$ individuals that are *a2/a2* homozygotes is b, the frequency of the *a2* allele (f_{a2}) is

$$f_{a2} = \sqrt{b}.$$

Since, according to the original assumption, there are only two alleles, *a1* and *a2*, and the sum of frequencies of all alleles must be 1.0,

$$f_{a1} + f_{a2} = 1.0$$
$$f_{a1} = 1 - f_{a2}$$
$$f_{a1} = 1 - \sqrt{b}.$$

Finally, since the frequency of heterozygotes is $2f_{a1} f_{a2}$, and both allelic frequencies are known, one can determine the genotypic frequencies of *a1/a1* homozygotes (f_{a1}^2), *a2/a2* homozygotes (f_{a2}^2), and *a1/a2* heterozygotes ($2f_{a1}f_{a2}$).

5.11 Family Studies

From the estimated genotypic frequencies, one may predict mating frequencies (f_m). To do this, a new assumption must be made—that mating is random with respect to the genotypes under study. According to this assumption, the mating frequency of any two genotypes equals the product of the frequencies of these genotypes. For example, the frequency of mating between *a1/a1* homozygotes and *a1/a2* heterozygotes is

$$f_{m\gamma} = f_{a1}^2 \times 2f_{a1}f_{a2}.$$

Knowing the mating frequencies, one can predict the frequencies of progeny that express (a1$^+$) or do not express (a1$^-$) the antigen detected by anti-a1. The predicted (expected) values can be compared with the actual (observed) values found by testing a large sample of families selected randomly from the population. In this step of the analysis, an assumption is made that the selected sample contains all possible mating combinations and that these matings are represented with the frequencies predicted theoretically. However, there is no real assurance that this is indeed the case. One may, by chance, select an excess of one mating, or, conversely, another mating may be underrepresented. If this occurs, the observed values may not coincide with the expected values. The same may happen if any of the previous assumptions were, in fact, incorrect—e.g., mating is not random or the population is not in equilibrium.

To determine whether the expected and observed values differ from each other by chance alone, a χ^2 test is used. In this method, an assumption called the **null hypothesis** is made—that observed and expected values are identical or more precisely, that they do not differ significantly. The value of χ^2 is calculated from the formula

$$\chi^2 = \Sigma \; \frac{(O - E)^2}{E} \, ,$$

where O represents observed and E represents expected values. Once χ^2 is calculated, it is transformed into the probability (p) that the null hypothesis is correct and may be accepted. In general, the smaller χ^2 is, the larger p is. As a rule, when χ^2 corresponds to p = 0.05 or less, one must reject the null hypothesis. By doing so, one must accept the notion that expected and observed values are significantly different and, therefore, that one of the original assumptions made to derive the expected values might be incorrect.

The analysis involving multiallelic or multigenic systems employs a similar approach. However, the complexity of the formulas increases significantly, and computations may require sophisticated computer programs. A detailed description of such formulas and their applications lies beyond the scope of this book and can be found in statistics textbooks.

6 / *Biochemical Methods*

GENERAL ANALYTICAL AND PREPARATIVE METHODS

6.1 Enzymes as Tools for Molecular Biology

Restriction endonucleases are enzymes that cleave double-stranded (duplex) DNA at a specific base sequence. There are two types of restriction endonucleases. Type I enzymes recognize and bind to a specific DNA sequence but cleave the DNA at a random site other than the recognition sequence. Type II enzymes also recognize a base sequence, but the cleavage site is either within this recognition sequence or at a constant distance from the enzyme binding site. The recognition site, in most cases, is an inverted repeat of four or six bases in length.

Type II enzymes are particularly useful for analyzing gene structures and for work with recombinant DNA. These enzymes (see Table 6.1) produce three types of product termini:

5′ overhang:	—GAATTC—	Eco R1	—G	pAATTC—
	—CTTAAG—	⟶	—CTTAAp +	G—
3′ overhang:	—GGTACC—	Kpn I	—GGTAC	pC—
	—CCATGG—	⟶	—Cp +	CATGG—
Blunt end:	—AGCT—	Alu I	—AG	pCT—
	—TCGA—	⟶	—TCp +	GA—

The two overhangs, called **sticky ends**, can be exploited to recombine specifically two unrelated DNA molecules. Any combination of blunt ended molecules can be ligated together. There are over 100 known restriction endonucleases for which sequence specificities have been determined (Table 6.1).

Nucleic acid **polymerizing** and **joining enzymes** make up another set of enzymatic tools of the molecular biologist. These enzymes are required for the synthesis and modification of DNA and RNA and the ligation of recombinant DNA molecules (Table 6.2).

6.2 Electrophoresis

Most biological macromolecules carry basic or acidic groups that result in a pH-dependent net charge. The placement of these molecules in an electric field will result in their movement toward either the anode or the cathode, depending on their net charge. Several support media for electrophoresis—e.g., paper, agarose, polyacrylamide, or starch—are used, depending upon whether the purpose of the procedure is analytical or preparative. In the absence of a physical constraint on movement, the rate of movement in an electric field is dependent upon the ratio of charge to mass of the molecule. However, in most practical applications of electrophoresis, free

TABLE 6.1. Some Restriction Endonucleases

Enzyme	Source (microorganism)	Sequence 5'→3'[a]
Alu I	*Arthrobacter luteus*	... AG↓CT ...
Bam HI	*Bacillus amyloliquefaciens* H	... G↓GATCC ...
Eco RI	*Escherichia coli* RY13	... G↓AATTC ...
Hae III	*Haemophilus aegyptius*	... GG↓CC ...
Hind III	*Haemophilus influenzae* R_d	... A↓AGCTT ...
Hinf III	*Haemophilus influenzae* R_f	... G↓AN[b]TC ...
Hpa II	*Haemophilus parainfluenzae*	... C↓CGG ...
Kpn I	*Klebsiella pneumoniae*	... GGTAC↓C ...
Pst I	*Providencia stuartii*	... CTGCA↓G ...
Pvu II	*Proteus vulgaris*	... CAG↓CTG ...
Sal I	*Streptomyces albus*	... G↓TCGAC ...
Sau 3AI	*Staphylococcus aureus* 3A	... ↓GATC ...
Taq I	*Thermus aquaticus*	... T↓CGA ...

[a]Arrow indicates cleavage position and the periods indicate bases that are irrelevant for enzyme activity.
[b]N = any base.

TABLE 6.2. Some Polymerizing and Joining (ligating) Enzymes

Common Name	Activity	Function	Other Characteristics
E. coli DNA polymerase I	Polymerase	DNA replication and repair	3' OH requirement; 3' → 5' and 5' → 3' exonuclease activities
Klenow fragment of DNA polymerase I	Polymerase	DNA replication	3' OH requirement; lacks 5'→3' exonuclease activity
T4 DNA polymerase	Polymerase	DNA replication	3' OH requirement
Reverse transcriptase	Polymerase	Synthesis of DNA complementary to an RNA template	3' OH requirement; dependent on RNA
Terminal deoxynucleotidyl transferase	Polymerase	Adds dNMP to DNA or RNA	
Polynucleotide phosphorylase	Polymerase	Links dNMP	Template independent
E. coli DNA ligase	Ligase	Covalently closes nicks in double-stranded DNA	NAD dependent
T4 DNA ligase	Ligase	Joins 5' P-DNA fragments in double-stranded DNA; will also ligate blunt-ended DNA molecules	ATP dependent
T4 RNA ligase	Ligase	Joins 5' P-RNA fragments	

movement is prevented to eliminate diffusion. This technique is routinely employed for molecular weight determinations, which require this sieving effect.

An empirical relationship exists between the mobility (migration distance in an appropriate medium) and the $\log_{10}$ of the molecular weight of nucleic acids or proteins. Prior to electrophoresis, proteins are dissociated by boiling in sodium dodecyl sulfate (SDS) and treatment with 2-mercaptoethanol. SDS denatures the proteins by binding to their hydrophobic cores, and 2-mercaptoethanol reduces disulfide bonds. For most proteins, the amount of SDS bound is directly related to the size of the protein. Since SDS carries a strong negative charge, the mobility of the protein in a gel will be determined by the SDS charge and, thus, will be related to the size of the polypeptide chain. A measure of the mobility of the protein of interest, and its comparison with that of standard protein markers provides a measure of the molecular weight of the protein (Fig. 6.1**C & D**). In addition to molecular weight determinations, SDS gel electrophoresis provides a means of separating proteins into their subunits; thus complex proteins composed of distinct subunits can be identified, and the molecular weights and stoichiometry of these subunits can be determined. Agarose or polyacrylamide gels are employed to separate RNA or DNA molecules or their fragments according to size (Fig. 6.1**A & B**). The mobilities of the nucleic acids in the gel are measured, and the apparent molecular weights of the nucleic acids are determined from a standard curve that is derived from mobilities of molecules of known molecular weight. The most reliable measurements are made when the DNA or RNA samples are denatured prior to and during separation in gels containing 99 percent formamide, 6–8 M urea, methylmercuric hydroxide, or glyoxal.

6.3 Isotope Labeling

Most studies on the rate of synthesis, maturation, or degradation, as well as primary structure determinations of macromolecules, require radioisotopic labeling either in vivo or in vitro. Radioactive amino acids, nucleosides, and sugars are employed to label proteins, nucleic acids, and polysaccharides, respectively.

The rate of synthesis of a macromolecule can be measured by analyzing the level of radioactivity in the molecules at various times after a short-term addition (**pulse**) of an

---

FIG. 6.1. Gel electrophoresis of DNA, RNA, and protein. (**A**) DNA of plasmid pBR322 separated in 0.5 percent agarose-2.5 percent acrylamide gel, stained and observed by UV fluorescence: **1** = circular; **2** = linear; **3** = supercoiled. (**B**) RNA of *E. coli* separated in 0.5 percent agarose-2.5 percent acrylamide gel, stained and observed as above: **1** = 23S rRNA; **2** = 16S rRNA; **3** = 5S rRNA and tRNA. (**C**) Proteins boiled in SDS and 2-mercaptoethanol, separated in a 10 percent polyacrylamide gel, and stained with Coomassie blue: **1** = phosphorylase (molecular weight of 92,000); **2** = bovine serum albumin (molecular weight of 64,000); **3** = glyceraldehyde 3-phosphate dehydrogenase (molecular weight of 36,000); **4** = myokinase (molecular weight of 22,000). (**D**) Molecular weight standard curve plotted from distances measured in C.

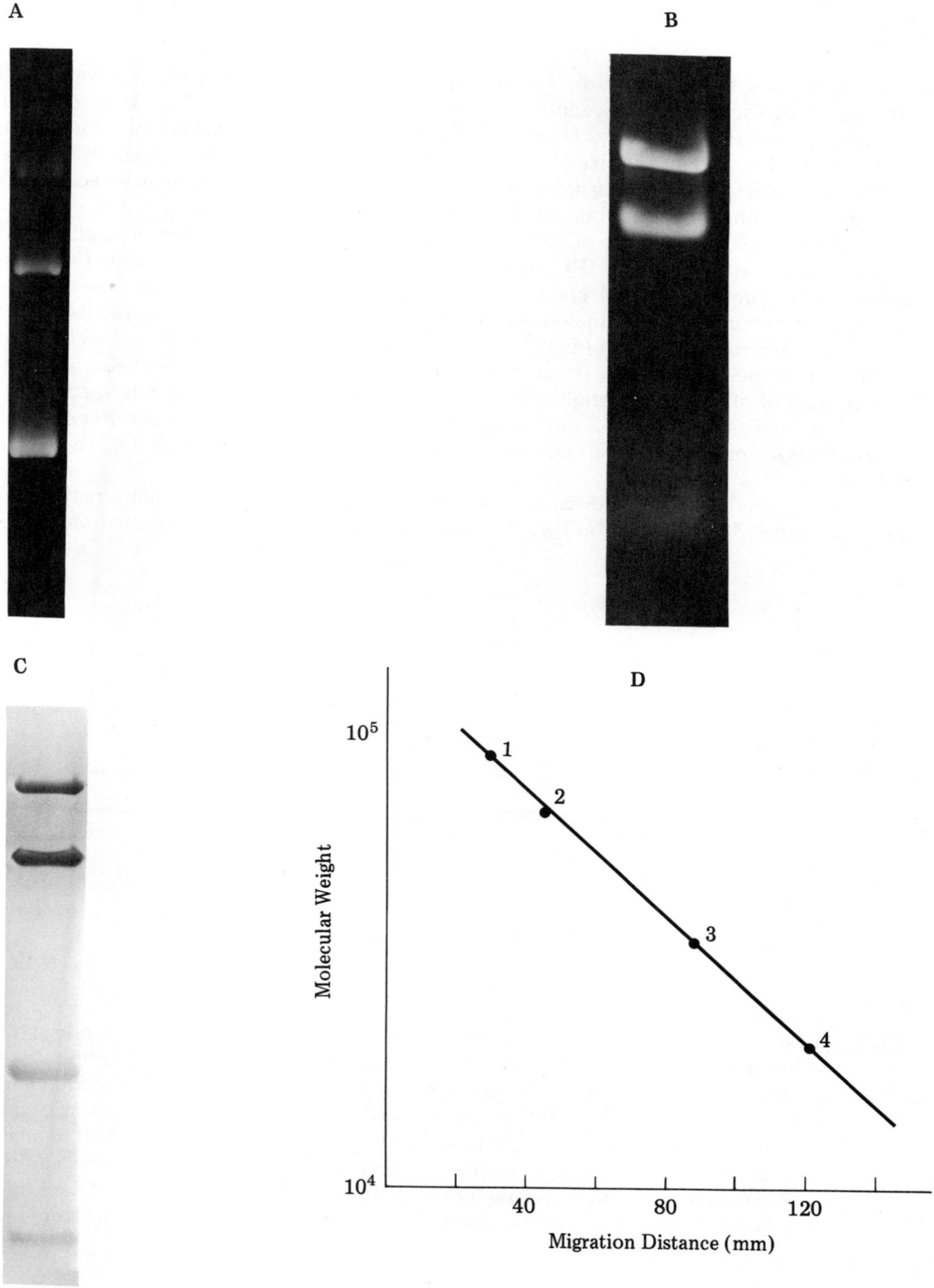
A
B
C
D
10^5
1
2
3
4
Molecular Weight
10^4
40
80
120
Migration Distance (mm)

appropriate radioactive precursor. The addition of nonradioactive precursors at various times after initiating the labeling procedure will reduce the specific activity of the labeled precursor and, thus, stop the incorporation of radioactivity into the macromolecules that are being synthesized. By analyzing the size of the different molecular forms of the molecule of interest, at various times after adding the nonradioactive precursor, the reduction in specific activity permits one to **chase** an initial molecular species into a subsequent form.

An example of this type of analysis is presented in Fig. 6.2. In this case, all forms of a protein—the initial precursor (P), an intermediate (I), and the mature form (M)—can be precipitated by antibodies to M, and the components in the immune precipitate can be analyzed by gel electrophoresis. The immune precipitates of radioactively labeled cell extracts can be analyzed to determine the size of the initial protein and the processing pathway that leads to the production of the mature form. In this case, P has a molecular weight 68,000 and is converted to a product M of molecular weight 45,000 via a 55,000 molecular weight intermediate I.

The change in the level of radioactivity in M, measured at various times after cessation of radioactivity incorporation, is a measure of the rate of disappearance of M, i.e., the **turnover rate**.

Long-term labeling of M, rather than pulse labeling, will yield a highly radioactive M. This radiolabeled compound can then be used for primary structure determination.

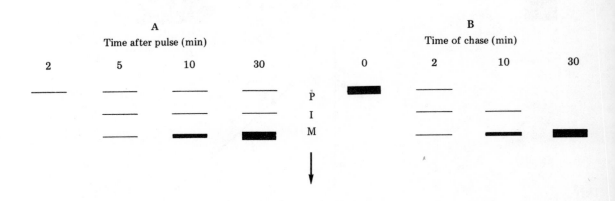

FIG. 6.2. Gel electrophoresis of immune precipitates of three forms of a protein; precursor (**P**), intermediate (**I**), and mature (**M**) present in the cell extract. Precipitates were obtained by addition of antibodies to the mature product. (**A**) ³⁵S-methionine was added at time 0, and samples were removed at various times after addition of labeled amino acid. (**B**) The cells were pulse labeled for two minutes. At time 0, nonlabeled amino acid was added, and samples were removed at various times after addition of nonlabeled amino acid. **Arrow** indicates direction of electrophoresis. **Black bands** indicate the position and the quantity of radioactive proteins after electrophoresis.

METHODS FOR STUDIES OF PROTEINS

6.4 Protein Isolation

Proteins can be isolated from whole cell homogenates or subcellular fractions by a series of procedures that select for molecules of a particular size, net charge, or binding capacity.

Chromatographic resins have been developed that can separate proteins on the basis of these three properties. Gel permeation chromatography separates proteins according to their size. Resins are available that can separate macromolecules over a range of molecular weights, from a few hundred to more than 10^7. A specific resin possesses pores that permit molecules of a given size to enter and totally exclude larger molecules. Proteins applied to a column are then eluted, with the largest components eluting first and followed by proteins of lower molecular size.

Proteins have a net charge that is dependent on their amino acid composition and the pH of the solution. Cationic (+) and anionic (−) resins will bind proteins differentially according to their charge. Proteins are selectively eluted from these resins by either pH or salt concentration gradients. Salts act as eluents by decreasing the electrostatic interaction between the protein and the resin, whereas a pH gradient alters the net charge on the protein. In each case, proteins that have the weakest affinity for the resin will elute first.

Proteins that are capable of binding strongly to another molecule—i.e., an enzyme to its substrate or an antibody to its antigen—can be purified by affinity chromatography. The substrate or antigen can be linked chemically to a resin, and the resin can be allowed to interact with the corresponding enzyme or antibody. Ideally, only proteins that display an affinity for the substance linked to resin will bind strongly. An enzyme bound to a resin-linked substrate can be subsequently eluted by competition induced by the addition of large amounts of substrate. Antibodies can only be dissociated from their antigens by being partially denatured.

6.5 Protein Sequence Determination

The primary sequences of many proteins of up to 1,000 amino acids in length have been determined. The general approach employed is the same whether the protein is large or small. The first step is the selective and quantitative cleavage of the protein into unique smaller polypeptide chains. Proteins are selectively cleaved either chemically (e.g., at methionine residues by cyanogen bromide [CNBr]) or enzymatically (e.g., by trypsin or chymotrypsin). Trypsin cleaves selectively at the basic residues arginine and lysine, whereas chymotrypsin cleaves preferentially at the hydrophobic residues: tryptophan, tyrosine, and phenylalanine. Since these cleavage reactions are highly specific, a unique set of polypeptide fragments will be generated. These peptides are then separated either by gel chromatographic techniques, as described above, or by a combination of electrophoresis in one direction followed by chromatography at a 90° angle to the direction of electrophoresis.

This **tryptic peptide mapping** permits a rapid and highly reproducible separation of protein fragments. Since the amino acid sequence of a protein is unique, its tryptic peptide fragments remain constant. Thus, the degree of similarity of two proteins can be determined on the basis of the number of identical tryptic cleavage products.

The amino acid sequences of the individual peptides are then determined either manually or automatically by an amino acid sequencing machine. Each approach requires the selective modification of the N terminal residue by the Edman reagent phenyl isothiocyanate, followed by cleavage of that N terminal amino acid derivative. The released amino acid is identified by thin layer or high pressure liquid chromatography, and the cycle is repeated with the next amino acid in the chain. After the sequence of each peptide generated by one cleavage method is determined, the order of these peptides in the protein chain is determined by identifying the amino acid sequence of overlapping peptides generated by another cleavage approach.

In recent years, the sensitivity of the sequencing techniques has been enhanced by new developments in instrumentation and the application of radioisotopic techniques to the sequencing problem. When proteins of interest can be labeled in vivo with amino acid precursors, the position of each radioactive amino acid in the polypeptide being sequenced can be determined simply by identifying the cleavage step in which the radioactive derivative of that amino acid is released.

METHODS FOR STUDIES OF NUCLEIC ACIDS

6.6 Labeling Nucleic Acids In Vitro

High specific activity nucleic acids are required for nucleic acid sequencing and hybridization studies. There are several methods employed to generate highly radioactive DNA, cDNA (complementary DNA), and RNA in vitro. **Nick translation** is one method in which double-stranded DNA can be made radioactive to a level of 10^8 dpm/μg* by employing two enzymes and high activity α^{32}P deoxynucleoside triphosphates (dNTP). One enzyme is pancreatic DNAse, which is used at low levels to generate a limited number of nicks in the DNA of interest. The other enzyme is *E. coli* DNA polymerase I, which possesses two activities employed in this method. The activity of a $5' \rightarrow 3'$ exonuclease removes bases in a 5' to 3' direction; and after initiating at a nick, its DNA polymerase activity fills in the gap generated by the $5' \rightarrow 3'$ exonuclease activity. If radioactive dNTP are employed, the gaps are filled with labeled nucleoside monophosphates (NMP) and the DNA becomes radioactive. A radioactive copy of an mRNA—i.e., cDNA—can be made by using the enzyme–reverse transcriptase in the presence of an oligo-deoxythymidine (dT) primer and radioactive dNTP. The 5' and 3' termini of RNA or DNA can be specifically labeled by using a number of enzyme activities and radioactive substrates. For example, T4 polynucleotide kinase catalyzes the transfer of the γ phosphate of ATP to a free 5' hydroxyl group on RNA or DNA. This reaction is often employed in generating a uniquely labeled end for DNA sequence analysis by the Maxam-Gilbert technique (Section 6.10). Terminal transferase can be employed to attach radioactive dNMP onto the 3' end of an

*A dpm = disintegration per minute.

RNA or DNA molecule. T4 RNA ligase can be employed to label specifically the 3' end of an RNA by attaching to it ^{32}P (nucleoside diphosphate).

6.7 Nucleic Acid Hybridization

Nucleic acids possess the property of complementarity. The base sequence in one strand of DNA is complementary to the base sequence in its sister strand, while RNA base sequence is complementary to the base sequence of the coding strand of the DNA template. When separated in solution, double-stranded nucleic acids—DNA, RNA, or RNA plus DNA hybrids— will, under appropriate conditions, search out and find their complementary sequences and re-form a duplex structure, i.e., **reanneal**. This process follows second-order kinetics, which is dependent upon the initial concentration of the complementary nucleic acid sequences present in solution (Fig. 6.3).

One can measure the rate of reannealing of duplex DNA in a solution containing separated DNA single strands by observing any of several physical properties of DNA—e.g., the sensitivity of the DNA solution to a single-stranded specific nuclease S1. At "zero" time in the reannealing process, all of the DNA is single-stranded; therefore, all or nearly all will be cleaved by S1. When hybridization is complete and all of the nucleic acid is in a duplex form, it will be entirely resistant to digestion with S1 nuclease.

The reannealing kinetics for duplex formation vary depending on the type of DNA (Fig. 6.3). As one would predict, simple sequence DNA reassociates most readily, and as the DNA sequence becomes more complex, the rate of reassociation slows considerably. The reassociation kinetics of eukaryotic DNA vary depending on the sequences of DNA involved. There are repeated DNA sequences that reanneal readily and unique or single-copy DNA sequences that reassociate only very slowly. Most structural genes are single-copy or unique sequences.

The size of the DNA fragments of a gene of interest, generated by digestion of a DNA preparation with a restriction endonuclease and separated by gel electrophoresis, can be determined by the hybridization of the DNA fragments with radioactive mRNA or cDNA. This process has been greatly simplified by the development of the **Southern transfer method**. In this procedure, the cleaved DNA is separated in an agarose gel according to the size of the fragments. The DNA in the gel is denatured in situ and after neutralization is transferred quantitatively to a nitrocellulose paper. The paper is treated with a radioactive probe, i.e., single-stranded mRNA or cDNA, and the sites of hybridization are determined by autoradiography after removing any unhybridized probe.

An analogous procedure called the **Northern transfer method** can be employed to identify and determine the sizes of mature RNA molecules, their precursors, and processing intermediates. Total RNA can be separated by size in denaturing agarose gels, and the RNA can be quantitatively transferred onto a nitrocellulose paper. A cDNA probe to the mature mRNA can be employed in a hybridization reaction to identify RNA molecules related to the mature mRNA. The positions of the RNA species and their molecular weights can be determined by analysis of the autoradiograph of the nitrocellulose filter on which hybridization took place (Fig. 6.4).

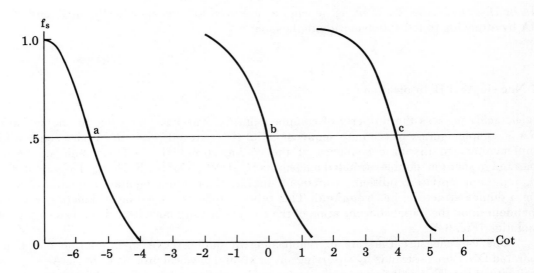

FIG. 6.3. Reassociation curves of 400 nucleotide fragments of DNA of different degrees of sequence complexity: **a** = poly(U) + poly (A); **b** = bacteriophage T4; **c** = nonrepetitive fraction of calf thymus. Ordinate: fraction of remaining single-stranded (f_s). Abscissa: **Cot** = product of initial concentration (**Co**) and time (**t** in seconds).

6.8 Physical Map of a DNA Molecule

The physical structure and conformation of single- and double-stranded DNA or RNA can be observed with an electron microscope. A nucleic acid solution can be spread on the surface of a low salt solution and picked up onto an electron microscope grid. The nucleic acid, coated with a basic substance, i.e., the protein cytochrome C, can be stained with uranyl acetate or shadowed with platinum atoms, to make an electron-dense surface that takes the shape of the DNA or RNA molecule (Fig. 6.5). The size of a molecule can be calculated by comparison of length measurements with those of a standard molecule of known molecular weight.

    The physical map of a DNA molecule—i.e., the position of the DNA from which a given RNA is transcribed—can be determined by the **R-loop mapping** procedure. This method takes advantage of the fact that an RNA/DNA hybrid is more stable (resistant to melting) than duplex DNA. RNA is hybridized to DNA under partial denaturation conditions in which the stable RNA/DNA hybrid forms, and the resulting complex is prepared for examination under the

---

FIG. 6.4. Basic steps in Southern (DNA) and Northern (RNA) transfer methods. (**1**) Fragments of either DNA or RNA are separated into fractions (**a-g**) by electrophoresis in an agarose gel. (**2**) Fractions, after denaturation, are transferred to nitrocellulose paper. (**3**) Transferred fractions are hybridized with a labeled probe. (**4**) Formation of hybrids by fractions **a** and **c** is detected by autoradiography.

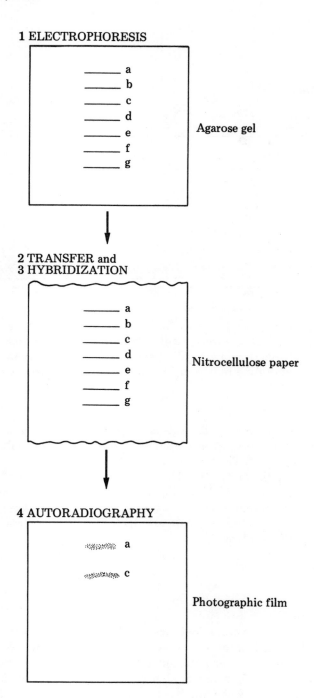

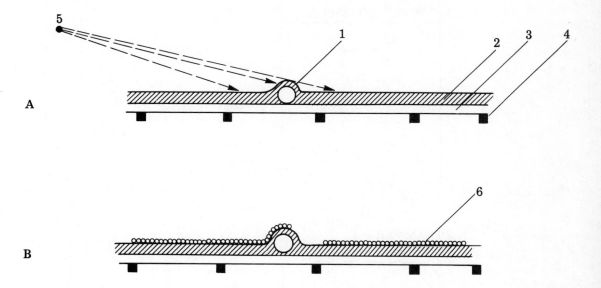

FIG. 6.5. Preparation of nucleic acid sample for examination under the electron microscope. (**A**) The DNA fiber (**1**) is covered with cytochrome C (**2**), which after spreading on supporting film (**3**) and on a grid (**4**) is stained with uranyl acetate. The preparation is exposed to evaporating platinum (**5**). (**B**) The platinum forms a layer of atoms (**6**) that outlines the DNA fiber.

electron microscope. Several distinct types of R-loops can be formed (Fig. 6.6). A simple R-loop (Fig. 6.6**A**) is formed between the RNA and partially denatured duplex DNA in which a single strand of DNA has been displaced. The position of the R-loop on the DNA can be determined by measuring the distances from the ends of the DNA to the loop. In the case of a more complex R-loop (Fig. 6.6**B**), there is, in the middle of the RNA/DNA hybrid, a looping out of single-stranded DNA owing to an intervening sequence that is present in the gene but absent from the mature mRNA. The same looping out (Fig 6.6**C**) of the intervening sequence DNA may find its complementary sequence in the displaced DNA strand and form a DNA/DNA duplex.

6.9 Recombinant DNA

An understanding of the basic principles of recombinant DNA methodology requires a discussion of several facets of the work: **vectors**, or the DNA that serves as a carrier of the foreign DNA; **gene isolation**, ligation to the vector, and **transformation** or **infection** of a bacterial host; and selection of the recombinant DNA-containing clone. For the sake of simplicity, only prokaryotic vectors and bacterial hosts will be discussed, but this technology employs the same basic concepts when applied to eukaryotic cells.

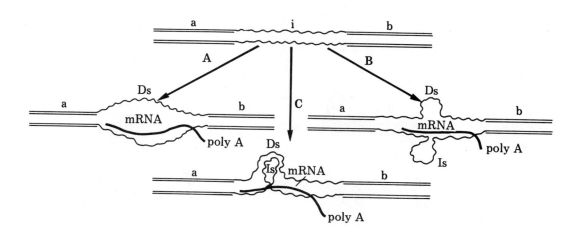

FIG. 6.6. R-loop mapping. The double-stranded DNA to be studied is inserted (**i**) between two arms (**a, b**) of bacteriophage λ DNA. After partial denaturation, two strands of the insert are dissociated, and one of the strands is hybridized with mRNA, while the second strand remains displaced (**Ds**). (**A**) Simple R-loop. (**B**) R-loop with looping out of the intervening sequence (**Is**) that lacks a complementary sequence in the mRNA. (**C**) R-loop in which the looped out intervening sequence (**Is**) reassociates with the complementary displaced DNA strand (**Ds**).

There are two types of vectors that are employed—**bacterial plasmid DNA** and the **bacteriophage λ**. The plasmid DNA vectors are useful for cloning and subcloning DNA fragments that represent a high percentage (>0.1 percent) of the total DNA. Modified λ vectors are useful for cloning DNA fragments that represent a small percentage (as low as 0.0001 percent) of the total DNA.

Plasmid DNA is extrachromosomal bacterial DNA. Plasmid vectors have been engineered so that they possess three useful properties: an independent origin of DNA replication, one or more antibiotic resistance genes, and several useful restriction endonuclease cleavage sites with known map positions (Fig. 6.7).

DNA of the bacteriophage λ possesses an internal region, approximately 30 percent of its length, that is nonessential and can be removed by endonuclease digestion (Fig. 6.8). Two peripheral regions (arms a and b of the DNA) can be isolated and then religated to foreign DNA. This DNA recombinant can now be used to infect bacteria, and viable phage that carry a foreign insert can be identified.

Several approaches to gene isolation can be attempted. Recombinant DNA technology has reached a point in which the selection techniques are so sensitive that, in most cases, prior partial isolation of a gene is unnecessary. If purified mRNA from the gene of interest can be

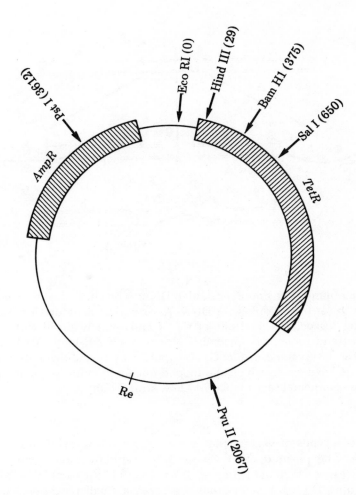

FIG. 6.7. Physical map of the plasmid pBR322: **Re** = origin of replication; **AmpR** = ampicillin resistance; **TetR** = tetracycline resistance. **Arrows** and **symbols** indicate sites of cleavage by restriction nucleases (for symbols see Table 6.1). The numbers in parentheses correspond to map positions of the cleavage sites.

obtained, a double-stranded cDNA copy can be synthesized by employing reverse transcriptase and DNA polymerase I (Fig. 6.9). This double-stranded cDNA copy of the mRNA can be modified at the ends by one of two mechanisms to permit it to be ligated to a vector. The first mechanism involves the ligation of chemically synthesized **linker DNA** sequences, which possess a known restriction endonuclease cleavage site, to the ends of the double-stranded cDNA. These termini and the vector DNA are cleaved by the same restriction endonuclease, and the resulting sticky ends are joined together and ligated. A second approach employs the

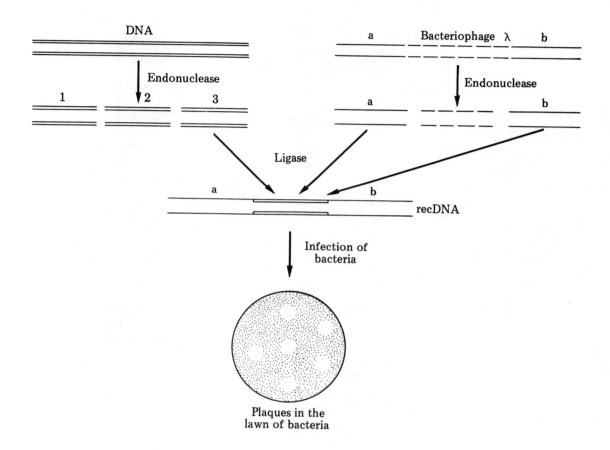

FIG. 6.8. Preparation of recombinant DNA (**recDNA**) using bacteriophage λ. DNA is digested with an endonuclease into fragments **1-3**, and the central nonessential segment from λ phage (**dashed**) is removed. Fragment **3** and purified phage arms **a** and **b** are ligated by DNA ligase. The recombinant DNA (arms and fragment 3) is used to infect bacteria. The infected bacteria are detected by formation of foci of bacteriolysis (**plaques**) in the lawn growth.

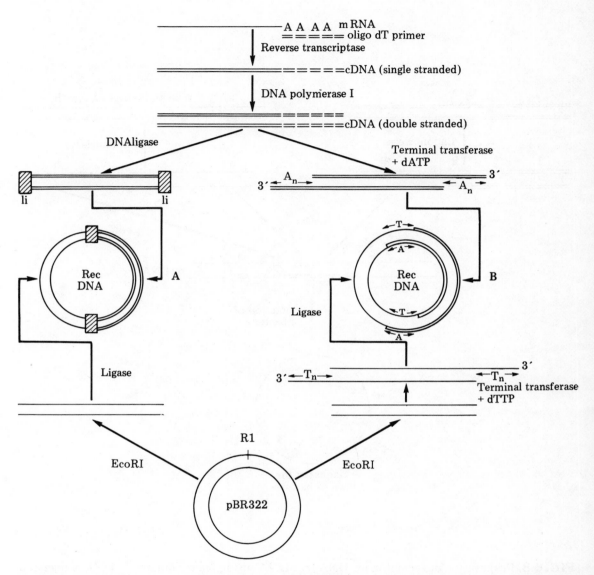

FIG. 6.9. Preparation of recombinant DNA (**recDNA**) using plasmid pBR322. The cDNA is prepared using mRNA as a template and the enzyme reverse transcriptase. It is ligated to the linear form of the plasmid through either (**A**) linker (**li**) attached by DNA ligase or (**B**) complementary ends created by terminal deoxynucleotidyl transferase. For details, see text.

enzyme terminal deoxynucleotidyl transferase, which is used to add dAMP residues to the 3′ end of the double-stranded cDNA and dTMP residues to the 3′ end of a linear form of the vector. Complementary tails can then be joined, and the resulting recombinant molecules are used to infect the bacteria.

Prior to ligation, the gene of interest can be partially purified by size, using velocity gradient sedimentation or agarose gel electrophoresis, or by base composition, employing equilibrium density gradient sedimentation. A combination of these procedures usually results in a 10- to 100-fold purification; however, if the gene of interest is a single-copy gene, it will still be only 0.01 percent pure.

To make **cloning** of single-copy eukaryotic genes manageable, an approach was developed to make a library of the total genome of an organism (Fig. 6.10). A special property of bacteriophage λ made this possible. Newly synthesized λ DNA is joined end to end in long concatamers, i.e., complexes containing 10 or more complete viral genomes. The ends of the λ DNA serve as recognition sites for the binding of empty viral heads and tails to the DNA in a first step of packaging the DNA into the virus. The empty tail binds to the linked ends of the concatameric DNA and draws the equivalent of one genome of λ DNA into its head. To produce a library, a partial digestion of total cellular DNA is carried out with an enzyme that recognizes a four-base sequence. Fragments of about 10,000 to 20,000 base pairs in length are selected, and a linker sequence is put on the ends. The foreign DNA is now mixed with purified λ arms a and b and ligated into long concatamers. Purified heads and tails of λ phage are added, and the heads are filled with DNA. If the length of the insert between the a and b arms is proper, a viable lytic phage is produced. These filled phage are used to infect a bacterial culture, and a population of phage is prepared that contains foreign DNA inserted between the a and b arms. This joined DNA, now inside the virus head, has the property of being able to be transferred to a bacterial recipient with a very high frequency. Sites of infection with virus can be identified, since the virus will lyse infected bacteria and produce plaques in the "lawn" of growing microorganisms. It takes about 10^6 recombinant DNA-containing phage particles prepared in this way to ensure that 99 percent of the genomic DNA has been inserted into the total population of these bacteriophages.

Various procedures have been developed for identification and selection of clones containing recombinant DNA. The bacterial plasmids possess one or more drug resistance genes. After infection of a competent bacterial host with a preparation of recombinant DNA-containing plasmids, the cells are spread on plates containing an antibiotic—e.g., ampicillin or tetracycline in the case of pBR322 plasmid. Under such conditions, only cells that have picked up the plasmid DNA with drug resistance genes will grow, while all other bacteria are eliminated (Fig. 6.11). The colonies that contain a DNA segment of interest are selected by one or more of the following methods.

When a radioactive mRNA or cDNA probe to a gene of interest is available, **colony hybridization** can be performed. Clones containing recombinant DNA are grown on agar plates. A portion of each colony is transferred to a nitrocellulose filter and lysed in situ, and the DNA is denatured and affixed to the filter. The filter is incubated with the radioactive probe, and after removing the unhybridized probe, the radioactive colonies—i.e., those containing recombinant DNA complementary to the probe—are identified by autoradiography (Fig. 6.11).

Another approach known as **hybrid arrested translation** requires a preparation of

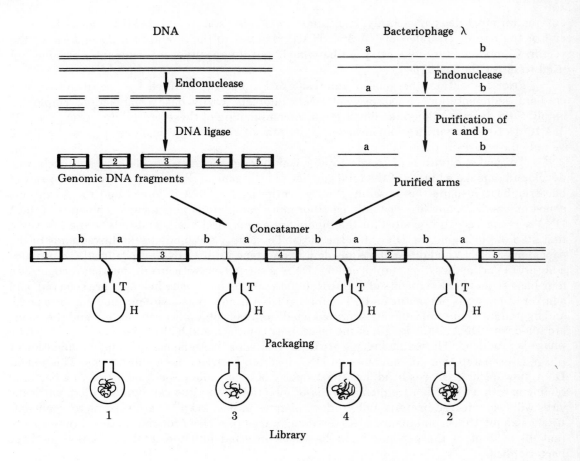

FIG. 6.10. Preparation of a library of genomic DNA using bacteriophage λ. Fragments (**1-5**) of genomic DNA with linker sequences (**black bars** at the ends) are ligated to the **a** and **b** arms of bacteriophage λ. After forming large concatamers, the DNA segments corresponding to one phage equivalent are packed into empty viral particles each consisting of a head (**H**) and a tail (**T**). The genomic DNA library consists of the population of viruses (**1, 3, 4,** and **2**), each carrying a segment of foreign DNA.

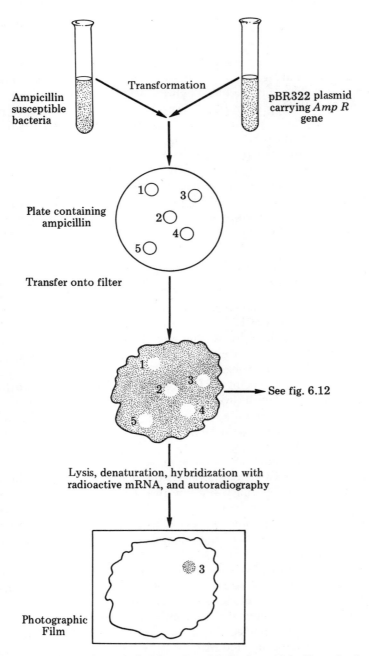

FIG. 6.11. An example of the colony hybridization method to identify colonies containing a specific recDNA. The ampicillin susceptible bacteria are transformed with recombinant DNA containing the pBR322 plasmid carrying a gene for ampicillin resistance (**AmpR**). Only transformed organisms will grow and produce colonies (**1-5**) on the agar containing ampicillin. Colonies are transferred onto a nitrocellulose filter and lysed; their DNA is denatured and hybridized with labeled mRNA for the gene of interest. The colony containing this gene (**3**) can be selected on the basis of positive autoradiography owing to hybridization with labeled mRNA.

translatable, but not necessarily pure, mRNA. Colonies of bacteria that contain recombinant DNA are grown, and plasmid DNA is prepared from a portion of the cells. This DNA is denatured and affixed to nitrocellulose and used as a hybridization probe to bind complementary mRNA present in the crude mRNA preparation. Translation is carried out both on the mRNA that remains in solution after hybridization and on the mRNA that, after binding to the filter, has been eluted. The translation products are separated by gel electrophoresis, and the protein products, including that from the gene of interest, are identified by autoradiography (Fig. 6.12).

Since bacteriophage will only package DNA of a certain size range and the arms a plus b alone are too small to be packaged; only viruses that have incorporated an insert of foreign DNA will grow and form plaques on a lawn of bacteria. Plaques that are produced by recombinant DNA-containing phage are screened by a method analogous to colony hybridization and hybrid arrested translation as in the case of plasmid DNA recombinants described above.

6.10 Nucleic Acid Sequencing

Two methods of nucleic acid sequencing, which permit the determination of the sequence of an unlimited number of base pairs of DNA, are currently employed.

In the procedure developed by Maxam and Gilbert, quantitative base-specific chemical cleavage reactions and labeling of a unique terminus of DNA (or RNA) are combined with separation by high resolution polyacrylamide gel electrophoresis. The procedure (Fig. 6.13) requires the labeling of a unique end of the DNA strand and the partial **modification** at G alone; A and G; T and C; or C alone. On the average, only one base per chain is modified, and the chain is quantitatively cleaved at the modified base. The products of partial cleavage reactions are separated by gel electrophoresis, and the base sequence of the DNA can be read directly from the autoradiograph of the gel.

Using the same basic approach, RNA sequence analysis can be carried out by enzymatic and chemical means. RNAse T1 cleaves after G, and pancreatic RNAse cleaves after U and C. RNAse Phy I cleaves after G, A, and U but not after C. The alkali, sodium hydroxide, cleaves after all bases. Therefore, base-specific cleavage reactions are available, and partial cleavage products can be generated, separated by gel electrophoresis, and identified by autoradiography. A set of chemical modifications and cleavages, similar to those employed in the DNA sequencing method, have also been developed for RNA sequencing.

The Sanger method of DNA sequencing employs enzymatic means to generate partial polymerization products that terminate at only one type of base in the sequence (Fig. 6.14). A primer with a free 3′ hydroxyl is annealed to a single-stranded DNA whose sequence is to be determined. The hybrid formed between the primer and DNA is divided into four aliquots, each containing four different deoxynucleoside triphosphates (dNTP) and one dideoxynucleoside triphosphate (ddNTP), which is labeled with ^{32}P. The latter, owing to the lack of a 3′ hydroxyl, stops polymerization whenever it is incorporated into a growing chain. As a result, four sets of partial elongation products are generated, with each set containing the products terminated at the 3′ end by the labeled dideoxynucleoside that was present in the reaction mixture. High resolution polyacrylamide gel electrophoresis is employed to separate the products according to their

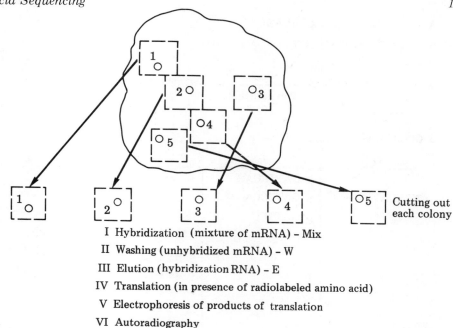

I Hybridization (mixture of mRNA) – Mix

II Washing (unhybridized mRNA) – W

III Elution (hybridization RNA) – E

IV Translation (in presence of radiolabeled amino acid)

V Electrophoresis of products of translation

VI Autoradiography

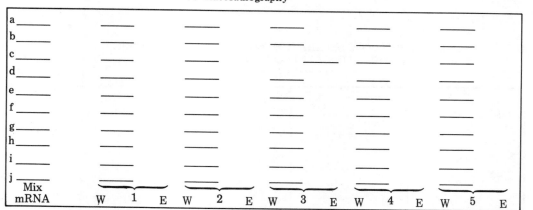

Photographic film

FIG. 6.12. Hybrid arrested translation and hybrid selected translation. A mixture of mRNA (**Mix**) is translated, in the presence of a labeled amino acid, into 10 distinct (**a-j**) products that are separated by electrophoresis. The same products are obtained by translation of the mix mRNA nonhybridized to plasmid DNA from colonies **1, 2, 4,** and **5** and washed (**W**) from filters. The mRNA nonhybridized with DNA from colony **3** and washed from filter (**W**) gives all products (of the mix mRNA) except **c**. The product c is synthesized by eluting (**E**) the hybridized mRNA bound to the filter with DNA from colony 3. The product c is encoded by DNA carried by the plasmid that transformed colony 3.

A   LABELING AT 5¹ END

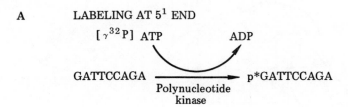

B′ CLEAVING AT MODIFIED BASE

G	A and G	T and C	C
	p*GATTCCAG		
p*GATTCCA	p*GATTCCA		
	p*GATTCC		
		p*GATTC	p*GATTC
		p*GATT	p*GATT
		p*GAT	
		p*GA	
	p* G		
P*	P*		

C   ELECTROPHORETIC SEPARATION AND AUTORADIOGRAPHIC IDENTIFICATION OF CLEAVAGE PRODUCTS

Deduced base sequence *

A
G
A
C
C
T
T
A
G

FIG. 6.13. Maxam and Gilbert procedure of nucleic acid sequencing. (**A**) 5′ end of DNA molecule is labeled with ^{32}P. (**B**) DNA is modified and cleaved, at the base indicated, yielding mixture of cleavage products. (**C**) Products are separated by electrophoresis and identified by autoradiography owing to 5′ end label. The base sequence is deduced from the autoradiograph as follows. Band **1** is present among products of cleavage at A and G and cleavage at G; hence cleavage had to involve G. Band **2** is present among products of cleavage at A and G but not G alone; hence cleavage had to involve A. Likewise, band **3** is present in the products of cleavage at C and T but not C alone; therefore, it must represent T.

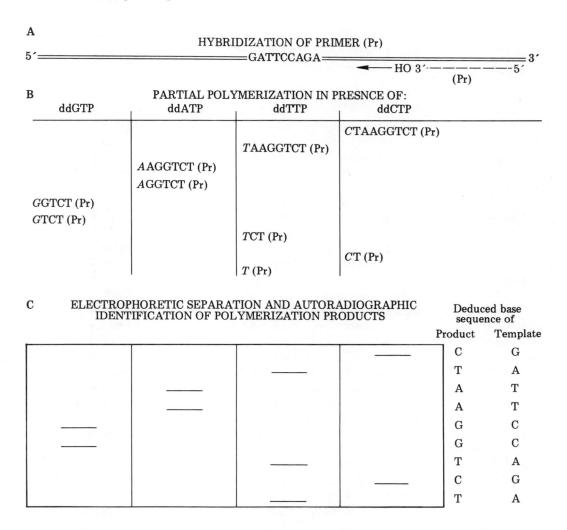

FIG. 6.14. Sanger procedure of nucleic acid sequencing. (**A**) Hybridization of primer (**Pr**) with free OH group at 3′ end. (**B**) Polymerization of four aliquots, each containing *all* four deoxynucleoside triphosphates (**dNTP**) and *one* of four dideoxynucleoside triphosphates (**ddNTP**). (**C**) Separation by electrophoresis of products of polymerization and their identification by means of autoradiography that detects labeled ddNTP. Base sequence of products is deduced from autoradiography, since each product must have at the 3′ end a labeled ddNTP present in the aliquot. The sequence of products is converted into the sequence of the template DNA.

length, and the elongation products are identified by autoradiography. The base sequence of each product can be easily converted into template sequence.

6.11 Determination of a Restriction Endonuclease Cleavage Map of a Gene

Through the use of DNA sequence-specific type II restriction endonucleases, it is possible to develop a physical map of a gene in which the precise locations of the cleavage sites for several restriction endonucleases are determined. Several approaches have been developed, all of which require determinations of DNA fragment size by analytical electrophoresis in agarose or polyacrylamide gels.

For the determination of a simple map consisting of only a few DNA fragments, the sizes of the products of a complete digestion can be compared with the sizes of partial digestion products (Fig. 6.15A). For example, total digestion of DNA of 10 Kb* in length yields five unique fragments: a, b, c, d, and e. Partial digestion yields these same five fragments plus a series of partial digestion products, P_1–P_7. Each partial product is a combination of two or more of the five unique fragments of DNA obtained after total digestion. From the molecular weights of these partial products, one or more possible map orders can be determined.

Often the DNA is digested simultaneously with two enzymes of different base sequence specificity. If the map order is known for one enzyme, the analysis of the molecular weights of the **double digestion products** will yield information on the map order of the DNA fragments generated by the second enzyme (Fig. 6.15**B**). For example, two enzymes, 1 and 2, separately cleave the DNA. In double digest by enzymes 1 and 2, the 4 Kb fragment is missing and is replaced by a 3.5 Kb fragment. Since enzyme 2 produces only 4 Kb and 6 Kb fragments and enzyme 1 generates several other fragments, the 4 Kb fragment produced by enzyme 1 must include the site recognized by enzyme 2.

Still another method involves end labeling and partial digestion. One can specifically label the termini of the DNA, separate the two labeled terminal fragments (e.g., the 6 Kb and 4 Kb products of enzyme 2 digestion), carry out a partial digestion reaction with enzyme 1, and separate the partial digestion fragments. The partial products will be labeled only at the end. Therefore, every radioactive component must contain the end fragment. The size of the partial digestion products will be the sum of the molecular weights of the terminal fragment plus one or more additional DNA fragments (Fig. 6.15**C**). The 4 Kb fragment yields the 0.5 Kb fragment of enzyme A and the undigested 4 Kb from enzyme B. The 6 Kb fragment yields a 3 Kb and 1 Kb fragment from enzyme A, and so on. The unequivocal map order is presented in Fig. 6.15**D**.

If a purified mRNA or a cDNA clone to an mRNA of interest is available, it is possible to map the position of the transcribed portion of a gene using the Southern transfer method or the S1 nuclease mapping method. In the Southern transfer method, radioactive mRNA or cDNA is hybridized to restriction fragments of DNA separated by gel electrophoresis, denatured, and affixed to nitrocellulose. One can use the map generated in Fig. 6.15**D** and locate the map position of a 1.0 Kb mRNA, which possesses 0.2 Kb of poly A tail in Fig. 6.16**A**, **B**. The

---

*Kb = kilobase (1,000 bases).

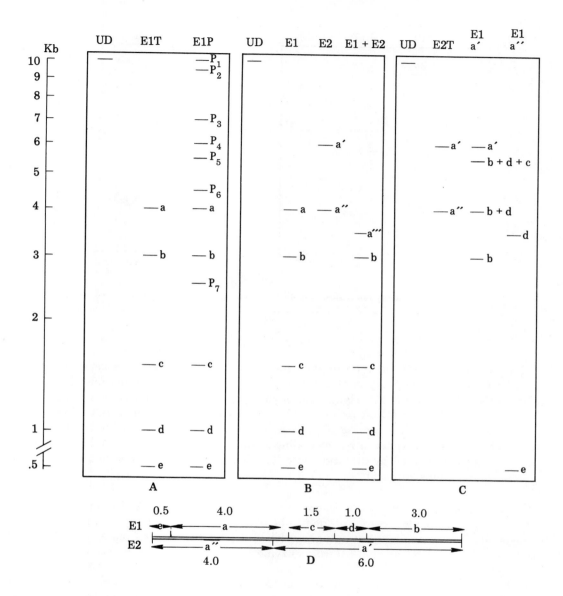

FIG. 6.15. Determination of a physical map of an undigested (**UD**) DNA fragment of 10 Kb in length. (**A**) Total (**T**) and partial (**P**) digestion with enzyme (**E1**). (**B**) Digestion with two enzymes (**E1** and **E2**) separately or together. (**C**) Total (**T**) digestion of terminally labeled DNA with one enzyme (**E2**) and partial digestion of fragments a′ a″ with another enzyme (**E1**). (**D**) Map of DNA deduced from comparison of fragments obtained by digestion with **E1** or **E2**.

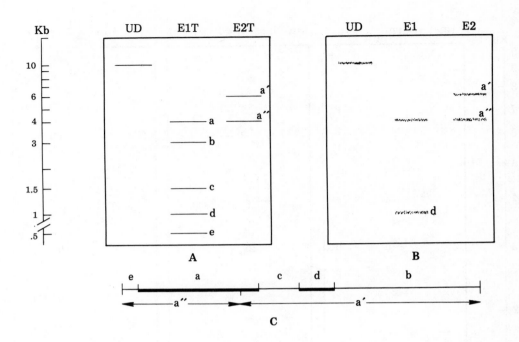

FIG. 6.16. Southern transfer method applied for mapping the position of a gene on a DNA fragment. (**A**) Separation of products of total digestion with either one (**E1**) or the other (**E2**) enzyme. (**B**) Hybridization of separated digestion products with a radioactive mRNA or cDNA probe by the Southern transfer method. (**C**) Sequence of fragments deduced in Fig. 6.15**D** with segments forming hybrids indicated by **thicker lines**. Apparently, the coding sequence for mRNA is located in fragments **a** and **d** produced by digestion with E1. Fragment **c** may correspond to an intron (intervening sequence).

complete digestion of the 10 Kb fragment is presented in Fig. 6.16**A**. It can be seen that hybridization of the complete cDNA probe can be observed with the undigested DNA and with both fragments from enzyme 2, but only the 4 Kb and 1 Kb fragments from enzyme 1 exhibit radioactivity. The 1.5 Kb fragment (d) from enzyme 1 may be part of an intervening sequence.

A very precise mapping method can be employed to determine the exact location on the map of the 5′ and 3′ termini of the mature mRNA. In this method, nick-translated DNA is cleaved with a restriction endonuclease to generate radioactive restriction fragments. The isolated DNA fragments are denatured and reannealed to the purified nonradioactive mRNA probe under conditions that favor RNA/DNA hybrid formation. The single-stranded RNA and DNA tails are removed by digestion with nuclease S1, the RNA/DNA hybrids are denatured, and the size of the fragment protected from digestion by nuclease S1 is determined (Fig. 6.17). In addition, R-loop mapping can be employed to gain further information on the structure of a gene.

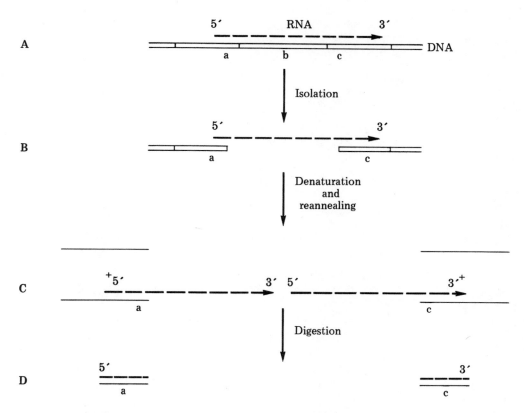

FIG. 6.17. S1 nuclease mapping method. (**A**) Transcription map of a gene composed of fragments **a**, **b**, and **c** of double-stranded DNA (**double line**). The position of mRNA (**dashed line**) is indicated. (**B**) Isolation of restriction fragments **a** and **c**. (**C**) Reannealing of denatured fragments **a** and **c** of DNA (**single lines**) to RNA (**dashed lines**) to form a stable RNA/DNA hybrid. (**D**) Single-stranded regions of DNA and RNA are digested with S1 nuclease to obtain only RNA/DNA hybrids. The precise location of the 5′ and 3′ ends of the RNA in fragments a and c, respectively, can be determined by measuring the length of the fragments protected from S1 digestion.

It should be obvious from the preceding discussion that current biochemical methods provide immunogeneticists with powerful tools for the most sophisticated research. Intensive application of these methods will resolve several controversial issues posed by results of classic immunologic and genetic studies.

II / *Suggested Supplementary Readings*

The following list of publications has been compiled to provide the reader with a source of specific references. It consists predominantly of the most recent textbooks, monographs, reviews and some selected original papers. Each publication listed has an extensive list of references that may be useful for the reader who desires to pursue in depth some of the topics discussed in the preceding section.

Altman, P. L., Katz, D. D. (eds.), *Inbred and Genetically Defined Strains of Laboratory Animals*. Federation of American Societies for Experimental Biology, Bethesda, 1979.

Bailey, D. W., How pure are inbred strains of mice. Immunol. Today **3**: 210–214, 1982.

Cavalli-Sforza, L. L., Bodmer, W. F., *The Genetics of Human Populations*. W. H. Freeman & Co., San Francisco, 1971.

Dun, O. J., *Basic Statistics: A Primer for Biomedical Sciences*. J. Wiley & Sons, New York, London, Sydney, 1964.

Festing, M. F. W., *Inbred Strains in Biomedical Research*. Oxford University Press, New York, 1979.

Fudenberg, H. H., Stites, D. P., Caldwell, J. L., Wells, J. V. (eds.), *Basic and Clinical Immunology*. Lange Medical Publications, Los Altos, California, 1976.

Golub, E. S., *The Cellular Basis of the Immune Response. An Approach to Immunobiology*. Sinauer Associates, Sunderland, Massachusetts, 1977.

Green, F. L., *Genetics and Probability in Animal Breeding Experiments*. Oxford University Press, New York, 1981.

Grossman, L., Moldeve, K. (eds.), *Methods in Enzymology LXV Nucleic Acids*. Part I. Academic Press, New York, 1980.

Jerne, N. K., Nordin, A. K., Plaque formation in agar by single antibody producing cells. Science **140**: 495–497, 1975.

Klein, J., *Biology of the Mouse Histocompatibility-2 Complex.* Springer-Verlag, New York, Heidelberg, Berlin, 1975.

Klein, J., *Immunology: the Science of Self-Nonself Discrimination.* Wiley-Interscience, New York, 1982.

Köhler, G., Milstein, C., Continuous cultures of fused cells secreting antibody of predefined specifity. Nature **256**:495–497, 1975.

Lefkovits, I., Pernis, B., (eds.), *Immunological Methods.* Academic Press, New York, London, Toronto, Sydney, San Francisco, 1981.

Lehninger, A. L., *Biochemistry.* Worth Publishers, New York, 1982.

Loveland, B. E., McKenzie, I. F. C., Which T cells cause graft rejection? Transplantation **33**: 217–220, 1982.

Milgrom, F., Abeyounis, C. J., Kano, K. (eds.), *Principles of Immunological Diagnosis in Medicine.* Lea & Febiger, Philadelphia, 1981.

Rose, N. R., Friedman, H., *Manual of Clinical Immunology.* American Society for Microbiology, Washington, D.C., 1976.

Rose, N. R., Milgrom, F., van Oss, C. J. (eds.), *Principles of Immunology.* Macmillan, New York, 1979.

Rosenthal, A. S., Determinant selection and macrophange function in genetic control of the immune response. Immunol. Rev. **40**: 136–152, 1978.

Walsh, K. A., Ericsson, L. H., Parmelee, D. C., Titani, K., Advances in protein sequencing. Ann. Rev. Biochem. **50**: 261–284, 1981.

Weir, D. M. (ed.), *Handbook of Experimental Immunology.* Third Edition. Blackwell Scientific Publications, Oxford, London, Edinburgh, Melbourne, 1978.

Wu, R. (ed.), *Methods in Enzymology LXVIII Recombinant DNA.* Academic Press, New York, 1979.

Zaleski, M. B., Abeyounis, C. J., Kano, K. (eds.), *Immunobiology of the Major Histocompatibility Complex.* S. Karger, Basel, 1981.

III / Genetics of Immunoglobulins

7 / *Structure and Phylogeny of Immunoglobulins*

HISTORICAL BACKGROUND

7.1 Theories of Antibody Formation

The primary structure of polypeptide chains, the building blocks of immunoglobulin molecules, is encoded in the genome. All genes coding for the synthesis of one immunoglobulin chain appear to be arranged in tandem on one segment of a chromosome. A recombination mechanism selects genes that are to be expressed phenotypically. This mechanism requires a minimum of DNA material for the generation of a maximum number of different immunoglobulin molecules (Chapter 8). Initially, immunoglobulin molecules are synthesized without the intervention of the antigen and form receptors on the surface of the uncommitted B cells. When antigen is encountered, it combines with these cell-surface receptors; this event provides the stimulus for cell differentiation and proliferation and, eventually, for antibody formation by plasma cells.

The entire sequence of events leading to the synthesis of specific antibodies has only recently been elucidated in its general outline. Still, many "blanks" remain; the mechanisms of some events are still ambiguous and others are totally obscure.

Because the role of antigen in the immune process is so apparent, much more attention was given in early investigations to the **antigen-driven** events than to the events preceding the encounter with antigen. Therefore, one has to admire the genius of Paul Ehrlich who, in 1900, proposed his theory of antibody formation, known as the **side chain hypothesis**. Ehrlich's concept was based on the presence of **preformed cell-surface receptors**. To emphasize that these receptors are not the result of encounter with the antigen, Ehrlich proposed that they may play a role in the cell's metabolism. By virtue of their configuration, receptors combine with those antigen molecules that are able to penetrate near the receptor-bearing cell. After combination with the antigen, the complex of receptor and antigen separates from the cell surface so that the cell receives a "biochemical injury." This "wound" is healed by overproduction of identical receptors, i.e., antibodies that in the process are sloughed into the circulation (Fig. 7.1).

Unfortunately, Ehrlich's hypothesis fell victim to the rapid progress in immunology and biochemistry during the next five decades. From the works of Karl Landsteiner and others, it became clear that one can induce the formation of antibodies against almost any chemical configuration. The concept of receptors or antibodies preformed to react with a synthesized compound that does not exist in nature seemed totally unacceptable. To explain this paradox, **"instructive" theories** were introduced by Breinl and Haurowitz, Pauling, and others proposing that antigens are directly involved in the formation of antibodies and in determining their specificity.

Pauling postulated that the antigen directs the folding of the antibody molecule in such a way that the combining sites of antibody become mirror images of the antigenic determinants. This concept proved to be too simplistic, and when attempts failed to confirm Pauling's concept that an antibody molecule can be reshaped in vitro by exposure to antigen, the theory itself was no longer tenable. Haurowitz postulated that antigen is incorporated into the antibody synthetic machinery and that it controls the primary structure of engendered antibody molecule. The crucial point in this hypothesis was the requirement for persistence of antigen for as long as the

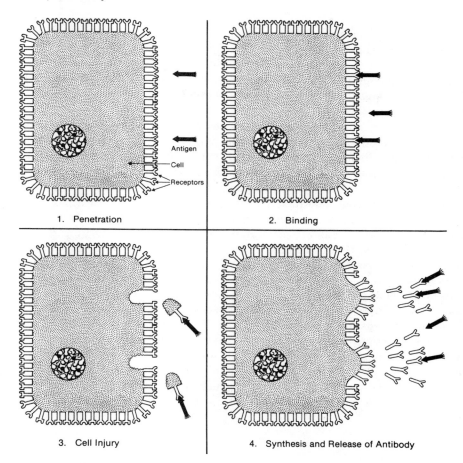

Labels within figure:
Antigen
Cell
Receptors

1. Penetration
2. Binding
3. Cell Injury
4. Synthesis and Release of Antibody

FIG. 7.1. Ehrlich's theory of antibody synthesis as outlined by Hirszfeld. (**1**) Penetration of antigen. (**2**) Antigen binds to cell surface receptors. (**3**) Antigen causes biochemical injury. (**4**) Overproduction of receptors; receptors released into the circulation.

immunological memory lasts. Presently, it is not possible to prove or to disprove that minute amounts of antigen persist for any period of time.

After more than five decades of banishment, the concept of preformed antibody molecules was resurrected by Niels Jerne in 1955. Jerne pointed out the presence of **natural antibodies*** and their wide spectrum of specificities. According to Jerne, antibody formation is triggered by the combination of antigen with a molecule of natural antibody of matching specificity. The complex is taken up by macrophages and constitutes a stimulus for the

*The term natural antibodies refers to antibodies that are seemingly produced without intentional challenge with the corresponding antigen.

synthesis of more of the same antibody molecules. The hypothesis was a retrograde step in relation to Ehrlich's initial thesis, since it did not explain the origin of the natural antibodies or the mechanism by which more of the same antibody is made after the antigen-antibody complexes had been taken up by the cells. Two years later, in 1957, Burnet formulated the first version of his **clonal selection theory**, a hypothesis that forms the basis of our modern concept of immunity.

The basic difference between the hypotheses of Ehrlich and Burnet is that the latter postulates that one antibody-forming cell is capable of producing antibody molecules of only one type. Accordingly, cells display receptors on their surfaces identical in specificity to the antibody molecules that they are capable of manufacturing. Combination of antigen with cell-surface receptor triggers proliferation of the cell that carries the affected receptor. A **clone** of identical daughter cells is formed, each of which synthesizes antibody of identical specificity that is capable of combining (binding) with the antigen that stimulated the mother cell. A large number of different clonal precursor cells are generated early during ontogeny by a random process equivalent to multiple **somatic mutations**. Cells that, during this process, develop autoimmune receptors are eliminated as **forbidden clones** by early encounter with "self" antigens. Soon after Burnet's theory had been outlined, it received very strong experimental backing: individual cells were shown to make antibody of only one specificity and **myeloma proteins** were found to be monoclonal, i.e., products of one clone of plasma cells derived from a single mother cell that underwent malignant transformation, resulting in a disease known as **multiple myeloma**.

The clonal selection theory had an unprecedented fertilizing effect on immunological research and on the development of new ideas in theoretical immunology. Single cell techniques, elucidation of immunoglobulin structure, research on tolerance and immunity, and, last but not least, the great controversy of the 1970s on the generation of diversity of antibodies all either owe their existence to Burnet's hypothesis or have been at least partly stimulated by this hypothesis.

7.2 Development of Basic Concepts

During the first 30 or so years of modern immunology, antibodies were described by their functions—i.e., precipitation, agglutination, binding of complement, etc.—but the molecular basis of these phenomena was unclear. The evidence that antibodies are proteins and belong to the globulin fraction of serum was provided in 1938 by Breinl and Haurowitz, and by Marrack. In 1939 Tiselius and Kabat used the recently developed electrophoretic technique (Section 6.2) and showed that antibodies are located in the **gamma globulin fraction**. Further progress was hindered by the extreme heterogeneity of antibodies; whereas other proteins—e.g., enzymes—can be purified, or even crystallized, gamma globulins showed continuous distribution when attempts were made to fractionate them by any chemical or physical method. Attempts to raise **anti-antibodies** also failed when specifically purified antibodies were used for immunization; the resulting anti-antibodies reacted with all gamma globulins, irrespective of their antibody specificity.

An era of very rapid progress began in the late 1950s when it was found that **Bence Jones proteins**, myeloma proteins, and normal gamma globulins share antigenic determinants. Two classes of globulins, **IgG** and **IgM** (formerly known as 7S and 19S molecules, respectively), were described. Bence Jones proteins, although of much lower molecular weight, were found to share antigenic determinants with both IgG and IgM molecules. In 1960 Heremans proposed the name **immunoglobulins** (Ig) for all these antigenically related proteins.

In 1956 Grubb and Oudin independently described intraspecies antigenic differences within classes of immunoglobulins in man and in the rabbit. Oudin created the term **allotypy** (Chapter 9) for this type of genetic polymorphism. Research conducted during the next 15 years by Dubiski, Dray, Kelus, Herzenberg, and others laid the foundations for this new branch of immunogenetics. At the same time, improvements in biochemical methods made it possible to study the structure of immunoglobulins. In 1959 Porter reported the splitting of immunoglobulins into three fragments that can be subsequently separated by chromatography. Two of these fragments (Fab) retain their antigen-binding capacity; the third (Fc) does not combine with antigen, is homogeneous, and crystallizes readily. This was the first significant step toward the elucidation of the structure of immunoglobulins. Porter's paper was quickly followed by other reports. The outcome of this unprecedented qualitative jump was the emergence, by 1962, of the classic four-chain model of the immunoglobulin molecule.

In spite of the rapid progress in understanding immunoglobulin structure and function, it was still not certain as to what determines the conformation of the antigen-combining site of antibody. In 1964 Haber showed that completely denatured antibody molecules can refold and regain their function without the intervention of the corresponding antigen. Haber's report removed any remaining doubt that the combining capacity of antibodies depends solely on the primary structure of their polypeptide chains. For this reason, determination of the amino acid sequence of antibody molecules (Section 6.5), or rather of their component chains, became the next major goal of molecular immunology. Owing to the heterogeneity of immunoglobulins, this task would have been next to impossible if not for the myeloma proteins. It had just been realized that these proteins can be regarded as monoclonal antibodies in terms of the clonal selection theory. These highly homogeneous proteins proved to be ideal for structural studies, since they were available in large quantities and could be easily purified. Manual, and later automated, sequencing of myeloma proteins interpreted by specially designed computer programs and aided by X-ray crystallography resulted in the elucidation of immunoglobulin structure and promoted the understanding of many aspects of immunoglobulin function and phylogeny and, to a large extent, genetic control of immunoglobulin formation. As more and more immunoglobulin sequence data were accumulated, it was realized that the variability of sequences is virtually infinite. The question next raised was whether this diversity was generated during evolution and is now encoded in the genome or whether it had to be reinvented by every individual during ontogeny. This fascinating problem can only now be approached with the help of recently developed DNA sequencing technology (Section 6.10).

The structural diversity of antibodies is reflected by the diversity of their antigenic determinants associated with antigen-combining properties. The term **idiotypy** (Chapter 10) was coined by Oudin in 1966 for this type of polymorphism. Research by Oudin, Kelus and Gell, and later by Nisonoff, who was the first to use inbred strains of mice in research on idiotypy, laid the foundation for the **idiotype network theory** proposed in 1974 by Jerne (Chapter 10).

BASIC STRUCTURE OF IMMUNOGLOBULINS

An IgG molecule is an example of the structural unit of all immunoglobulin molecules (Fig. 7.2**A**). It is composed of two pairs of polypeptide chains, **heavy** (H) and **light** (L), with molecular weights of 52,000 and 22,500, respectively. The four chains are held together by disulfide bonds as well as by noncovalent interactions. Electron microscope and X-ray crystallography studies show that the shape of the molecule resembles the letter Y. For historical reasons, the upper arms of the letter are called **Fab** (fragment antigen binding) portions, and the stem of the Y is the **Fc** (fragment crystalline) portion. An entire light chain and the amino terminal half of a heavy chain form each of the two Fab portions. The Fc portion is formed by the carboxy terminal halves of the two heavy chains. The antigen-combining site, a depression measuring approximately $3.4 \times 2.0 \times 0.7$ nm, is located at the tip of each Fab portion. Both the heavy and the light chain contribute to its formation. A longitudinal axis of symmetry divides the molecule into two identical halves, each consisting of one light and one heavy chain and each possessing an identical combining site.

The part of the molecule where the two Fab portions and the Fc portion are joined together is called the **hinge region**. Because of its primary structure, this part is extremely flexible; segmental flexibility between the Fab and Fc is essential for the function of the antibody molecule.

Comparison of the amino acid sequences of a large number of immunoglobulin (Ig) chains shows a number of regularities. The amino terminal sequences of L chains (half) and of H chains (one fourth or one fifth) vary markedly from one antibody to another. For these reasons, these parts of the Ig polypeptide chains are designated **variable** (V) regions. Sequences of the rest of the Ig chains are much less variable and are designated **constant** (C) regions. On the basis of the sequences of their constant regions, Ig chains can be classified into discrete groups. L chains exist in two different **types**: κ (kappa) and λ (lambda); among the H chains five **classes** are known to exist: γ (gamma), μ (mu), α (alpha), δ (delta), and ε (epsilon). The first three classes, γ, μ, and α are further divided into **subclasses**, which are designated by numerals, e.g., γ1.

Closer analysis of the H and L chains revealed the existence of a certain periodicity of amino acid sequences within their C regions. Each of the units, defined by such periodicity of sequence, is called a **domain** and consists of approximately 100 amino acid residues. Sequences of various domains show considerable homology with each other. Within C_γ, C_α, and C_δ, three domains can be distinguished; C_μ and C_ε each has one additional domain; C_L is composed of a single domain. Each V region is also a separate domain (Table 7.1). The sequences of immunoglobulin domains show considerable homology with the sequence of β_2 microglobulin (Chapter 18).

During comparison of variable sequences of many light and heavy chains, it was found that their variability is confined to certain "hot spots" called **hypervariable** (HV) regions. The remainder of the domain, called a **framework**, shows relatively little variability. Both heavy and light chains have three hypervariable regions. Hypervariable regions are confined to amino acid residues 24–37, 50–56, and 89–97 of the light chains and to residues 31–35, 51–68, and 84–110 of the heavy chains. Needless to say, hypervariable regions take part in shaping the antigen-combining site of an antibody.

Domains, chains, and immunoglobulin units are the building blocks of immunoglobulin

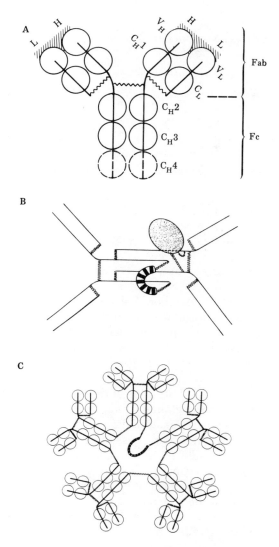

FIG. 7.2. Schematic models of immunoglobulin molecules. **(A)** Basic four-chain (L H)$_2$ unit (monomer of IgG, IgA, IgM, IgD, and IgE): **heavy lines** = longitudinal axes of polypeptide chains; **circles** = domains; **broken line circles** = C$_H$4 domains present only in μ and ε chains; **wavy line** = interchain disulfide bond(s); intrachain bonds are not shown; **shaded area** = antigen-combining site. **(B)** Secreted molecule of IgA dimer. Heavy and light chains are represented as **lines**; domains are not shown; the J chain is represented as a **C-shaped structure**; the secretory component is shown as an **oval structure**; the drawings do not represent the real shapes of these components. Note the presence and localization of disulfide bonds (**wavy lines**). **(C)** Pentameric molecule of IgM. Note the presence of the J chain and the disulfide bonds (**wavy lines**) that connect the units. The presence of the second set of disulfide bonds between C$_H$3 domains (not shown) is controversial.

TABLE 7.1. Nomenclature of Immunoglobulin Domains

Chain	Regions & domains
Light	V_L; C_L (C_κ, C_λ)
Heavy	V_H; C_H1: $C_\gamma1$, $C_\gamma2$, $C_\gamma3$
	$C_\mu1$, $C_\mu2$, $C_\mu3$, $C_\mu4$
	$C_\alpha1$, $C_\alpha2$, $C_\alpha3$
	$C_\delta1$, $C_\delta2$, $C_\delta3$
	$C_\varepsilon1$, $C_\varepsilon2$, $C_\varepsilon3$, $C_\varepsilon4$

molecules (Table 7.2). The class or subclass of the heavy chain determines the class or subclass of the immunoglobulin molecule: γ heavy chains participate in the formation of IgG molecules, α in **IgA**, μ in IgM, δ in **IgD**, and ε in **IgE** formation. Each class has two types of molecules, containing either two κ or two λ light chains but never one of each. IgG, IgD, and IgE are monomeric molecules, consisting of only one basic four-chain; IgM molecules are pentamers (Fig. 7.2**C**); and IgA immunoglobulins are either monomers or dimers. Disulfide bonds hold the chains of the monomer molecule together. Polymeric immunoglobulins contain an additional component, a **J chain,** * which is linked with the rest of the molecule by means of disulfide bonds. IgA can exist in two forms: **serum IgA** and **secretory IgA**. The secretory form is a dimer associated with an additional polypeptide chain, the **secretory component**, which is synthesized by epithelial cells and added to the IgA molecule during its passage through the mucous membrane (Fig. 7.2**B** and Table 7.2).

The domains are tightly folded portions of the polypeptide chain; their structure and the overall configuration of the immunoglobulin molecule are maintained by a number of intra-domain, interdomain, and interchain disulfide bonds. The number and location of these bonds vary with class and type and will not be discussed here.

Fragments of immunoglobulin molecules can be obtained by cleavage with proteolytic enzymes and other agents, e.g., cyanogen bromide (CNBr). Invariably, the cleavage occurs between the domains. By using appropriate cleaving agents and conditions, almost every domain or group of domains can be isolated.

IMMUNOGLOBULINS AS ANTIGENS

Differences in amino acid sequences between immunoglobulin classes or types determine the antigenic specificities or determinant(s) of immunoglobulins. Antisera, specific for a given class or type of immunoglobulin molecule, can be raised when the molecule is injected into an individual who lacks this particular determinant. Immunoglobulin molecules carry three categories of antigenic determinants: **isotypic**, **allotypic**, and **idiotypic**.

Isotypic determinants reflect differences between the various classes and types of immunoglobulin polypeptide chains within a given species. Since every normal individual possesses all the classes and types characteristic for its species, antisera directed against

---

*This J chain is the product of a separate gene and should not be confused with the J region of each light and heavy chain gene (Chapter 8).

TABLE 7.2. Human Immunoglobulin Classes—Their Composition and Function

Immunoglobulin Class	Heavy Chain Class or Subclass[a]	Number of Basic Units	Approximate Molecular Weight $\times 10^{-3}$	Carbohydrate Content (percent)	Mean Serum Content (mg/ml)	Main Function
IgG	$\gamma 1$ $\gamma 2$ $\gamma 3$ $\gamma 4$	Monomer	145	2.5	12	Humoral antibody
IgM	μ	Monomer	190(?)	?	—	Cell surface receptor;
		Pentamer[b]	900	5–10	1	Natural antibody; early humoral response
IgA	$\alpha 1$ $\alpha 2$	Monomer	160	5–10	2	Serum antibody;
		Dimer[b]	300		—	Antibody in
		Dimer[c]	—	—	—	external secretions
IgD	δ	Monomer	180	10	.03	Cell surface receptor
IgE	ε	Monomer	190	12	.0003	Immunity to parasites; fixing to mast cells; mediating allergic reactions

[a]Each heavy chain class or subclass can occur with κ or λ light chain type.
[b]Contains one J chain per polymeric molecule.
[c]Contains one J chain and one secretory component per polymeric molecule.

isotypic determinants can only be raised by **heteroimmunization**, i.e., by injection of material from one species into an animal belonging to another species. Only exceptionally will isotypic antibodies be formed as a result of immunization within a species. Individuals with an IgA deficiency are not only unable to synthesize IgA but also do not recognize IgA as "self." Blood transfusion or attempts to reconstitute these individuals with normal plasma usually result in formation of antibodies directed against IgA isotypic determinants.

Allotypic determinants reflect the genetic polymorphism of immunoglobulins within one immunoglobulin class and within one species (Section 9.1). Thus, individuals of a given species possess a given immunoglobulin class that either does or does not carry a certain allotypic determinant. The best way to raise antibodies directed against allotypic determinants is

alloimmunization, i.e., immunization in which both the donor and the recipient of the immunizing material belong to the same species but possess different allotypic determinants. Antibodies to allotypic determinants are also formed as a result of heteroimmunization, but the predominant antibodies formed in this situation are directed against isotypic determinants. To reveal the allotypic antibodies in heteroimmune sera, antibodies to isotypic determinants have to be removed by absorption. During this process, the allotypic antibodies may also be lost, particularly when their initial concentration is low or when a cross-reaction occurs between these antibodies and structurally related determinants. In spite of these limitations, some antiallotype immune sera of heterologous origin are being successfully prepared and used for characterization of some human and murine allotypes and have also been raised against some rabbit allotypes.

Idiotypic determinants reflect antigenic differences related to the configuration of the antigen-combining sites of antibody molecules (see Chapter 10). This does not mean, however, that antibodies of the same specificity must have the same idiotypic determinant. Even if a relatively simple molecule, having only one or very few antigenic determinants, is used for immunization, numerous cell clones are usually activated. Products of different clones will have different idiotypes, even if their antigen-combining specificities are similar. Only products of the same clone will be identical, both in terms of their amino acid sequences and idiotypes.

Antibodies directed against idiotypic determinants can best be elicited by immunization within the species. Preferably, all allotypic determinants of the immunogen donor and the immunized animal should be matched, so that no antiallotype antibodies can be formed. However, heteroimmunization is also a practical method of raising anti-idiotypic antibodies, especially those directed against human or murine myeloma proteins.

Allotypic and idiotypic determinants are, as a rule, very weak immunogens; their immunogenicity is considerably increased if they are allowed to form complexes with the antigen against which the antibodies carrying these determinants are directed. A low degree of aggregation of immunoglobulin molecules—e.g., by treatment with glutaraldehyde—has a similar effect.

FUNCTION OF IMMUNOGLOBULINS

Each immunoglobulin class performs two separate functions that are carried out by distinct regions of the antibody molecule. The first function, specific binding of antigen, is executed by the two combining sites. These sites are located on the tips of the Fab portions of the molecule and are formed cooperatively by the hypervariable regions of heavy and light chains. An antibody molecule that has combined with antigen can now exert its other biological functions. These functions are carried out by the Fc portion of the molecule. Fc domains of immune complexes acquire the ability to combine with the C1q component of complement and with various cellular receptors (Table 7.3). Some functions of the Fc domains (e.g., interaction with trophoblast or mast cell receptors or control of the catabolic rate) do not require activation.

TABLE 7.3. Functions of IgG Domains

Function	Domains Involved
Antigen binding	$V_H + V_L$
Subunit interaction	
H-L	$V_H + V_L, C_\gamma1 + C_L$
H-H	$C_\gamma3$
Complement (C1q) binding	$C_\gamma2$
Interaction with cellular receptors of:	
Macrophages	$C_\gamma3$
Neutrophils	$C_\gamma2 + C_\gamma3$
K cells	$C_\gamma2 + C_\gamma3$
Trophoblasts	$C_\gamma2 + C_\gamma3$
Control of catabolic rate	$C_\gamma2$

PHYLOGENY OF IMMUNOGLOBULINS

7.3 Humoral Immunity in Invertebrates

The sequence homologies between immunoglobulin domains suggest that both heavy and light chains might have evolved from a common ancestor, a **protoantibody** molecule equal in size to the currently envisioned domain. Should efforts that are aimed at elucidation of the phylogeny of immunoglobulins concentrate on the search for such primitive antibody molecules? Combining sites of the present-day antibody molecules are formed in cooperation between light and heavy chains; the capacity to bind antigen disappears almost completely when the chains are separated. It is difficult to imagine that the affinities of the hypothetical protoantibody molecules could have been much higher than those of the separated contemporary heavy or light chains. Molecules of such low affinities could not contribute significantly enough to the body defense mechanisms to warrant their preservation in evolution. However, a large number of low affinity molecules acting together as receptors on the surface of a primitive immunocyte would enable the cell to bind antigen with reasonable avidity. Only after their efficiency was considerably improved by natural selection could antibody molecules function in the circulation. Therefore, a priori we can expect that even the first antibody molecules to be found in the circulation would be reasonably efficient in binding antigen and that the **primordial antibody** molecule most likely would be found on the cell membrane rather than in the circulation.

There is no clear-cut evidence for the presence of humoral antibody molecules in **invertebrates**. However, even such primitive animals as sponges possess an efficient self-recognition system. **Annelides** (earthworms) recognize "nonself" and reject xenografts from related species and some allografts from individuals of the same species that belong to geographically distant races. The rejection is clearly a cellular phenomenon and involves free-moving **coelomocytes**.

Agglutinating and opsonizing substances have been found in the hemolymph of the horseshoe crab (*Limulus polyphemus*), in an echinoderm (*Asterias forbesii*), in the spiny lobster, and in some mollusks. There is no evidence that these substances are structurally related to vertebrate immunoglobulins. "Agglutinin" from the horseshoe crab has been studied in considerable detail. The molecule is a large (400,000 molecular weight) polymer composed of 18 subunits. It is a cylindrical toroid, which looks like a stack of donuts, each donut composed of six subunits. Only noncovalent bonds are involved in the formation of toroids. Agglutinin molecules from other species mentioned above are probably very similar.

7.4 Immunoglobulins of Vertebrates

All existing vertebrate species, including the primitive lampreys and hagfishes, seem to be able to form circulating antibodies in response to stimulation with a variety of antigens (Fig. 7.3). Antibodies raised in lampreys have been isolated and studied in considerable detail. They are composed of light and heavy chains; the molecules are polymeric, have a sedimentation coefficient of 14S, and can be dissociated, without reduction, into subunits. Each subunit has a sedimentation coefficient of 6.6S and consists of two heavy and two light chains. The homology with human IgM is remarkable: judged by amino acid composition, lamprey antibody and human IgM are more closely related than lamprey and human hemoglobins.

Lamprey serum also contains another protein molecule that, to some extent, resembles the natural agglutinin of the horseshoe crab. It thus appears that Cyclostomata, which form a phylogenetic bridge between prevertebrates and vertebrates, share some of the immunologic characteristics of both.

An important achievement of the true vertebrates is the acquisition of the disulfide bonds in their immunoglobulins. IgM-like immunoglobulins of all vertebrate species are held together by covalent bonds and form tetramers, pentamers, or even hexamers (Fig. 7.3). Why different vertebrate groups favor different polymers is not known. The polymerization seems to involve the J chains. Characterization of these prototype J chains may shed some light on the mechanism of polymerization. Whatever the mechanism of polymerization, immunoglobulins of early vertebrates are predominantly polymeric. Monomers appeared in the circulation later during evolution, probably as a consequence of improvements in the design of the combining sites, when antibodies developed affinity sufficiently high to make multiple binding sites unnecessary for strong combining with antigen. Monomeric antibodies first appear in sharks, but they are of the same class as the polymers. These monomeric antibodies, perhaps being the first secretory immunoglobulins, are also found in body fluids other than blood.

The lungfish can be credited with the "invention" of a new immunoglobulin class. Besides pentameric IgM antibodies, the lungfish makes monomeric molecules, the heavy chains of which are distinct not only from μ but also from γ. This new class has been tentatively called **IgN**. IgN molecules are formed by amphibians, reptilians and birds and possibly also by some mammals. IgG antibodies are first found in anuran amphibians. The kinetics of antibody response in amphibians closely resembles that of mammals: IgM antibodies are formed early in the immune response and are subsequently replaced by IgG antibodies, which are formed later. Another immunoglobulin class, tentatively called **IgY**, is found in reptilians and in birds.

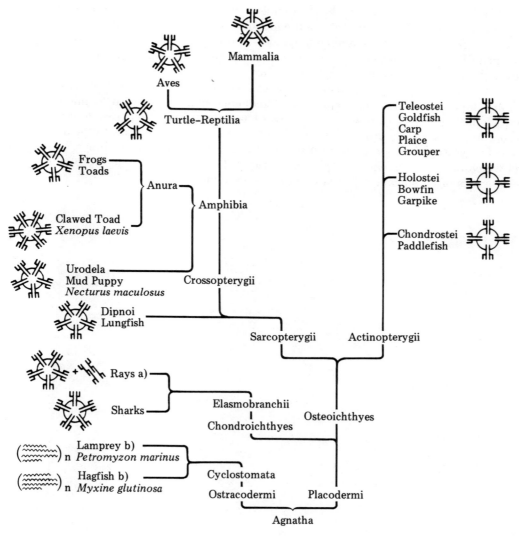

FIG. 7.3. Evolutionary tree of IgM immunoglobulins. For discussion of evolution of other immunoglobulin classes, see text. The figure shows phylogenetic relations between various vertebrate groups and the form of the prevalent circulatory IgM-like molecules in each of these groups. (**a**) In *Dasyatis centrura* the prevalent form of IgM-like molecules is a dimer; in *D. americana*, the IgM is pentameric. (**b**) Immunoglobulins of *Petromyzon marinus* are polymers of units composed of two heavy and two light chains. The number of units in a polymeric molecule has not been determined. No disulfide bonds are present in this species. (Modified from: Marchalonis, J. J. (ed.), *Comparative Immunology*. Blackwell Scientific Publications, Oxford, 1976, p. 248, used with permission.)

The above is only a very brief summary of the subject of immunoglobulin evolution. Present knowledge of the phylogeny of the immune system is far from being complete; evolution of the antigen-combining site and complement-binding sites, the presence and role of J chains, and the occurrence of antibodylike receptors on the cell surface are the most fruitful, but by no means the easiest, directions for future studies.

The immune system and its evolution can be considered in a much wider context: human immunoglobulin domains show amino acid sequence homologies with β_2 microglobulin, with haptoglobin, and with two so-called **acute-phase proteins**, C-reactive protein and α_1 acid glycoprotein. C-reactive protein, in turn, bears a number of similarities to the agglutinin of the horseshoe crab and to some serum proteins that occur naturally in lampreys, sharks, and eels and which bind some mono- and polysaccharides. Thus, the acute-phase proteins of man may be the relics of an ancient "alternate" humoral immune system.

8 / *Structure of the Immunoglobulin Genes*

A genetic analysis of immunoglobulin allotypes (Section 9.4) has identified a minimum number of genes determining the constant regions of light and heavy chains. In mice there is a single C_κ gene for the constant region of the κ light chains and as many as four C_λ genes for the constant region of λ light chains. Furthermore, single genes determine the constant regions of the μ, α, ε, γ_1, γ_{2b}, γ_{2a}, γ_3 and δ heavy chains. Six of these genes display a certain degree of polymorphism. Amino acid sequence analyses of the constant regions of both heavy and light chains have confirmed the genetic observations that there are relatively few (13) genes that determine constant regions. These genes belong to three linkage groups (families): λ, κ, and H; and in mice the genes are called *Igl-C*, *Igk-C*, and *Igh-C*, respectively (Section 9.7)., and are assigned to chromosomes 16, 6, and 12.

In contrast to these data, amino acid sequence analysis of a large number of variable regions, from either heavy (V_H) or light (V_L) chains, revealed that there are numerous V_H and V_L genes. Such an analysis of more than 20 murine λ chains showed that they can be assigned to two families of related sequences. Murine κ chain sequences can be divided into more than 30 such families of closely related sequences. A similar situation was observed for V_H amino acid sequences. Therefore, there may be a minimum of 2 V_λ, 30 V_κ, and 30 V_H genes in the murine genome. However, since these data are derived from the amino acid sequences of a relatively small number of immunoglobulins, they may have identified only a small fraction of the entire repertoire of V_L and V_H genes. All V genes are linked with corresponding C genes and in mice are referred to as *Igl-V*, *Igk-V*, and *Igh-V*, respectively (Section 9.7). Although this chapter discusses murine *Ig* genes, most of the basic information applies to various other animal species. With this in mind, a general and noncommittal nomenclature—V_L(V_λ and V_κ), C_L(C_λ and C_κ), V_H, and C_H (C_μ, C_α, etc.)—will be used in preference to specific nomenclature (Section 9.7).

These facts bring to mind several basic questions that must be answered to arrive at a full understanding of the genetic determination of the structure of the immunoglobulins. The most fundamental questions are: How can the gene products of multiple variable region genes be linked to the product of a single constant region gene? How does the immature B lymphocyte choose only a single V_H gene and a single V_L gene? How does the cell exclude expression of the other allele and of the other genes? How does the plasma cell switch from the production of one class of heavy chain to another? Finally how does the enormous degree of antigenic-binding diversity in one individual result from the limited number of antibody genes?

In this chapter, a portion of the veritable explosion of information on the structure of the immunoglobulin light and heavy chain genes will be presented. This information has been obtained using induced tumors of plasma cells, **plasmacytomas**, which secrete a single class of immunoglobulin molecule (myeloma protein), or a monoclonal antibody (Section 4.9 and 7.2). These cell lines provide a rich source of protein for amino acid sequence analysis and also provide a large supply of mRNA and DNA for studies on the structure and expression of immunoglobulin genes. In addition, recombinant DNA techniques have allowed the isolation of both **germ line** and plasmacytoma forms of the immunoglobulin genes (Section 6.9). Germ line DNA refers to the completely unrearranged DNA found in germ cells (spermatozoa or ova). In contrast, the embryonic DNA found in cells after fertilization may be partially rearranged, whereas the DNA of plasmacytoma cells that actively produce an immunoglobulin, by definition, has to be fully rearranged (see below). Application of rapid DNA sequencing techniques has permitted a detailed structural analysis of these genes (Section 6.10). The information gathered so far, although incomplete, creates a reasonable basis for an attempt to answer the crucial questions posed in the preceding paragraph. The discussion of specific genes should be facilitated by a brief outline of the ontogenesis of immunoglobulin-secreting cells.

ONTOGENESIS OF B CELLS

Two stages can be distinguished during the development of cells that secrete immunoglobulins (Fig. 8.1). In an antigen-independent stage, the immature B lymphocyte differentiates from a stem cell and develops the capacity to synthesize a light chain of either the λ or κ type and a μ heavy chain. The light chain and the heavy chain each possesses one of the many possible variable regions linked to the constant region. The light and heavy chains join to form a membrane-bound type of immunoglobulin M, **mIgM**,* which serves as a cell surface receptor for binding an antigen. An additional cell surface antigen-binding receptor, **mIgD**, is coexpressed on the majority of B lymphocytes that bear mIgM molecules.

During the early development of the B lymphocyte, only one V_L and one V_H gene are selected for expression. In addition, only one allele for the constant region of each chain is expressed, while the other alleles are excluded (Section 9.22).

The second, antigen-dependent stage of differentiation begins after stimulation of mature B cells by an antigen that binds to the mIgM or mIgD receptor. Morphologically, cell proliferation results in an expansion of the stimulated clone and differentiation into immunoglobulin-secreting plasma cells. At this time, the production of membrane-bound mIgM ceases and synthesis of a soluble **sIgM** begins. Subsequently, sIgM is secreted and along with the J chain forms the pentameric sIgM found in serum. During further differentiation of the B cell (Fig. 8.2), the variable (V_H) region found in the sIgM is switched to a constant region of a different class of heavy chain. Thus, production of sIgM or sIgD is replaced by production of a different class of immunoglobulin, e.g., IgG, IgA, or IgE still bearing the same V region and, thus, displaying the same antigen-binding specificity. This change in synthesis from IgM to another immunoglobulin class is called the **heavy chain switch**.

LIGHT CHAIN GENES

The structure of the λ type of light chain genes was the first to be studied in detail and seems to be the simplest of all immunoglobulin genes. Most of the principles of immunoglobulin gene structure and rearrangement can be illustrated employing the example of C_λ and V_λ genes.

8.1 Genes for the λ Light Chain

In each λ chain, the variable (V) region comprises the amino terminal 110 amino acids, and the constant (C) region comprises the carboxyl terminal 110 amino acids. Protein sequence data for

---

*Other authors use the designation sIgM for surface immunoglobulin and plain IgM for serum immunoglobulin.

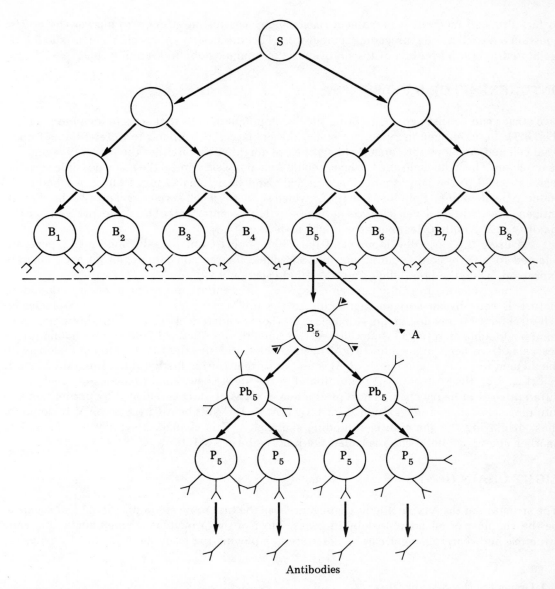

FIG. 8.1. Antigen-independent differentiation of B cells from stem cell (**S**) and antigen-dependent differentiation of specific clone(s) of plasma blasts (**Pb**) and plasma cells (**P**) that secrete antibodies. Antigen (**A**)-specific receptors are indicated by various structures on the surface of B cells.

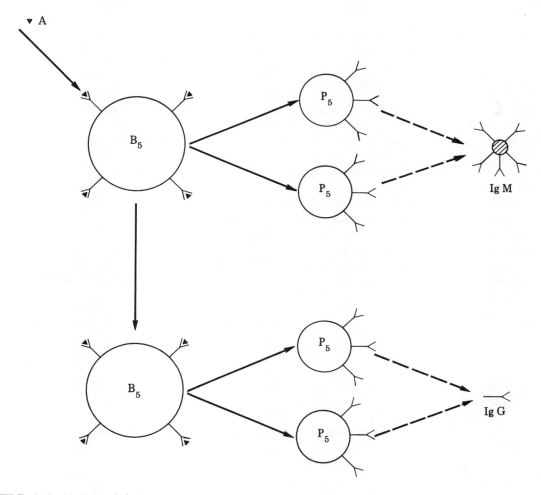

FIG. 8.2. Antigen (**A**)-dependent differentiation of a B cell (**B**) from Fig. 8.1 that initially results in the development of plasma cells (**P**) that secrete sIgM. Subsequently, owing to the heavy chain switch, plasma cells (**P**) that secrete IgG develop.

more than 20 different λ chains reveal that there are 4 subtypes of λ chains distinguishable by their unique constant region sequences. There are also two different variable region sequences with defined hypervariable subsequences.

Initial RNA/DNA hybridization studies demonstrated that in germ line DNA there are only a few C_λ genes. This fact eliminated from consideration for immunoglobulin gene structure an early model that required one gene for each different light or heavy chain synthesized. According to this model, the 20 different sequences of λ chains would require an equal number of genes. More recent analysis by hybridization to DNA cleaved with restriction endonucleases, using the Southern transfer method, demonstrated that cell lines that secrete immunoglobulins possess light and heavy chain genes that are rearranged from the germ line gene configuration. This observation indicates that, in cells secreting immunoglobulins, a single C_λ and C_H gene may be linked to any of a number of V_λ and V_H genes, respectively.

Genes for a murine λ light chain were isolated from embryonic DNA and from a λ-secreting plasmacytoma. A physical map of both the germ line and rearranged gene was constructed and their complete DNA sequence determined (Fig. 8.3). From a comparison of the amino acid sequence with the DNA sequence, several remarkable facts about the genes for the λ light chain were deduced. In the germ line DNA, the two genes for λ chains, the V_λ and C_λ, are separated by an undetermined distance. The V_λ gene has a leader (L_λ) region in which the N terminal hydrophobic segment of the λ chain, consisting of 19 amino acids, is encoded. It is proposed that the leader segment permits secretion of the λ light chain. The exon that encodes the leader segment permits secretion of the λ light chain. The exon that encodes the leader is separated from the exon determining variable region by a 93 base intervening sequence I_1. The variable region exon codes for amino acid -4 ($+1$ is the N terminal amino acid found in the mature λ light chain) through $+97$. The region that encodes amino acids 98–109 is separated from the C_λ gene determining the constant region by a intervening sequence, I_2, which is about 1,250 bases long. The DNA sequence that encodes amino acids 90–109 is the site at which the rearranged gene the V_λ gene is joined to the C_λ gene. This sequence is called the J_λ region. Finally, the C_λ gene codes for amino acids 110 to the C terminus.

Further analysis of protein sequences and DNA clones has led to the identification of two V_λ genes and four sets of J_λ–C_λ genes. Their arrangement on the chromosome is:

$$\cdots\cdots V_{\lambda I} \cdots\cdot [J_{\lambda 3}-C_{\lambda 3}] \cdots [J_{\lambda 1}-C_{\lambda 1}] \cdots\cdot V_{\lambda II} \cdots\cdot [J_{\lambda 2}-C_{\lambda 2}] \cdots [J_{\lambda 4}-C_{\lambda 4}] \cdots\cdot$$

The $V_{\lambda I}$ gene has been shown to rearrange preferentially at the $J_{\lambda I}$–$C_{\lambda I}$ set, but a recombinant between $V_{\lambda i}$ and $J_{\lambda 3}$–$C_{\lambda 3}$ has been identified. In addition, $V_{\lambda II}$ has been shown to rearrange at the $J_{\lambda 2}$–$C_{\lambda 2}$ set only.

The expression of the rearranged gene for the λ chain (Fig. 8.4) involves its transcription into a large preRNA, which is then processed by RNA splicing and RNA modification reactions to form the mature mRNA. The mRNA is then translated, and the hydrophobic segment L_λ is removed as the polypeptide chain is transported into endoplasmic reticulum.

FIG. 8.3. Amino acid sequence of a λ chain and nucleotide sequence of a murine λ gene deduced from the DNA sequence analysis of the unrearranged V_λ and C_λ genes and the rearranged V_λ gene: L_λ = the exon that encodes hydrophobic leader sequence; V_λ = the exon for variable region; J_λ = the exon for the joining site of V_λ and C_λ regions; C_λ = the exon that encodes constant region; I_1 and I_2 = introns; **HV1**, **HV2**, and **HV3** = hypervariable regions. (Modified from Bernard et al. Sequences of mouse immunoglobulin light chain genes before and after somatic changes. Cell **15**:1133–1144, 1978. Used with permission.)

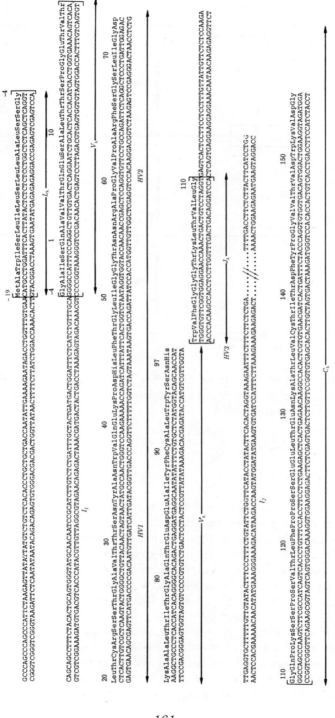

161

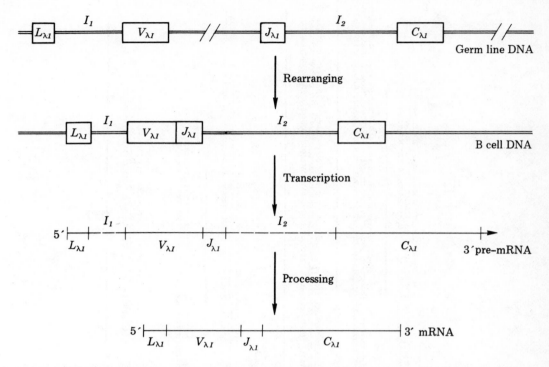

FIG. 8.4. Rearrangement of the murine germ line λ chain genes during differentiation from a stem cell. The rearrangement is followed by transcription and processing that produce the mature mRNA.

8.2 Genes for the κ Light Chain

In mice about 95 percent of the light chains produced belong to the κ type. Partial and complete amino acid sequence data revealed that there are about 30 different sequences of amino acids 1–97 of the V_κ region. In addition, four distinct sequences could be distinguished between amino acids 98–110. Only a single C_κ region sequence was found. In light of our knowledge of the λ light chain gene structure, the amino acid sequence data suggest that the family of genes determining the κ chain consists of at least 30 V_κ genes corresponding to the subtypes, 4 or more J_κ gene segments, and a single C_κ gene. Indeed, nucleic acid hybridization data demonstrated that there is a single C_κ gene.

Since four to six related V_κ genes can be identified for each V_κ probe employed in hybridization experiments, there may be as many as 100–200 V_κ genes in germ line DNA. Recombinant DNA technology has permitted the isolation of several clones that contain germ line V_k, J_κ, and C_κ sequences as well as the isolation of the active rearranged form of the gene from plasmacytoma cell lines. Nucleotide sequence analysis of the cloned V_κ genes demonstrates that each

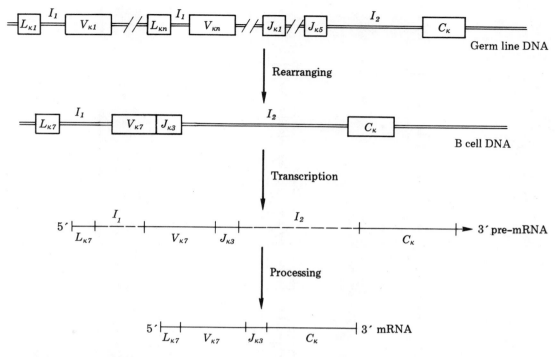

FIG. 8.5. Rearrangement of the murine germ line κ chain genes during differentiation from a stem cell to a B cell. The rearrangement is followed by transcription and processing that yield the mature mRNA. Arbitrarily, the selected gene is shown to consist of a particular combination of *L*, *V*, and *J* sequences.

gene consists of a L_κ portion encoding the hydrophobic leader peptide, which is separated from the V_κ gene by an intervening sequence I_1. The V_k gene encodes amino acids -4 to $+97$ of the V_κ region. At an unknown distance from the V_κ genes, there is a set of five J_κ segments of which only four appear to be functional. The J_κ sequence closest to the C_κ gene is separated by the intervening sequence, I_2, about 2,400 base pairs long.

In contrast to the λ chain in which the number of combinations of V_λ and C_λ regions is highly restricted since there is only one V_λ gene per two C_λ genes, in the κ chain case, there is a large potential for random generation of diversity. If there are 200 different V_κ genes and 5 J_κ sequences, up to 1,000 different κ chains could potentially be generated.

HEAVY CHAIN GENES

At least eight classes and subclasses of immunoglobulins can be identified in mice on the basis of the different amino acid sequences of the constant regions of their heavy chains μ, δ, γ1, γ2a,

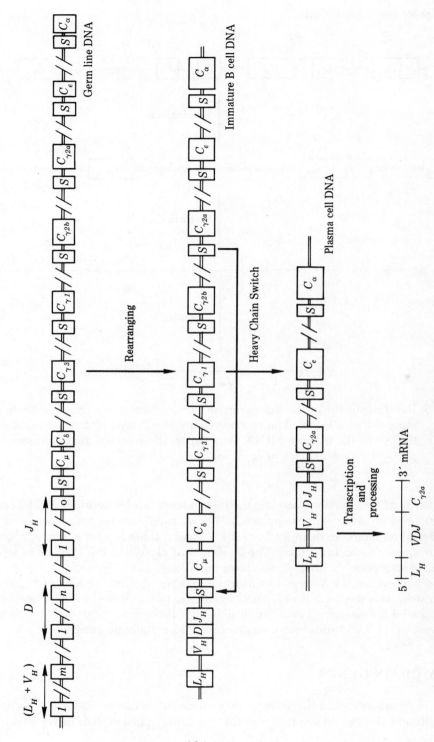

FIG. 8.6. Family of heavy chain genes in germ line DNA, in an immature B cell that expresses mIgM, and in a plasma cell secreting IgG2a immunoglobulin.

TABLE 8.1. Highly Preserved Hepta- and Decanucleotides (italicized) Found in the Vicinity of *V* and *J* Genes and Separated by Nonhomolgous Sequences of 10–23 Nucleotides

Gene	Preserved	Nonhomologous	Preserved
V	*CACAGTG*	ATACAAATCAT	*AACATAAACC*
	CACAGTG	ATTCAAGCCAT	*GACATAAACC*
	CACAGTG	ATTCAAGCCAT	*GACATAAACC*
	CACAGTG	CTCAGGGCTG	*AACAAAAACC*
	CACAGTG	AGAGGACGTCATTGTGAGCCCA	*GACACAAACC*
	CACAATG	ACATGTGTAGATGGGGAAGTAG	*ATCAAGAACA*
J	*GGTTTTTGTA*	GAGAGGGGCATGTCATAGTCCT	*CACTGTG*
	GGTTTTTGTA	AAGGGGGGCGCAGTGATATGAAT	*CACTGTG*
	GGGTTTTGTG	GAGGTAAAGTTAAAATAAAT	*CACTGTA*
	AGTTTTTGTA	TGGGGGTTGAGTGAAGGGACAC	*CAGTGTG*
	GGTTTTTGTA	CAGCCAGACAGTGGAGTACTAC	*CACTGTG*
	AGTTTTAGTA	TAGGAACAGAGGCAGAACAGA	*GACTGTG*
	GGTTTTTGTA	CACCCACTAAAGGGGTCTATGA	*TAGTGTG*
	GGTTTTTGCA	TGAGTCTATAT	*CACAGTG*

SOURCE: Early, P., et al. An immunoglobulin heavy chain variable region gene is generated from three segments of DNA: V_H, D, and J_H. Cell **19**: 981–992, 1980, used with permission.

$\gamma 2b$, $\gamma 3$, α, and ε. The constant regions of class-specific heavy chains display a high degree of amino acid sequence homology with each other. Three or four homology units, or domains, of about 110 amino acids can be distinguished within the constant region of each class or subclass. Amino acid sequence analysis of the variable region of many heavy chains has revealed that, similar to V_κ, there are multiple V_H regions that are associated with four distinct J_H sequences.

Each cell contains one C_H gene for each class or subclass. The structure of the linkage group of heavy chain genes and the rearrangements that occur during B lymphocyte development are shown in Fig. 8.6. Several genes for heavy chains have been isolated from germ line DNA and from plasmacytoma DNA by recombinant DNA technology. Each of the multiple V_H genes possesses a leader sequence (L_H) that codes for hydrophobic amino acids −19 through −5. The leader sequence is separated from the V_H sequence by an intervening sequence I_1. The V_H DNA codes for amino acids −4 to +97 at which point the coding portion ends. The heavy chain genes possess four J_H sequences, two of which are shown in Fig. 8.6. In contrast to the light chain genes, DNA sequence studies showed that V_H is not directly joined to J_H (Fig. 8.6). There is an additional segment of DNA, called *D* for diversity, which in germ line DNA is present in about 10 copies. Thus, DNA rearrangement of the heavy chain genes requires two steps and generates a *VDJ* sequence. The J_H region is separated from the C_H gene by an intervening sequence I_2. The C_H genes are arranged on the chromosome in the following order: C_μ, C_δ, $C_{\gamma 3}$, $C_{\gamma 1}$, $C_{\gamma 2b}$, $C_{\gamma 2a}$, C_ε, and C_α. The structure of these genes is similar, but it may be noteworthy that the hinge regions of Cδ, Cγ, and Cα chains are encoded by separate exons.

Analysis of the DNA sequence in the vicinity of several V_L and V_H genes and the J_L and J_H segments shows a remarkable conservation of hepta- and decanucleotides (Table 8.1). These are separated by a 10–11 or 21–23 base pair nonhomologous stretch of nucleotides. Presumably,

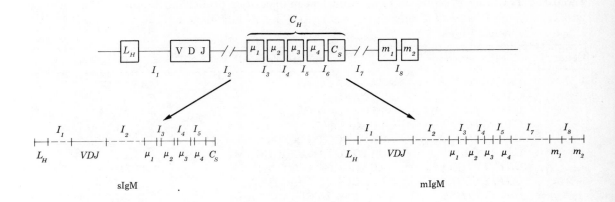

FIG. 8.7. Rearranged μ chain gene consisting of sequences for leader (**L$_H$**), variable (**V**), diversity (**D**), joining (**J**), constant domains (**C$_{H\mu}$1-C$_{hm}$4**), secreted terminus (**C$_s$**) and hydrophobic membrane-anchoring sequences (**C$_{m1}$** and **C$_{m2}$**) is drawn. The pre RNA is processed to yield mRNA either for sIgM containing C$_s$ but lacking C$_m$ sequence or for mIgM containing C$_m$ but missing the C$_s$ sequence. (Modified from: Early, P., et al. Two mRNAs can be produced from a single immunoglobulin μ gene by alternative RNA processing pathways. Cell **20**: 313–319, 1980. Used with permission.)

similar sequences are found in the vicinity of *D* regions of the heavy chain genes. An appealing model for recombination between *V* and *J* regions proposes that these sequences serve as recognition sites for specific proteins that bind to these sequences and cut and splice the corresponding segments of the DNA in a precise order. The model could be operative in rearrangement of both the heavy and light chain genes.

8.3 Structure and Expression of Genes for the μ Chain

Physical mapping and nucleotide sequence analysis of the C_μ gene have revealed several interesting features. The C_μ chain can be divided into four domains based upon amino acid sequence analysis. R-loop mapping of cloned germ line DNA for C_μ with mRNA for the μ chain revealed that the C_μ region of the DNA is divided into four coding domains (about 330 bases in length), each separated by a short intervening sequence (100 to 300 bases). Each coding domain in the C_μ gene corresponds to a homology unit of the constant region within the μ heavy chain. This observation is also true for other C_H genes.

As mentioned above, IgM is initially formed as a monomeric membrane-bound receptor, mIgM. After antigen stimulation, a soluble form, sIgM, is synthesized and secreted as a pentamer held together by J chains. Amino acid sequence analysis of μ_m and μ_s reveals that they are identical through the fourth domain (C$_H$4). Beyond this point μ_s has a stretch of 21 amino acids at the carboxyl terminus. This sequence of amino acids (C_s) is encoded in the DNA adjacent to the C_H4 region. The μ_m instead has a sequence of 41 hydrophobic amino acids at the carboxyl terminus (C_m). This sequence is encoded in two blocks of DNA separated from the coding sequence of the C_H4 by an intervening sequence of 1,600 bases (Fig. 8.7). The two different chains, μ_s and μ_m, are synthesized from two different mRNA molecules that are derived from a common preRNA via alternate RNA processing pathways. Therefore, one important signal regulating the expression of the gene determining IgM is mediated by modulation of the splicing pattern of mRNA for the μ chain. A similar C_m segment is also found in membrane-bound mIgD.

8.4 Heavy Chain Switch

As mentioned above, in addition to the conversion from μ_m to μ_s, a given V_H region may be switched to one or possibly more different C_H regions. This occurs by at least two mechanisms.

During the course of maturation of most B cells, the two membrane-bound immuno-globulins, mIgM and mIgD, can be simultaneously expressed. This simultaneous synthesis of both μ_m and δ_m chains is believed to be accomplished by alternative processing of a single large precursor mRNA that contains transcript of both the C_μ and the C_δ regions of the chromosome.

The antigen-dependent switch of the heavy chain variable region, V_H, from C_μ to another C_H region requires a different type of mechanism. Hybridization studies demonstrated that the C_μ gene is deleted in cell lines after switching to a C_H gene of another class. Further analysis showed that for cell lines expressing one C_H class, the genes located between the J_H region and the C_H gene being expressed are deleted. These data have led to a model for the heavy chain switch, which requires an additional DNA rearrangement in the C_H gene region and a deletion of a segment of DNA. Nucleotide sequence analysis of DNA on the 5' sides of the C_μ gene and of the $C_{\gamma1}$, $C_{\gamma2b}$, $C_{\gamma3}$, and C_α genes has revealed a series of homologous, tandemly repeated sequences. These sequences have been shown to be the sites of the recombination event responsible for the heavy chain switch and are referred to as **switch (S) sequences**. It is believed that during plasma cell differentiation a unique set of proteins must recognize these DNA sequences and perform the recombination event. This model accounts for both the specificity of the switch event and the loss of intervening DNA during the process (Fig. 8.6).

8.5 Allelic Exclusion

In immunoglobulin-producing cells or plasma cells, only one member of each pair of alleles is involved in the synthesis of the immunoglobulin being expressed. In other words, correct rearrangement of only one chromosome is needed for the generation of each expressed light or heavy chain gene.

Structural analyses of germ line and plasmacytoma DNA showed that in some cases, indeed, only one chromosome is rearranged, while in other cases both homologous chromosomes undergo rearrangements, but alleles from only one chromosome are expressed. In the case where only one rearrangement occurs, expression of the alternate allele is excluded owing to a lack of a contiguous VJ or VDJ joining. In cases where rearrangements occur in both chromosomes, any of several types of abnormality may occur and result in the nonexpression of one allele. These abnormalities include improper VJ or VDJ joining, loss of an RNA-splicing site, formation of an mRNA sequence in which the codons are out of phase, or generation of a translation stop codon.

It is implicit that productive rearrangements in the light and heavy chain genes must have taken place in a cell that can be selected from a heterogeneous population of lymphoid cells on the basis of immunoglobulin synthesis. The productive rearrangements of DNA involve only one set of genes encoding light and one set of genes encoding heavy chains, and it is these two sets that are eventually expressed. The other sets remain unexpressed, presumably owing to nonproductive rearrangements. In fact, there may be a large number of B cells in which all sets are rearranged unproductively. Obviously, these cells are unable to synthesize immunoglobulins and, therefore, are undetectable by the selection procedure.

GENETIC BASIS OF ANTIBODY DIVERSITY

Two models have been proposed to explain the structure of the immunoglobulin genes and the molecular basis of antibody diversity. The first model stated that each antibody heavy and light chain is encoded by a unique germ line gene. During B lymphocyte development, one light and one heavy chain are selected for expression, while others are suppressed. The model seems to be untenable in light of data presented above. The somatic mutation model postulates that in the germ line DNA there is only a single or a very small number of light and heavy chain genes for each class, subclass, type, or subtype of immunoglobulin. During B cell development, alterations in the DNA sequence encoding the variable regions might occur, resulting in somatic mutant genes that determine light and heavy chains with different variable region amino acid sequences.

Nucleotide and protein sequence analyses of the many light and heavy chain genes and gene products have permitted the identification of several mechanisms that contribute to the origin of antibody diversity. Three basic mechanisms, taken together, can account for the production of about 10^9 distinct antibody molecules.

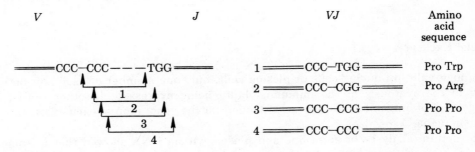

FIG. 8.8. Relationship between the site of recombination of *V* and *J* genes during rearrangements and nucleotide and amino acid sequences of **VJ** segment.

8.6 Direct Combinatorial Basis

One can assume that any possible light chain can combine with any possible μ_m chain to generate an active mIgM molecule. This assumption is supported by the finding of an extreme degree of conservation of amino acid sequences in the constant region of all light and heavy chains. The constant regions are the major sites of interaction between the two chains. In mice there are two V_λ genes, each associated with two C_λ genes. Therefore, there are four possible λ light chains. If there are 200 V_κ genes and 5 J_κ regions, there are 1,000 possible κ light chains. If there are 200 V_H genes, 10 D sequences, and 4 J_H regions, there are 8,000 possible μ heavy chains. Assuming that each of the 1,004 light chains can combine with the 8,000 possible H chains, one can envision the potential for 8×10^6 different immunoglobulins based simply on the number of possible rearranged light and heavy chain genes in mice.

8.7 Recombination-Generated Alterations

The VJ and VDJ joining sites are located in the third hypervariable region (HV3) of the light and heavy chains, respectively. A comparison of the DNA sequence in the J region with the protein sequence in the variable region of either light or heavy chains demonstrates that the amino acid encoded at the point of DNA joining in the rearranged DNA sequence is variable and depends upon the precise site of ligation of the DNA after rearrangement (Fig. 8.8). In other words, each J sequence can potentially encode several V amino acid sequences in HV3. This could significantly increase the antibody diversity, possibly increasing the number of potential light and heavy chains by a factor of 10 or more, i.e., to 8×10^7.

8.8 Somatic Mutations

An early hypothesis, proposed to explain antibody diversity (see above), stated that the V genes undergo a high rate of mutation during B lymphocyte development, and that this results in the production of a large number of different V region sequences. It was calculated above that about 10^8 different antibodies can be produced by the random combination of variable regions with D or J segments in the immunoglobulin heavy and light chains. Recently obtained data on the amino acid sequence of V_H regions for immunoglobulins that bind phosphoryl choline (PC) and nucleotide sequence data on their V_H genes suggest that a high degree of somatic mutation may also take place. It was shown that, of the 19 different immunoglobulins that bind PC, 10 possess an identical V_H amino acid sequence and the other 9 differ from this prototype V_H sequence by one to eight amino acid residues. After isolating and analyzing the DNA sequence of several germ line V_H genes that were likely to encode these V_H regions, it was concluded that all 19 PC-binding antibodies are the product of a single V_H gene. Thus, the cell lines that produce the nine immunoglobulins with an altered V_H amino acid sequence must possess V_H genes with altered DNA sequences derived from the prototype V_H sequence by somatic mutation.

Therefore, the total number of possible immunoglobulin chains that an individual can produce can be estimated by multiplying the number of light and heavy chain gene combination by the number of possible amino acid sequence changes produced by VJ and VDJ joining, and by the probability of somatic mutation occurring during B lymphocyte development; 10^9 being not an unreasonable estimate.

9 / *Allotypy of Immunoglobulins*

HUMAN IMMUNOGLOBULIN ALLOTYPES

It has been known for some time that sera of patients suffering from **rheumatoid arthritis** contain anti-immunoglobulin antibodies with a wide spectrum of specificities. These antibodies can be demonstrated by precipitation of heat-aggregated immunoglobulins, by agglutination of sheep erythrocytes "sensitized" with subagglutinating doses of rabbit or horse antibody, or by agglutination of latex particles coated with rabbit or human immunoglobulins. Some rheumatoid arthritis sera are also capable of agglutinating human Rh-positive erythrocytes coated with certain "incomplete" anti-Rh antibodies (Section 11.3). Some of these reactions require the immunoglobulin that functions as antigen to be aggregated either by heating or by combining with antigen. In these cases, the native immunoglobulin does not inhibit the reaction. Other human sera are inhibitable by native immunoglobulins.

When individual normal human sera were tested for their ability to inhibit the agglutination of erythrocytes coated with anti-Rh antibodies by rheumatoid arthritis antiglobulin sera, it was observed that some sera of normal individuals inhibited agglutination, whereas some other sera had no inhibitory capacity. It was soon found that this inhibitory capacity of normal sera is due to the presence of certain antigenic determinants, i.e., allotypic specificities that are inherited in a Mendelian fashion. The importance of the discovery of human immunoglobulin allotypes cannot be overestimated. In 1956 red cell antigens (blood groups) were practically the only polymorphic traits in man that were known to be under simple genetic control and at the time were not directly related to pathology. Polymorphisms of haptoglobins, enzymes, and, of course, MHC-related molecules were described *after* the discovery of immunoglobulin allotypes.

9.1 Allotypic Markers

The "new" polymorphic system of human immunoglobulins was designated Gm^a. The two variants, originally called Gm(a+) and Gm(a−) were distinguished by their capacity to inhibit the agglutination of anti-Rh-sensitized erythrocytes by rheumatoid arthritis sera; Gm(a+) inhibits, whereas Gm(a−) does not. In the intervening years, a large number of related allotypic markers have been described. Table 9.1 presents a summary of the notation of these markers and of their identification with immunoglobulin classes and/or subclasses and polypeptide chains.

In the notation proposed at a World Health Organization (WHO) meeting (1976) the first capital letter indicates the class (or type) of the immunoglobulin chain: G for IgG (γ), A for IgA (α), K for κ, etc. The number following the letter indicates the subclass of the heavy chain. The letter m has no special meaning other than relating the notation to the original Gm notation and indicating that a given symbol identifies a human immunoglobulin *m*arker. The number in parentheses identifies the allotypic marker (or specificity).

The chemical basis is known for a number of human allotypic specificities. So far, all have been determined by the primary structure of the respective chain (Table 9.2). However, some of the specificities are detectable only in an intact molecule. G1m(3) and G1m(17) are located on the C region of the Fab fragment and cannot be detected on separated heavy or light chains. The allotypic determinant lost by separation is restored by rejoining G1m(3)- or G1m(17)-bearing

TABLE 9.1. Notation of the Currently Testable Human Allotypic Specificities

Location	Notation		Antisera	Detection Method
	WHO	Previous		
IgG1	G1m(1)	a	N, R, H	HI
	(2)	x	N, R	HI
	(3)	f, b^w, b^2, 4	N, R	HI
	(17)	z	H	HI
IgG2	G2m(23)	n	H	PG, HI
IgG3	G3m(11)	b^β, b^0	N	HI
	(5)	b, b^1, b^γ, 12	N, R, H, P	HI
	(13)	b^3, Bet, 25	N	HI
	(14)	b^4	N	HI
	(10)	b^α, b^5	N	HI
	(6)	Gm-like, c, c^3	N, R	HI
	(24)	Gm-like, c^5	N, R	HI
	(21)	g	R, H	HI, PG
	(15)	s	R	HI
	(16)	t	N	HI
	(26)	Pa, u	R, H	HI
	(27)	Ray, v	—	HI
	(28)	Ber	N	HI
IgA2	A2m(1)	Am(1), Am_2	ID	HI, PG
	(2)		ID	HI
V_H (variable portion)	Hv(1)		H	HI
κ light chains	Km(1)	InV(1)	N	HI
	(2)	(2)	N, TR	HI
	(3)	(3)	N	HI

R = Sera from patients suffering from *r*heumatoid arthritis.

N = Sera from *n*ormal individuals.

TR = Sera from individuals given blood *tr*ansfusions.

H = Antibodies raised by *h*yperimmunization of rabbits or primates with myeloma proteins.

ID = Sera from patients suffering from IgA *i*mmuno*d*eficiency; patients were given transfusions in the past.

P = Naturally (?) occurring antibody found in the serum of one chimpanzee.

HI = *H*emagglutination *i*nhibition.

PG = *P*recipitation in *g*el.

Source: Notation recommended by the participants of the World Health Organization (WHO) Meeting on Human Immunoglobulin Markers, J. Immunogen. **3**: 357, 1976.

TABLE 9.2. Known Amino Acid Residues Responsible for Various Allotypic Markers of Human Immunoglobulin Allotypes

Allotypic Specificity	Amino Acid Residue	Position	Chain
G1m(1)	Asp-Glu-Leu-Thr-Lys	356–360	γ1
nG1m(1)	Glu-Glu-Met-Thr-Lys	356–360	γ1, γ2, γ3, γ4*
G1m(3)	Lys	214	γ1
G1m(17)	Arg	214	γ1
G3m(5)	Phe ... Phe	296 ... 436	γ3
G3m(21)	Tyr ... Tyr	296 ... 436	γ3
nG4m(a)	Val-Leu-His	309–311	γ4
nG4m(b)	Val ... His	309–311	γ4
A2m(2)	Met	131	α2
Km(1)	Val ... Leu	153 ... 191	κ
Km(1, 2)	Ala ... Leu	153 ... 191	κ
Km(3)	Ala ... Val	153 ... 191	κ

*The same amino acid residues are present on γ4, but the specificity is not serologically detectable.

heavy chains with unrelated light chains. Thus, although these specificities are determined by the primary structure of the heavy chain, they depend on the conformation brought about by the combination with a light chain. Light chain specificities, although detectable on isolated light chains, require heavy chains for full expression. The recently described Hv(1) marker common to all classes is located on the variable portion of the heavy chain. All remaining allotypic specificities are located on the Fc portion of the respective heavy chains.

9.2 Isoallotypic Markers

A special feature of human allotypes, so far not encountered in other species, is the existence of **isoallotypes** that were previously called **non-markers**. An isoallotype behaves as if it was an allotype of one of the immunoglobulin subclasses, but at the same time it is present on one or more other subclasses of all individuals, like an isotype. According to the present convention, isoallotypes are designated by the letter n, followed by the symbol of the marker for which it appears to be allelic. The discovery of isoallotypes resulted from studies on the structure of purified myeloma proteins. A pentapeptide, Asp-Glu-Leu-Thr-Lys, was found to be associated with G1m(1) specificity, whereas another pentapeptide, Glu-Glu-Met-Thr-Lys, was reported to be associated with non-G1m(1), i.e., G1m(1)-negative, molecules. Immunization of primates and rabbits with G1m(1)-negative purified myeloma proteins and absorption of collected antisera samples with G1m(1)-positive purfied myeloma proteins yielded antisera of a very peculiar specificity. As expected, the antisera reacted with all G1m(1)-negative IgG1 myeloma proteins but did not react with G1m(1)-positive myeloma proteins. Significantly, the antisera reacted also with purified myeloma proteins of IgG2 and IgG3 sublasses. Thus, the nG1m(1) determinant

TABLE 9.3. Notation and Distribution of Isoallotypic markers of Human Immunoglobulins

Notation		Distribution					
WHO	Previous	IgG1	IgG2	IgG3	IgG4	IgA1	IgA2
nG1m(1)	non-a	G1m(3):+ G1m(1):−	I	I	I*	0	0
nG1m(17)	non-z	G1m(3):+ G1m(17):−	0	I	I	0	0
nG3m(11)	non-b0	I	I	G3m(21):+ G3m(11):−	0	0	0
nG3m(5)	non-b1	I	I	G3m(21):+ G3m(5):−	0	0	0
nG4m(a)		I	0	I	G4m(b):+ G4m(a):−	0	0
nG4m(b)		0	I	0	G4m(a):+ G4m(b):−	0	0
nA2m(2)		0	0	0	0	I	A2m(1):+ A2m(2):−

0 = The isoallotypic marker does not occur on molecules of this subclass.

I = The marker behaves as an isotype and occurs on all molecules of this subclass.

+ or − = In this subclass, the marker behaves as an allotype and is either present or absent on molecules; the allelic markers are identified opposite the "+" or "−" sign, which refers to the presence or absence of a given isoallotypic marker.

Source: Notation recommended by the participants of the World Health Organization Meeting on Human Immunoglobulin Allotypic Markers, J. Immunogen., **3**: 357, 1976.

was found to be present not only in G1m(1)-negative IgG1 molecules but also in *all* IgG2 and IgG3 molecules, irrespective of their allotypes. IgG2 and IgG3 molecules are *always* nG1m(1)-positive, whether the individual's IgG1 molecules are G1m(1)-negative or G1m(1)-positive. Sera from normal, nonmyelomatous individuals react in the same manner; immune sera directed against nG1m(1) react with all immunoglobulin molecules of IgG2 and IgG3 subclasses and with IgG1 molecules of G1m(1)-negative individuals. Subsequently, other isoallotypic markers were descibed and assigned to various Ig subclasses, as shown in Table 9.3.

The presence of identical amino acid sequences on chains belonging to different subclasses suggests that these chains were derived by gene duplication and that this event was relatively recent. Since anti-non-marker immune sera react with sera of all normal individuals, the isoallotypes cannot be used in population or family studies. However, the isoallotypes provide useful landmarks in the determination of the fine structure of purified myeloma proteins and in attempts to correlate the presence of various alleles with the primary structure of the respective polypeptide chains.

9.3 Isotypic Markers of Human λ Chains

Constant regions of human λ chains occur in three isotypic variants (subtypes). This indicates that man must have at least three discrete C_λ genes. All three subtypes are present in the sera of normal individuals; only one subtype is present in any particular myeloma protein. These subtypes are defined by the presence or absence of two markers, **Oz** and **Kern**, detectable by heterologous immune sera. Monoclonal λ chains can be Oz(+)Kern(−), Oz(−)Kern(+), or Oz(−)Kern(−). Oz(+) and Oz(−) are correlated with the interchange of lysine for arginine at position 188; Kern(+) and Kern(−) are correlated with the interchange of glycine for serine at position 157. Another pair of λ chain isotypes, **Mcg(+)** and **Mcg(−)**, are correlated with interchanges of Asp, Thr, and Lys for Ala, Ser, and Thr at positions 111, 113, and 167, respectively. The Mcg type suggests that there may be at least four, but possibly six, subtypes of the human λ chain and a similar number of corresponding C_λ genes.

9.4 Genetics of Human Allotypes

Human allotypic markers belong to two linkage groups. The first linkage group determines the **Km** markers of κ light chains. The allotypic specificities Km(1), Km(2), and Km(3) are controlled by three codominant alleles $Km^{1,2}$, Km^3 (relatively frequent), and Km^1 (relatively rare). One, two, or three Km allotypic specificities may, therefore, be present in an individual. The second linkage group includes all heavy chain markers (**Gm, Am,** and **Hv**) and is linked to the locus determining the polymorphism of α_1 antitrypsin.

    Markers of the heavy chain linkage group determined by alleles located on one chromosome are inherited as a haplotype, in a manner similar to antigens controlled by the major histocompatibility complex (Chapter 15). Anthropologic surveys of various populations showed the existence of a large number of haplotypes, some occurring only in individuals belonging to one race or sometimes only in a single isolated population. Table 9.4 lists some haplotypes encountered in different racial groups.

    Studies of normal and myeloma proteins show clearly that a single immunoglobulin chain can contain more than one marker. Specificities that can simultaneously occur on the same chain must, therefore, be controlled by pseudoalleles, since true alleles by definition cannot determine the same molecule. For instance G1m(1) and G1m(17), or G3m(5), G3m(11), G3m(13), and G3m(14), respectively, cannot be controlled by true alleles, whereas G1m(1) and nG1m(1) or G1m(3) and G1m(17) appear to be mutually exclusive and are, very likely, controlled by true alleles for which the term **homoallele** has been coined. Population studies provide probable, but not definite, answers to the question regarding which markers are mutually exclusive. Definitive answers can only come from studies of amino acid sequences.

    Analysis of peculiar Gm haplotypes, thought to result from recombination of the chromosomes carrying the Gm genes, has led to a conclusion that the genes controlling different human IgG subclasses are arranged on the chromosome in the following sequence: $C_{\gamma 4}$-$C_{\gamma 2}$-$C_{\gamma 3}$-$C_{\gamma 1}$.

    An individual whose IgG was deficient in some allotypic markers normally associated with IgG1 or IgG3 has been described. The IgG1 molecules of this person lacked any allotypic

TABLE 9.4. *Gm* Haplotypes Commonly Present in each of Several Races[1]

Race	Haplotypes
Caucasoid	*(1,17,21,26), (1,2,17,21,26), (3,5,10,11,13,14,26)*
Negroid	*(1,5,10,11,13,14,17,26), (1,5,10,11,14,17,26), (1,5,6,11,17,24,26), (1,5,6,10,11,14,17,26)*
Mongoloid	*(1,17,21,26), (1,2,17,21,26), (1,10,11,13,17)[2], (1,3,5,10,11,13,14,26)*
Ainu	*(1,17,21,26), (1,2,17,21,26), (1,10,11,13,17)[2], (2,17,21,26)*
Khoisan	
San (Bushmen)	*(1,17,21,26), (1,10,11,13,17)[2], (1,5,10,11,13,14,17,26), (1,5,13,14,17,21,26)[3], (1,5,11,17,26)*
Khoikhoi (Hottentots)	*(1,2,17,21,26), (1,5,10,11,14,17,26), (1,10,11,13,17)[2], (1,5,10,11,13,14,17,26)*
Pygmy	*(1,5,6,11,17,24,26), (1,5,10,11,13,14,17,26)*
Micronesian	*(1,17,21,26), (1,3,5,10,11,13,14,26)*
Melanesian	
New Guinea	*(1,17,21,26), (1,2,17,21,26), (1,3,5,10,11,13,14,26), (1,5,10,11,13,14,17,26)*
Bougainville	*(1,17,21,26), (1,2,17,21,26), (1,3,5,10,11,13,14,26)*

[1]When tested for Gm (1,2,3,5,6,10,11,13,14,17,21,24,26).

[2]When tests for Gm (15) and Gm(16) are done the haplotype is $Gm^{1,10,11,13,15,16,17}$ among Mongoloids and Ainu, but it may be also $Gm^{1,10,11,13,15,17}$ among the Khoisan.

[3]Not tested for Gm(10) and Gm(11). Gm(10) is probably present, but Gm(11) may not be.

Source: Reproduced, with permission, from Steinberg, A.G., Cook, C.E. *The Distribution of the Human Immunoglobulin Allotypes.* Oxford University Press, Oxford, 1981.

markers normally associated with IgG1, although his IgG3 molecules contained some determinants. To explain these findings, it has been proposed that a recombination fused part of the chromosome that controls the C1 domain of the γ1 chain with the part that controls the C2 and C3 domains of the γ3 chain. During this fusion, parts of the chromosome containing sequences that encode G1m(1), G3m(5), and G3m(11) were eliminated. Similar recombination between genes controlling two different heavy chains has been described in the mouse. This type of recombination is referred to as **Lepore type**, since it resembles the crossing-over mechanism that led to the formation of the **Lepore hemoglobin**.

Other individuals with unusual chromosomes have been described; the formation of their chromosomes can be explained by crossing-over leading either to gene duplication or to gene deletion. For instance, gene duplication might have generated a chromosome that appears to have two $C_{\gamma 1}$ genes (one carrying $G1m^{1,17}$, the other $G1m^{n1,3}$). An individual who possesses the latter chromosome inherits and transmits an unusual haplotype, i.e., one that contains genes that normally should be mutually exclusive, e.g., $G1m^{17}$ and $G1m^3$. Similarly, lack of any detectable *Gm* genes of one of the subclasses of immunoglobulin can be explained by a deletion.

Intragenic recombinations might have generated some of the contemporary haplotypes; in Mongoloids, $G1m^1$ and $G1m^3$ are commonly parts of the same haplotype, whereas in Caucasoids they occur in different haplotypes, namely, either $G1m^{1,17}$ or $G1m^{n1,3}$. The separation of $G1m^1$ and $G1m^3$ could have occurred by intragenic crossing-over. Intergenic crossing-over might have been responsible for the association of $G1m^1$ with $G3m^{21}$ in Caucasoids or with $G3m^5$ in Negroids.

Studies on the frequencies of various Gm markers in different populations are of great interest to anthropology. Unfortunately, the knowledge of Gm distribution is still fragmentary; since only a few markers have been used, small numbers of individuals have been tested, and only a few populations have been surveyed.

9.5 Biologic Role of Allotypy

The existence of an extensive Gm polymorphism raises a question concerning the forces that maintain such polymorphism. Most of the Gm markers are located on the Fc portion of the immunoglobulin molecule. Thus, an association between Gm markers and the biologic function of antibody molecules seems very likely. In fact, there are many reports indicating that the presence of some Gm markers may influence immune responses. Individuals possessing G1m(1) and G3m(21) were found to be "high responders" to the flagellin antigen of *Salmonella adelaide*, whereas G1m(3), G3m(5) persons were "low responders." High responders were reported (over a six-year period of observation) to have an increased overall survival rate (life expectancy) as compared with low responders. On the other hand, the G1m(3), G3m(5) phenotype has been associated with an increased risk of autoimmune thyroid disease. Moreover, another report associated the genotype $Gm^{1,17;21}/Gm^{3;5,13,14}$ with a low immune response against meningococcal polysaccharide A.

There are reports that antibodies to some antigens, e.g., dextran, are predominantly, if not exclusively, of a single immunoglobulin subclass. It would be interesting to determine the Gm markers of such antibodies.

Allotypic specificities also appear to regulate the normal total concentrations of immunoglobulins of particular subclasses. Concentrations of IgG3 in individuals possessing G3m(5) are twice as high as those found in individuals carrying G3m(21). Higher levels of IgG2 and IgG4 are associated with the presence of G2m(23), as compared with levels associated with the absence of this marker. Finally, levels of IgG2 are higher in persons homozygous for $G1m^4$, $G2m^{23}$, and $G3m^5$ than in those homozygous for $G1m^{1,17}$, $G3m^{21}$.

An issue undoubtedly related to the association of Gm allotypes with enhanced immunity, or greater susceptibility to certain diseases is the problem of the formation of anti-Gm antibodies. In normal individuals, anti-Gm antibodies may be formed as a result of an unintentional or unexpected antigenic stimulus, e.g., blood or plasma transfusion. Also, exchange of immunoglobulins during pregnancy has been shown to stimulate both the mother and the fetus. Finally, normal healthy persons may form anti-Gm antibodies without apparent antigenic stimulus. All the above antibodies are always formed against allotypic markers not present in the serum of the recipient that makes the antibody.

Anti-Gm antibodies may also be formed in a variety of pathological conditions such as Still's disease, coal workers' pneumoconiosis, tuberculosis, leprosy, cryoglobulinemia, etc., but predominantly in rheumatoid arthritis. Sera of patients suffering from these diseases contain, besides the anti-Gm antibodies, a variety of antibodies with a wide spectrum of specificities. Usually, these sera react not only with human but also with animal immunoglobulins and may preferentially react with aggregated immunoglobulins. Although antibodies directed against self Gm markers cannot be detected in the circulation, there is ample evidence that auto-anti-Gm antibodies are being formed. These antibodies form complexes with immunoglobulins (antigen), are eliminated from the circulation, and are deposited in tissues.

The antigenic stimulus responsible for the formation of anti-immunoglobulin antibodies in pathological conditions is not known. The prevalent view is that the pathological processes lead to structural changes of autologous immunoglobulins, which, as a result, acquire "nonself" determinants. It is known that immunoglobulin molecules may acquire new determinants by aggregation, partial denaturation, combination with antigens, or partial digestion with proteolytic enzymes.

9.6 Human Allotypic Specificities in Primates

An indication that some of the human Gm specificities evolved from a common ancestral structure was provided from structural studies on primate immunoglobulins. A peptide, called the **OWM peptide** (OWM = Old World monkeys), was found to be closely related to the two peptides found in human immunoglobulins and associated with allotypic markers G1m(1) and nG1m(1):

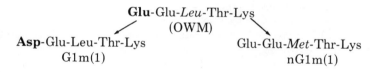

In addition, some human allotypic markers are serologically detectable and polymorphic in primates; Km markers are polymorphic in chimpanzees; and some G3m markers are polymorphic in chimpanzees and orangutans. Some other human allotypic markers appear to be isotypic in primates. Human markers are not detectable in monkeys of species lower than the Old World monkeys (Cercopithecoidea). The studies in nonhuman primates are fragmentary; small numbers of individuals have been tested, and the possibility that the results are biased by the fact that the animals tested might have belonged to a nonrepresentative group, or race, cannot be excluded at the present time.

MURINE IMMUNOGLOBULIN ALLOTYPES

9.7 Nomenclature and Genetics

Murine immunoglobulin genes belong to three linkage groups: heavy chain, kappa light chain, and lambda light chain. Each of these groups has genes for constant and variable regions of immunoglobulin molecules (Table 9.5).

So far no allotypic variants of the κ chain constant region have been described. An allotypic marker of the λ chain constant region has been characterized by alloantisera raised in

TABLE 9.5. Murine Immunoglobulin Genes

	Linkage Group		
Region	Heavy Chain (class or subclass)	κ Chain (type or subtype)	λ Chain (type or subtype)
Constant	Igh-C	Igk-C	Igl-C
	Igh-1 (γ2a)	Igk-1	Igl-1 (λ1)
	Igh-2 (α)		
	Igh-3 (γ2b)		
	Igh-4 (γ1)		
	Igh-5 (δ)		
	Igh-6 (μ)		
Variable	Igh-V	Igk-V	Igl-V
	Igh-Ars*	Igk-Ef1**	Igl-Lo+
	and numerous others	Igk-Pc**	
		Igk-Trp**	

*No variable framework region allotypes (analogous to the *Aa, Ax, Ay,* or *Aw* of the rabbit) have been found in the mouse. Genes determine idiotypes.

**May be identical with each other (see text).

+It is not known whether *Igl-Lo* is in the variable or constant region. It is closely linked to *Igl-1.*

Notation proposed under the aegis of the Committee on Standardized Genetic Nomenclature for Mice and recommended by a group of scientists, Immunogenetics, **8**:89, 1979.

SJL mice by immunization with BALB/c myeloma protein. The alloantisera detect a marker, Igl-1a, present in the prototype strain BALB/c and determined by the allele *Igl-1ᵃ*. The product of the other allele, *Igl-1ᵇ*, present in the prototype strain SJL has not been identified.

The locus *Igl-1* is closely linked to *Igl-Lo*, and the allele *Igl-Loᵃ* has the same strain distribution as the allele *Igl-1ᵃ*. The *Igl-Loᵃ* allele determines a normal serum concentration of λ1, whereas *Igl-Loᵇ* determines a level of λ1 which is one-fiftieth of a normal in the SJL strain. The mechanism of action of this regulatory gene is not clear; similar regulatory functions of some *Gm* genes were discussed earlier in this chapter.

Most of the known allotypic variants are controlled by the heavy chain constant group (*Igh-C*). Separate loci control each of the six immunoglobulin subclasses; these six loci were given consecutive numbers in order of their discovery: *Igh-1* for γ2a, *Igh-2* for α, etc. Several (2–14) alleles have been described at each locus. Since all the *Igh-C* loci are closely linked (no recombinants have been observed in more than 5,000 offspring of special crosses), the alleles at all six loci occur in clusters (haplotypes) characteristic for a given inbred strain. So far, 14 different haplotypes have been encountered—11 in inbred laboratory strains and the remaining 3 in outbred wild mice. Only limited surveys of wild mice populations have been performed so far. One can expect that considerably more haplotypes will be described in wild mice, since most of the inbred strains have common ancestors and are probably less polymorphic than the wild population.

An *Igh-C* haplotype is designated by a lowercase letter (*a-n*) superscript. A prototype strain has been assigned for each haplotype. Alleles included in each of the haplotypes are listed in Table 9.6. For example, haplotype *d*, which is characteristic for AKR mice, includes the following alleles: *Igh-1ᵈ, Igh-2ᵈ, Igh-3ᵈ, Igh-4ᵃ,* and *Igh-5ᵃ*. No allele of the *Igh-6* locus has been identified in association with this haplotype.

Unfortunately, the above notation is potentially confusing because the same symbols were chosen for haplotypes as for alleles; all alleles included in the *a* and *b* haplotypes were designated *a* and *b*, respectively. However, this regularity no longer holds for the haplotypes *c* to *n*. For example, haplotype *c* includes alleles *Igh-1ᶜ, Igh-2ᶜ, Igh-3ᵃ, Igh-4ᵃ,* and *Igh-5ᵃ* (Table 9.6).

Several markers of the variable portion of the heavy chain have been described. At the present time, it is not known whether these markers are determined by allelic genes. None of these markers are analogous to the rabbit variable framework markers, i.e., Aa, Ax, Ay, and Aw allotypes. Instead, they are closely associated with the antibody combining site and with the hypervariable regions. Because of this association, they fall under the definition of idiotype and will be discussed in Chapter 10.

Three pairs of markers are associated with the variable portion of the κ light chain. The allele *Igk-Ef1ᵃ* determines the presence of bands 58, 61, and 66 in an isoelectro focusing pattern of the protein from AKR, RF, PL, and C58 mice. The other allele, *Igk-Ef1ᵇ*, occurs in all other tested inbred strains and determines the presence of bands 25 and 60 in the isoelectro focusing pattern. The allele *Igk-Pcᵃ* determines a lower isoelectric point, and the other allele, *Igk-Pcᵇ*, determines a higher isoelectric point of the light chain preparation. Finally, the alleles *Igk-Trpᵃ* and *Igk-Trpᵇ* determine, respectively, the presence and absence of the peptide I_B in a tryptic digest from the light chain preparation. The *a* alleles of all three genes have the same strain distribution. This strongly suggests that all three *a* alleles are identical and determine the same primary structure, which, in each case, is detected by a different method. It is not known

TABLE 9.6. Haplotypes and Alleles at the Murine *Igh-C* Loci

Prototype Strain	Haplotype	Alleles at Locus (Chain)					
		Igh-1 (γ2a)	*Igh-2* (α)	*Igh-3* (γ2b)	*Igh-4* (γ1)	*Igh-5* (δ)	*Igh-6* (μ)
BALB/c	a	a	a	a	a	a	a
C57BL	b	b	b	b	b	b	b
DBA/2	c	c	c	a	a	a	—
AKR	d	d	d	d	a	a	—
A	e	e	d	e	a	e	e
CE	f	f	f	f	a	a	—
RIII	g	g	c	g	a	a	—
SEA	h	h	a	a	a	a	—
CBA/H	j	j	a	a	a	a	a
KH-1[a]	k	k	c	a	a	—	—
KH-2[a]	l	l	c	a	a	—	—
Ky[a]	m	m	b	b	b	—	—
NZB	n	e	d	e	a	a	e

[a]Wild mice.

Notation proposed under the aegis of the Committee on Standardized Genetic Nomenclature for Mice and recommended by a group of scientists, Immunogenetics, **8**:89, 1979.

whether the markers are located in the hypervariable regions or in the framework part of the variable portion. The importance of the *Igk-Trp* locus for the expression of the idiotype ARS will be discussed in Chapter 10.

9.8 Typing Sera and Allotypic Specificities

Antisera directed against the heavy chain allotypic markers are raised by alloimmunization in carefully chosen combinations of donors and recipients so as to obtain antisera of the desired specificity. To increase immunogenicity, the immunizing immunoglobulins are usually administered as antigen-antibody complexes, e.g. complexed with *Proteus vulgaris* cells. Alternatively, the immunogen can be administered after mild aggregation with glutaraldehyde. Some of the murine antiallotype antibodies are of the precipitating quality and can be used in gel precipitation tests or in radioimmunoassay (Section 4.4). In the latter, precipitation of radioactively labeled purified myeloma protein of known allotype by the typing antiserum is inhibited by an unlabeled serum of unknown allotypes. Less potent antisera can be used to inhibit the hemagglutination of erythrocytes coated with an appropriate purified myeloma protein in a procedure similar to that used in human Gm typing.

Each marker, determined by a given *Igh-C* allele, is comprised of a number of antigenic determinants (allotypic specificities) that may be shared by the products of different alleles at the same locus (chain class). These specificities are denoted by numbers preceded by the locus designation—e.g., the specificity Igh-1.1 is one of the specificities determined by the allele *Igh-1ᵃ*. The inclusion of the designation of the locus is important, since determinants of different classes may have the same numbers. For instance, Igh-1.1 and Igh-3.1 are discrete determinants controlled by *Igh-1ᵃ* and *Igh-3ᵃ* alleles, respectively. If more than one determinant of the same allelic product is to be listed, the locus designation has to appear only once: Igh-1.1,2,6,7,8,10,12 or Igh-2.1,3,7, etc. Table 9.7 lists some of the specificities determined by the genes at various *Igh-C* loci.

TABLE 9.7. Allotypic Specificities Controlled by Different Murine *Igh-C* Haplotypes

Locus	Chain[a]	Allele	Specificities or determinants	
Igh-1	γ2a (γG)	a	1,2,6,7,8,10,12	(1,6,7,8,26,28,29,30)
		b	4,7	(2,27,28)
		c	2,3,7	(3,8,29)
		d	1,2,5,7,12	(4,6,7,8,26,29)
		e	1,2,5,6,7,8,12	(4,6,7,8,26,28,29,30)
		f	1,2,8,11	(5,7,8,26,30)
		g	2,3	(3,8,26)
		h	1,2,6,7,10,12	(1,6,7,8,28,29)
		j	—	(1,6,7,8,28,29,30)
		k	—	(3,5,7,8)
		l	—	(3,5,8)
		m	—	(1,2,6,7,8)
Igh-2	α (γA)	a	2,3,4	(12,13,14)
		b	—	(15)
		c	1,3	(35)
		d	3	(13,17)
		f	4	(14)
Igh-3	γ2b (γH)	a	1,2,4,7,8	(9,11,22,31,33,34)
		b	4,7,8,9	(9,16,22,33,34)
		d	1,3,7,8	(4,23,31,32,33,34)
		e	1,3,7	(4,23,31,32,33)
		f	1,2,3,4	(9,11,31,32)
		g	1,2,4	(9,11,31)
Igh-4	γ1 (γF)	a	1	(8,19)
		b	2	(42)
Igh-5	δ (γD)	a	1	(36)
		b	2	(37)
		e		
Igh-6	μ (γM)	a	1,2	(38,39)
		b	2,4	(40,41)
		e	3,4	(39,41)

[a]Potter-Lieberman notation is given in parentheses.

NOTE: The Herzenberg (H) and the Potter-Lieberman (P-L) notation systems are not fully overlapping. The following specificities of the H system have been identified with the following specificities of the P-L system (numerals in parentheses): Igh-1: 1(7), 2(8), 10(1), 12(6); Igh-2: 2(12), 3(13), 4(14); Igh-3: 2(11), 4(9).

The above system of notation has been proposed by Herzenberg. An alternative system, based on consecutive numbering of determinants, has been proposed by Potter and Lieberman. The two systems are not fully overlapping, so that some determinants defined in one system have no analogues in the second system. It is of some interest that in the Potter-Lieberman system two different heavy chain subclasses share two determinants: determinant 4 found on both γ2a and γ2b heavy chains, while determinant 8 is present on γ2a and γ1 chains. This identity or similarity of determinants located on chains of different subclasses may be explained by a recent duplication.

The homology between human Gm and mouse heavy chain allotypes is striking. Similar to Gm markers, mouse determinants most likely reflect single amino acid substitutions. Obviously, the mouse model offers unique opportunities for correlating serologic markers with amino acid sequences and determining which of the markers are controlled by true alleles. Because there is much knowledge about the immunoglobulins and genetics of the mouse, it is hard to understand why more advantage has not been taken of these opportunities. So far, not even a single amino acid substitution has been correlated with a murine allotypic marker.

RABBIT IMMUNOGLOBULIN ALLOTYPES

9.9 Nomenclature of Rabbit Allotypes

Polymorphism of rabbit immunoglobulins has been extremely useful in solving a number of problems related to mechanisms of immunoglobulin synthesis and the regulation of the immune response. Rabbit allotypes belong to four linkage groups: κ light chain, λ light chain, heavy chain, and the secretory component linkage group (Table 9.8). Distinct specificities or determinants are designated by numbers, which are preceded by at least one lowercase letter that identifies the locus. According to an international agreement, it is advisable to add a capital letter (A for allotype, M for IgM) before the locus designation. These letters are frequently omitted to avoid repetition. Alternatively, although this is not internationally approved, the locus designation might include an indication of its location. Thus variable portion loci Aa, Ax, Ay and Aw might alternatively be designated V_Ha, V_Hx, V_Hy, V_Hw respectively. Constant portion heavy chain loci Ad, Ae, Af, Ag, and Ms might be designated $C_\gamma d$, $C_\gamma e$, $C_\alpha f$, $C_\alpha g$, and $C_\mu n$, respectively. Finally, the Ab and Ac genes for light chain markers might become κb and λc, respectively.*

Because of the complexity of the subject, the following discussion will be concerned only with the noncontroversial markers that currently can be tested. The heavy chain linkage group is the largest and comprises $C_H\gamma$, $C_H\mu$, and $C_H\alpha$ genes for Fcγ, Fcμ, and Fcα constant portion specificities, respectively, variable portion specificities V_Ha, and "alternate" (a-negative) variable portion specificities V_Hx, V_Hy, and V_Hw.

---

*The letters A and M will be used only when referring to the entire set of markers, but, for the sake of convenience, they will be omitted in a case of specific markers or corresponding loci or alleles.

9.10 Specificities of the γ Chain

Two subloci*, d and e, have been described, each having two alleles, d^{11}, d^{12} and e^{14}, e^{15}, respectively. The d11 specificity correlates with the presence of methionine at position 225 (hinge region), while d12 corresponds to the presence of threonine at the same position. The specificities e14 and e15 correlate, respectively, with the presence of threonine and alanine residues at position 309 ($C_\gamma 2$ domain). Anti-d and anti-e sera are obtained by alloimmunization. The antibodies directed against these specificities usually do not form visible precipitates with the respective IgG molecules. Therefore, typing is normally done by inhibition of passive hemagglutination; alternatively, double diffusion (precipitation) (Section 4.4) in agar containing 2 percent polyethylene glycol (PEG) can be used for testing of some antisera. Frequencies of d11 and d12 vary in different breeds, and e14 is very rare in most populations. The Ad and Ae markers seem to be the closest analogues of the human Gm allotypes.

9.11 Specificities of the IgM Molecules

Allotypes of the IgM class were first described in 1965 and are serologically the most complex of all rabbit markers. Because of this complexity, the complete picture of IgM allotypes has begun to emerge only during the past few years. At present, there seem to be only two IgM markers coded by alleles at the n (or μ or Ms) locus. The two markers are designated Ms16 and Ms17, or n81 and n80, respectively. There are several other IgM determinants that depend on conformational changes induced by pairing of particular constant and variable portions of the μ chain or of μ chains with particular κ chains (Table 9.9). When the constant portion that carries the allotype Ms16 is paired with the variable portion that carries the a1 determinant (see below), a new distinct determinant, Ms21, is created in addition to the Ms16 and a1, which are still detectable. Similarly, pairing of Ms17 and a1 creates Ms24. Pairing of μ and certain κ light chains results in the formation of two new conformational determinants. The b4 marker of κ chains (see below) occurs in two variants, b4.1 and b4.2 (or b4var), which correlate with amino acid substitutions at positions 121 and 124. When a κ chain with the b4.1 marker is used to assemble an immunoglobulin molecule with μ or with γ chains, two conformational markers, Ms3 or Gs3, respectively, are formed. Combination of b4.2 κ chains with μ or γ chains results in the formation of Ms7 or Gs7 determinants, respectively (Table 9.9).

9.12 Allotypes of the α Chains

Rabbit secretory IgA molecules occur as two subclasses, IgA_f and IgA_g. The former subclass is resistant to cleavage by papain in the absence of cystein, whereas the latter is susceptible. The determinants of the α_f chains are defined by five antisera: anti-f69, anti-f70, anti-f71, anti-f72,

---

*The term sublocus is a misnomer and in reality corresponds to a different portion of a single locus carrying the gene for the Cγ region.

TABLE 9.8. Rabbit Immunoglobulin Allotypes

Linkage Group	Chain Class or Type	Locus	Specificities	Remarks
Heavy chain	$C_H\gamma$	d	d11, d12	Correlated with single amino acid substitution; located at position 225 (hinge region)
	$C_H\gamma$	e	e14, e15	Correlated with single amino acid substitution; located at position 309
	$C_H\mu$	$n, \mu,$ or Ms	n80(Ms17), n81(Ms16)	
	$C_H\alpha_f{}^a$	f	f69, f70, f71, f72, f73	Each specificity has multiple determinants; some may be shared with other specificities
	$C_H\alpha_g{}^a$	g	g74[b], g75[b], g76, g77	Each specificity has multiple determinants; some may be shared with other specificities
	V_H	a	a1, a2, a3	—
	V_H	x	x32, x32$^-$	—
	V_H	y	y30, y33, y$^-$	y33 and y30 are most likely controlled by pseudoalleles[c]
	V_H	w	w34, w35	—
κ chain	κ	b	b4, b5, b6, b9, bbas	—
λ chain	λ	c	c7, c21	c7 and c21 are most likely controlled by pseudoalleles
Secretory component		t	t61, t62	—

[a]α_1 (α_1) subclass is resistant to proteolysis; α_g (α_2) is cleaved by proteolytic enzymes.

[b]The g74 and g75 have been divided into subspecificities, g74.1, g74.2 and g75.1, g75.2, respectively. The .1 specificities were found on the $C_\alpha 1$ domain; the .2 specificities, on the Fc portion.

[c]$y^{33.30}$, $y^{30.-}$, and y^{--} haplotypes have been found.

and anti-f73; the determinants of the α_g chains are detected by four antisera: anti-g74, anti-g75, anti-g76, and anti-g77. However, each antiserum must detect more than one determinant, because antisera within each subclass show extensive cross-reactions and because determinants of both IgA$_f$ and IgA$_g$ subclasses are on the Fab portions ($C_\alpha 1$ domain) as well as on the Fc portions. It is presumed that at least some of these antigenic determinants reflect differences in amino acid sequences, but neither the involvement of carbohydrate moieties nor the presence of conformational determinants has been excluded.

9.13 Allotypes of the Variable Portion of the Heavy Chains

These markers, like the human Hv(1) marker, are shared by all immunoglobulin classes. Finding the same marker on all immunoglobulin classes of a given individual aided in the understanding

TABLE 9.9. "Conformational" Allotypes of Rabbit Immunoglobulins

Determinant of		Formed in the Presence of	Synonym	Linkage Group
IgG	IgM			
Gs3	Ms3	b4.1 + μ or γ	b4.1	κ light chain[a]
Gs7	Ms7	b4.2 + μ or γ	b4var	κ light chain[a]
—	Ms23	a3+Ms16[b]	n85	Heavy chain
—	Ms24	a1+Ms17	n83	Heavy chain
—	Ms21	a1+Ms16	—	Heavy chain
—	Ms25	a2+Ms17	n82	Heavy chain
—	Ms22	a2+Ms16	—	Heavy chain[c]
—	Ms26	a3+Ms17	n86	Heavy chain

[a]Correlate with the following amino acid residues at positions 121 and 124 of the κ chain: Gs3 = Ala ... Gln; Gs7 = Ser ... Leu.

[b]Ms16 = n81; Ms17 = n80.

[c]Existence of this determinant has been predicted but not shown.

of the now generally accepted mechanism of splicing variable and constant genes during immunoglobulin synthesis.

Aa specificities occur on a major subtype of the variable portion of the heavy chain, they are determined by the gene at the a locus. The a1, a2, and a3 markers have been known since 1956 and have been the subject of particularly extensive research. Yet, relatively little is known about them. Unlike the Ad or Ae markers of the constant region, the Aa allotypes seem to be correlated with extensive amino acid substitutions, probably as many as 12 to 15 residues. So far, few of these differences have been confirmed by sequence studies (Table 9.10). For example, Thr-Glu at position 84–85 was found to correlate with a1, Ala-Gln with a2, and Ala-Ala with a3. Further indications of the complex, multideterminant nature of the Aa markers are observations of cross-reactivity of some anti-a3 antisera with a1-positive molecules and the observation that some antibodies of restricted heterogeneity lack some of the a1 determinants that are regularly found on "normal" a1-positive immunoglobulins. Each of the Aa markers may represent a number of subspecificities similar to human or mouse markers occurring on one constant portion subclass. If this were the case, one would expect the subspecificities to be more separable, i.e., to occur in more than just three fixed sets. Although only three markers are found in domesticated rabbits, additional markers of the Fd portion* have been found in wild European and Tunisian rabbits (Table 9.11). The a100, a101, A102, A103, and A104 markers are detected by alloantisera raised in domestic rabbits by immunizaton with a1-, a2-, and a3-negative immunoglobulins obtained from wild rabbits. Binding assays show that these markers cross-react with the "conventional" a1 and a3 allotypes so that a multideterminant nature of the Aa specificities similar to that of Gm allotypes cannot be completely dismissed.

---

*The Fd portion corresponds to the enzymatically separated V region of the heavy chain.

TABLE 9.10. Possible Correlations of Aa Allotypes with Amino Acid Sequences of the V_H Region

Allotype	Position								
	4	7	9	11	12	15	16	84	85
a1	Glu	Gly	**Arg**	Val	**Thr**	**Pro**	**Gly**	**Thr**	**Glu**
a2	**Lys**	**Glu**	**Gly**	**Phe**	Lys	**Asp**	**Thr**	Ala	**Gln**
a3	Glu	Gly	**Asp** **Val**	Val	Lys	**Ala**	**Ser**	Ala	**Ala**

NOTE: Residues in bold print represent substitutions.

The formation of the major subtype of the variable portion of the heavy chain carrying the Aa specificities may be suppressed by treatment of newborn rabbits with antiserum directed against the Aa specificities (Section 9.20). When this happens, a compensatory mechanism increases the synthesis of minor subtypes, so that the total immunoglobulin concentration in the suppressed animals is unaffected. These minor subtypes, "alternative" to the major subtype that carries the Aa markers, were originally called **a-negative**. Antibodies of restricted heterogeneity, which consisted of a-negative V_H regions, were formed by one rabbit in response to immunization with streptococcal carbohydrate antigen. The a-negative heavy chains were found to differ from the Aa (a-positive) chains by their amino terminal amino acid sequences. Appropriate immunizations with a-negative immunoglobulins obtained from Aa-suppressed a-negative rabbits revealed that the alternate V_H portions carry three groups of allotypic markers, Ax, Ay, and Aw. So far five markers have been characterized: x32, y33, y30, w34, and w35. The rabbits were found to be either x32-positive or x32-negative, which suggests that the x^{32} gene has at least two alleles. With regard to Ay markers, $y^{33.30}$, $y^{33.-}$, and y^{--} haplotypes were observed. All tested rabbits were found to be either w34-positive or w35-positive. The w34 and w35 markers appear to be structurally related; they are characterized by differences in their

TABLE 9.11. Allotypic Markers Found in Wild Rabbits

Linkage Group	Designation	Remarks
Heavy chain (Fd portion)	a100, a101, A102, A103, A104	Found in *Oryctolagus cuniculus cuniculus* (indigenous to Europe) and in Tunisian rabbit (*O. cuniculus algirus*); cross-reactions with a1 and a3 observed
κ light chain	A93, A94, A96, b95	Occurs in wild rabbits from a Tunisian island (*O. cuniculus algirus*); cross-reactions with "conventional" b series allotypes observed
	b98	Found in *O. cuniculus* in Portugal; requires association with heavy chains for expression; cross-reactions observed

reactions with the same antibody. Antiserum directed against w34 and w35 was raised in an individual whose preimmunization serum sample contained a low concentration of the Aw subclass immunoglobulins; thus, this antiserum is an autoantibody. Aw markers are normally expressed on a very small proportion of immunoglobulin molecules, far smaller than the Aa markers and even smaller than the "minor" Ax and Ay markers. Concentration of w34 can increase substantially as a compensation following suppression of other V_H markers; w35 does not seem to have similar compensatory ability. There are some indications that the list of alternative V_H markers is not yet complete. It is interesting to note that in spite of the high number of possible combinations of the heavy chain markers, the number of actually observed haplotypes seems to be limited to not much more than 10.

9.14 Allotypes of the κ Chains

The b4, b5, b6, and b9 specificities are excellent markers of rabbit immunoglobulin molecules and B cells, mainly because κ chains occur in most of the rabbit's immunoglobulin molecules (>90 percent) and all Ab allotypic specificities are good immunogens that stimulate formation of potent precipitating antisera. The fifth κ marker, bbas (for *Basilea*), has only recently been added to the Ab series. It was first thought that b^{bas} was a "silent" allele at the b locus that probably resulted from a recent mutation. Later, the product of this allele was identified as a κ marker. The reason why b^{bas} was thought to be silent is its remarkably low penetrance. In homozygotes, the bbas marker is expressed on fewer than 10 percent of the immunoglobulin molecules, the balance being molecules carrying λ chains. In heterozygous individuals, the bbas marker can only be detected by the sensitive inhibition of hemagglutination assay and is probably present on approximately 1 percent of the molecules.

Recent studies on sera from feral rabbits have indicated that the *bas* gene is not allelic to the b series, but is closely linked to the b locus. The bas(+) phenotype can be detected in a proportion of feral, but not domestic rabbits, that are heterozygous at the b locus. So far, no recombinations between the b and the *bas* locus have been observed. It has been postulated that rabbit κ chains exist in the two isotypic forms, κ1 and κ2 and that these isotypes are controlled by closely linked genes. The κ1 molecules carry allotypes of the Ab series, the κ2 molecules carry the bas(+) or, alternatively, its allelic form, the bas (−) marker, So far, no antisera against this form of κ2 chains have been raised.

Two subtypes, $κ_a$ and $κ_b$, of the rabbit κ chain have been proposed. The prevalent $κ_b$ chains have seven, instead of five, half-cysteine residues. The two extra half-cysteines form an intrachain disulfide bond that links the V_L and C_L domains. Remarkably, the Ab markers occur on both subtypes. Alternatively, it was proposed that $κ_a$ and $κ_b$ merely reflect the difference in the degree of reduction of the same chain.

A large percentage of amino acid residues, perhaps as much as 30 percent, seems to be related to differences in Ab allotypes (Table 9.12). Whether all of these differences indeed correlate with Ab allotypic markers remains to be seen. From the serologic data alone, it is obvious that the Ab markers are complex multideterminant antigens. The fine specificity of anti-Ab antisera depends on the Ab allotypes of the immunized animal. For instance, if an anti-b5 or anti-b6 antiserum is raised in a rabbit that does not possess either b5 or b6, the antiserum will

TABLE 9.12. Amino Acid Sequences of C_κ Rabbit Chains and Correlations with Ab Allotypes

Allotype — Position

Allotype	108	109	110	111	112	113	114	115	116	117	118	119	120	121	122	123
b4	Asp	Pro	Val	[ ][a]	Ala	Pro	Thr	Val	Leu	Ile	Phe	Pro	Pro	Ala	Ala	Asp
b5				—	Ala	—	—	—	—	—	—	—	—	—	Ser	Ala
b6	Ala	Thr	Leu	[ ]	—	—	—	—	—	—	—	—	—	Ser	Ser	Ala
b9	—	—	Pro	Ile	—	—	—	—	—	Leu	—	—	—	Ser	—	—

Allotype	124	125	126	127	128	129	130	131	132	133	134	135	136	137	138	139
b4	Gln	Val	Ala	Thr	Gly	Thr	Val	Thr	Ile	Val	Cys	Val	Ala	Asn	Lys	Tyr
b5	—	Leu	—	—	—	—	—	—	—	—	—	—	—	—	—	—
b6	Glu	Leu	—	—		Ala	—	—	—	—	—	—			—	—
b9	—	Leu	Thr	—	Glx	—	—	—	—	—		—	—	—	—	Phe

Allotype	140	141	142	143	144	145	146	147	148	149	150	151	152	153	154	155
b4	Phe	Pro	[ ]	Asp	Val	Thr	Val	Thr	Trp	Glu	Val	Asp	Gly	Thr	Thr	Gln
b5	—	—	[ ]	—	Gly	—	—	—	—	—	—	—	—	Lys	Pro	Leu
b6	—	—	[ ]	—	Gly	—	—	—	—	Lys	—	—	—	—	Ile	—
b9	Arg	—	Asp	—	Ile	—	—	—	—	Lys	—	—	Asp	Glu	Ile	—

Allotype	156	157	158	159	160	161	162	163	164	165	166	167	168	169	170	171
b4	Thr	Thr	Gly	Ile	Glu	Asn	Ser	Lys	Thr	Pro	Gln	Asp	Ser	Ala	Asp	Cys
b5	—	—	—	—	—	Thr	—	—	—	—	—	Asn	—	Asp	Asx	—
b6	Ser	Ser	—	—	Asn	—	—	—	—	—	—	Asn	Gly	—	—	—
b9	Gln	Ser	—	—	—	—	—	Thr	—	—	—	Ser	Pro	Glu	—	—

Allotype	172	173	174	175	176	177	178	179	180	181	182	183	184	185	186	187
b4	Thr	Tyr	Asn	Leu	Ser	Ser	Thr	Leu	Thr	Leu	Thr	Ser	Thr	Gln	Tyr	Asn
b5	—	—	—	—	—	—	—	—	—	—	Gln	Lys	Ser	Asn	—	—
b6	—	—	—	—	—	—	—	—	—	—	—	—	—	—	—	—
b9	—	—	?	—	—	—	—	—	Ser	—	—	Lys	Ala	—	—	—

Allotype	188	189	190	191	192	193	194	195	196	197	198	199	200	201	202	203
b4	Ser	His	Lys	Glu	Tyr	Thr	Cys	Lys	Val	Thr	Gln	Gly	Thr	Thr	Ser	Val
b5	—	—	Asn	Gln	—	—	—	Gln	Leu	Pro	—	—	Ala	Gly	—	—
b6																
b9	—	—	Ser	[ ]	—	—	—	Gln	—	His	Asn	Ser	Ala	(Gly	—)[b]	Ile

Allotype	204	205	206	207	208	209	210	211	212
b4	Val	Gln	Ser	Phe	Asn	Arg	Gly	Asp	Cys
b5	—	—	—	—	Ser	—	Lys	Asn	—
b6							Lys	Ser	—
b9	—	Glx	—	—	—	—	—	—	—

[a]Brackets indicate deletions that were introduced to maximize homology of the sequences compared. Dash indicates identity of residues, the blank spaces indicate undetermined residues.

[b]Indicates that more than one residue was identified at these positions. The most prevalent residue is indicated.

SOURCE: Reprinted, with permission, from *CRC Critical Reviews in Immunology*, **2**(4). Copyright © Chemical Rubber Co., CRC Press Inc.

show extensive cross-reactivity with b6 and b5, respectively. If, on the other hand, an anti-b5 antiserum is raised in a b6-positive rabbit, or anti-b6 in a b5-positive animal, the resulting antisera will not cross-react. Thus, b5 and b6 must share some determinants. Similarly, there is evidence that b4 and b6 also have some determinants in common. These, and other more subtle cross-reactions, seem to be consistent with the minimum number of determinants involved, being 10 or even more.

Most of the commercially available rabbits or rabbits bred at large research institutions are b^4/b^4 homozygotes. The frequencies of b^5, b^9, and b^6 alleles (in decreasing order) are very low. These rare allotypes can be found in rabbits bred in small colonies or by hobby breeders. Interestingly enough, they are also found in Australian feral rabbits. Wild rabbits from Tunisia carry a number of specificities that have not been encountered in domestic animals. Allotype b95 has been shown to be controlled by an allele at the b locus. Others such as A93, A94, and A96 are also very likely alleles at this locus (Table 9.11).

9.15 Allotypes of the λ Chains

The λ type chains in rabbits occur in not more than 10 percent of the immunoglobulins. It becomes a major light chain only in b^{bas} homozygotes (see above) or in rabbits in which synthesis of κ type chains has been suppressed as a result of neonatal treatment with anti-κ allotype immune serum. Two markers of λ chains have been described: c7 and c21. Both occur in very high frequencies in most rabbit populations. Since they are not mutually exclusive, they are probably controlled by pseudoalleles. No allelic variants of c7 or c21 have been described.

9.16 Allotypes of the Secretory Component

Two allotypic variants of the rabbit secretory component, t60 and t61, have been described (Table 9.8).

9.17 Latent Allotypes

The preceding discussion has been based on the concept that allotypes are encoded by structural genes inherited according to Mendelian principles. Although the majority of the family data support this, there are several reports that rabbit sera may sometimes contain allotypes not expected according to this concept. These unexpected allotypes are referred to as **latent**, as opposed to "normal" allotypes, which are referred to as **nominal**. It must be emphasized that antigenically latent and nominal allotypes are identical. The serum levels of latent allotypes tend to fluctuate and, as a rule, are lower than those of the nominal allotypes. Hyperimmunization of an animal usually results in an increase of the concentration of latent allotypes. Latent allotypic specificities that belong to the heavy chain and to the κ chain linkage groups have been described. Careful studies have excluded several trivial explanations for the latent allotype phenomenon. Among the explanations ruled out are the presence of rheumatoid-type factor, presence of antiallotype antibodies, maternal transfer of immunoglobulins, maternal transfer of stem cells with consequent chimerism, cross-reactivity, the presence of additional antibodies in the antiallotype immune sera, etc. Immunoglobulin molecules carrying latent allotypes have been isolated and found to be indistinguishable from molecules carrying the respective nominal allotypes.

At the cellular level, latent allotypes are expressed on the surface of the same cells that express the nominal allotypes. Similar studies, not as carefully documented, showed the occurrence of latent allotypes in species other than the rabbit. Thus, the finding of latent allotypes forces one to modify, or at least to question, not only the conventional concept of Mendelian structural genes coding for allotypes but also the central dogma of the clonal selection theory, the **one cell-one antibody** postulate (Section 7.1).

Synthesis of latent allotypes may be triggered by exposure of lymphoid cells to antiallotype antibody. The specificity of the synthesized allotype appears to depend on the specificity of the antiallotype antibody and on the allotype carried by the donor of the antiallotype antibody. On the basis of these observations, it has been suggested that nominal and latent allotypes and their respective antibodies are involved in a regulatory network, analogous to the idiotype-anti-idiotype network proposed by Jerne (Chapter 10).

9.18 Pepsin Agglutinators

The sera of several mammalian species contain natural antibodies directed against hidden allotypic determinants, which can be revealed after enzymatic digestion of immunoglobulins. Because the phenomenon was first observed after the digestion of immunoglobulins with pepsin, the antibodies are called **pepsin agglutinators**. Pepsin agglutinators do not react with intact immunoglobulins. They belong to IgG or IgM classes and have been detected in man, in the rabbit, and in several nonhuman primates. They react with fragments of autologous immuno-globulins as well. The biologic function and significance of pepsin agglutinators are obscure, as is the mechanism of their formation. It is likely that the antigenic stimulation that results in production of pepsin agglutinators occurs during the breakdown of antigen-antibody complexes.

9.19 Function of Rabbit Allotypes

For any genetic polymorphism, including allotypy, to evolve and be maintained through natural selection, it must provide some selective advantage(s) for the individual. Feral rabbit popula-tions possess a much more complex allotype polymorphism as compared with that of rabbits bred by commercial establishments or by research institutions. This suggests that allotype polymorphism may indeed offer selective advantages that are particularly important under conditions of very intensive selective pressures. A selective role of allotypes is also suggested by the finding of linkage disequilibrium between V_H and C_H allotypic genes; in a study of a fairly large population of domestic rabbits in Canada, the a^3; e^{14} haplotype was never found, even though e^{14} was found in coupling with other V_H allotypes. In the same population, an excess of double heterozygotes—namely, rabbits carrying a^1/a^2 and e^{14}/e^{15} alleles—was found.

Allotypes of the C_H portion of the immunoglobulin molecule may facilitate or regulate their biologic functions; those of the V_H portion or of light chains may be involved in antigen capture by cellular receptors or in binding of antigen by free immunoglobulin molecules. At present, the mechanisms of most of these regulatory influences can only be the subject of speculation. The charges of the antigen are known to determine the charge of the resulting antibody molecules. Antigen molecules are more likely to be captured by cellular receptors carrying charges opposite to those of the antigen than by receptors carrying charges similar to those of the antigen. Thus, antibody molecules formed in response to negatively charged antigens are predominantly positively charged and vice versa. Allotypic markers determine, to some extent, the charges of the immunoglobulin molecules; molecules carrying b4 markers are relatively heterogeneous in their charges as opposed to molecules carrying b9 markers, which are more homogeneous and relatively negatively charged as compared with b4 molecules. It was shown that, in response to negatively charged antigens b^4/b^4 homozygotes make significantly more antibody than b^9/b^9 homozygous rabbits, whereas there are no such quantitative differences in the response to positively charged antigens. Clearly, the heterogeneity of allotype-dependent charges of the cell surface receptors must be a factor that determines the probability of antigen capture by an individual cell and, consequently, the overall number of cells making antibody to a particular antigen.

In heterozygotes the allotypic alleles are usually unequally expressed on immunoglobulin molecules and on cell surface receptors. This phenomenon is known as the **pecking order**. For the alleles of the *Ab* series, the pecking order is:

$$b^4 > b^6 > b^5 > b^9 > b^{bas}.$$

It means that in any heterozygote the b^4 allele is always expressed on a larger proportion of molecules than the other allele. Conversely, in a b^{bas} heterozygote, the proportion of molecules carrying the bbas allotype is always smaller than the proportion of cells carrying the product of the other allele. The unequal expression of allotypic genes may be determined by differences in the probability of antigen capture, because the pecking order appears to develop under the control of environmental factors. For example, in very young b^4/b^9 heterozygotes, the proportions of cells bearing b4 and b9 surface immunoglobulins are equal; only as the animals grow older does the percentage of b4-positive cells increase until the b4:b9 ratio reaches 2.5, a value characteristic for adult b^4/b^9 heterozygotes.

Involvement of charges in the control of expression of b^4 and b^9 genes does not mean that the relative expression of other allotypic genes must also be determined by the same mechanism. By the same token, charges may not be the only mechanisms involved in determining the expression of b^4 and b^9 genes.

PHENOMENA RELATED TO ALLOTYPY

9.20 Allotype Suppression

Injection of newborn rabbits or mice with antiserum directed against their genetically determined allotype results in suppression of the synthesis of immunoglobulin bearing this allotype.

Rabbits that are successfully suppressed usually never recover the normal level of their synthetic ability. Suppression can be induced only during approximately the first two weeks of life, and only antibodies with an intact Fc portion of rabbit origin are effective in inducing suppression. Induction of suppression does not require the presence of a complete hemolytic complement system, since in mice it is possible to suppress animals that are deficient in C5. The presence of circulating immunoglobulins of the type being suppressed interferes with the induction of suppression. Because rabbits are born with relatively high concentrations of maternal immunoglobulins that have been transferred during fetal life, it is easier to induce suppression of the paternal, rather than the maternal, allotype. When the maternal transfer is reduced or eliminated either by using a suppressed heterozygous female as a mother or by transferring homozygous embryos into a foster mother, suppression can be induced even in homozygous animals.

Induction of suppression clearly involves the immature B cells, which display immuno-globulin receptors on their surface (e.g., mIgM) (Chapter 8). Rabbits are born with an immature immune system, and after the B cells have differentiated past the stage that is susceptible to suppression, injections of antiallotype serum have no effect. B cell mitogens that increase the rate of cell differentiation seem to shorten the period during which the young rabbits can be suppressed. Only markers of Fab and IgM—i.e., those that are part of the mIgM receptors—can be suppressed. Suppression of any one marker affects the entire linkage group, resulting in suppression of all other markers whose genes are in a *cis* position with respect to the gene coding for the suppressed allotype

The mechanism of induction of suppression has not yet been elucidated, but it is thought that the combination of antibody with Ig receptors provides a signal similar to that generated when immunological tolerance is induced. Conceivably, this signal, when transmitted to the interior of the affected B cells, arrests their differentiation. Once suppression is induced, it is then maintained by mechanisms that are not completely clear. A number of contributing mechanisms may be involved, the simplest one being competition between differentiating cells. Cells committed to the expression of the gene coding for the suppressed marker are arrested in their differentiation, while cells committed to the expression of the other allele are unhindered in their differentiation and soon populate the immune system, leaving no need and no space for the suppressed cells. Experimental support for this concept comes from an observation that partial recovery from suppression is triggered by X-irradiation. By destroying a proportion of cells in the immune system, irradiation stimulates cell differentiation and division. Subsequently, uncommitted, dormant stem cells are activated, and a proportion of them may commit themselves to the synthesis of the previously suppressed allotype. Hyperimmunization, as opposed to X-irradiation, does not lead to recovery from suppression and, therefore, must activate other cells already committed to this antigen.

The **allogeneic effect*** is instrumental in terminating suppression in mice; injection of parental type thymus cells into suppressed F1 mice results in an increased synthesis of the suppressed allotype. The mechanism of this phenomenon is not yet known.

---

*The allogeneic effect refers to a phenomenon of increased response in animals undergoing GVHR (Section 4.11).

A possibility that suppression might be maintained by the presence of specific suppressor T cells has been raised by experiments that employed (BALB/c × SJL) F1 hybrid mice. Normally, mice exposed to antiallotype antibodies develop suppression lasting for only 8-10 weeks. However, progeny of BALB/c females and SJL males exposed to antibodies directed against the Igh-1b allotype develop **chronic suppression**, which lasts for six months or more. Reconstitution of X-irradiated, chronically suppressed (BALB/c × SJL) F1 hybrids with spleen cells from normal BALB/c mice failed to terminate the suppression. When transferred into irradiated BALB/c recipients, spleen or bone marrow cells from suppressed F1 donors also failed to "release" the transferred cells from suppression. Finally, when the suppressed cells were transferred together with cells from normal donors of the genotype identical to that of the suppressed hybrids, they prevented normal cells from expressing the Igh-1b allotype. This suppressor activity is associated with T cells. However, the existence of this interesting regulatory mechanism can only be demonstrated in the above strain combination, and it affects only the Igh-1b allotype. Igh-4b, another allotype characteristic for the SJL strain, is not affected by this mechanism and can only be suppressed for short periods of time. It should be noted that SJL mice have a highly abnormal immune system, i.e., a high frequency of gammopathies and reticulum cell sarcomata, an enlargment of lymph nodes, a low tolerance inducibility owing to insufficient suppressor cell capacity, etc. Chronic allotypic suppression may be caused by the same defects in the regulatory mechanisms controlling the immune system that are responsible for the other abnormalities.

9.21 Crossing-over and Somatic Recombination

The large number of markers belonging to the rabbit heavy chain linkage group makes this species an ideal subject to study the frequency of recombinations. Although specially intended studies have never been done, the recombinations between V_H genes encoding Aa and C_H genes determining Ad and Ae allotypes have been observed and are well documented. The estimated frequency of recombinations between V_H and C_H genes is 0.003 (0.3 percent).

Normally, the allotypes present on a given heavy chain correspond to either the maternal or the paternal haplotype, since the V_H and C_H genes are expressed in *cis* configuration. However, approximately one percent of circulating immunoglobulins express the V_H and C_H genes in *trans* configuration, so that one heavy chain carries a maternal V_H and a paternal C_H portion, or vice versa. This phenomenon was first recognized qualitatively, then confirmed by intracellular flourescent staining of immunoglobulins and by isolation of recombinant molecules from serum. The mechanism of this somatic recombination phenomenon and its importance remain obscure.

Recently, it has been shown that the concentrations of such recombinant molecules may increase as a result of a **transchromosomal allotype suppression**, i.e., suppression by antibodies directed against maternal V_H *and* paternal C_H allotypes (or vice versa). For instance, in one report a rabbit of the genotype $a^1; e^{15}; n^{81}/a^2; e^{14}; n^{80}$ was exposed to anti-a2 and anti-n81 antibodies. As a result of this treatment, the ratio of recombinant (i.e., a1-e14) to normal (i.e., a1-e15) immunoglobulin molecules was higher than that observed in untreated heterozygotes.

9.22 Allelic Exclusion

As it was discussed in Chapters 7 and 8, according to the clonal selection theory, each antibody-producing cell commits itself to the synthesis of antibody of only one specificity. This crucial postulate has been tested and confirmed by a number of ingenious single-cell experiments and by studies of myeloma proteins. To translate this tenet into genetic terms, one may say that the one cell-one antibody postulate requires that only one haplotype, out of the two that code for each of the immunoglobulin chains, can be expressed in any one single cell. This mechanism is known as allelic exclusion.

Allelic exclusion has also been demonstrated for genes located on the X chromosome, but immunoglobulin synthesis remains a unique case of **autosomal allelic exclusion**. In a number of synthetic events controlled by autosomal genes, the absence of allelic exclusion has been clearly demonstrated. For instance, in a person heterozygous for an abnormal hemoglobin gene, individual red blood cells have been shown to synthesize both normal and abnormal hemoglobin molecules.

In view of the confirmed linkage between idiotypic markers of the hypervariable portion of the immunoglobulin chain and the genes controlling the variable and constant portions of this chain (Section 8.3), one would expect allelic exclusion not to be limited to the antigen-combining site but also to affect allotypic specificities. Thus, one cell would be expected to display membrane immunoglobulin receptors (mIg) and to secrete immunoglobulin molecules (sIg) that carry only one allotypic marker from each group. There is overwhelming evidence in favor of this view. However, there are a few reports claiming that a proportion of cells may either display membrane immunoglobulin or secrete immunoglobulin molecules with markers that are products of two mutually exclusive haplotypes. At least some of these findings cannot be dismissed as merely being due to technical errors. Until recently, these reports have been describing "double producer" cells that carried or released markers controlled by nominal genes, i.e., genes transmitted from the parents in a Mendelian fashion. Recently, however, a new dimension has been added to his problem; now double producer cells have been described that carry both nominal and latent allotypic markers.

It seems likely that a B cell, during its differentiation, might go through stages in which it is a double producer of membrane receptors or even of circulating immunoglobulin molecules. However, it is almost certain that allelic exclusion is operative during most of the cell's period of synthetic activity.

10 / Idiotypy

THE CONCEPT OF IDIOTYPY

10.1 Definition and Detection of Idiotypes

The unique configuration of the antigen-combining site determines not only its specificity for antigen binding but also its own antigenic specificity. Therefore, it is possible to raise antibodies directed against the antigen-combining site of an antibody molecule. As expected, such anti-antibodies are of unique specificity and react only with antibody molecules that carry antigen-combining sites of the appropriate configuration. Some of these antibodies may inhibit binding of antigen by their target antibodies; others do not have such inhibitory capacity. This inhibitory effect, as in reactions between antienzymes, enzymes, and substrates, depends on the spatial relationship between the reactants and on the localization of the antigenic determinant (the target of the anti-antibody) in relation to that part of the hypervariable portion that actually comes in close contact with the antigen molecule or particle.

Engendering anti-antibodies, as defined above, was an elusive dream of the early immunologists, a dream that became a reality in the early 1960s when attempts in raising such antibodies finally succeeded and showed that antibody molecules, indeed, possess individually specific antigenic determinants associated with their antigen-combining sites. At the same time, it became clear that the antigenic individuality of myeloma proteins must also reflect the individuality of their antigen-combining sites (Section 7.1). The term idiotype or idiotypic specificity was coined for those individually specific determinants that reflect the unique configuration of the antigen-combining site. Anti-antibodies were consequently named **anti-idiotypes** or **anti-idiotypic** antibodies. This, fortunately, ended a confusion, since the term **anti-antibody** was originally used to define antibodies to those conformational determinants that appear on antibody molecules as the result of the antibodies' combination with the antigen.

Anti-idiotypic antibodies can be raised by xeno-, allo-, and autoimmunization. Sera containing antibodies of heterologous origin raised by xenoimmunization with a myeloma protein usually have to be absorbed with other myeloma proteins and/or normal immunoglobulins. After such an absorption, residual antibodies, with rare exceptions, react only with the myeloma protein used as an immunogen. Isologous anti-idiotypic antibodies are best raised by injections of antigen-antibody complexes into an allotypically matched recipient. Usually, such immune sera do not require any absorption. Autologous anti-idiotypic antibodies can be raised by a two-step procedure. First, an animal is injected with an antigen, and the serum is collected and antibody purified. Next, the animal is rested until the antibodies are no longer detectable in the circulation. At this moment, the second phase, immunization with autologous antibody, preferably in the form of antigen-antibody complexes, can be initiated, and it usually leads to the formation of auto-anti-idiotypic antibodies. Auto-anti-idiotypic antibodies are formed in the course of immunization with some antigens and were shown to coexist with antibodies in the circulation, partly in the form of antigen-antibody complexes. Monoclonal anti-idiotypic antibodies can be produced using the hybridoma technique (Section 4.9).

10.2 Time-Related Changes in the Synthesis of Idiotype

Prolonged and frequent exposure of immunocompetent cells to an antigen may lead to exhaustion of old clones and subsequently to stimulation of new clones. Such **clonal replacement** is reflected in the changes in idiotypes or **idiotype replacement**. This has been shown by raising two anti-idiotypic antibodies of different specificities directed against antibodies made by the same rabbit that had been immunized for a period of more than 17 months, always with the same antigen. One anti-idiotype was raised by immunization with "early" antibodies obtained two months after the start of immunization; the other, by immunization with "late" antibodies obtained eight months after the start of immunization. Concentrations of early and late idiotypes were then measured in a number of antibody samples taken from the same animal during the course of immunization. The early idiotype was present only in the first three samples (obtained two, three, and four months after the start of immunization). The fourth sample contained only traces of the early idiotype. The late idiotype, on the other hand, could not be detected in the first three samples but was present in all subsequent bleedings. Clone and idiotype replacement appear to be much slower if the animal is immunized less frequently: a major idiotype formed during the first series of immunizations was still present in bleedings taken a year or two later, after a second series of immunizations, if the animal was allowed to rest during the intervening period.

CHARACTERIZATION OF IDIOTYPES

10.3 Specificity and Cross-Reactivity of Idiotypes

The specificity of anti-idiotypic antibodies—and, thus, of idiotypes—should be discussed in terms of the specificity and heterogeneity of the antigen-combining sites. Stimulation, with even the simplest antigen carrying only a minimum number of determinants, results in an antibody response of considerable heterogeneity, i.e. in the synthesis of a wide range of antibody molecules of different specificities and affinities. Consequently, even antibodies directed against a single determinant will carry a large number of different idiotypes. On the other hand, one hypervariable region may be used for the assembly of more than one antigen-combining site. As a consequence, antibodies directed against seemingly unrelated antigens may show idiotypic similarities. The above general conclusions are based on a large body of experimental evidence, some of which is summarized in the following.

Rabbit anti-idiotypic antibodies show an astounding specificity; ordinarily, these antibodies do not react with other normal immunoglobulins of the donor animal, with antibodies of another specificity raised in the same donor animal, or with antibodies of the same specificity but raised in different individuals, even though these animals may be close relatives, siblings, or offspring of the donor animal. However, cross-reacting idiotypes occasionally do appear. Usually, these are carried by antibodies that are identical in their specificity with the immunizing antibodies and are likely to appear in rabbits genetically related to the donor of the immunizing antibody.

In mice cross-reacting or even identical idiotypes can be raised regularly in individuals of the same inbred strain. Antibodies raised in BALB/c mice by injections of killed rough pneumococci react with the phosphorylcholine (PC) determinant and carry a major idiotype that is designated T15. A myeloma tumor (TEPC15) that originated in the BALB/c strain was found to secrete immunoglobulins with PC-binding activity. Amazingly, this myeloma protein was found to carry the idiotype characteristic for the anti-PC antibodies raised in BALB/c mice. The T15 idiotype is also present in low concentration in the normal sera of BALB/c mice, probably as a consequence of exposure to environmental antigens. Another idiotype, U10-173, is characteristic for both natural and immune antibodies against levan from *Aerobacter levanicum* and for myeloma protein that binds levan. Since U10-173 is present on approximately 1 percent of normal immunoglobulin, it may be associated with a framework rather than with a hypervariable sequence of the variable region. Idiotype J558 is characteristic for antidextran antibodies and for myeloma protein that binds dextran.

Another classic example of cross-reacting idiotype is the ARS idiotype carried by anti-*p*-azophenylarsonate (anti-Ar) antibodies raised in A/J mice immunized with Ar conjugated with keyhole limpet hemocyanin (KLH). All immunized A/J mice express this idiotype, which is found on 30 to 70 percent of the antibody molecules. Similarly, A/J mice immunized with group A streptococcal polysaccharide (S-A-CHO) synthesize antibodies carrying a major idiotype called A5A. Immunization of BALB/c mice with S-A-CHO results in the appearance of another idiotype, S117. Two other idiotypes, A5Acr and S117cr, that are raised in different strains and considered distinct entities are antigenically similar to A5A and S117, respectively. Another idiotype in this group has been designated as ACH^d and has been raised in AKR mice. Several established idiotypes are listed in Table 10.1.

10.4 Idiotypes Associated with Antibody Affinity

The idiotypes discussed above were characterized by their unique antigenic determinants and were detected by anti-idiotypic antisera raised in rabbits, guinea pigs, or mice. A number of other idiotypes (Table 10.1) are characterized by the differences in their affinities against the homologous or the cross-reacting antigen. Affinity is the basis for classification of antibodies against *p*-azobenzenearsonate coupled to the carbon atom 5 of hydroxyphenylacetic acid (ABA-HOP) as well as antibodies against [(4-hydroxy-5-bromo-3-nitrophenyl)acetyl] (NBrP). Differences in affinities of antibodies raised in different strains can be as large as 100-fold. Antibody titers and the relative affinities are used to calculate **fine specificity indices** (FSI), which are characteristic for the producer strain and for the idiotype. Upon immunization with hydroxy-3-nitrophenyl (NP), C57BL mice make **heteroclitic** antibodies, i.e. antibodies whose affinity toward the related compound is higher than the affinity for the immunizing antigen (NP).

10.5 Idiotypes Associated with Antibody Specificity

Some idiotypes are defined by the specificity of the antibodies raised against certain antigens. Some inbred strains of mice, when immunized with staphylococcal nuclease, make antibodies

TABLE 10.1. Mouse Idiotypes

Idiotype Designation	Antigen	Method of Detection	Reference Immunoglobulin	Reference Strain	Locus Designation
ABA-HOP-b	ABA-HOP	AFF	SA	C57BL/6	Igh-Aa1
ABA-HOP-c	ABA-HOP	AFF	SA	A/J	Igh-Aa2
ABA-HOP-j	ABA-HOP	AFF	SA	CBA/H	Igh-Aa3
ARS	Arsanyl-p	ID	SA	A/J	Igh-Ars
J558	α-1,3-dextran	ID,Q	MP	BALB/c	Igh-Dex
Inuldx	Inulin	SP	MP	BALB/c	Igh-Inu
U10-173	Levan	ID*	MP	BALB/c	Igh-Lev
NBrP-a	NBrP	AFF	SA	BALB/c	Igh-Nbp
NP	NP	AFF	SA	C57BL/6	Igh-Np
Nase-A	Nuclease (1–99)	SP,ID	SA	A/J	Igh-Ns1
Nase-B	Nuclease (1–99)	SP,ID	SA	SJL	Igh-Ns2
Nase-C	Nuclease (1–99)	SP,ID	SA	C57BL/10	Igh-Ns3
Nase-D	Nuclease (99–149)	SP,ID	SA	A/J	Igh-Ns4
Nase-E	Nuclease (99–149)	SP,ID	SA	SJL	Igh-Ns5
T15	PC	ID*	MP	BALB/c	Igh-Pc
A5A	S-A-CHO	ID	SA	A/J	Igh-Sa1
A5Acr**	S-A-CHO	ID	SA	C57L	Igh-Sa2
S117	S-A-CHO	ID	MP	BALB/c	Igh-Sa3
S117cr**	S-A-CHO	ID	MP	DBA/2	Igh-Sa4
ACH[d]	S-A-CHO	ID	SA	AKR	Igh-Sa5
ESE	SRBC	SP	SA	C57BL/6	Igh-Src

*Immunoglobulin carrying this idiotype is also present in low concentrations in normal sera.
**A5 Acr and S117 cr idiotypes cross-react weekly with A5A and S117, respectively.

The notation used in Tables 10.1–10.3 has been proposed under the aegis of the Committee on Standardized Genetic Nomenclature for Mice and recommended by a group of scientists, Immunogenetics, **8**:89, 1979.

NOTES: Antigens: ABA-HOP = p-azobenzenearsonate coupled to the carbon atom 5 of hydroxyphenylacetic acid; arsanyl-p = azophenylarsonate; inulin = β-2,1-fructosan; levan = from *Aerobacter levanicum*; NBrP = [(4-hydroxy-5-bromo-3-nitrophenyl)acetyl]; nuclease (1-99) or nuclease (99-149) = staphylococcal nuclease fragments comprising amino acid residues 1–99 or 99–149, respectively; PC = phosphorylcholine; S-A-CHO = group A streptococcal carbohydrate; SRBC = sheep red blood cells. Reference immunoglobulins: SA = serum antibody: MP = myeloma protein. Method of detection: AFF = differences in affinity of antibodies; ID = anti-idiotype antibody; Q = differences in the quantity of antibodies; SP = differences in the specificity of antibodies.

that react with the peptide comprised of the first 99 amino acid residues; the antibodies raised in other strains react with the peptide comprised of the residues 99-149. These genetically controlled strain-related differences are the basis of defining five different Nase idiotypes (Table 10.1). Another idiotype, ESE, is defined by the specificity of antibodies raised by immunization with sheep red blood cells. C57BL/6 mice are able to make antibodies to "extra" antigens found on red blood cells only from some sheep, whereas other strains are able to respond only to antigens normally present on all sheep red blood cells, irrespective of the origin of the red cells.

10.6 Antigenic Complexity of Idiotypic Determinants

With accumulation of more data, the previous concept of idiotype as representing a unique configuration of the antigen-binding site has had to be somewhat modified. The same idiotype can be raised by immunization of mice of different strains. Some idiotypes, e.g., A5A, are limited to only a few closely related strains; others, e.g., U10-173, are found widely distributed among many inbred strains (Table 10.2). Thus, anti-A5A detects only a small number of determinants specific exclusively for anti-S-A-CHO antibodies, whereas antibody to U10-173 idiotype most likely recognizes determinants common to a number of distinct antibodies specific for a group of related antigens, perhaps even framework determinants. This does not exclude the possibility that U10-173 in addition to the "public" determinants also possesses some "private," idiotypic, in the strict sense, determinants. The detection of the latter is made difficult by the presence of public determinants.

The existence of public idiotypic determinants has actually been documented for human cold agglutinins of the IgM class. These antibodies were also shown to have, in addition to their private idiotypic determinants, cross-reacting idiotypes shared by all antibodies of this category. This also seems to be true for IgM from patients with Waldenström's macro-globulinemia* and for IgM with anti-IgG activity present in patients with rheumatoid arthritis (Section 9.1).

So far, idiotypes have been discussed as antigenic determinants that reflect the configuration of the antigen-binding site or some other V_H structures that are intimately related to this site and to its specificity. However, antibodies of completely different specificity can carry similar or identical idiotypes. For example, it is possible to split an ovalbumin molecule into two fragments, each containing a different and non-cross-reacting determinant. Immunization of rabbits with the native ovalbumin results in the formation of antibodies directed against both fragments. These antibodies, in spite of the apparent differences in their specificities, share the same idiotype. The same idiotype is also found on immunoglobulins that have formed as a result of immunization with ovalbumin but that lack any specificity for this antigen. It must be stressed that although the antiovalbumin idiotype fulfills all the criteria for an idiotype, it is not detected in sera obtained prior to immunization and it is individual-specific.

STRUCTURAL BASIS OF IDIOTYPY

From their close correlation with antibody specificity, one would expect that idiotypic determinants are localized on the variable portion of the immunoglobulin molecule and determined by the variable sequences. This is, indeed, the case. However, it has not been possible to associate unequivocally idiotypic specificities with either H or L chains alone. In general, most idiotypic reactivity is associated with an intact antibody molecule. Isolated H and L chains react with anti-idiotypic antibody less strongly, or sometimes not at all. Apparently, upon separation of the H and L chains, some idiotypic determinants are lost. It is not yet known whether these

---

*Waldenström's macroglobulinemia is a neoplastic proliferation of plasma cells producing mono-clonal IgM. It is thus analogous to multiple myeloma producing monoclonal IgG or other immunoglobulins.

TABLE 10.2. Strain Distribution of Murine Idiotypes

Strain	Igh-C Haplotype	ABA-HOP	ARS	J558	Inuldx	U10-173	NBrP-a	NP	Nase	T15	A5A	A5Acr	S117	S117cr	ESE
BALB/c	a	b	–	+	+	+	+	–	A,B,D	+	–	–	+	–	–
129	a		–	+	+	+				+	–	–	+		+
C58	a			+	+	+				+	–	–	+		
C57L	a			+	+	+	+(?)			+	–	+	+		
ST	a			+			+(?)			+					+
IAH	a			+			+(?)								
CBA	a	j	–	–	+	–								–	+
C3H	a	j	–	–	+	–				–				–	–
C57Br	a		–	+	+	+									+
MA	a			+											
A/J	e	c	+	–	+	+	+(?)		A,D		+		–		–
A/He	e		+	–							+		–		–
A/WySn	e		+												
NZB	e		–			+									+
AL/N	d		+		+	+									
AKR	d		–			–	–								+
C57BL/6	b	b	–			+	–	+		–	–		–	–	+
C57BL/10	b						–	+					–	–	+
C57BL/Ka	b						–	+							+
C57BL/Ks	b						–	+							
SJL	b	b				+	–		B,E						+
LP	b					+	–	+							+
SM	b														
DBA/1	c													+	–
DBA/2	c		–	–	–	+	+(?)	–				+		+	–
RF	c			+	+	+	+(?)					+		+	
SWR	c		–	–							–				
CE	f		–	–		+	+(?)								–

+ = Immunization with an appropriate antigen results in the production of a given idiotype.

– = Animals of a given strain are unable to raise antibodies that carry this idiotype.

Blank space = The strain has not been tested for its ability to produce the idiotype.

NOTES: For characterization of idiotypes, see Table 10.1. In ABA-HOP and Nase idiotypes, the letters identify the idiotype produced as a result of immunization with an appropriate antigen.

determinants depend on specific amino acid sequences of H, of L, or of both chains (see the discussion of "conformational" allotypic determinants in Section 9.11). In most cases, the idiotypic determinants can be restored by recombination of homologous H and L chains, but in some experiments, the recombination of H chains with nonspecific L chains, or vice versa, also results in restoration of some of the original idiotypes.

One of the goals of molecular immunology is the breaking of the "immunologic code," i.e., assigning particular hypervariable sequences to antibody specificities. Since immunization with even a very simple antigen results in a highly heterogeneous antibody response, this goal cannot be achieved by straightforward sequence analyses. From the preceding considerations, it is clear that at least some idiotypes are intimately related to the antigen-binding property of the antibodies and, consequently, to the structure of the hypervariable regions. Thus, one can expect that antibodies of the same specificity that share an identical idiotype will very likely have one or more hypervariable regions in common. This indeed, seems to be the case, although a true "dictionary" of the immunologic code is still very far away.

Sequence analysis of idiotype-specific antibodies of the ARS system has shown that their variable regions of heavy chains are homogeneous. While some of the framework sequences are similar to those of the ARS-negative anti-Ar antibodies, the hypervariable regions of the ARS-positive antibodies are unique and specific. The light chains of the ARS-positive antibodies show some differences, but only within the framework structures. Their hypervariable sequences are identical. ARS-positive anti-Ar antibodies uniformly belong to only one immunoglobulin subclass, IgG1. Thus, in the ARS system, the idiotype is associated with more than one framework structure, but with only one constant heavy chain region. This, however, does not seem to be a general rule, since an idiotype, unique for rabbit antibodies against *Salmonella typhi*, was found in association with both IgG and IgM classes. Similarly, an idiotype characteristic for group C streptococcal carbohydrate in an individual rabbit was found associated with two different variable regions, one carrying the heavy chain a3 allotypic marker, the second being the 'alternative', 'a-negative' variable portion (Section 9.13).

10.7 Idiotypes of Monoclonal Antibodies

Although the conventional immune response is known to be extremely heterogeneous, only a major idiotype can be detected and characterized in any one antiserum. Many minor idiotypes, also present in the antiserum, escape detection because each of them is expressed only on a small proportion of antibody molecules. In idiotype suppression (Section 10.9), some of these minor idiotypes compensate for the loss of the suppressed major idiotype and become expressed on a larger proportion of antibody molecules, which allows for their detection and characterization. An idiotype is defined by its reaction with an anti-idiotype, and, therefore, what is regarded as a major idiotype may in fact be a collection of fairly heterogeneous molecules that share only one idiotypic determinant. Because of these limitations of conventional antibodies, the deciphering of the immunologic code may only be possible if the studies are extended to monoclonal antibodies. Monoclonal antibodies may express any idiotype, even a minor one that cannot normally be detected in serum. This and the fact that each hybridoma line produces homogeneous antibody molecules make monoclonal antibodies an almost ideal model for the study of the structural basis of antibody specificity and of idiotypy. One can expect that by the monoclonal antibody technique a whole array of idiotypic specificities can be obtained in a system where conventional immunization normally results in the formation of only one major idiotype.

Several Ar-binding and dextran-binding hybridomas have been studied. In both systems, new idiotypes not detected by conventional immunization have been encountered. It is clear that some hybridomas possess truly unique determinants, while some others share determinants with other hybridomas. This heterogeneity is reflected in the heterogeneity of amino acid sequences.

In the antidextran system, the individual idiotypic specificity (called IdI) seems to be determined by amino acid residues at positions 100 and 101 (located within the third hypervariable region of the heavy chain). Two hybridomas that carry identical or similar idiotypes may have identical residues at these two positions. A difference in one of the two residues may result either in a complete loss of the idiotype or in possession of an antigenically similar idiotype.

Positions 54 and 55, located within the second hypervariable region, seem to determine the presence or absence of a determinant called IdX. IdX can be detected in a majority of dextran-binding hybridomas and is correlated with the presence of a carbohydrate moiety that attaches itself to the heavy chain at position 55. Substitution at this position destroys the attachment site for the carbohydrate. Thus, it is possible that IdX is in fact determined by the carbohydrate moiety itself. The first hypervariable regions of the heavy chains as well as the entire light chains of all dextran-binding hybridomas appear to be identical. Therefore, it would be attractive to think that the light chain and the first hypervariable region of the heavy chain control the gross specificity of the antibody molecule, whereas the second and the third hypervariable regions control the more subtle differences of antibody, and of idiotypic, specificity.

GENETICS OF MURINE IDIOTYPES

The first reports on idiotypes stressed their unique nature. An idiotype raised in one animal could not be duplicated in another individual, even when the same antigen was used and the two animals were closely related. These initial observations did not support the possibility of genetic control over idiotypes. Later, however, it was observed that mice of the same inbred strain may develop identical or very similar cross-reactive idiotypes (CRI). Similarly, closely related rabbits immunized with specially chosen antigens may develop, although infrequently, cross-reacting idiotypes associated with the heavy chain allotypes. These findings provided the necessary stimulus for genetic studies.

Today, practically all of the information on the genetic control of idiotypes is based on studies in inbred strains of mice (Table 10.1). All idiotypic determinants are encoded by genes of the heavy chain linkage group and are linked to the Igh-C genes, which are identifiable by allotypes (Section 9.7, Table 9.5). A linkage disequilibrium (Section 1.5) between Igh-C and Igh-V genes is reflected in the finding that in different strains the same idiotypes are associated with different Igh-C phenotypes. This also indicates that the linkage between the V_H and C_H genes is weaker than that between various genes of the *Igh-C* haplotype.

In similarity to the genes controlling allotypic determinants, genes that encode idiotypes seem to be codominant and can be expressed in the heterozygotes. It has been assumed that each idiotype is controlled by a gene at a specific locus (Table 10.1), although this has been shown for only a few idiotypes. Some idiotypes might be controlled by allelic genes, but it is a general feeling that this may well be an exception rather than a rule. The V_H segment, compared with its C_H equivalent, is much longer and therefore more likely to be subject to recombination. As a result of chromosomal rearrangements, the length of the chromosomal fragments and the relative positions of various loci may not be identical in different strains of mice. As a consequence of this instability, no truly allelic idiotypic genes may ever be found. So far at least three recombination events have been documented. Analysis of one of the recombinant strains is summarized in Table 10.3. Information provided by analyses of the recombinant strains may be used for construction of the following tentative genetic map:

$$A5A - A5Acr - ARS - T15 - Igh\text{-}C - Pre*$$

ABA-HOP	*NP*	*J558*
ESE	*NBrP*	*S117*
	Inuldx	

10.8 The Role of Light Chains

Experiments on the structure of idiotypes show that light chains frequently contribute to the expression of the idiotype. However, in genetic studies association has only been established between the idiotypes and C_H loci. This apparent paradox was resolved when it was shown that the ARS idiotype can only be expressed in the presence of one particular type of light chain, the occurrence of which is correlated with the presence of the *Igk-Trp*^{b}, but not the *Igk-Trp*^{a}, allele of the *Igk-V* gene (Section 9.7, Table 9.5). The *Igk-Trp*^{a} allele controls the presence of, and *Igk-Trp*^{b} the absence of, the I_B peptide demonstrable after tryptic digestion of light chains. All strains except AKR, RF, PL, and C58 carry the *Igk-Trp*^{b} allele. In studies in which both parental strains are homozygous with respect to *Igk-Trp*^{b}, only the requirement of the heavy chain gene for the expression of the idiotype is apparent. The requirement for the I_B-negative light chain (its presence being determined by the *Igk-Trp*^{b} allele) can be shown only if A/J mice (*Igh-Ars*$^+$/*Igh-Ars*$^+$ and *Igk-Trp*^{b}/*Igk-Trp*^{b} double homozygotes) are mated with PL or C58 mice (*Igh-Ars*$^-$/*Igh-Ars*$^-$ and *Igk-Trp*^{a}/*Igk-Trp*^{a} double homozygotes). Those of the F2 progeny that lack *Igk-Trp*^{b} do not express ARS even if they possess the heavy chain gene, *Igh-Ars*$^+$. Thus, it appears that light chain genes are required for the expression of idiotypes in mice; however, these requirements appear much less specific than those for the heavy chain genes because of the similarities of light chain gene repertoires in many strains of mice.

---

*The *Pre* gene controls polymorphism of the prealbumin.

TABLE 10.3. Recombination between Idiotypic and Allotypic Loci in the Heavy Chain Chromosomal Region

Strain	Idiotype						Igh haplotype	Pre*
P1 A/J	**A5A**	**ABA-HOP**	**ARS**	—	—	—	*Igh-1e*	o
P2 BALB/c	—	—	—	S117	J558	T15	*Igh-1a*	a
R BB7	**A5A**	**ABA-HOP**	—	S117	J558	T15	*Igh-1a*	a

P1 and P2 = Parental strains.
R = Recombinant individual.
Pre gene controls prealbumin polymorphism in serum.
NOTES: Markers characteristics for the A/J mice are printed in bold face. The vertical line indicates the location of the crossing-over.

IDIOTYPE SUPPRESSION

10.9 Conditions for Inducing Idiotype Suppression

Expression of idiotypes, like expression of allotypes, can be suppressed by the administration of antibodies of the appropriate specificity. Anti-idiotype antibodies of mouse and rabbit origin have been successfully used to induce **idiotype suppression** in mice. Guinea pig antibodies of the IgG2 subclass are also capable of inducing idiotype suppression in mice, whereas guinea pig anti-idiotype antibodies of the IgG1 subclass enhance idiotype expression. It must be noted that in contrast to IgG2 guinea pig IgG1 antibodies are incapable of activating the classical complement sequence and of adhering to macrophages.

There is no reason to assume that the mechanism of idiotype suppression differs qualitatively from the mechanism of allotype suppression (Section 9.20). In allotype suppression, it is believed that combination of the suppressing antibody with the cell surface receptor arrests the differentiation of the affected cell. After the cell passes the critical period, during which its differentiation can be arrested, it can no longer be suppressed. In both rabbit and mouse, cells producing natural antibodies differentiate shortly after birth. This seems to be responsible for the differences in susceptibility to induction of suppression between neonatal and adult animals. Mice do not make natural antibodies to Ar, so even in adult animals the differentiation of anti-Ar cells has not progressed past the critical stage beyond which suppression by antibody is impossible. Indeed, suppression of the ARS idiotype can be successfully induced in adult animals. It was mentioned before that small quantities of natural antibodies bind levan and phosphorylcholine (PC) and carry idiotypes U10-173 and T15, respectively. Thus, cells with antilevan and anti-PC receptors must differentiate early after birth. Consequently, suppression of the T15 idiotype can only be induced in neonatal animals. If the above reasoning is correct, one would expect that induction of suppression of the U10-173 idiotype is also possible only in neonates.

The suppression of idiotypes in mice lasts considerably longer than allotype suppression and can be reinforced by subsequent contact with the antigen, which should occur preferably two weeks or more after the injection of the anti-idiotype. Suppression can also affect the expression of an idiotype in the antibodies produced as a result of a secondary challenge with antigen.

The effect of the exposure to the anti-idiotype can only be assessed after challenge with an antigen. In most systems, the major (predominant) idiotype is carried only by a proportion of antibody molecules (usually 20 to 70 percent but sometimes as much as 90 percent). Also, suppression of a given idiotype does not interfere with the ability to synthesize antibodies against the immunizing antigen. In all successfully suppressed animals, after challenge with an antigen only the major idiotype is not detectable in the serum. However, suppression of the T15 idiotype abolishes not only the ability to produce this particular idiotype but also the ability to make antibodies to PC.

In the ARS idiotypic system, an attempt was made to characterize the idiotypes of anti-Ar antibodies raised in mice after the ability to synthesize the major ARS idiotype had been suppressed. It appeared that after the suppression of the major ARS idiotype each animal compensated by making its own, "private" idiotype. Thus, A/J mice are capable of producing anti-Ar antibodies with a very broad spectrum of idiotypic specificities, but, for some reason, the entire spectrum is never expressed in a normal individual; instead, the "major" idiotype ARS is expressed on most antibody molecules. When the ability to synthesize this preferred idiotype is suppressed, the remaining idiotypes have approximately equal chances of being expressed, so that in each mouse a different clone may be activated with equal probability. It remains to be seen whether this type of compensation is also characteristic for other idiotypic systems.

In an inbred strain of mice, the synthesis of a given idiotype, after an injection of certain antigens, is highly predictable. Thus, evaluation of the effects of the suppressing antibody is relatively simple. In the rabbit, however, the specificity of the idiotype produced as a result of antigenic stimulation cannot be predicted. Therefore, it is impossible to prepare the suppressing antibody ahead of time. This difficulty in inducing idiotype suppression in rabbits has been cirumvented in the following experiment. Several rabbits were immunized with *Salmonella* organisms. Antisera from individual animals were collected, and individual anti-idiotype antisera were prepared. After a 10-month rest period, during which no antigen was administered, the experimental rabbits were injected with antiserum directed against their own idiotype, and after three weeks they were challenged with the same strain of *Salmonella* organisms. The control rabbits that did not receive anti-idiotype antiserum were similarly challenged with the same *Salmonella* preparation. Sera from the experimental rabbits taken after the antigenic challenge did not contain the original idiotype that was present after the initial immunization and could be detected by the specific anti-idiotype antibody. Notably, sera from control rabbits did contain their respective original idiotypes. By repeating the experimental procedure (and raising an anti-idiotype antibody against the second idiotype), it was also possible to suppress the idiotype formed as a result of the second challenge with the immunogen. In these experiments, idiotype suppression lasted for the life of the animal.

10.10 The Mechanism of Idiotype Suppression

The mechanism of idiotype suppression in mice appears to be analogous to the mechanism of chronic allotype suppression (Section 9.20). Similar to allotype suppression, idiotype suppression may be induced by transfer of cells from a suppressed to a normal recipient. Immunization of the suppressed donor with the appropriate antigen is essential; the X-irradiation of the recipient is not necessary. Induction of suppression by cell transfer is a rather slow process; a period of six weeks is required between the cell transfer and the antigenic challenge of the recipient. Suppression can be serially transferred to as many as four successive recipients by immunizing the recipient with the antigen and then transferring its cells into the next recipient.

Recent studies on suppression in the ARS idiotypic system have revealed very interesting cellular mechanisms. Suppression of the ARS idiotype results in (1) a failure to synthesize circulating antibodies carrying the major ARS idiotype and (2) the suppression of the cell-mediated delayed hypersensitivity response to the p-azophenylarsonate (Ar) haptenic group. Whereas in the humoral response suppression affects only the synthesis of antibody molecules carrying the ARS idiotype, and does not affect the antibody response to Ar, in a cell-mediated response the suppression is manifested by a greatly diminished delayed hypersensitivity response. Both the cellular response and the synthesis of circulating antibodies with the ARS idiotype were found to be regulated by two types of suppressor T cells, T_{s1} and T_{s2}. Both types of cells can be generated by injection of anti-idiotypic antibody, followed by immunization with the antigen; however, T_{s1} cells are induced by the anti-idiotype, while T_{s2} cells are elicited by T_{s1} cells rather than by the anti-idiotype. Apparently, T_{s1} cells carry the idiotype, whereas T_{s2} cells have anti-idiotype, through which T_{s2} cells may directly interact with the cell surface idiotypes of T and B cells and induce the suppression. Most recent results indicate that an interaction of a third cell, T_{s3}, with T_{s2} may be required for suppression. A T_{s3} cell possesses idiotype determinants and requires both the ligand and the T_{s2} cell (or its product) for expression. Once activated, T_{s3} cells may be idiotype and antigen nonspecific.

The situation is further complicated by the possibility that two different suppression pathways exist: in the first pathway, described above, T_{s1} is idiotypic, T_{s2} is anti-idiotypic, and T_{s3} is idiotypic. In the second pathway, T_{s1} appears to be anti-idiotypic, T_{s2} idiotypic, and T_{s3} is anti-idiotypic. The second pathway would affect an idiotype-bearing effector cell and thus should be idiotype specific.

T_{s1} and T_{s2} cells release effector molecules (factors), TsF_1 and TsF_2, respectively (Table 10.4). The two factors are very similar in their properties except that TsF_1 carries idiotype determinants and TsF_2 carries anti-idiotype. The factors are not conventional antibodies because (1) no other determinants characteristic for immunoglobulin molecules are associated with either of them, (2) the generation of TsF_1 does not require the presence of the *Igk-Trp^b* allele that is required for the expression of the ARS idiotype, and (3) the TsF possess antigenic determinants controlled by the *I–J* subregion of the mouse MHC (Section 16.16). The spatial relationship between the idiotype or anti-idiotype, on the one hand, and the I-J determinants, on the other, is still unresolved. One would expect that the suppressor factor should consist of more than one polypeptide chain since it carries products of two completely unrelated genes located on two different chromosomes. However, recent but unconfirmed studies found both the *H-2* encoded determinants and the antigen-binding site on a single polypeptide chain. A hybridoma cell line that produces TsF_1 has recently been obtained.

T_{s2} and TsF_2 may also be induced by injection of lymphocytes conjugated in vitro with idiotype-carrying immunoglobulin molecules. Apparently, the recognition mechanism cannot discriminate between naturally induced idiotypes of T_{s1} cells and artificially created "decoy" determinants.

TABLE 10.4. Properties of Suppressor Cells and Suppressor Factors in the ARS Idiotype
System

Factor or Cell	Property
T_{s1}	Induced by injection of anti-idiotype serum or by i.v. injection of lymphocytes conjugated with Ar; T-derived; effect abolished by treatment with anti-Thy-1.2; has Lyt-1 $^{+}2.3^{-}$ characteristics; possesses idiotypic determinants; generates or releases TsF_1 (probably receptor of T_{s1})
TsF_1	Possesses idiotypic determinants; possesses antigenic determinants controlled by the *I-J* subregion of the *H-2* MHC; molecular weight = 33,00–100,000; induces formation of T_{s2}
T_{s2}	Induced by TsF_1 or by injection of lymphocytes conjugated with the idiotype; has Lyt-1 $^{+}2^{+}$ characteristics; possesses anti-idiotype; generates or releases TsF_2 (probably receptor of T_{s2})
TsF_2	Possesses anti-idiotype determinants; other properties are very similar to those of TsF_1; interacts with idiotype on T and B cells and induces suppression of delayed-type hypersensitivity and suppression of idiotype synthesis

T_{s1} and T_{s2} suppressor cells can induce suppression upon adoptive transfer into irradiated recipients. The effectiveness of a T_{s1} transfer is restricted by the *Igh-C* allotype, but it is not restricted by differences in the *H-2* or *Igh-V* genotypes. The T_{s2} cells are effective only in H-2 compatible recipients.

The BALB/c mice, although *Igh-Ars*-negative and unable to synthesize the ARS idiotype, are nevertheless capable of generating such suppressor cells. These cells can be detected by an adoptive transfer into an H-2 compatible, *Igh-Ars*-positive recipient.

THE REGULATORY ROLE OF IDIOTYPES—IDIOTYPE NETWORKS

In 1974 Jerne formulated his idiotype network hypothesis in which he proposed that the immune system is regulated by a network of idiotypes and anti-idiotypes. The idiotypes on the cell surface and the anti-idiotypes in the circulation recognize each other and, through this recognition, regulate the quality and magnitude of the immune responses. Small amounts of anti-idiotype may stimulate the proliferation of cells, while high concentrations of anti-idiotypic antibodies may suppress the formation of a given idiotype; T cells with anti-idiotypes may actually kill the cells displaying the corresponding idiotype.

The Jerne concept is based upon two cardinal postulates: (1) the formation of self anti-idiotypes and (2) the existence of self idiotypes and self anti-idiotypes in an interacting network. Both of these postulates have been demonstrated experimentally; therefore, the network theory is no longer a speculative hypothesis but may be subjected to experimental scrutiny. **Auto-anti-idiotype** (AAI) has been raised by immunization of a rabbit with an antigen followed by reinjection of its own antibodies directed against the original antigen. Antibodies against self idiotypes are also formed in mice upon prolonged immunization with PC and other antigens. In mice immunized with trinitrophenyl-lysine-ficoll, the formation of the AAI is exceptionally rapid and reaches its peak between four and seven days after a single intravenous injection of the antigen. The AAI is responsible for an apparent decrease in the number and affinity of plaque-forming cells (Section 4.7) during this time interval. It has also been shown that the potential plaque-forming cells are "blocked" with AAI. Thus, by in vivo blocking of the antibody-forming cells, AAI may suppress the humoral immune response.

An experimental model of the network postulated by Jerne has been created in an allogeneic situation by immunization of a series of animals. The first animal is immunized with an antigen and produces the first antibody (Ab1). This antibody (Ab1) is then injected into a second animal, and an anti-idiotype (Ab2) is produced. Next, immunization of another animal with Ab2 leads to the formation of an anti-anti-idiotype (Ab3), etc. Thus, Ab1, Ab3, etc., can be compared with a photographic negative and Ab2, Ab4, etc. with the photographic positive of the object (antigen). Components of this experimental network display two interesting properties.

1. Anti-idiotype antibodies (Ab2) may *sometimes* mimic antigen. For example, mice immunized with Ab2 directed against an idiotype associated with antibodies to tobacco mosaic virus (TMV) produced Ab3 antibodies, a proportion of which reacted with both Ab2 and TMV, even though the mice were never exposed to TMV. In other systems, however, Ab3 do not react with the original antigen.
2. In rabbits, Ab1 are antigenically similar to Ab3, and Ab2 are similar to Ab4. Statistically, the chances of raising the same, or even similar, idiotype in two unrelated animals are very small. Thus, the enormously large idiotype repertoire of the rabbit can be considerably reduced by idiotype-anti-idiotype interactions. This controlling role of the network has been shown also in an experiment in which female rabbits were injected with Ab2 and formed Ab3. When these rabbits and their progeny were given the original immunogen, the resulting antibodies (Ab1') in all female rabbits and in 40 percent of their progeny were found to be idiotypically similar to the original Ab1. Again, such similarity is highly unlikely unless one assumes that the specificity of Ab2 determines the specificity of Ab1.

It remains to be seen whether the reduction of idiotypic heterogeneity in the above experiments was exercised by summary suppression or by selective promotion of the respective clones. Regulation through suppression has been fairly well documented in the ARS system. Although possible involvement of a promoting mechanism has not been explored to a comparable degree, some observations indicate that such a mechanism may also be involved in the regulatory network. For example, DBA/2 mice are normally unable to make the idiotype that is associated with antibodies directed against dinitrophenol-conjugated ovalbumin (DNP-ovalbumin) and raised in BALB/c mice. DBA/2 mice, however, make the BALB/c-associated idiotype if the immunization with DNP-ovalbumin is preceded by immunization with Ab2 and the consequent production of Ab3. Thus, treatment with Ab2 causes an overriding of the genetic control of idiotype expression. It is not clear whether this override acts through suppression or through promotion; the elucidation of this phenomenon would be of great importance for an understanding of the entire network concept.

The mechanisms described above function under experimental conditions; however, the regulatory role of the idiotype network under normal physiologic conditions is far from being understood and proven. In addition to its perennial "housekeeping" role, outlined in the original

Jerne concept, the network system may be involved in the regulation and conservation of the enormous germ line repertoire of antibody specificities. Interactions between autologous Ab1, Ab2, Ab3, etc., similar to such interactions between experimentally raised allogeneic Ab1, Ab2, Ab3, etc., may be essential for maintaining a pool of seemingly useless genes that code for antibodies directed against "never-to-be-encountered" antigens. Thus, the ability to make exotic Ab1 may be conserved throughout the individual's lifetime and, possibly, throughout evolution, because these Ab1 may function, in the idiotypic network, as Ab3 directed against some autologous immunoglobulins.

III / *Suggested Supplementary Reading*

The following list of publications has been compiled to provide the reader with the source of specific references. It consists predominantly of most recent textbooks, monographs, reviews, and some selected original papers. Each publication listed has an extensive list of references that may be useful for the reader who desires to pursue in depth some of the topics discussed in the preceding section.

Alt, F. W., Bothwell, A., Knapp, M., Siden, E., Mather, E., Koshland, M.. Baltimore, D., Synthesis of secreted and membrane-bound immunoglobulin μ heavy chains is directed by mRNAs that differ at their 3' ends. Cell **20**: 293–301, 1980.

Altman, P. L., Katz, D. D. (eds.), *Inbred and Genetically Defined Strains of Laboratory Animals.* Parts I and II. Federation of American Societies for Experimental Biology, Bethesda, 1979.

Bell, G. I., Perelson, A. S., Pimbley, G. H., (eds.) *Theoretical Immunology*, Marcel Dekker, New York, Basel, 1978.

Bernard, O., Hozumi, H., Tanegawa, S., Sequences of mouse immunoglobulin light chain genes before and after somatic changes. Cell **15**: 1133–1144, 1978.

Blomberg, B., Traunecker, A., Eisen, H., Tonegawa, S., Organization of four mouse λ light chain immunoglobulin genes. Proc. Natl. Acad. Sci. USA **78**: 3765–3769, 1981.

Brack, C., Hirama, M., Lenhard-Schuller, R., Tonegawa, S., A complete immunoglobulin gene is created by somatic recombination. Cell **15**: 1–14, 1978.

Crews, S., Griffin, J., Huang, H., Calame, K., Hood, L., A single V_H gene segment encodes the immune response to phosphorylcholine: Somatic mutation is correlated with the class of the antibody. Cell **25**: 59–66, 1981.

Dubiski, S., Genetics and regulation of immunoglobulin allotypes. The Medical Clinics of North America. Symp. Clin. Immunol. **56**: 557–575, 1972.

Early, P., Rogers, J., Davis, M., Calame, K., Bond, M., Wall, R., Hood, L., Two mRNAs can be produced from a single immunoglobulin μ gene by alternative RNA processing pathways. Cell **20**:313–319, 1980.

Early, P., Huang, H., Davis, M., Calame, K., Hood, L., An immunoglobulin heavy chain variable region gene is generated from three segments of DNA: V_H, D and J_H. Cell **19**: 981–992, 1980.

Fougereau, M., Dausset, J. (eds.), *Immunology 80, Progress in Immunology IV* (3 volumes). Academic Press, London, New York, 1980.

Fudenberg, H. H., Pink, J. R. L., Wang, A-C., Douglas, S. D., *Basic Immunogenetics.* Oxford University Press, New York, 1978.

Fudenberg, H. H.,Stites, D. P., Caldwell, J. L., Wells, J. V. (eds.), *Basic and Clinical Immunology.* Lang Medical Publications, Los Altos, California, 1976.

Giblett, E. R., *Genetic Markers in Human Blood.* Blackwell Scientific Publications, Oxford, 1969.

Greene, M. I., Sy, M. S., Nisonoff, A., Benacerraf, B., The genetic and cellular basis of antigen and receptor stimulated regulations. Molec. Immunol. **17**:857–866, 1980.

Grubb, R., Samuelsson, G. (eds.), *Human Anti-Human Gammaglobulins.* Pergamon Press, Oxford, 1971.

Grubb, R., *The Genetic Markers of Human Immunoglobulins.* Springer Verlag, Berlin,

Hildeman, W. H., Clark, E. A., Raison, R. L., *Comprehensive Immunogenetics.* Elsevier, New York, 1981.

Honjo, T., Kataoka, T., Organization of immunoglobulin heavy chain genes and allelic deletion model. Proc. Natl. Acad. Sci. USA **75**: 2140–2144, 1978.

Honjo, T., Packman, S., Swan, D., Leder, P., Quantitation of constant and variable region genes for mouse immunoglobulin λ chains. Biochemistry **15**: 2780–2785, 1976.

Janeway, C., Sercarz, E. E., Wigzell, H. (eds.) *Immunoglobulin Idiotypes*, Academic Press, New York, 1981.

Jerne, N. K., Toward a network theory of the immune system. Ann. Immunol. **125C**: 373–389, 1974.

Kataoka, T., Kawakami, T., Takahashi, N., Honjo, T., Rearrangement of immunoglobulin γ_1-chain gene and mechanism for heavy-chain class switch. Proc. Natl. Acad. Sci. USA **77**: 919–923, 1980.

Kehry, M., Ewald, S., Douglas, R., Sibley, C., Raschke, W., Fambrough, D., Hood, L., The immunoglobulin μ chains of membrane-bound and secreted IgM molecules differ in their C-terminal segments. Cell **21**: 393–406, 1980.

Kindt, T. J., Rabbit immunoglobulin allotypes: Structure, immunology and genetics. Adv. Immunol. **21**: 35–86, 1975.

Liu, C., Tucker, P., Mushinski, J. F., Blattner, F. R., Mapping of heavy chain genes for mouse immunoglobulins M and D. Science **209**: 1348–1352, 1980.

Marchalonis, J. J., *Immunity in Evolution.* Harvard University Press, Cambridge, Massachusetts, 1977.

Marchalonis, J. J. (ed.), *Comparative Immunology.* Blackwell Scientific Publications, Oxford, 1976.

Max, E., Seidman, J. G., Leder, P., Sequences of five potential recombination sites encoded close to an immunoglobulin κ constant region gene. Proc. Natl. Acad. Sci. USA **76:** 3450–3459, 1979.

Miller, J., Bothwell, A., Storb, U., Physical linkage of the constant region genes for immunoglobulins λ_I and λ_{III}. Proc. Natl. Acad. Sci. USA **78:** 3829–3833, 1981.

Natvig, J. B., Kunkel, H. G., Human immunoglobulins: Classes, subclasses, genetic variants, and idiotypes. Adv. Immunol. **16:** 1–59, 1973.

Nisonoff, A. Bangasser, S. A. Immunological suppression of idiotypic specificities. Transplantation Reviews, **27:** 100–134, 1975.

Nisonoff, A., Hopper, J. A., Spring, S. B., *The Antibody Molecule.* Academic Press, New York, 1975.

Perry, R. P., Coleclough, C., Weigert, M., Reorganization and expression of immunoglobuin genes: Status of allelic elements. Cold Spring Harbor Symp. Quant. Biol. **45:** 925–933, 1980.

Perry, R. P., Kelley, D., Coleclough, C., Seidman, J., Leder, P., Tonegawa, S., Matthyssens, G., Weigert, M., Transcription of mouse κ chain genes: Implications for allelic exclusion. Proc. Natl. Acad. Sci. USA **77:** 1937–1941, 1980.

Review for the notation for the allotypic and related markers of human immunoglobulins. J. Immunogenetics., **3:** 357–362, 1976.

Rose, N. R., Bigazzi, P. E., Warner, N. L. (eds.), *Genetic Control of Autoimmune Disease.* Elsevier North-Holland, New York, 1979.

Rose, N. R., Friedman, H. (eds.), *Manual of Clinical Immunology.* American Society for Microbiology, Washington, D.C., 1976.

Seidman, J. G., Leder, P., The arrangement and rearrangement of antibody genes. Nature **276:** 790–795, 1978.

Seidman, J. G., Max, E., Leder, P., A κ-immunoglobulin gene is formed by site-specific recombination without further somatic mutation. Nature **280:** 370–375, 1979.

Seidman, J. G., Nau, M., Norman, B., Kwan, S., Scharff, M., Leder, P., Immunoglobulin V/J recombination is accompanied by deletion of joining site and variable region segments. Proc. Natl. Acad. Sci. USA **77:** 6022–6026, 1980.

Sela, M. (ed.), *The Antigens.* Academic Press, New York, 1973 (pp. 161–298; 299–371).

Steinberg, A. G., and Cook, C. E., *The Distribution of the Human Immunoglobulin Allotypes.* Oxford University Press, Oxford, 1981.

Tonegawa, S., Brack, C., Hozumi, N., Schuller, R., Cloning of an immunoglobulin variable region gene from mouse embryo. Proc. Natl. Acad. Sci. USA **74:** 3518–3522, 1977.

Tonegawa, S., Maxam, A., Tizard, R., Bernard, O., Gilbert, W., Sequence of a mouse germ-line gene for a variable region of an immunoglobulin light chain. Proc. Natl. Acad. Sci. USA **75:** 1485–1489, 1978.

Tucker, P., Liu, C., Mushinski, J. F., Blattner, F. R., Mouse immunoglobulin D: Messenger RNA and genomic DNA sequences. Science **209:** 1353–1360, 1980.

Weir, D. M. (ed.), *Handbook of Experimental Immunology.* Third Edition. Blackwell Scientific Publications, Oxford, London, Edinburgh, Melbourne, 1978.

IV / Genetics of Blood Groups

11 / The Major Human Blood Groups

INTRODUCTION

It might be difficult to justify setting aside blood groups as a separate subdivision of immuno-genetics. After all, an argument could well be made that since blood is often considered to be a subtype of connective tissue, blood group substances are actually tissue-restricted allo-antigens.

What then is meant by the term **blood group antigens**? In normal usage, the term applies to those alloantigens that are principally, but not exclusively, found on erythrocytes and, hence, must be considered in the ordinary practice of blood transfusion. In fact, these antigens play a major role in determining the outcome of a blood transfusion, which is the most common form of transplantation and is performed thousands of times each day in the United States alone. Thus, one may agree that the term blood group antigens is introduced for pragmatic reasons rather than for filling a basic need for a unique term that describes a strictly defined subdivision of immunogenetics. Still, it is worthwhile to remember that the discovery of the first blood group—a genetic trait demonstrable by immunologic methods—is assumed to mark the birth of immunogenetics as a subdivision of both genetics and immunology.

In the field of blood groups and transfusion, some terms are used in a somewhat different context that in conventional genetics. In fact, it is not too strong to say that occasionally the nomenclature of human blood groups, since it has grown along with their discovery, is just short of chaotic. Historical precedent and common clinical usage frustrate attempts to change names or introduce new symbol conventions. Nevertheless, because of the urgent need for a simple and uniform nomenclature amenable for use in computerized analysis, a new terminology for various blood groups was recently proposed (Table 11.1). The reader who intends to embark on immunohematologic studies or to master the immunology of blood transfusion would do well to press on with learning the traditional, though often unconventional, nomenclature as well as the new one.

11.1 Genetic Determination of Blood Groups

Blood group antigens are inherited in one of the several patterns described earlier (Section 1.2). In general, they are determined by polymorphic genes that occupy specific loci. The detection of blood groups and genetic analysis of their inheritance are made possible by their polymorphism, i.e., the presence of variants, each variant being determined by a distinct allele. The different blood groups are determined by distinct allelic series at discrete loci. The loci for two distinct groups may be either independent (i.e., located on different chromosomes) or linked to various degrees (i.e., present on the same chromosome). The linkage strength between genes for any two blood groups ranges between two extremes. In one extreme, alleles at two loci remain inseparable by crossing over for many generations and thus appear as alleles at a single locus. In another extreme, actual linkage can be proven only indirectly by demonstration of linkage to some other gene located between the two blood group genes in question. In this case the two genes are often called **syntenic** in distinction from genes for which linkage can be demonstrated directly. In the case of two linked genes, it may be important to distinguish whether particular alleles at linked loci are in *cis* (coupling) or *trans* (repulsion) position. This is because the relative positions of two alleles may affect the immunologic properties of their products.

    In contrast to histocompatibility antigens (Chapter 15), the blood group phenotype of an individual often differs from the genotype. This is because some blood group alleles are recessive, i.e., are not expressed in heterozygotes, or are silent (**amorphic**) and are not expressed in either heterozygotes or homozygotes. In these cases, obviously, direct testing for the phenotype does not permit determination of the genotype; to do so, progeny (family) studies are needed (Section 5.11). These studies may be complicated by the occasional polygenic nature of some blood groups. In these cases, genes at two or more loci determine the actual phenotype and various combinations of alleles at the loci involved determine the corresponding phenotypic variants. Considering the broad variability in the genetic determination of various blood groups, the term **blood group system** was introduced some time ago. It should be understood that this is a very loose term, and its precise definition is best left unattempted. In some instances, the term simply stands for all alleles at a given locus, while at other times it includes both all the alleles and all serologically detectable products. In still other instances, the term blood group system refers to a set of distinct linked genes whose products interact to generate the final blood group antigen and its phenotypic variants.

11.2 Principle of Blood Group Determination

It is important to know that the detection of products of blood group genes depends on serologic tests. This, in turn, means that usually only those products that can evoke an antibody

TABLE 11.1. Uniform Numerical Nomenclature of Human Erythrocyte Antigens (blood group antigens)

Traditional Blood Group	Letter Symbol	Number Symbol	Antigen Symbols (traditional)
ABO	ABO	1	1 (A)
			2 (B)
			3 (AB)
			4 (A$_1$)
			5 (H)
MNSs	MNS	2	1 (M)
			2 (N)
			3 (S)
			4 (s)
			5 (U)
P	P	3	1 (P$_1$)
Rhesus	RH	4	1 (D)
			2 (C)
			3 (E)
			4 (c)
			5 (e)
Lutheran	LU	5	1 (a)
			2 (b)
Kell	KEL	6	1 (K)
			2 (k)
Lewis	LE	7	1 (a)
			2 (b)
Duffy	FY	8	1 (a)
			2 (b)
Kidd	JK	9	1 (a)
			2 (b)

response will be recognized as allelic variants. Since the determination of human blood groups and their genetic analysis mainly depends on serologic reactions between erythrocytes expressing antigens and antibodies (specific for these antigens) that are found in certain human sera (alloantibodies), a brief review of principles and specific problems is in order. With few exceptions, the antisera employed in blood group studies are obtained from donors with high titers of alloantibodies resulting from earlier transfusion or pregnancies. Furthermore, to define the mode of inheritance, it is essential to identify the informative families and test serologically as many members of such families as possible.

In the interpretation of a blood group determination, it is presumed that cells that react with a given antiserum possess an antigen against which the antiserum contains specific antibodies. Conversely, cells that do not react are presumed to lack the antigen. The cardinal assumption is made that—except in unusual circumstances—the individual who produces antibodies does not possess the antigen with which the antibodies specifically combine. This assumption applies to all the different antibodies that may happen to be present in a given antiserum. Indeed, more often than not, a given antiserum contains several antibodies induced by multiple transfusions of blood from different individuals. To determine the specificity of any serum, it must be tested against a panel of erythrocytes, each with a known combination of blood group antigens. The pattern of reaction with the cells of a sufficient number of individuals usually will permit the assignment of specificities of antibodies present in a serum (Table 11.2). The assignment can then be confirmed by proper absorption.

Conversely, to determine the antigenic composition (phenotype) of erythrocytes of a particular individual, one must test that person's erythrocytes with a panel of antisera containing antibodies of known specificities.

If an antiserum is encountered that gives, with the erythrocytes of certain individuals, a pattern of reaction incompatible with the distribution of all known antigens, there is a high degree of probability that the antiserum contains an antibody to a new blood group antigen. One, however, must be extremely cautious in reaching such a conclusion. Specifically, it is imperative to eliminate the chance that an unusual pattern is due to the presence of multiple antibodies against known antigens (see above).

11.3 Serologic Tests Used for Blood Group Determination

The serologic test most commonly employed in studies of blood groups is hemagglutination (Section 4.6). However, the detection of the antibodies to blood group antigens does not always lend itself to a simple procedure; often more sophisticated procedures are required. This is at least partially due to the particular properties of blood group antibodies.

Antibodies to blood group antigens may belong to either the IgM or IgG class or they may be a mixture of both classes. IgM antibodies react better at lower temperatures (18°C or less),

TABLE 11.2. Principle of Assigning Specificity to an Antiserum

Individuals of Panel	Reactions with Antisera to												Reaction of Antiserum Tested*
	M	N	S*	C	D	E	c	e	K	k	Le^a	Le^b	
1	+	+				+	+		+			+	+
2	+			+	+		+		+			+	
3	+			+	+	+			+		+		+
4	+	+		+	+		+		+			+	+
5	+			+	+	+			+		+		
6		+			+	+			+			+	
7	+				+	+			+			+	+

*Apparently, tested serum reacts with erythrocytes of the same individuals that react with anti-N serum (see outlined columns). For the sake of simplicity only positive (+) reactions are indicated.

whereas IgG antibodies react better at higher temperatures (37°C). Thus, testing must be carried out at two different temperatures to provide the optimal conditions for these two different classes of antibodies.

IgM antibodies readily agglutinate erythrocytes that are suspended in saline, whereas IgG antibodies are often unable to produce agglutination under these conditions. In such a suspension, erythrocytes have a net negative charge that causes them to repel each other to a distance too large to be spanned by the relatively small IgG molecules (Section 7.2). On the other hand, the rather large IgM molecules are able to bridge repelled erthrocytes. Hence, IgG antibodies that react with individual erythrocytes but that do not agglutinate them are called **incomplete antibodies**. Significantly, after combining with antigens of individual cells, IgG antibodies cover these antigens and make them inaccessible to IgM antibodies that otherwise would produce agglutination. Because of this, IgG antibodies are occasionally referred to as **blocking antibodies**. The electrostatic forces that repel erythrocytes and prevent agglutination by IgG antibodies can be reduced by the addition to the medium of certain high molecular weight compounds (proteins, dextran, polyvinylpyrrolidone). These compounds are used routinely in serologic procedures employing IgG antibodies. Alternatively, erythrocytes can be treated with certain proteolytic enzymes before being tested with IgG antibodies. When performed properly, such a pretreatment reduces the net charge of erythrocytes; but when performed incorrectly, it may destroy antigens or induce nonspecific agglutination of cells.

In addition to the above modifications of simple agglutination, the most popular method used to detect IgG antibodies is the indirect antiglobulin (Coombs') test (section 4.6). All these methods may be employed for detection and determination of any blood group. Among the numerous blood group systems of man, the ABO and Rh have been most extensively studied and dealt with on a day-to-day basis. These two systems will be discussed separately from all other systems (Chapter 12). This arrangement, however, is not meant to imply that the other systems are of no importance; the antigens and antibodies of any of the systems can be of vital significance in a certain situation.

THE ABO BLOOD GROUP SYSTEM

Because the discovery of the human ABO system heralded the birth of immunogenetics, it is worthwhile to retrace the footsteps of those who at the beginning of this century laid the groundwork of the field.

11.4 The Discovery and Definition of the ABO System

In 1900 Landsteiner undertook studies to confirm earlier reports that certain pathological sera contained lytic antibodies (**lysins**) against normal human erythrocytes. During his studies, Landsteiner failed to demonstrate the presence of lysins associated specifically with febrile diseases but noticed that apparently healthy individuals have in their sera agglutinins directed against the erythrocytes of some other humans. Interestingly, this observation was relegated to a footnote in the original report.

Nevertheless, Landsteiner realized that his incidental observation suggested the presence of antigens that can distinguish one individual from the other within the same species. Such antigens were then called **isoantigens** but now are referred to as alloantigens. To investigate more systematically the possibility of the existence of erythrocytic alloantigens, Landsteiner obtained cells and sera from himself and five of his colleagues and mixed a saline suspension of erythrocytes of each individual with the serum of each individual. The results, which are shown in Table 11.3, led to the following explanation and the concept of what was to become the ABO system.

Apparently, both sera and erythrocytes could be divided into three distinct groups, initially called A, B, and C. The sera of group A agglutinated erythrocytes of group B, whereas the sera of group B agglutinated the erythrocytes of group A. The sera of group C agglutinated erythrocytes of both A and B groups, but the erythrocytes of this group were not agglutinated by either serum A or B. To interpret these observations, Landsteiner proposed that the sera of normal individuals contain two types of agglutinins that are present either separately as in groups A and B or together as in group C. Furthermore, two antigens, A and B, present individually or totally absent from erythrocytes had to be postulated to explain the observed reactions. Perhaps the most important observation was that agglutinins and antigens were present in completely normal individuals and disease had little, if any, bearing on the pattern of reactions. However, it is to the credit of Landsteiner that he realized the potential clinical importance of his discovery as evidenced by the concluding remark in his paper:

> "Finally, it must be mentioned that the reported observations allow us to explain the variable results in therapeutic transfusions of human blood."

Follow-up studies revealed that essentially every individual could be classified into one of the three groups, A, B, or C (now A, B, and O). The only discrepancy was demonstrated with umbilical cord blood in which antigens could be shown on erythrocytes, but no agglutinins in the serum were ever found. We now know that this is easily explained by the fact that cord blood belongs to the fetus, which at birth is immunologically immature and has no antibodies other than those received from its mother via the placenta.

It remained for the students of Landsteiner to discover the fourth and rarest blood group that is characterized by the simultaneous presence of both antigens and the absence of both agglutinins. This group was originally termed D (now AB). Unfortunately, in those early days some investigators failed to realize the relationships among the four groups, and this led temporarily to a great deal of confusion and to several terminologies. Even more important, the resulting confusion resulted in serious transfusion errors until an international nomenclature was adopted using the original Landsteiner notation for the antigens. The contribution of Landsteiner that originally was reported in a footnote ultimately was recognized as a significant breakthrough, and Landsteiner was awarded the Nobel Prize in 1930.

11.5 Genetics of the ABO System

It is noteworthy that much excitement was created by the suggestion that blood groups may be genetically controlled. However, such excitement becomes understandable when one realizes

TABLE 11.3. Results of Original Experiment of Landsteiner in which Blood of Six Apparently Healthy Men was Tested

Sera	Group	Erythrocytes of					
		St.	Plecn.	Sturl.	Erdh.	Zar.	Landst.
St.	C	−	+	+	+	+	−
Plecn.	A	−	−	+	+	−	−
Sturl.	B	−	+	−	−	+	−
Erdh.	B	−	+	−	−	+	−
Zar.	A	−	−	+	+	−	−
Landst.	C	−	+	+	+	+	−

that at that time eye color was the only normal trait in man known to be inherited according to Mendelian principles. Proof for the genetic inheritance of the ABO system came from family studies that showed that antigens A and B are always dominant and can be demonstrated in children only when present in at least one of the parents. It was originally hypothesized that there are two independent genes, each with two alleles: *A* and *a*, and *B* and *b*; the first allele in each case would determine the antigen, whereas the second would not. According to the hypothesis, nine polygenotypes should be identifiable, leading to four polyphenotypes. The hypothesis postulated that the mating of an individual O (genotype *a/a b/b*) with an individual AB (genotype *A/a B/b*) would produce all four phenotypes: O, A, B, and AB. However, in reality such matings yielded only two phenotypes—A (50 percent) and B (50 percent)—and never the phenotypes O and AB. In view of this observation, the original hypothesis had to be rejected.

The presently accepted concept for the inheritance of the ABO system was proposed in 1925 by Bernstein (Table 11.4). He proposed that there is a single locus* with three alleles: *A, B,* and *R. R* represented a recessive allele and is presently designated *O.* The three alleles yield six genotypes determining four distinct phenotypes. The alleles *A* and *B* are codominant, and both are fully dominant over the *O* allele. The latter is now often considered amorphic or silent. Since, as will be seen later, the blood group substances are glycoproteins and glycolipids and their antigenic specificity resides in the carbohydrate, it must be assumed that such antigenic determinants are the secondary products of the *A* and *B* alleles. If this is the case, the *A* and *B* alleles must have a primary product other than the blood group antigens themselves. Indeed, it has been universally accepted that the *A* and *B* alleles determine specific glycosyl transferases that catalyze a glycosylation reaction converting the specific substrate substance (see below) into the corresponding antigens.

The primary product of the *A* allele is **N-acetyl galactosaminyl transferase**, which attaches one molecule of α-D-N-acetyl galactosamine to the substrate substance and by doing so generates the determinant of the **A antigen**.

---

*The locus is sometimes designated by a letter *I* and the alleles are denoted I^A, I^B, and I^O. However, this designation has not been universally accepted and may be confused with the I blood group (Chapter 12).

TABLE 11.4. The Genotypes of ABO Blood Groups and Corresponding Phenotypes Defined by Anti-A and Anti-B Sera

Alleles*	Genotype	Reaction with		Phenotype*
		Anti-A	Anti-B	
O (R)	*O/O*	−	−	O (C)
A (A)	*A/O, A/A*	+	−	A (A)
B (B)	*B/O, B/B*	−	+	B (B)
	A/B	+	+	AB (D)

*Original designations are given in parentheses.

The product of the *B* allele is **galactosyl transferase**, which catalyzes the attachment of an α-D-galactose molecule to substrate substance and thus converts this substance into B antigen.

Apparently, the silent allele *O* does not encode any enzyme; therefore, in *O/O* homozygotes, no specific antigen is formed.

11.6 The *H* Gene and Its Alleles

This model of the genes and their primary products requires that the expression of either allele is contingent on the presence of a substrate substance. Indeed, there is a glycoprotein that displays the property of the substrate for enzymes determined by the *A* and *B* alleles. This property is associated with a particular carbohydrate **precursor** consisting of β-galactosyl-N-acetylglucosamine disaccharide. The attachment of an α-L-fucose converts the precursor substance into **H substance**, which serves as substrate for the enzymes determined by the *A* or *B* alleles. The fucose attachment is catalyzed by the enzyme **fucosyl transferase**, which is genetically determined by the dominant allele designated *H* at a locus independent of the locus carrying the *A*, *B*, and *O* alleles.

The vast majority of people are *H/H* homozygotes and only occasionally *H/h* heterozygotes; and because of the full dominance of the *H* allele, they are capable of synthesizing H substance. However, in rare instances, the individual may be a recessive homozygote *h/h* and thus lack this specific fucosyl transferase. Such a condition leads to lack of H substance, and this, in turn, precludes the expression of the *A* and *B* alleles. As a result, the *h/h* homozygotes express neither A nor B antigens even though they may have the appropriate alleles. Phenotypically, these individuals appear as belonging to the O blood group, but in contrast to ordinary O individuals who cannot have a child of group AB, the former individuals may have such a child if they actually carry either *A* or *B* or both alleles that are not expressed owing to the absence of precursor substance. In a child who receives the dominant *H* allele from another parent, the nonexpressed allele can be normally expressed. The *h/h* homozygous individuals are known as having the so-called **Bombay phenotype**, first described in 1952. This phenotype has been the subject of extensive family studies. The phenotypes are designated O_h^O, O_h^A, O_h^B, or O_h^{AB}, where the superscript indicates the *ABO* alleles, if they are known, from family studies, and the subscript indicates homozygosity for the *h* allele. Interestingly, the absence of A and B antigens in Bombay individuals seems not to be absolute inasmuch as the erythrocytes of such individuals, while not agglutinated by the corresponding antibodies, in some instances, can absorb the antibodies directed against their "suppressed" A, B, or H antigen.

11.7 ABO Agglutinins and Their Determination

The regular presence of IgM alloagglutinins that are specific for the A or B antigens is a relatively unique situation among various blood groups of man and other mammals. Ordinarily, only xenoantigens (antigens of other species) are defined by naturally occurring antibodies, whereas alloantigens (antigens of a given species) are defined by antibodies induced by deliberate immunization with an alloantigen.

The presence of natural agglutinins (anti-A or α and anti-B or β) in the absence of apparent antigenic stimulation prompted theories that these antibodies may be inherited in a manner similar to the inheritance of antigens. However, none of these theories found experimental support, and at present the consensus is that only the ability to produce agglutinins is inherited, whereas the actual antibody is the result of appropriate antigenic stimulation. The most likely sources of antigenic stimulation seem to be enteric bacteria or their products, which have some antigenic determinants identical or similar to those found in A and/or B antigens. The bacteria are present as part of the normal microbial flora of the gastrointestinal tract or are ingested with food. Still, the affinity of various agglutinins appears to be influenced by the particular ABO phenotype of the individual who produces these agglutinins. The mechanism of these influences is at present poorly defined and even less understood.

In addition to anti-A and anti-B agglutinins, certain human sera contain agglutinins specific for H substance (anti-H). These agglutinins (also called $\alpha2$) are capable of agglutinating essentially any human erythrocyte, but they do so preferentially with erythrocytes of group O. This apparent affinity of certain human sera for O erythrocytes led originally to the proposition that, in fact, the allele *O* determines its own specific product, "antigen O," analogous to the antigens A and B. However, this proposal was found untenable when it was discovered that erythrocytes expressing simultaneously both A and B antigens, i.e., erythrocytes of individuals lacking allele *O*, are also agglutinated by certain human sera that contain putative "anti-O" agglutinins. Today it is clear that preference for O erythrocytes of the sera containing anti-H is due to the fact that such indidividuals have an excess of H substance, because they cannot convert it into either A or B antigen. In fact, it was demonstrated that the amount of H substance present on erythrocytes depends on the ABO phenotype and this relationship can be expressed as follows:

$$O > A_2 > B > A_2B > A_1 > A_1B.$$

11.8 Subgroups of A

In the early studies of the ABO system, it was noticed that certain anti-A sera appeared to contain two distinct agglutinins that could be separated by sequential absorption with different erythrocytes of the A or AB phenotype. One agglutinin (anti-A or α) reacted with all group A and AB erythrocytes, whereas the second agglutinin (anti-A1 or $\alpha1$) reacted only with erythrocytes of some individuals of the A or AB phenotype. On the basis of this observation, it was postulated that there are two distinct but cross-reactive variants of the A antigen: A_1 that reacts with both agglutinins (α and $\alpha1$) that recognize the A and A_1 determinants; and A_2 that reacts with one agglutinin (α) that recognizes only the A determinant. The two antigens, A_1 and A_2, appear to be products of two distinct alleles, A_1 and A_2. Thus, the ABO system must be expanded into four alleles, A_1, A_2, B, and O, forming 10 genotypes and 6 phenotypes (Table 11.5). This concept has been convincingly supported by numerous family studies and is presently accepted fully. However, even today the qualitative difference between A_1 and A_2 antigens is occasionally challenged. The challengers raise the possibility that A_1 and A_2 do reflect quantitative differences between cells expressing significantly more antigen (A_1) and cells expressing relatively small amounts of the same antigen (A_2). In support of this concept are experiments in which large numbers of A_2 cells (presumably reacting with only α agglutinin) did absorb not only α but also $\alpha1$ agglutinins with which these cells should not react. However, close examination of such experiments reveals that they cannot be interpreted in a straightforward manner. The eluates of antibodies absorbed by A_1 and A_2 cells are not equally reactive with the A_2 cells. Specifically, eluates from A_1 cells agglutinate both A_1 and A_2, whereas eluates from A_2 cells agglutinate A_1 but not A_2 cells. Perhaps the most convincing evidence in favor of qualitative differences between A_1 and A_2 is the finding that 1 to 2 percent of A_2 individuals and about 26 percent of A_2B individuals have natural $\alpha1$ (anti-A_1). This finding refutes the thesis that A_2 represents a smaller amount of A_1; the presence of $\alpha1$ (anti-A_1) in A_2 would have to represent autoantibody.

TABLE 11.5. The Expanded ABO Blood Group System as Defined by Anti-A, Anti-A_1, and Anti-B Agglutinins

Phenotype	Frequency in Caucasoids	Reaction with			Genotype
		Anti-A (α)	Anti-A_1 ($\alpha1$)	Anti-B (β)	
O	0.45	−	−	−	O/O
A_1	0.35	+	+	−	A_1/O, A_1/A_1, A_1/A
A_2	0.09	+	−	−	A_2/O, A_2/A_2
B	0.08	−	−	+	B/O, B/B
A_1B	0.02	+	+	+	A_1/B
A_2B	0.01	+	−	+	A_2/B

The concept attributing the serologic distinction of A_1 and A_2 variants to merely quantitative differences of a single substance should not be confused with the well-established fact that the concentrations of the A_1 and A_2 antigens vary significantly. These differences, established using rabbit anti-A heteroantibodies, are as large as fivefold (Table 11.6).

While the vast majority of human group A erythrocytes can be classified as either A_1 or A_2, there are rare exceptions of erythrocytes that appear to be A_2 but that can react weakly, albeit definitely, with $\alpha 1$ (anti-A_1). These individuals give a reaction with α (anti-A) that is intermediate between A_1 and A_2 and thus are designated as A_{int}. Interestingly, the reaction of these erythrocytes with anti-H is not intermediate, since they react definitely stronger than normal A_2. A plausible explanation for the A_{int} erythrocytes defines these cells as A_1 with a quantitatively reduced number of accessible A determinants that are shared by A_1 and A_2 cells and react with the α (anti-A) agglutinin. This creates the impression of an intermediate reactivity with α.

11.9 Variants of the A Antigen

In addition to the easily determined A_1 and A_2 subgroups, there exist several rare variants of the A antigen. Some of these variants appear to be products of very rare alleles; some do not seem to be allelic. The three most common variants are A_3, A_x, and A_m.

A_3 cells are easily identified since even with the most potent antisera only a small fraction of cells forms agglutinates and the cells do not react with $\alpha 1$ (anti-A_1). Interestingly, A_3 individuals secrete A substance in their saliva (Section 11.11).

A_x cells react either weakly or not at all with α (anti-A). On the other hand, the same cells react strongly with sera of group O individuals (so-called anti-A+B sera). Genetically, A_x people group as O, but they do not possess anti-A in their sera. A_x individuals do not secrete A, but they produce H substance and their erythrocytes react strongly with anti-H.

A_m cells are never agglutinated by α (anti-A) antibodies, though they can adsorb them. A_m individuals appear as O, but their sera do not have the natural antibodies to A normally present

TABLE 11.6. Estimated Number of the A_1 and A_2 Determinants on the Surface of Human Erythrocytes of Various Phenotypes and of Various Origins

Phenotype	Source of Erythrocytes	Molecules A_1	A_2
A_1	Peripheral blood	800,000–1,200,000	—
A_1	Cord blood	250,000–350,000	—
A_1B	Peripheral blood	450,000–850,000	—
A_2	Peripheral blood	—	240,000–300,000
A_2	Cord blood	—	140,000
A_2B	Peripheral blood	—	120,000
A_2B	Cord blood	—	220,000 (?)

in O individuals. Their saliva contains A and H substances. It is believed that A_m is an extremely rare allele.

There are still rarer A variants—A_{end}, A_{finn}, A_{el}, and A_{bantu}— and some extremely rare B variants. At present, these variants are of interest only to the blood group specialist.

11.10 Tissue Distribution of A, B, and H Antigens

Although by definition blood group substances are associated with erythrocytes, they may also be present on cells of other tissues as well as in body fluids and secretions. Indeed, because soon after their initial discovery on erythrocytes the presence of A and B antigens was also demonstrated in serum, an extensive search for these antigens in other tissues and fluids ensued.

Generally, different methods of extraction (alcohol or water) and different methods of testing for antigen content (complement fixation or absorption of specific sera) were used in this search. Regardless of the method employed, it was demonstrated clearly that extracts of many organs including liver and kidney, but not brain and testes, contain A or B antigens. In addition, various body fluids and secretions (saliva, gastric juice, semen, milk, urine, tears) were found to contain the corresponding antigens. The amount of antigen in different fluids, and also the amount in a particular fluid from different individuals, displays broad variability.

Saliva has been employed most extensively owing to its easy availability in quantities amenable to extensive testing. Most commonly, the presence of A and B antigens in saliva is determined on the basis of the capacity of saliva to inhibit (absorb) the agglutinating activity of anti-A or anti-B serum. The presence of the H antigen (substance) is usually assessed on the basis of the capacity of saliva to inhibit the activity of **anti-H lectins** (agglutinins from plants). The latter are substances that, by combining with the saccharides of H substance, cause specific agglutination of erythrocytes expressing this substance. Using these assays, it was soon realized that the saliva of about 80 percent of individuals contained the appropriate antigens, whereas the remaining 20 percent did not. The presence or absence of antigens in saliva is controlled by alleles of a gene that is independent of both the *ABO* and the *H* genes.

11.11 *Secretor* Gene

The gene controlling the secretion of ABH antigens into saliva was designated the **secretor gene**, and two alleles have been identified. The fully dominant allele *Se* (formerly *S*), with a frequency of 0.52 in Caucasoids, permits the secretion of the antigens. The recessive allele *se* (formerly *s*) is found with a frequency of 0.48. When an individual is an *se/se* homozygote, there is no secretion of antigens in either saliva or other fluids. The two alleles are inherited in a straightforward Mendelian manner. Because *se/se* homozygotes can be identified unequivocally in a given population, it is relatively easy to determine the frequency of the *se* allele; because the system has only two alleles, finding the frequency of one permits estimation of the frequency of the other. Subsequently, applying the Hardy-Weinberg equation, it is possible to estimate the genotypic frequencies of *se/se* as 0.23, *Se/se* as 0.50, and *Se/Se* as 0.27. These frequencies are consistent with the observed phenotypic frequencies of secretors (0.80) and nonsecretors (0.20).

It is believed that the dominant allele *Se* in some manner controls the activity of the fucosyl transferase encoded by the *H* allele or regulates the transcription of the *H* allele. However, the activity of the secretor gene affects only the conversion of cell-free (water-soluble) precursor substance and not the cell-bound substance. Thus, the *Se* allele permits the production and secretion of antigens in the fluids, whereas the *se* allele precludes this process in body fluids but does not affect production of the antigens in the erythrocyte membrane.

11.12 The Lewis (Le) Blood Group System

To understand the chemistry of and relationship between A, B, and H antigens one must become familiar with still another system, in addition to the three already discussed: ABO, H, and secretor. This system, called the Lewis blood group system, was originally defined by two antisera detecting two antigens, Le^a and Le^b, found in random populations in 22 percent and 78 percent of individuals, respectively. Although originally believed to be the products of two alleles, both antigens are actually determined by a single allele called *Le* (formerly *L*). This allele encodes the enzyme **fucosyl transferase** that catalyzes the transfer of α-L-fucose from fucosyl-GDP to N-acetylglucosamine of the precursor substance. It should be noted that the fucosyl transferase determined by the *Le* allele is different from the fucosyl transferase encoded by the *H* allele. Since precursor substance serves as a substrate for the fucosyl transferase, the reaction is independent of the allele at the *H* locus; the reaction takes place in *H/H* homozygotes and *H/h* hetrozygotes as well as *h/h* homozygotes. The product of this reaction is a Le^a substance, initially present in plasma and body fluids and subsequently passively adsorbed on the surface of erythrocytes where it is detected as a blood group substance. The fucosyl transferase determined by the *Le* allele also catalyzes the attachment of α-L-fucose to H substance in the presence of both the *Se* allele and the *H* allele (which encodes a different fucosyl transferase that permits conversion of precursor substance into H substance). This transfer converts the H substance into Le^b substance, originally present in plasma but ultimately adsorbed on erythrocytes where it is detected as a blood group antigen.

Since both Le^a and Le^b substances may be formed in the presence of *H* and *Se* alleles, the phenotype of erythrocytes changes during early life. Because the Le^a substance is formed directly from precursor substance, initially erythrocytes are Le(a+b−). In the next stage, the H substance is converted to Le^b, resulting in the transient phenotype Le(a+b+). This phenotype is ultimately replaced at the age of three to six years by the final phenotype Le(a−b+) in 78 percent of individuals. In the presence of an *Se* allele, both Le^a and Le^b substances are found in secretions. In the absence of the *Se* allele, the transformation stops at the first stage, and in 22 percent of individuals the erythrocytes have the Le(a+b−) phenotype permanently. When an individual is homozygous for the amorphic allele *le*, neither Le^a nor Le^b substance can be formed and the individual has the phenotype Le(a−b−). Table 11.7 briefly summarizes the relationships among the four genetic systems involved in the formation and distribution of the A, B, H, and Le substances in tissues and body fluids.

TABLE 11.7. Relationship between Genotypes and Phenotypes of ABO(H) and Lewis Blood Groups among Caucasoids in North America

Genotypes and Allelic Frequencies	A	B	H	Le^a	Le^b	Blood Groups*	
H/H or H/h — Se/Se or Se/Se — Le/Le or Le/le — A/A or A/O	+		+	+	+	A	
A/B	+	+	+	+	+	AB	Le(a−b+)
B/B or B/O		+	+	+	+	B	
O/O			+	+	+	O	
le/le — A/A or A/O	+		+			A	
A/B	+	+	+			AB	Le(a−b−)
B/B or B/O		+	+			B	
O/O			+			O	
se/se — Le/Le or Le/le — A/A or A/O				+		A	
A/B				+		AB	Le(a+b−)
B/B or B/O				+		B	
O/O				+		O	
le/le — A/A or A/O						A	
A/B						AB	(Le(a−b−)
B/B or B/O						B	
O/O						O	
h/h — Se/Se or Se/se — Le/Le or Le/le — A/A or A/O				+		O_h^A	
A/B				+		O_h^{AB}	Le(a+b−)
B/B or B/O				+		O_h^B	
O/O				+		O_h^O	
le/le — A/A or A/O						O_h^A	
A/B						O_h^{AB}	Le(a−b−)
B/B or B/O						O_h^B	
O/O						O_h^O	
se/se — Le/Le or Le/le — A/A or A/O				+		O_h^A	
A/B				+		O_h^{AB}	Le(a+b−)
B/B or B/O				+		O_h^B	
O/O				+		O_h^O	
le/le — A/A or A/O						O_h^A	
A/B						O_h^{AB}	Le(a−b−)
B/B or B/O						O_h^B	
O/O						O_h^O	

$H \approx 1.0$ $Se = .52$ $Le = .82$ $A = .28$
$h =$ very $se = .48$ $le = .18$ $B = .06$
low $O = .65$

*O_h corresponds to the so-called Bombay phenotype.

Source: Milgrom, F., Flanagan, T. D., (eds.), Medical Microbiology, 1982. Used with permission.

11.13 Chemical Structure of Blood Group Substances

Although chemical studies began soon after Landsteiner's initial report, they were thwarted by difficulties in obtaining the blood group substances in a serologically useful form. Aqueous extraction yielded only minimal amounts, whereas extracts made with organic solvents, although rich in activity, were difficult to assay or chemically characterize. Extensive chemical studies became possible only after the discovery of blood group substances in the secretions. Further progress was made after the discovery of A-like and B-like substances in the mucous membranes of various animals (swine, horses, etc.) from which they could be extracted in a high yield. Studies carried out primarily with the material isolated from secretions revealed that various blood group substances of the ABO and Lewis systems are surprisingly similar in spite of their apparent antigenic differences.

The basic analysis showed that the substances are glycoproteins of widely ranging molecular weights (300,000–1,000,000), depending on their source, and consist of 15 percent protein and 85 percent carbohydrate. At present, nothing is known about the genetic determination and structural variability of the protein component of blood group substance. The protein constitutes a backbone supporting a large number of oligosaccharide side chains that determine serologic specificities. The oligosaccharides are composed of five sugars: D-galactose (GAL), L-fucose (FUC), N-acetyl-D-glucosamine (GLU-N), N-acetyl-D-galactosamine (GAL-N), and N-acetylneuraminic acid (SIAL) (sialic acid). The proportion of sugars varies slightly, and the specificity of a given antigen is usually determined by a single sugar and/or its position within the chain (see below).

The role of individual sugars in determining the antigenic specificity was established by two approaches. In the first approach, single sugars inhibited the activity of antisera, suggesting that specific antibodies combine with that particular sugar. In the second, using certain bacterial and protozoan enzymes, it was shown that in vitro removal of specific sugars and their accumulation in the medium could be correlated with the loss of immunogenicity of the substance treated with the enzyme. These studies ultimately led to the finding that even precursor substance has its own antigenic specificity, which is similar, if not identical, to that of type XIV pneumococcus capsular carbohydrate.

11.14 Synthesis of Blood Group Substances

The biosynthesis of the H, Le, A, and B substances occurs in several consecutive steps, each of which is catalyzed by a specific glycosyl transferase. The primary substrate for the entire chain of reactions is a precursor substance that contains a disaccharide, galactosyl-N-acetylglucosamine. There are two types of precursor substance: type I in which the two sugars are linked by a $1 \rightarrow 3$ bond and type II in which a $1 \rightarrow 4$ bond is found.

In the first step, α-L-fucose is attached to the galactose of either type of precursor substance. The linkage is by a $1 \rightarrow 2$ bond, and H substance is formed as the result of the reaction.

GDP –(FUC) + (GAL)1 (GLU-N)1 (GAL)1 (GAL-N) Type I (or Type II) R

↓ Fucosyl transferase (H)

GDP + (GAL)1 (GLU-N)1 (GAL)1 (GAL-N) H Substance R
       2
   (FUC)1

The reaction is catalyzed by the fucosyl transferase encoded by the *H* allele.

Alternatively, in the absence of the *Se* allele, another fucosyl transferase encoded by the *Le* allele may attach, by a $1 \rightarrow 4$ bond, an L-fucose to the N-acetylglucosamine of the precursor substance, converting it to the Le^a substance.

GDP –(FUC) + (GAL)1 (GLU-N)1 (GAL)1 (GAL-N) Type I R

↓ Fucosyl transferase (Le)

GDP + (GAL)1 4(GLU-N)1 (GAL)1 (GAL-N) Le^a Substance R
               (FUC)1

In the second step of biosynthesis, the H substance becomes the substrate for one of the three enzymes.

The *Le*-determined fucosyl transferase attaches fucose by a $1 \rightarrow 4$ bond to N-acetylglucosamine of the H substance, converting the latter into the Le^b substance. However, this reaction can take place only in the presence of the *Se* allele; the absence of the *Se* allel precludes formation of the Le^b substance.

GDP–(FUC) + (GAL)1 (GLU-N)1 (GAL)1 (GAL-N) H Substance R
         2
     (FUC)1

↓ Fucosyl transferase (Le)

GDP + (GAL)1 4(GLU-N)1 (GAL)1 (GAL-N) Le^b substance R
       2   2
   (FUC)1 (FUC)1

Alternatively, H substance may serve as the substrate for an N-acetylgalactosaminyl transferase, encoded by the *A* allele, or for galactosyl transferase, determined by the *B* allele. In

the first case, N-acetylgalactosamine is attached by a 1 → 3 bond to the terminal galactose, and the H substance is converted into A substance. In the second case, galactose is bound by a 1 → 3 bond to the terminal galactose, and, as a result, B substance is formed.
result, B substance is formed.

Naturally, both reactions take place simultaneously, and both substances are formed in an individual of the *A/B* genotype. The reactions that lead to synthesis of the H, Le^b, A, and B substances in body fluids and secretions may take place only when the *Se* allele is present, whereas formation of the H, A, and B substances in the erythrocyte membrane occurs regardless of the *Se* genotype.

CLINICAL SIGNIFICANCE OF THE ABO SYSTEM

The antigens of the ABO system play an important role in several distinct areas of clinical medicine.

11.15 ABO Groups in Blood Transfusion

A transfusion of erythrocytes bearing A and/or B antigens into a recipient that does not have these antigens almost invariably produces a severe and often life-threatening **transfusion reaction**. This reaction is caused by the binding of natural anti-A or anti-B agglutinins present in the recepient's plasma with the corresponding antigens on the surface of the donor erythrocytes. This binding leads to intravascular agglutination and, subsequently, owing to activation of complement, to intravascular hemolysis of the transfused erythrocytes. In addition, transfusion of blood containing antibodies directed to antigens on the recipient's erthrocytes may also cause a reaction but does so only rarely. This is because the transfused antibodies are quickly diluted in the plasma of the recipient to an ineffective concentration. In the past, blood from individuals of group O (**universal donors**) was occasionally transfused into individuals of group A, B or AB, whereas blood from individuals of group O, A, or B was transfused into individuals of group AB (**universal recipients**). This practice has been abandoned to avoid a transfusion reaction; presently donor and recipient are almost always ABO compatible, i.e., have the identical ABO group. Although antigens of the ABO system are of primary importance in transfusion reactions, such reactions can be produced by antigens and antibodies of numerous other systems. To eliminate the possibility of such an unexpected reaction, a **major crossmatch** between the serum of the prospective recipient and the erythrocytes of the prospective donor is performed immediately prior to transfusion. In principle, the crossmatch consists of testing for a reaction between the erythrocytes of the donor and serum of the recipient under three conditions: in a saline medium at room temperature, in a high protein medium at $37°C$, and with an antiglobulin serum (Coombs' reagent) (Section 4.6). The first test primarily detects IgM antibodies, while the other two tests detect predominantly IgG antibodies. It is beyond the scope of this book to describe the technical details of the tests employed in the crossmatch. From a practical point of view, however, it is important to realize that a positive reaction in the major crossmatch, regardless of the conditions under which it occurs, indicates the presence of antibodies against the donor erythrocytes in the serum of a prospective recipient and, therefore, precludes transfusion of the blood from this particular donor. An important point to remember is that the crossmatch detects the presence of antibodies but *does not* identify their specificities.

11.16 ABO Incompatibility as a Cause of Hemolytic Disease of the Newborn

Anti-A and anti-B agglutinins, if they belong to the IgG class, may cross the placenta in pregnant women and enter the fetal circulation. Once in the fetal circulation, these antibodies may combine with the corresponding antigens of fetal erythrocytes and cause various degrees of hemolysis. Indeed, about 20 percent of babies of group A or group B born to mothers of group O display some signs of hemolytic disease. Among such infants, the vast majority are group A_1 and only occasionally group A_2 or B. **Hemolytic disease of the newborn** due to ABO incompatibility is usually mild and, in most instances, requires no treatment. In rare cases, however, severe disease may develop with symptoms even more pronounced than seen in the disease caused by anti-Rh antibodies (Section 11.27). In these cases, exchange transfusion may be required to save the life of the child. Because the serologic diagnosis of hemolytic disease elicited by anti-A and/or anti-B antibodies is technically difficult with direct procedures, one must employ indirect testing, e.g., Coombs' test, elution of antibodies from fetal erythrocytes, etc.

11.17 ABO System in Paternity Testing and Forensic Medicine

The A and B antigens were the first to be used in tests concerning disputed paternity (Section 20.6). However, the efficiency of such testing proved to be relatively low owing to several factors. The limited polymorphism of the system makes proof of paternity essentially impossible, while exclusion of paternity is limited by the fact that the heterozygotes *A/O* and *B/O* cannot be distinguished phenotypically from homozygotes *A/A* and *B/B*, respectively. For example, a child of group B cannot be fathered by a man of genotype *A/A* but could be fathered by a man of genotype *A/O*.

   The principle of paternity exclusion is based on two cardinal rules. First, a man cannot father a child that has *two* antigens of which neither is present in the man, e.g., a group O man cannot be the father of a group AB child. Second, a man cannot father a child that lacks both the antigens present in the man, e.g., a group AB man cannot have a group O child.

   Although the ABO system is routinely used for resolving cases of disputed paternity, testing for other more polymorphic antigens, especially those of the HLA system, is currently often employed, also (Section 20.6).

   The antigens of the ABO system of a suspect and of blood stains found at the scene of a crime are used routinely to link or dissociate a suspect with the crime under investigation. The presence of antigens in blood stains, saliva, or semen is usually detected by the ability of such materials, if they contain antigens, to inhibit (absorb) the corresponding antisera. In these procedures, advantage is taken of the fact that the antigens of the ABO system are remarkably stable and can be demonstrated in specimens collected many months or even years after a crime. Also, anti-A and anti-B antibodies appear to be relatively stable and can be recovered from the dried material after several weeks. One must, however, remember that because many tests commonly used in forensic medicine are subject to errors and misinterpretations, appropriate controls must always be used.

11.18 ABO System in Organ Transplantation

Because A and B antigens are present on the cells of many organs, their binding with natural antibodies present in the plasma of a recipient may cause injury to grafted organs. This is especially true in the case of bone marrow and kidney grafts. In fact, some investigators believe that the ABO system determines a set of major histocompatibility antigens (Section 20.5). This unfortunate use of the term major histocompatibility led to a great deal of confusion. Indeed, while the ABO-incompatible kidney grafts are rapidly or hyperacutely rejected, the possibility has never been formally excluded that the gene that carries *A, B,* or *O* alleles is linked to a distinct minor histocompatibility gene (Section 21.3).

THE Rh BLOOD GROUP SYSTEM

The first antigen of what was to become the highly complex Rh system was discovered by Levine and Stetson in 1939 using antibodies found in the serum of a mother who had just delivered a child that was suffering from hemolytic disease of the newborn (Section 11.27). Had these investigators given their newly discovered antigen a name, today we would be using an entirely different designation for the Rh system. As it happened, the antigen was found also to react with antibodies that Landsteiner and Wiener had produced by injecting rabbits and guinea pigs with erythrocytes of a Rhesus monkey. The latter investigators showed that after suitable absorption these antibodies reacted not only with Rhesus monkey erythrocytes but also with the erythrocytes of about 85 percent of Caucasoids. Since the antibodies were named anti-Rhesus and seemed to react with the antigen discovered by Levine and Stetson, the antigen was named the **Rhesus factor** or, abbreviated, **Rh antigen**.

Subsequently, erythrocytes from members of several families were examined with antibodies from the two different sources; i.e., the serum of the mother of the child with hemolytic disease and absorbed sera of rabbits immunized with Rhesus monkey erythrocytes. The results supported the idea that the Rh antigen is a dominant trait and obeys the Mendelian rules of inheritance. Subsequently, it was clearly shown that the Rh antigen is inherited independently of the ABO blood groups and, hence, is a member of an unrelated alloantigenic system. It should be mentioned that during the ensuing years it became recognized that the specificity of the rabbit and guinea pig antibodies is not exactly the same as that of the antibodies produced by humans following transfusion or pregnancy. Thus, there are some investigators who distinguish two discrete systems: one detectable by xenoantisera, which is called anti-LW (anti-Landsteiner-Wiener), and the other defined by human alloantisera, which is referred to as anti-Rh (anti-Rhesus). Very soon after the discovery of the first Rh antigen, other antibodies were encountered in the sera of different patients. These sera seemed to detect antigens that—although apparently related to the original Rh and belonging to the same system—were distinctly different from each other.

11.19 Genetics of the Rh System

Shortly after the discovery of the Rh antigens, two schools of thought arose concerning the structure and inheritance of what is now called the Rh system.

In 1943 the British statistician Fisher proposed that the Rh antigens are determined by pairs of alleles at three very closely linked loci. The loci were called *C, D,* and *E* and were thought to comprise the *Rh* complex. In fact, the three putative loci are so closely linked that, thus far, no crossing-over between them has been found. Each locus would carry two alleles: *C* and *c* at the *C* locus; *D* and *d* at the *D* locus; and *E* and *e* at the *E* locus. Except for *D* and *d*, the alleles are codominant. The alleles at the three loci of a given chromosome form the *Rh* haplotype, which, because of the close linkage of the loci, is inherited as a block. If one accepts the concept that there are three loci and that each has two alleles, there should be eight haplotypes representing all possible combinations of the alleles. In fact, these haplotypes have been identified; their frequencies vary over a broad range with some being relatively common, while others are exceedingly rare (Table 11.8). Furthermore, the frequencies of the *Rh* haplotypes vary in different human populations.

In proposing his three-gene concept, Fisher had available the results of tests employing four antisera that serologically seemed to identify four distinct but related antigens. Two of those antisera recognized seemingly antithetical antigens, which prompted Fisher to consider

TABLE 11.8. The *Rh* Haplotypes (Alleles) as Designated by the Two Nomenclature Conventions

Rh Haplotypes (Fisher-Race)	*R* Alleles (Wiener)	Frequency in Caucasoids
CDe	R^1	0.408
cde	*r*	0.389
cDE	R^2	0.141
cdE	*r″*	0.012
Cde	*r′*	0.010
CDE	R^z	Rare
CdE	r^y	Rare
cDe	R^o	0.026

these antigens as products of two alleles at a single locus—*C* and *c*. Since the other two sera reacted with antigens that were not antithetical, and one of them apparently was the Rh antigen, Fisher proposed that the Rh antigen should be called D and the other antigen E and their corresponding alleles *D* and *E*. Furthermore, Fisher predicted that with a more extensive search antisera detecting the antithetical antigens d and e would be found. Eventually, anti-e serum was found, but anti-d serum thus far has not been encountered. Apparently, the *d* allele is silent and does not encode a detectable molecule. Fisher's concept, and its notation, is presently known as the Fisher-Race notation and will be used throughout this chapter.

An alternative concept of the Rh genetics was proposed by Wiener in 1943. According to the Wiener concept, there is a single gene, *Rh*, that determines a complex molecule that carries several antigenic determinants (factors). The gene has multiple alleles, each determining an allelic product possessing a particular combination of determinants. At least eight alleles can be distinguished (Table 11.8). The alleles R^1, R^2, R^z, and R^o determine molecules that have a determinant corresponding to the original Rh antigen, while the alleles *r*, *r′*, *r″*, and r^y determine molecules that do not possess the Rh antigen. Wiener's determinants correspond to Fisher's antigens and are designated by combination of letters. Many investigators believe that the Wiener genetic concept is most likely correct although years of work has not provided the ultimate proof, i.e., isolation of a single molecule. It is unfortunate that Wiener's notation is so unwieldly. In fact, for those who have only an occasional need to consider the Rh system, the Wiener notation is simply too complicated to keep it at one's fingertips.

The usefulness of the two notations discussed above is greatly limited by striking differences in the nomenclatures for the different antigenic determinants. The two notations are a source of annoyance, if not confusion, to the novice in the field. Still, to be capable of following further discussion, a serious student is advised to master at least the more common symbols of the two notations. Perhaps the most important fact to remember is that as a matter of practicality when one speaks about Rh(+) and Rh(−) individuals, one actually refers to the presence or absence of the D antigen of Fisher or the Rh_o factor of Wiener. This factor is by far the most important in day-to-day clinical practice; the other actors are of importance in only relatively complicated cases (see below).

11.20 Variants of Common Antigens of the Rh System

The simple concepts of Rh genetics became significantly complicated by finding that in addition to the common antigens C, D, E, c, and e several variants can be identified serologically. Some of these variants are of practical importance and are discussed briefly here.

The first variant of the D antigen was described in 1946 by Stratton and named D^u. This variant is found more frequently in Negroids than in Caucasoids. In most instances, the D^u antigen appears as an allelic form of D distinguishable by its agglutinability with IgG, but not by IgM, anti-D sera. In some individuals, the D^u antigen reacts with IgG antibodies only in the presence of antiglobulin (Coombs') reagent (Section 4.6). However, upon standard typing, these individuals all appear as Rh(−). In some other rare instances, a standard D antigen appears to behave as a D^u variant. Typically, such cases involve individuals with the genotype *CDe/cde*. Presently, D^u is considered to be a quantitative, rather than qualitative, variant of D. It has been demonstrated that the concentration of the D antigen on D^u erythrocytes is appreciably lower than the concentration on ordinary Rh(+) cells.

The D^u variant has received wide attention because it has been reported to elicit production of anti-D antibodies in Rh(−) individuals. For these reasons, it became common practice to examine individuals who were originally defined as Rh(−) for the presence of the D^u antigen. This is done by using IgG anti-D and Coombs' reagent and is intended to avoid inadvertent immunization of an Rh(−) recipient by erythrocytes of a D^u donor that upon standard testing appears as Rh(−). However, some investigators question the advisability of this practice since the detection of the D^u variant heavily depends on the choice of a particular serologic reagent. Indeed, it is quite common for one laboratory to define an individual as possessing D^u and for another laboratory to type the same individual as not having D^u antigen, i.e., as D negative or Rh(−). Nevertheless, it should be kept in mind that erythrocytes carrying D^u may be susceptible to the effects of anti-D; therefore, a D^u infant may suffer from hemolytic disease of the newborn.

There are some other variants of the D antigen—e.g., D^w and D^{Cor} (Go^a)—but their low frequency and minimal clinical significance do not justify discussion here.

The complexity of the D antigen is not limited to the three variants mentioned above. This is obvious from the well-documented observations that some individuals carrying the D antigen may produce anti-D antibodies when immunized with erythrocytes of some other Rh(+) individuals. Since these antibodies do not react with erythrocytes of the responding person, an autoimmune response can be ruled out. Even more surprising, anti-D antibodies produced by an Rh(+) individual may react with erythrocytes of some other Rh(+) individuals who also have produced anti-D. In fact, an exhaustive cross comparison of Rh(+) individuals reveals six definite patterns of reactions. The patterns range from those individuals who react with anti-D antibodies of all sources, except their own, to those who react with anti-D antibodies produced only by certain Rh(+) individuals. This fact led to the proposition that the D̄ antigen is in fact a mosaic structure from which various parts can be deleted and, thus, render the cells nonreactive with certain anti-D sera. The most important implication of this idea is that any antiserum designated anti-D may contain a mixture of antibodies directed to different discrete determinants of the D antigen. Consequently, the D antigen itself would be a composite of different determinants rather than a strictly defined entity. The production of a series of monoclonal antibodies should be of great importance in resolving the apparent complexities of the D antigen.

Almost simultaneously with the discovery of the D^u variant, a variant of C antigen, C^w, was reported. The antibody that identified this variant, which behaves as an allele to the C and c antigens, was found in the serum of a *CDe/CDe* homozygous patient who received a blood transfusion from a seemingly Rh-identical donor. Subsequent studies revealed that most anti-C sera also contain anti-C^w antibodies; these two antibodies can be separated by proper absorption. It has been shown that anti-C^w is responsible for some cases of hemolytic disease of the newborn. There are other variants of C, such as C^x, C^u, and C^a, but they are so rarely encountered that their nature remains uncertain.

The E and e antigens also have rare variants (E^w, E^T, e^s, e-like) of which e^s is relatively common in Negroids and is responsible for the formation of one of the compound antigens discussed below.

11.21 Compound Antigens of the Rh System

Perhaps the most striking feature of the Rh system is the formation of unique serologic determinants by combination of two common antigens.

The most frequent **compound antigen**, called f, is generated when *c* and *e* alleles are present in the *cis* position. The f antigen, therefore, may be justifiably considered a result of *cis* complementation (Section 1.2) of *c* and *e* alleles or of interaction of c and e determinants. It is still unresolved whether anti-f serum, produced by immunization with erythrocytes expressing f antigen, reacts simultaneously with the c and e molecules (determinants) or with a unique determinant created by interaction of these two molecules. The f antigen is inherited as an allele with respect to f(−). However, anti-f (or anti-ce) antibodies present in anti-c and anti-e sera are relatively rare and of little clinical importance. Nevertheless, anti-f is an important tool in testing for disputed paternity, since it permits clear-cut distinction between the genotype *CDe/cDE*, which does not determine the f antigen, and the genotype *CDE/cde*, which does. In the absence of an anti-f reagent, the distinction of the above genotypes would have to rely on family studies; for that matter, only in certain families would such studies provide valid information.

Another compound antigen, common in Negroids but rare in Caucasoids, is called V. It is related to the f antigen since it is generated by interaction of c and e^s determinants, the latter being relatively common in Negroids.

By means of carefully selected antisera, it can be shown that C and E determinants form another compound antigen (CE), whereas C and e determinants form yet another compound antigen (Ce). Occasionally, erythrocytes of apparently Rh(−) individuals of the genotype *cde/cde* unexpectedly react with antisera that contain anti-D and anti-C antibodies simultaneously. Such sera are commonly called anti-CD. The reactivity of anti-CD with cells that apparently lack both C and D is explained by the supposition that these cells express an antigen called G. The nature of the G antigen is an enigma. There is no compelling evidence that the G antigen is a typical compound antigen. However, the presence of G antigen could account for various rather perplexing observations. On the one side, anti-CD activity has been reported in sera of pregnant *cde/cde* women in spite of the fact that the father of the child lacked C antigen even though he did possess D antigen. Apparently, the anti-CD in this case was in fact composed of anti-D (against the father) and anti-G against the fetus. On the other side, pregnant *cde/cde* women may have anti-CD after carrying a *Cde/cde* fetus. In this case, the "anti-CD" is apparently composed of anti-C and anti-G.

11.22 Uniform Nomenclature of Rh Antigens

Defining the compound antigens as well as variants of the basic antigens complicated the nomenclatures proposed originally by Fisher and by Wiener. To alleviate the situation, Rosenfield and his collaborators proposed a unified nomenclature (Table 11.9). The nomenclature assigns a sequential number to any serologically identifiable antigenic determinant, whether basic, variant, or compound. In fact, a number is often assigned not so much to an antigen as to an antiserum with characteristic reactivity. The nomenclature concerns phenotypic entities exclusively and is applicable to either of the genetic concepts described earlier. The notation proposed by Rosenfield has met with unexplainable reluctance and is used only occasionally. This is rather unfortunate since, being relatively simple and noncommittal, it circumvents the increasing complexity of the Fisher notation and the extremely complicated notation of the Wiener proposal. A recent initiative to develop a uniform terminology of human blood groups (Table 11.1) may be viewed as a continuation and extension of the Rosenfield idea.

11.23 Incomplete Rh Phenotypes

The first example of an Rh phenotype that lacked some antigens was described in 1950. The individual was the offspring of a consanguineous marriage, and his erythrocytes apparently expressed D antigen but completely lacked the antigens of the Ee and Cc series. Interestingly, these erythrocytes were readily agglutinated by many IgG anti-D sera even when suspended in saline, though normally such sera agglutinate only in the presence of a medium containing a high molecular weight substance (Section 11.3). It was postulated that, being the product of a consanguineous marriage, the individual was a homozygote for a rare Rh haplotype, -D- ("blank D blank"). This notion was supported subsequently by the finding of other examples of such phenotypes, most of which were expressed in offspring of intrafamily marriages. However, this simple explanation appears untenable in the light of the fact that -D- individuals have significantly higher than the expected number of siblings who are also -D-. Since the parents of -D- individuals have a complete Rh phenotype, they must be presumed to be heterozygotes carrying only one -D- haplotype; thus, only 25 percent of their children should be -D-. In reality, significantly more than 25 percent of children of such marriages are -D-. Therefore, one must consider that the expression of -D- may involve a more complex mechanism than merely a partial

TABLE 11.9. Unified Nomenclature of the Serologic Determinants of the Rh System as Proposed by Rosenfield

Rosenfield Notation	Fisher-Race Antigens	Wiener Factor	Type of Determinants (symbol)
Rh1	D	Rh_o	Basic
Rh2	C	rh'	Basic
Rh3	E	rh''	Basic
Rh4	c	hr'	Basic
Rh5	e	hr''	Basic
Rh6	ce	hr	Compound (f)
Rh7	Ce	rh^i	Compound
Rh8	C^w	rh^w	Variant of c
Rh9	C^x	rh^x	Variant of c
Rh10	ce^s	hr^v	Compound (V)
Rh11	E^w	rh^{w2}	Variant of E
Rh12	—	rh^G	G antigen
Rh13	—	Rh^A	Variant of D
Rh14	—	Rh^B	Variant of D
Rh15	—	Rh^C	Variant of D
Rh16	—	Rh^D	Variant of D
Rh17	D	Hr_o	Variant (D of -D- phenotype)
Rh18	d	Hr	Actually absence of antigen
Rh19	e-like	hr^s	Variant of e in Negroids
Rh20	e^s	—	Variant of e
Rh21	C^G	—	Variant of C
Rh22	CE	—	Compound
Rh23	D^w	—	Variant of D
Rh24	E^T	—	Variant of E
Rh25	LW	—	Different System?
Rh26	c-like	—	Variant of c
Rh27	cE (in *cis* position)		Compound
Rh28	—	hr^H	Variant of Rh10 (ce^s) in Negroids
Rh29	—	RH (total)	Unknown
Rh30	$D^{Cor}(Go^a)$	—	Variant of D
Rh31	—	hr^B	Variant of e in Negroids
Rh32	—	R^N	Variant of D in Negroids
Rh33	—	R_o^{Har}	Variant of D
Rh34	—	Bas	—
Rh35	—	1114	Variant of Rh32 in Negroids

deletion of a haplotype inherited in a Mendelian fashion.

The -D- individuals have a high degree of risk of being immunized against various Rh antigens since they express only two antigens, D and possibly G, and therefore are capable of responding to all other antigens of the Rh system. Interestingly, they do not form antibodies that react against other incomplete phenotypes, e.g., C^wD-, cD-. These incomplete phenotypes were also found in consanguineous families; in both instances, the expression of D antigen was unusually strong, while the expression of C^w or c was apparently reduced. It is notable that no phenotype in which E or e is present in the absence of D or C has been found. This suggests that formation of E or e antigens may require the presence of alleles at either *C* or *D* or both loci.

Perhaps the most informative cases, with respect to the genetics and expression of the Rh antigens, are examples of the total lack of Rh antigens or so-called Rh_{null} phenotypes, which were formerly designated −−−. The first case of an Rh_{null} phenotype was reported in 1961. At that time, it was suggested that this phenotype represented the lack of a gene that determines a precursor substance for the Rh antigen, the condition analogous to the absence of precursor or H substance in the ABO system. In the absence of the precursor substance, the genes of the *Rh* complex would not be expressed, and thus the individual would appear as Rh_{null}. Indeed, the second case of an Rh_{null} individual confirmed this supposition since the woman who was Rh_{null} delivered a child who had the CDe/cde phenotype. Since the father was a *cde/cde* homozygote, the child's *CDe* haplotype had to be obtained from the mother. The *CDe* haplotype, although not expressed in the mother, was expressed in the child presumably owing to a normal paternal gene for the precursor.

This type of Rh_{null} is called **regulator type** since it is due to a gene X_r^o inherited independently of the *Rh* complex. This more common type of null phenotype, in addition to the Rh system, is also observed to have an effect on some other blood group antigens such as s and U antigens of the MNS system (Section 12.1) and the En^a antigen.

There is another type of Rh_{null} phenotype called the **amorphic type** caused by the presence of one or more amorphic or silent alleles (*rh*) in the *Rh* complex. In either case, Rh_{null} individuals suffer from an anemia of varying severity. The anemia is believed to reflect the fact that the Rh molecules are integral components of the erythrocyte membrane; the absence of these molecules results in a defect of the membrane and an ensuing susceptibility of such erythrocytes to damage and lysis.

11.24 Relationship between Rh and LW Systems

It was originally believed that the alloantibodies to Rh antigens produced by Rh(−) individuals immunized with Rh(+) cells detect an antigen identical to that detected by xenoantibodies produced by rabbits or guinea pigs immunized with erythrocytes of the rhesus monkey. More recent data strongly indicate that in fact these two antibodies detect two distinct antigens; Rh and LW, respectively. The evidence that the two antigens are actually distinct comes from several observations. First, anti-Rh alloantisera distinguish Rh(+) from Rh(−) individuals, whereas anti-LW xenosera do not. Second, extracts of Rh(−) cells can elicit anti-LW responses in animals. Finally, human Rh(+) erythrocytes, after being coated with IgG anti-Rh, are not agglutinated by IgM anti-Rh but are still agglutinated by anti-LW. All these observations indicate that the LW antigen is distinct from the Rh and that the LW antigen is present on the erythrocytes of most people. Such erythrocytes do elicit an anti-LW response when injected into the occasional individuals who are LW(−).

Taking these facts into consideration, it was postulated that the LW system is determined by two alleles: the *LW* allele, which is responsible for the LW(+) phenotype, and the recessive *lw* allele, which produces the LW(−) phenotype. The two alleles segregate independently of the *Rh* alleles or haplotypes. Still, the two systems appear to be interrelated since all Rh_{null} individuals are also LW(−). It was suggested that LW might be a precursor substance for Rh in a manner similar to the H substance for the ABO antigens. This explanation, although generally consistent with the available data, does not account for all known facts. For example, some anti-LW sera react with LW(−) erythrocytes (as determined with other anti-LW sera), suggesting that the LW substance may be carrying multiple determinants and, accordingly, that the corresponding antisera are polyspecific.

11.25 Chemistry of Rh Antigens

Numerous attempts to determine the chemical nature of the Rh antigens have been largely unsuccessful, and the results of various tests have been at best equivocal. The major problem faced by the immunochemist is the fact that the Rh antigens, which are an integral component of the erythrocyte membrane, cannot be isolated by aqueous solvents. On the other hand, extraction with organic solvents often destroys the antigenic properties of the Rh substance(s). On the basis of the limited available data, it has been proposed that the Rh antigen is a protein that requires association with a lipid moiety for its serologic integrity.

CLINICAL SIGNIFICANCE OF THE Rh SYSTEM

The Rh system, similar to the ABO system, plays an important role in several areas of clinical medicine.

11.26 Rh Antigens in Blood Transfusion

Although there are no natural antibodies to Rh antigens, such antibodies can be elicited by a single transfusion of Rh-incompatible blood. Among the various Rh antigens, the D antigen is the strongest immunogen, but others can and do elicit specific responses. The exception, of course, is the d antigen. The following order of antigenicity of Rh antigens has been established:

$$D > c > C > E > e.$$

As a rule, to avoid undesirable immunization against Rh antigens following transfusion, the prospective recipient and donor should be Rh compatible. However, in practice only compatibility for the D antigen is routinely established, whereas compatibility for other antigens is ignored except in unusual instances. This is to say that no attempt is routinely made to match the Rh phenotype of the donor and recipient exactly except in the case of Rh(−) individuals. The convention has been to avoid transfusion of D-positive blood to D-negative individuals, and thus D(−) recipients of transfusions were presumed to be cde/cde and were cross-matched only with donor bloods of this phenotype. This practice, however, has been challenged in recent years.

In the case of D(+) recipients, on the other hand, no attempt is made to match phenotypes of the donor and recipient. Thus, any D(+) donor would be selected regardless of his antigens C or E. Once elicited, anti-Rh antibodies may cause transfusion reactions that consist of intravascular sensitization of donor's erthrocytes but not intravascular hemolysis since anti-Rh antibodies do not activate complement. Usually, the reaction is characterized by premature removal of the antibody-coated erythrocytes rather than by a frank hemolytic reaction.

11.27 Rh Antigens as a Cause of Hemolytic Disease of the Newborn

Although antibodies to virtually any Rh antigen can cause hemolytic disease of the newborn, the most frequently encountered are anti-D antibodies. In a typical case, an Rh(−) mother carrying an Rh(+) fetus becomes immunized during the late stages of pregnancy and/or at labor owing to the leakage of fetal blood into the maternal circulation. Since the immunization occurs late in pregnancy, the first Rh(+) baby is usually spared the disease. However, the residual IgG anti-D antibodies are often present in the maternal circulation from the onset of subsequent pregnancies. These antibodies cross the placenta and enter the fetal circulation where they injure fetal erythrocytes if the erythrocytes are Rh(+). As the result of the massive onslaught of antibodies, a severe anemia ensues, followed by a reparative erythroblastic reaction and jaundice. If untreated, the disease may cause death or severe neurologic damage (**Kernicterus**).

The treatment in each case depends on the severity of the disease. Two problems must be managed: the anemia must be corrected and the quantity of the serum bilirubin must be reduced. In the mild cases, simple transfusion may be all that is required. In more severe cases, an exchange transfusion is necessary to combat anemia and reduce circulating bilirubin. In recent years, the technique of intrauterine transfusion has been introduced. The decision to perform intrauterine transfusion is based on the results of examination of amniotic fluid obtained by amniocentesis at the third trimester of pregnancy. A high concentration of pigments in amniotic fluid constitutes an indication for intrauterine transfusion.

To prevent hemolytic disease of the newborn, it is now common practice to administer to the Rh(−) mother a measured amount of potent anti-D antibodies after each delivery of an Rh(+) baby. It is believed that these antibodies bind to the fetal erythrocytes that have leaked into the maternal circulation. The antibody-coated erythrocytes are then sequestered in the spleen before they can immunize the mother. This highly effective procedure is widely used to prevent hemolytic disease caused by D incompatibility, but so far no prophylactic antisera to other Rh antigens are available.

11.28 Rh System in Paternity Testing and Forensic Medicine

The determination of the *Rh* haplotypes is widely used in cases of disputed paternity. However, since the *d* allele is silent, it is impossible to distinguish between *D/d* heterozygotes and *D/D* homozygotes. In some instances, the distinction can be attempted on the basis of probability of a given haplotype in a particular population (Table 11.8). For example, in Caucasoids the genotype *CDe/cde* is significantly more frequent than is *CDe/cDe*, while among Negroids the situation is reversed.

Owing to their labile nature, Rh antigens are easily decomposed and, thus, have only limited usefulness in forensic medicine.

11.29 Association of the Rh Antigens with Autoimmune Hemolytic Anemia

An individual who has antibodies directed against his own erythrocytes is said to be suffering from autoimmune hemolytic anemia. The antibodies can be classified as either **cold** when they react best at temperatures lower than $22°C$ or **warm** when they react optimally at $37°C$. Interestingly, among the latter, antibodies specific for Rh antigens are frequently encountered. Anti-e antibodies are perhaps the most common, but other specificities are also found. The mechanism of these hemolytic anemias and their clinical significance are discussed extensively in various textbooks of hematology.

12 / Some Clinically Important Blood Group Systems in Man

A large number of blood group systems have been identified in man. Although all of them may be of interest to immunogeneticists, only some of them have appreciable clinical importance. In this chapter, only the latter will be discussed briefly, and the others will be omitted. The interested reader may find more detailed information about all of the systems in the specialized textbooks and monographs listed in the references for this section.

THE MNS BLOOD GROUP SYSTEM

The MNS system, according to the new terminology MNS-2, was originally identified by a xenoantiserum obtained by immunization of rabbits with human erythrocytes. Upon proper absorption, this serum reacted with erythrocytes of some but not all individuals. The reaction was attributed to the binding of antibodies with an antigen designated M. Subsequently, an alternate antigen called N was identified.

12.1 Phenotypes and Genotypes of the MNS System

The early studies suggested that the M and N antigens are determined by two codominant alleles, *M* and *N*, at a single locus (*MN*). The two alleles produce three genotypes—*M/M, M/N,* and *N/N*—and their corresponding phenotypes. This simple picture, however, was not to last since subsequent studies identified two other antigens, S and s. These two antigens appeared to be products of two codominant alleles, *S* and *s*. The two alleles are believed to be at the *Ss* locus that is closely linked but distinct from the MN locus. With this in mind, the system had to be expanded into haplotypes consisting of *M* or *N* and *S* or *s* alleles. As a result, the number of phenotypes increased from three to six (Table 12.1).

Apparently, the *Ss* locus must carry a third allele, which appears to be silent since there are, especially among blacks, individuals whose erythrocytes do not have either S or s antigens.

In addition, there is another antigen called U that probably is the product of still another gene linked to the other two loci. Of the two putative alleles of this gene, one determines the U antigen, while the second either encodes an unidentifiable product or is actually silent. The phenotype lacking U is referred to as S^u. Since the relationship between the *MN, Ss,* and *U* genes remains poorly understood, one must, for the time being, accept a concept of three closely linked genes with alleles that comprise several haplotypes. In fact, even this concept is an oversimplification, since the MNS system consists of some 20 serologically identifiable determinants. While some of them appear to be rare alleles at the *MN* locus, the true nature of the others is still enigmatic.

12.2 Chemistry of the MN Antigens

The M and N substances are glycoproteins composed of a protein core and side chains made up of sugars and sialic acid. The molecular weight of the repeating units is estimated to be 50,000 to 53,000. The actual determinants are formed by the addition of neuraminyl groups to the side

TABLE 12.1. Genotypes and Phenotypes of the MNS System in Man

Genotype	Phenotype	Frequency in Caucasoids	Reaction of Erythrocytes with			
			Anti-M	Anti-N	Anti-S	Anti-s
MS/MS	MS	0.20	+		+	
MS/Ms			+		+	+
Ms/Ms	Ms	0.08	+			+
MS/NS	MNS	0.28	+	+	+	
MS/Ns			+	+	+	+
Ms/NS			+	+	+	+
Ms/Ns	MNs	0.22	+	+		+
NS/NS	NS	0.07		+	+	
NS/Ns				+	+	+
Ns/Ns	Ns	0.15		+		+

chains by appropriate neuraminyl transferases. During enzymatic degradation of M substance by neuraminidase, the specific determinants are lost and the M substance is converted into N substance. Upon continuing digestion, the latter is converted first into T substance and then into T_n.

$$M \xrightarrow{\text{SIAL}} N \xrightarrow{\text{SIAL}} T \xrightarrow{\text{GAL}} T_n$$

SIAL—sialic acid   GAL—galactose

On the basis of this observation, it is believed that the biosynthesis of M and N substances involves the conversion of N into M by an enzymatic process similar to that involved in the conversion of H substance into either A or B antigens (Section 11.14). Accordingly, the *M* and *N* alleles should determine specific enzymes catalyzing the conversion, while the actual substances would merely be secondary products of these alleles. In fact, one may speculate that the *N* allele is silent, i.e., does not encode any enzyme, whereas the *M* allele encodes an enzyme responsible for the conversion of N into M.

12.3 Clinical Significance of the MNS System

Natural anti-M or anti-N antibodies are rare; induced antibodies usually belong to the IgM class. Anti-M antibodies are more common than anti-N probably because N substance seems to be the precursor for M substance. An exceptional situation is encountered in individuals undergoing chronic hemodialysis; these individuals have a pronounced tendency to produce anti-N antibodies. Even when present, anti-M and anti-N do not cross the placenta and, thus, do not cause hemolytic disease of the newborn. However, although either antibody can cause transfusion reaction, their rare presence makes such a reaction an unusual event. One should still remember that exceptionally rare antibodies of the IgG class may cause a serious reaction.

In contradistinction to anti-M and anti-N, anti-S and anti-s may be either natural or induced and can cause both a transfusion reaction and hemolytic disease of the newborn.

Testing for the antigens of the MNS system is successfully used in excluding disputed paternity. Using anti-M, anti-N, anti-S, and anti-s sera, one can exclude paternity in about 24 percent of cases; the results are equivocal in the remaining 76 percent.

THE P BLOOD GROUP SYSTEM

The P system, according to the new terminology P-3, was discovered much the same way as the MNS system, using intentionally produced xenoantisera that detected an antigen that was named P. Soon thereafter, natural anti-P antibodies were found in normal human beings as well as in sera from pigs, cows, and horses.

12.4 Phenotypes and Genotypes of the P System

One of the current concepts of serology and genetics of the P system is summarized briefly in Table 12.2. There are five distinct phenotypes, but for all practical purposes only two of them, P_1 and P_2, are found in an appreciable proportion of people. The P_1 phenotype, characterized by the presence of determinants P and P_1, is demonstrable in 75 percent of the population, whereas the P_2 phenotype, which expresses only the determinant P, is found in 25 percent. The extremely rare phenotype p has no detectable antigenic determinant.

The genetic determination of phenotypes has not been definitely established. However, according to the most recently proposed model, alleles at two discrete loci are involved. One locus may have three alleles. The dominant P^k and P_1^k alleles are found with similar frequency of 0.5; they encode a galactosyl transferase that catalyzes the conversion of ceramide dihexoside (CDH) into ceramide trihexoside (CTH) or P^k antigen. The product of the P_1^k allele galactosyl transferase, also converts paragloboside into P_1 substance. The recessive and extremely rare p allele is silent; the individual homozygous for p forms neither P^k nor P_1 substance. The other locus could have two alleles. The dominant and frequent P_2 is believed to determine an N-acetylgalactosaminyl transferase. This enzyme catalyzes glycosylation of P^k substance (CTH) and converts it into P substance. The second, extremely rare allele, the recessive P_2^0, is silent and does not encode an enzyme. Thus, the p/p, P_2^0/P_2^0 homozygous individual cannot form any of the determinants and has the p phenotype.

An alternative model proposes three loci, each with two alleles of which one is dominant and the other recessive (silent). A p^k allele encodes galactosyl transferase that converts CDH into P^k substance. The P_1 allele at another locus encodes a regulatory molecule that allows the galactosyl transferase encoded by the p^k allele to convert paragloboside into P_1 substance.

TABLE 12.2. Phenotypes of the P Blood Group System in Man

Phenotype	Frequency in Caucasoids	Reaction of Erythrocytes with		
		Anti-P	Anti-P_1	Anti-PP_1P^{k}*
P_1	0.75	+	+	+
P_2	0.25	+	−	+
P_1^{k}	Very low	−	+	+
P_2^{k}	Very low	−	−	+
p	Very low	−	−	−

*Formerly called anti-Tj^a antibody, which regularly is found in serum of individuals with the phenotype p.

Finally, the P_2 allele at the third locus determines galactosaminyl transferase that is responsible for the conversion of the P^k substance into the P substance (globoside).

12.5 Chemistry of the P Substances

The presently available data are consistent with the concept that P antigens are either glycolipids or glycoproteins. The initial precursor substances are ceramide dihexoside (CDH) and paragloboside.* In the first case, CDH is converted into ceramide trihexoside (CTH) or P^k substance by the action of transferase encoded by the P^k or P_1^k alleles. The CTH becomes substrate for an N-acetylgalactosaminyl transferase encoded by the P_2 allele; glycosylation results in formation of globoside, i.e., the P antigen. In the second case, paragloboside is a substrate for α-galactosyl transferase, determined by the P_1^k allele, and is converted into the P_1 antigen.

In rare instances in which no CTH is formed owing to homozygosity for the *p* allele, the P_2 allele cannot be expressed even if present, whereas the P_1^k allele is expressed since it does not require the presence of CTH. Individuals with such a genotype will have a P_1^k phenotype characterized by the presence of P_1 and the absence of P antigens. On the other side, p^k homozygotes that are simultaneously P_2/P_2 homozygotes will have a P_2^k phenotype lacking both P_1 and P antigens. The two P^k phenotypes can be distinguished from the p phenotype by their reaction with anti-PP_1P^k (formerly anti-Tj^a) serum with which the p phenotype does not react.

12.6 Clinical Significance of the P System

Anti-P_1 antibodies are found commonly as natural antibodies in the sera of P_2 persons, and anti-PP_1P^k are regularly encountered in sera of individuals with the phenotype p. However natural

---

*Paragloboside is also a substrate for the fucosyl transferase encoded by the *H* allele (Section 11.14) and may be converted by this enzyme into the H substance.

antibodies do not cause a transfusion reaction. On the other hand, induced anti-P_1, i.e., developing after transfusion of P blood into P_1 recipients, can cause a transfusion reaction that includes intravascular hemolysis.

A special situation is encountered in the case of Donath-Landsteiner (DL) autoimmune antibodies, which may react with both P and P_1 antigens. These antibodies bind to the antigens at relatively low temperature; subsequently, when the temperature rises, they activate complement and cause massive hemolysis in situ. This phenomenon is responsible for a characteristic syndrome of paroxysmal cold hemoglobinuria.

Limited polymorphism and our current inability to determine genotypes directly make the P system unsuitable for paternity exclusion or for forensic studies.

THE KELL BLOOD GROUP SYSTEM

12.7 Phenotypes and Genotypes of the Kell System

The Kell system—or according to the new terminology, KEL-6—was originally considered a simple system consisting of two condominant alleles, K and k, and two corresponding antigens, K and k, the latter formerly called Cellano. In Caucasoids the phenotypic frequencies are K = 0.002, Kk = 0.08, and k = 0.92, corresponding to the three genotypes *K/K, K/k,* and *k/k*. Since the time of the original description, more than 18 rare alleles of the Kell system have been reported. It is currently believed that the Kell system may be similar to the Rh system (Section 11.9) with a bewildering array of alleles and determinants. This analogy became particularly obvious when it was realized that the Kell system consists of three pairs of antithetical antigens—K and k, Kp^a and Kp^b, and Js^a and Js^b. Recently, it was proposed to rename these antigens K_1 and K_2, K_3 and K_4, and K_6 and K_7, respectively. The three antigens may be determined by multiple alleles at a single locus or, alternatively, by pairs of alleles at three closely linked loci, forming a haplotype. Interestingly, the rare phenotype K_o was reported that, in similarity to Rh_{null}, has no known K antigens. Individuals with the K_o phenotype are capable of producing a variety of Kell-related antibodies after being transfused with blood from virtually any donor. In spite of a multitude of antigens assigned to the Kell system, the K and k antigens appear to be of the greatest importance.

Virtually nothing is known of the chemistry and biosynthesis of the Kell antigens. Since the synthetic pathways are speculative and disputed, they will not be addressed in this book.

12.8 Clinical Significance of the Kell System

Except for antigens belonging to the ABO and Rh systems, the K antigen is probably the most immunogenic of the remaining blood group antigens of man. A single transfusion of blood from a K+ donor into a K− recipient results in production of anti-K in about 5 to 10 percent of cases. Conversely, transfusion of blood from a k+ donor into a k− recipient often results in production of anti-k. Since the *K/K* homozygotes are extremely rare (0.002), it may be particularly troublesome to select a suitable donor that is K compatible in addition to being ABO and Rh compatible The induced antibodies are of the IgG class and can cause both transfusion reaction and hemolytic disease of the newborn.

Interestingly, a rare K_o phenotype is overrepresented among patients suffering from chronic granulomatous disease; it seems that there is a relationship between K_o and the disease.

THE DUFFY BLOOD GROUP SYSTEM

12.9 Phenotypes and Genotypes of the Duffy System

The Duffy system (new nomenclature, FY-8) consists of two principal antigens, Fy^a and Fy^b. However, since the original description of the system, the number of antigens has increased significantly by discovery of several rare antigens. Because the relationship between the rare and common antigens remains obscure, they will not be discussed here.

The four phenotypes (Table 12.3) are determined by three alleles, Fy^a, Fy^b, and Fy^x. The Fy^x allele, although rare in Caucasoids and Orientals, is found very frequently in Negroids. It may actually represent a variety of alleles still unidentified. Recently, the Fy gene has been assigned to human chromosome 1 where it is linked to the Cae gene that determines congenital cataract.

Considering the fact that the Fy^a antigen is particularly susceptible to proteolytic enzymes, it is tempting to speculate that the protein component is either directly or indirectly responsible for the antigenic properties of the antigen. Unfortunately, the postulated pathways of biosynthesis of Duffy antigens are highly speculative and modeled in analogy to ABO and Rh systems. There are no chemical data to support any of the proposed schemes.

12.10 Clinical Significance of the Duffy System

Anti-Fy antibodies develop almost invariably as the result of transfusion or pregnancy. Each of the two possible antibodies, anti-Fy^a and anti-Fy^b, may cause a transfusion reaction; however, only the former appears to be involved in hemolytic disease of the newborn.

TABLE 12.3. Genotypes and Phenotypes of the Duffy Blood Group System in Man

Genotype	Phenotype	Frequency in Caucasoids	Reaction of Erythrocytes with	
			Anti-Fy^a	Anti-Fy^b
Fy^a/Fy^a	Fy(a+b−)	0.17	+	−
Fy^a/Fy^b	Fy(a+b+)	0.49	+	+
Fy^b/Fy^b	Fy(a−b+)	0.34	−	+
Fy^x/Fy^x*	Fy(a−b−)	Very low	−	−

*The Fy^x allele may actually represent several different alleles or a single silent allele.

Although the Duffy system is used to exclude paternity, use is limited by constraints in acquiring or selecting specific and strong antisera.

Owing to its striking racial distribution, the Duffy system is an invaluable tool in the hands of anthropologists. For example, the Fy (a+b−) phenotype is very frequent in Orientals (0.996), less frequent in Caucasoids (0.17), and rare in Negroids (0.09), whereas the Fy(a−b−) phenotype in Negroids has a frequency of 0.68–0.90 and is rare in Orientals and Caucasoids.

THE KIDD BLOOD GROUP SYSTEM

12.11 Phenotypes and Genotypes of the Kidd System

The Kidd system (JK-9) consists of two antigens, Jk^a and Jk^b, that are products of two codominant alleles, *Jk^a* and *Jk^b*. The two alleles are responsible for three genotypes and their corresponding phenotypes, which are found in strikingly different frequencies in various racial groups. In Caucasoids, phenotypic frequencies are Jk(a+b−) = 0.28, Jk(a+b+) = 0.49, and Jk(a−b+) = 0.23. In contrast, in Negroids the corresponding frequencies are 0.54, 0.39, and 0.07. Furthermore, in non-Caucasoids, a fourth phenotype, Jk(−b−), was discovered, suggesting that there is a third allele (*Jk^o*) that is silent. Nothing is known about the chemistry or biosynthesis of these antigens. Interestingly, granulocytes and platelets may have an antigen that is cross-reactive when a mixture of anti-Jk^a and anti-Jk^b sera is used.

12.12 Clinical Significance of the Kidd System

Anti-Jk antibodies are induced by transfusion and by pregnancy. Once formed, these antibodies, which are usually IgG, may cause both transfusion reaction and hemolytic disease of the newborn. A particularly insidious problem encountered with anti-Jk antibodies is a delayed transfusion reaction. This reaction develops in people who were preimmunized with Kidd antigens but at the time of a second transfusion have no detectable antibodies. The second transfusion elicits a brisk secondary response with a rising titer of antibodies that may cause a reaction when such antibodies bind with transfused erythrocytes. The insidious delayed reaction, however, is rare because anti-Jk antibodies, once induced, usually persist for years.

The Kidd system may occasionally be employed to exclude paternity.

THE I BLOOD GROUP SYSTEM

The system consists of two antigens, I and i, detectable by antibodies that preferentially react at low temperatures and usually remain inactive at 37°C. Among adult Caucasoids, the vast majority of individuals are I(+), but in rare instances, an individual may be I(−). These individuals express an alternative antigen, i. The two antigens are determined by two corresponding alleles, *I* and *i*, of which the former is dominant—thus only *i/i* homozygotes will have the i phenotype. All newborns are phenotypically i, and their erythrocytes react with and anti-i but do not react with anti-I. During the newborn's first 18-24 months of life, its cells slowly develop reactivity with anti-I and simultaneously lose reactivity with anti-i, however, anti-i reactivity is never lost entirely. Apparently, I substance is synthesized at the expense of the i substance, but this process takes place only in individuals carrying the *I* allele. One is tempted to speculate that the i substance represents a precursor, analogous to H substance, from which the I substance is formed. Interestingly, most individuals in spite of being I(+) contain in their sera anti-I antibodies of the IgM class. Although these antibodies usually cause no reaction in vivo, owing to their poor reactivity at 37℃ , antibodies of certain individuals occasionally do become active at body temperature. This results in a hemolytic anemia known as the cold antibody type of acquired anemia.

PUBLIC AND PRIVATE ANTIGENS

Because certain antigens are found in a vast majority of individuals; these antigens are often considered species specific and are commonly referred to as **public**, especially if their frequency is 0.97 or higher. Being extremely frequent, they are discovered only by accidental finding an individual who lacks a given public antigen. As expected, the individual lacking a certain public antigen often produce antibodies upon transfusion or after pregnancy. These antibodies, once demonstrated, can be used to identify the antigen and its frequency. In addition, intentional immunization of such an individual with erythrocytes carrying public antigen induces production of antibodies to public antigens. Testing the population with these antibodies enables one to identify those individuals whose erythrocytes do not react with antibodies owing to the lack of the particular public antigen.

TABLE 12.4. Partial List of Public and Private Blood Group Antigens in Man

Public[a]		Private[b]	
At^a	(Augustine)	Be^a	(Berrens)
En^a		By^a	(Batty)
Ge^a	(Gerbich)	Becker	
Gn^a	(Gonsowski)	Job	(Jobbins)
Gy^a	(Gregory)	Levay	
Kn^a	(Knops-Helgensen)	Rm^a	(Romunde)
Lan	(Langereis)	Sw^a	(Swann)
Sd^a	(Sid)		
Vel$_1$	(Vel)		
Vel$_2$	(Vel)		

[a]Phenotypic frequency $\approx$ 0.97.
[b]Phenotypic frequency $\approx$ 0.0025.
NOTE: Each name is formed from the name of the individual (shown in parentheses) in whom the antigen was identified or in whose sera the first specific antibodies were found.

In contrast to public antigens are antigens that are extremely rare. Such antigens are identified by the accidental discovery of antibodies that react with these antigens. Because of their rarity, it is difficult to find individuals expressing these antigens and to test their erythrocytes extensively. Furthermore, when found, the antibodies are often in limited supply, and sometimes the entire pool of antiserum is exhausted before extensive testing is accomplished. These rare antigens are commonly referred to as **private**. The exact classification of an antigen as rare or private is a matter of judgment and usually is made arbitrarily. In several instances, after years of studies, private antigens are found to be rare variants of the antigens belonging to one of the established systems. For example, various antigens of the Kell system were originally considered as private antigens before they were assigned to the system.

Certain private and public antigens form distinct systems in which two antigens are products of alleles at the same locus that appear with strikingly different frequencies. To assign public and private antigens to a single system may be an arduous task. Such a system initially appears as nonpolymorphic, and from the point of view of formal genetics, it actually is (Chapter 1). However, the systems consisting of one public and one private antigen are important from a clinical point of view. For example, in rare instances the individual who carries a private antigen may require transfusion, which should be given with blood from a donor who also carries the same private antigen. Otherwise, the first transfusion will result in immunizing the individual against the antithetical public antigen and, as direct result, preclude future transfusions with commonly available blood. An abbreviated list of public and private antigens in man is given in Table 12.4.

13 / Blood Groups of Non-human Animal Species

The amount of attention devoted to the blood groups of a given species often is related to the economic and/or scientific importance of the species. Thus, some species have received a great deal of attention, while others have been only summarily examined or totally ignored. In addition, since many investigations have taken place in isolation by different groups of researchers, some antigens or entire sytems have been discovered independently by different laboratories and, unfortunately, named independently. Only recently have efforts been made to exchange typing antisera and to systematize and standardize the nomenclatures of different systems. However, the reader must be cautioned that no definite agreement has been reached in many cases; multiple notations are still in use and occasionally the description given below may seem to conflict with original reports found in the literature. In this chapter, a brief overview is given with the intention of presenting selected information. When considering the phenotypic or allelic frequencies of various animal blood group systems, one should also be aware that in most instances the breeding of domestic animals is far from random. Intentional selection for certain commercially desirable traits (body size, coat color, behavior, size of litter, etc.) may distort a random distribution of blood groups in various populations if the selection for the desired traits inadvertently also affects the blood group genes.

BLOOD GROUP SYSTEMS OF VARIOUS NON-HUMAN SPECIES

13.1 Mice (*Mus musculus*) and Rats (*Rattus norvegicus*)

By the virtue of being expressed on erythrocytes, some murine alloantigens are classified into a separate group called **erythrocyte alloantigens** (Ea). However, the name is grossly misleading since most of the Ea were subsequently also demonstrated on various nucleated cells. In fact, some of them were at one or another time considered to be histocompatibility antigens and assigned H notation (Chapter 21). Even today, the capacity to induce an HVGR by some Ea molecules remains the subject of dispute. It seems that the HVGR originally attributed to some Ea molecules is actually elicited by H antigens determined by the *H* genes, which are closely linked to the *Ea* genes. In other cases, no such linkage has been demonstrated, leaving open the issue of a possible involvement of Ea antigens in the rejection of allogeneic skin grafts.

Currently, eight distinct Ea systems are defined (Table 13.1). Each system consists of a relatively few (two to three) alleles; in some instances, one of the alleles is silent. Virtually nothing is known about the molecular products of the *Ea* alleles and their biologic function.

Even less is known about blood group systems in rats. So far, at least three systems—RT2, RT3, and RT4—have been defined (Table 21.4). Considering the phylogenetic relatedness of rats and mice, one would expect that rats should have blood group systems similar to those identified in mice. Indeed, a homology between the Ea-1 system of mice and the RT2 of rats has been reported some time ago. The rat systems are also considered minor histocompatibility antigens by some investigators. However, very recent studies show that rats do not reject grafts bearing incompatible RT2 and RT3 antigens despite a demonstrable production of antibodies against these antigens.

TABLE 13.1. Murine Erythrocyte Alloantigen (Ea) Systems Identified in Inbred Strains

Locus	Alleles	Antigens	Congenic Pairs	Tissue Distribution (other than erythrocytes)
Ea-1	*a*	1.1 (A)	—[a]	
	b	1.2 (B)		
	c (o)	None	—[b]	
Ea-2 (*R-Z,rho,H-14*)	*a* (1)	2.1 (R)	B10.F-*Ea-2*[a]	Brain, thymus, kidney, liver,
	b (2)	2.2 (Z)	B10[c]	lungs, spleen, testes
Ea-3 (λ)	*a*	3.1	B10.L	
	b	None	B10	
Ea-4 (*BL,D*)	*a*	4.1	C3H-*Ea-4*[a]	Kidney, lung, thymus
	b	4.2	C3H	
Ea-5 (α,*H-5*)	*a*	5.1		Brain, kidney, liver, lungs,
	b (o)	None		muscle, spleen, testes
Ea-6 (*H-6*)	*a*	6.1	C3H-*H-6*[a]	Brain, kidney, lungs, muscle,
	b	6.2	C3H-*H-6*[b]	spleen, testes
Ea-7 (*T*)	*a*	7.1	B10.129(5M)	Thymocytes
	b	7.2	B10	
Ea-8	*a*	8.1		
	b	?		

[a]Alleles *Ea-1*[a] and *Ea-1*[b] have been identified only in wild mice.
[b]All inbred strains carry the *Ea-1*[c] allele.
[c]Several other congenic pairs are available.
NOTE: The synonym notations are given in parentheses.

13.2 Rabbits (*Oryctolagus cuniculus*)

Although scores of papers have been published about the blood groups of rabbits, it seems that in most, if not all, instances the same system is rediscovered over and over again. This major system—called Hg—was originally discovered in the early 1930s and since then has been given no fewer than 10 different designations (Table 13.2). It is difficult to decide which of these nomenclatures is most appropriate, but in this discussion the most recent notation will be employed.

From the numerous studies reported in the literature, it seems to be well established that the Hg system is determined by three codominant alleles—Hg^A, Hg^D, and Hg^F—residing at a single locus *Hg*. The three alleles determine the corresponding products A, and D, and F, which can be detected by specific antibodies induced by intentional immunization. The antibodies are elicited by injection of erythrocytes into appropriate recipients, but, apparently, the effectiveness of the immunization depends on the Hg phenotype of both the donor and the recipient. Specifically, essentially all A(−) animals respond to the A antigen, but only a few D(−) rabbits

TABLE 13.2. Various Notations of the Phenotypes of the Hg Blood Group System of the Rabbit

Current Genotype Designation	(Cohen 1962)[a]	Phenotypic frequency[b]	(Ivanyi 1956)	(Dahr 1955)	(Heard 1955)	(Joysey 1955)	(Anderson 1955)	(Kellner 1953)	(Marcusen 1936)	(Fisher 1933)	(Castle 1933)
						Phenotype (author and year of introduction)					
A/A	A	0.12–0.31	Hcsch	V_1	Y	B	A	g	Kb	K_1	H_2
DJK/DJK	DJK	0.0–0.12	—	O	W	C	O	—	—	O	O
FK/FK	FK	0.06–0.52	HcN	R_1	Z	A	B	G	Ka	K_2	H_1
A/FK	AFJK	0.23–0.78	He	R_1r_1	YZ	BA	AB	gG	KbKa	K_1K_2	H_2H_1
A/DJK	ADIJK	?	—	r_1	YW	BC	A	—	—	K_1	H_2
FK/DJK	DFJK	?	—	R_1	ZW	CA	B	—	—	K_2	H_1

[a]See text for detailed descriptions.

[b]Random breeding colonies selected for high reproductive capacity.

262

will produce anti-D antibodies. The response to F antigen varies depending on the phenotype of the responder; A(+) animals respond frequently, whereas A(−) respond only occasionally. Notably, strong antibodies are also elicited by grafting skin between Hg-incompatible animals. This was originally assumed to be evidence that Hg antigens are expressed on skin cells and, thus, may represent minor histocompatibility antigens. However, currently most investigators regard the antibodies produced after skin grafting to be the result of stimulation by passenger erythrocytes present in the blood vessels of the graft. This conclusion is supported by the observation that anti-Hg antibodies do not cause skin graft rejection nor are they cytotoxic for nucleated cells. On the other hand, they are clearly responsible for transfusion reactions and, when injected into pregnant females, cause the abortion of fetuses that express the antigens for which the injected antibodies are specific.

The availability of specific antibodies permitted extensive studies of the allelic products of the Hg system. These studies revealed that two of the original antigens, D and F, share another determinant called K in addition to their unique determinants. Upon this discovery, the two alleles and two antigens were renamed DK and FK, respectively. Subsequently, it was demonstrated that the DK antigen has still another determinant, J, and accordingly should be renamed DJK. Apparently, the three antigens—A, DJK, and FK as they are presently known—are multideterminant and highly complex moieties. This unforeseen complexity was certainly responsible for the confusion that reigned over early studies of the Hg system. The complexity is further compounded by the presence of so-called **interaction** or **hybrid determinants**. These determinants are present in certain *Hg* heterozygotes but absent from parental homozygotes. For example, Hg^A/Hg^{FK} animals express the J determinant that is absent from either of the parents; the Hg^A/Hg^{DJK} heterozygotes express the I determinant. Taking into the account these various determinants, six distinct Hg phenotypes are presently recognized (Table 13.2). The phenotypic frequencies encountered in various colonies selected for high reproductive capacity varies over a broad range probably in part owing to an inadvertent selection for blood groups during intentional selection within the colonies. Interestingly, in a wild population living in isolation and under harsh environmental conditions, there is striking preference for heterozygosity; it remains to be seen whether this represents a biologically significant phenomenon or just fortuitous observation.

Nothing is known about the chemistry of the Hg antigens. Serologic studies suggest that the Hg antigens of the rabbit are not analogous with any known system of man, mice, or rats.

13.3 Cats (*Felix felix*)

Six antigenic systems designated A, B, C, D, E, and F have been identified in cats. The first four systems are defined by deliberately produced antibodies. These antibodies permit the distinction of allelic products determined by two codominant alleles within each system. In contrast, E and F system antigens are identified by natural antibodies found in the sera of the animals that lack the corresponding antigen. The two systems seem to be related to each other, since of the four phenotypes expected from the random assortment of alleles belonging to the two systems, one phenotype, E(+)F(+), has never been demonstrated. The serologic and/or genetic basis for this remains unknown.

13.4 Dogs (*Canis familiaris*)

Seven independent systems—A, B, C, D, F, Tra and He—have been identified in dogs (Table 13.3). Within most of the systems, animals can be divided into two phenotypic classes: one class that expresses serologically detectable antigen and a second class that lacks a given antigen. In the simplest terms, each system could be considered as consisting of two autosomal alleles, one dominant allele that encodes an antigen and a second allele that is recessive and silent. However, it should be kept in mind that products of the putative silent alleles may eventually be identified.

The A system appears to be an exception to the general pattern. In this system, the phenotypes Aa and Aa_1 are distinguished in addition to a phenotype that lacks detectable antigen. Therefore, the A system must have three alleles—A^1, A^2, and a—which can be arranged into six genotypes. The Tra system also seems to have three alleles—Tr, O, and $(-)$. The first two alleles determine substance that is synthesized in tissues and subsequently adsorbed on erythrocytes. The substance is chemically related to human A substance (Section 11.3) and A-like substances of animals (see below). The antigens are usually detected using intentionally induced antibodies that produce agglutination or hemolysis. An exception is the D system in which sera of D(−) animals may contain natural anti-D antibodies. The blood group antibodies of the dog can cause transfusion reaction, and numerous studies have been done using the dog as an experimental animal for research on transfusion incompatibility.

13.5 Horses (*Equus caballus*)

There is a great deal of confusion concerning the nomenclature of equine blood groups. The primary source of this confusion is the fact that the original studies were carried out independently in four countries, and in each country a different notation was proposed (Table 13.4). Most regretfully, the four notations have employed the same symbols (either capital letters or Arabic numerals) to denote entirely different systems or antigens. Therefore, care must be exercised to indicate which nomenclature is actually used. Furthermore, it must be kept in mind that the notations refer merely to the serologically identifiable antigens (determinants), and information is insufficient to arrange these antigens into distinct systems. The distribution of antigens in different populations of horses varies significantly. For example, the D antigen of the French notation is relatively frequent (0.44) in France, whereas it seems to have disappeared altogether in North Africa. Interestingly, in European race horses the D antigen is also rather infrequent (0.02).

The quantitative expression of some antigens in horses is influenced by the chromosomal position of the corresponding alleles. For example, antigen 1 of the British notation when inherited in a *trans* position with either antigen 2 or 5 has a strikingly reduced expression,

TABLE 13.3. Canine Blood Group Systems

System (synonym)[a]	Genotype	Phenotype[b]	Phenotypic Frequencies[c]	Method of Detection
Aa	A^1/A^1, A^1/A^2, A^1/a	Aa	0.45	Lysis
(CEA1, DEA1)	A^2/A^2, A^2/a	Aa$_1$	0.19	
	a/a	a	0.36	
Ba	B/B, B/b	B(+)	0.05	Agglutination
(CEA3, DEA3)	b/b	B(−) or b	0.95	
Ca	C/C, C/c	C(+)	0.98	Agglutination or
(CEA4, DEA4)	c/c	C(−) or c	0.02	antiglobulin test
Da	D/D, D/d	D(+)	0.20	Agglutination
(CEA5, DEA5)	d/d	D(−) or d	0.78	
Fa	F/F, F/f	F(+)	>0.99	Agglutination
(CEA6, DEA6)	f/f	F(−) or f	<0.01	
Tra	Tr/Tr, Tr/O, $Tr/-$	Tr(+)	0.50	Agglutination
(CEA7, DEA7)	O/O, $O/-$	O(+)		
	$-/-$	Tr(−)		
He	?	He(+)	0.40	Agglutination
(CEA8, DEA8)				

[a]Synonymous notations were introduced in 1973 (CEA = canine erythrocyte antigens) and in 1976 (DEA = dog erythrocyte antigens) and they were replaced by current notations in 1978.

[b]The minus sign (−) after a phenotype indicates that no antigen can be detected.

[c]In a random population of "street dogs" in the USA and the Netherlands.

whereas inheritance in a *cis* position results in normal expression of antigen 1. The mechanism of this phenomenon remains unclear.

The study of equine blood groups was in part stimulated by the fact that the first case of hemolytic disease of the newborn was actually observed in the horse. However, the disease, known as isohemolytic disease of the foal, differs from that of man—namely, the horse placenta is virtually impermeable to the antibodies present in the serum of the mare. Once born, the foal that is nursed by his own mare becomes exposed to the antibodies present in her colostrum. Within the first 24 hours of life, these antibodies can be absorbed through the stomach of the foal and may cause fatal disease owing to intravascular hemolysis.

TABLE 13.4. Different Notations for the Blood Group Antigens of Horses

Notation	Antigens																
French	A	C	D	E	F	H	I	J	L								
Rumanian	A	B	E			C		D		F							
Polish	1		2		3						4	5					
British	6		10					4		3	1	2	5	8	11	7	9

13.6 Pigs (*Sus scrofa*)

Currently, 10 distinct systems are recognized in this species (Table 13.5). The G system consists of two codominant alleles that determine corresponding products, whereas the A, B, F, H, I, and J systems, in addition to dominant alleles, have a recessive (silent) allele that does not encode a detectable product. The genetic determination of the E, K, and L systems is still the subject of controversy (see below).

The detection of blood group antigens in pigs is accomplished by use of various antibodies (alloimmune, heteroimmune, and natural) in direct agglutination, hemolysis, or antiglobulin (Coombs') tests. In addition, extensive studies using various lectins* have identified several moieties that do not belong to any known system.

Interestingly, the E system of pigs resembles the human Rh system (Section 11.19). The similarity in the pattern of inheritance of the Rh and E systems led to speculations concerning the genetics of the E system; these speculations parallel those discussed for the Rh system. There are two concepts (Fig. 13.1) that deserve a brief comment. According to one concept, there is a single E locus with at least five alleles. Each allele determines a product bearing three out of the six known antigenic determinants identifiable by proper antibodies. The second concept proposes that there are three very closely linked loci, E_1, E_2, and E_3; each locus bears at least two alleles. Each allele determines a product identifiable by a single antigenic determinant. Alleles at the three loci on a given chromosome form an E haplotype. Theoretically there should be eight distinct haplotypes, but currently only five have been found. It is unknown whether the three anticipated, but not yet identified, haplotypes actually exist in nature. In contrast to the human Rh system, no deletion or null E haplotypes are known.

Similar alternative concepts of single versus multiple loci have been proposed for two other swine systems: K and L.

13.7 Cattle (*Bos sp.*)

Probably because of their economic importance, cattle have been extensively studied for genetic markers. These studies resulted in the identification of a least 11 independent blood group systems (Table 13.6). Studies of cattle blood groups pose a unique problem since bovine erythrocytes can be classified as well agglutinated or poorly agglutinated regardless of the antigen and antibodies employed. The differences are most likely caused by a peculiar location of the antigens within the cell membrane; in poorly agglutinated cells, the antigen is located exceptionally deep in the membrane. Although this does not prevent the binding of the antigen with antibodies, it does interfere with bringing cells together in agglutination. Because of this, hemolysis rather than agglutination is routinely employed in studies of the bovine blood group systems. While some of the cattle systems are relatively simple and display limited polymorphism, others are bewilderingly complex. Among the latter, the B and C systems occupy unique positions and deserve more detailed discussion.

The B system is the first to be described in the species. Phenotypically, it consists of

---

*These are plant extracts that combine specifically with certain sugars of cell surface molecules.

TABLE 13.5. Summary of the Blood Group Systems of Domestic Pigs

System	Genotype	Allelic Frequencies		Phenotype*	Method of Detection
A	A/A, A/a a/a	A	0.08–0.49	A O or A(−)	Agglutination (natural antibodies) or hemolysis (heteroantibodies)
B	B^a/B^a, B^a/B^- B^-/B^-	B^a	0.72–0.92	Ba(+) Ba(−)	Agglutination
F	F^a/F^a, F^a/F^- F^-/F^-	F^a	0.07–0.34	Fa(+) Fa(−)	Agglutination
G	G^a/G^a G^a/G^b G^b/G^b	G^a G^b	0.13–0.62 0.38–0.87	Ga Gab Gb	Agglutination or antiglobulin test
H	H^a/H^a, H^a/H^- H^a/H^b H^b/H^b, H^b/H^- H^-/H^-	H^a H^b H^-	0.13–0.43 0.00–0.04 0.55–0.85	Ha(+) Hab(+) Hb(+) H(−)	Lysis or antiglobulin test
I	I^a/I^a, I^a/I^- I^-/I^-	I^a	0.40–0.48	Ia(+) Ia(−)	Antiglobulin test
J	J^a/J^a, J^a/J^- J^-/J^-	J^a	0.29–0.85	Ja(+) Ja(−)	Antiglobulin test
K	K^a/K^a, K^a/K^- K^{ad},K^{ad}, K^{ad}/K^a, K^{ad}/K^- K^b/K^b, K^b/K^- K^b/K^a K^b/K^{ad} K^-/K^-	K^a K^{ad} K^b	0.15–0.49 0.00–0.04 0.28–0.73	Ka(+) Kad(+) Kb(+) Kab(+) Kadb(+) K(−)	Agglutination or lysis
L	L^a/L^a L^a/L^b L^a/L^{bc} L^b/L^b L^{bc}/L^{bc}, L^{bc}/L^b	L^a L^b L^{bc}	0.2–0.8 0.03–0.51 0.17	La(+) Lab(+) Labc(+) Lb(+) Lbc(+)	Agglutination

*The minus sign (−) after the phenotype indicates that no antigen can be detected.

more than 40 serologically identifiable determinants (factors), and the number of determinants is still increasing with the development of new reagents.* Some of the known determinants appear to be allelic—e.g., "BGK" and O_1T_1—since when present in a given individual, they are never transmitted to the same offspring. Other determinants seem to be determined by closely linked genes and are transmitted together. The determinants that are transmitted as a block from a bull or cow to their offspring form a so-called **phenogroup**. There is good evidence that as many as 1,000 distinct phenogroups exist. Two parental phenogroups form the phenotype of

*A partial list of determinants consists of the following: A′, A′^{a}, B_1, B_2, B′, D′, E'_1, E'_2,E'^a_3, F′, G, G′, G′^{a}, I_1, I_2, I′, J′, K′, O, O_1, O_2, O_3, O_x, O′, O′^{a}, P, p′, Q, Q′, Q′^{a}, T′, T_1, T^a_1, Y, Y_1, Y_2, Y′, 7.

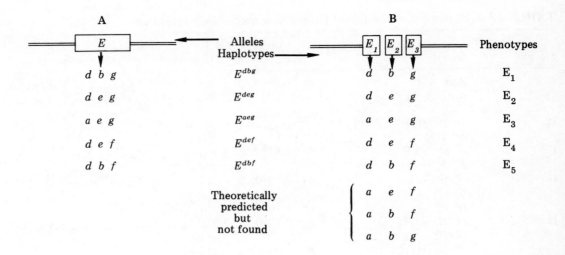

FIG. 13.1. Two models of the genetic determination of the E system in pigs. (**A**) Single locus concept with five alleles that determine multideterminant molecules. (**B**) Three loci (E_1, E_2, and E_3) concept with each locus carrying at least two alleles. The alleles at three loci on the given chromosome form the E haplotype.

TABLE 13.6. Summary of Blood Group Systems of Domestic Cattle

System	Number of Alleles or Haplotypes	Number of Phenotypes	Number of Antigens (determinants)	Known Antigens (determinants)
A(A-H)	10	13	5	A_1, A_2, D, D_2, Z'
B	1,000	15,000	~40	See text
C	100	300	15	C_1, C_2, C_1'', C_2'', E, L', R_1, R_2, W, X_1, X_2, F6, F10, F12, F15
F-V	4	9	5	F_1, F_2, V_1, V_2, V_3
J	4	4*	2	J, Oc
L	2	2*	1	L
M	3	4*	2	M_1, M_2
N	2	2*	1	N
S	5	12	6	S, H, H_1, U, U_1, U_2
Z	3	3*	2	Z, Z_2
R'S'	2	3	2	R', S'

*Includes a negative phenotype with no detectable product.

the offspring. There are close to 15,000 phenotypes. It should be kept in mind that some phenogroups may be "duplicates," since each laboratory currently uses its own battery of typing sera and some antisera with different designations may actually detect the same determinants. The enormous amount of information concerning cattle phenogroups was collected after it was agreed that all cattle belonging to a particular commercial breed (Angus, Hereford, Holstein, Jersey, Limousin, Maine-Anjou, etc.) should have its B phenotype registered. This typing revealed that each breed has certain characteristic phenogroups, and the sum of the frequencies of the 10 most common phenogroups in any given breed equals about 0.8, whereas the less characteristic phenogroups, numbering up to 50 in each breed, are responsible for the remaining 0.2. Some phenogroups appear to be limited to a single breed.

The genetics of the B system is the subject of heated debate among specialists. On the one side are the investigators who propose a multigenic model of the B system inheritance. To support their contention, these investigators bring forth numerous reports of "abnormal" transmission of the phenogroups with either loss or gain, or both loss and gain, of certain factors. Such abnormal transmissions are commonly interpreted as evidence of crossing-over between closely linked genes forming the B complex. The number of distinct genes postulated to form the B complex in the most extreme case was proposed to be as high as 22. However, the number is more likely closer to 6 or 12. The genes on a given chromosome would form a haplotype determining a particular phenogroup. The distance between the two most distal genes of the haplotype that presumably determine factors Q and I was estimated by various investigators to be between 0.4 and 0.34 cM. The extreme polymorphism and multigenic determination of the B complex bring into mind a homology with the MHC systems of various species (Chapter 17).

The alternative concept proposes that the B system is determined by multiple alleles at a single locus. According to the proponents of the single-locus model, the abnormal inheritance represents either intragenic crossing over (between exons) or random mutations or both. The available data do not permit distinction between the two concepts.

The C system consists of multiple factors that make up close to 100 phenogroups. The genetic determination of the C system remains unresolved; and, again, two concepts—multigenic and single gene—are considered. In the first case, the most distal genes of the C haplotype that presumably encode determinants X and L are believed to be about 0.4 cM apart.

Some antigens of the various blood group systems of domestic cattle are apparently shared by phylogenetically related species such as the elk and bison.

13.8 Sheep (*Ovis aries*)

There are two sets of blood group systems of sheep proposed by two different groups of investigators. One set consists of 10 systems designated by the capital letters A-K. However, except for the A system (see below), it is unknown whether these are indeed separate and independent systems or actually different allelic products of a single or only a few systems. The other set consists of eight defined systems, each with several alleles (Table 13.7). Five of these systems are relatively simple and consist of two to three dominant and recessive alleles inherited in a straightforward Mendelian fashion. The remaining three systems are more complex.

The RO or Rr system consists of two alleles R and r^o at a single locus R. The R allele

TABLE 13.7. Summary of Blood Group Systems of Sheep

System	Genotype	Phenotype*	Phenotypic Frequencies	Method of Detection	Related to Bovine System
A	A/A, A/a	A(+)	0.5–0.8	Hemolysis	
	a/a	A(−)	0.2–0.5		
B	Multiple	52 phenotypes	—	Hemolysis	B
C	C/C, C/C^x, C/c	C	0.0–0.9	Hemolysis	C
	C^x/C^x, C^x/c	Cx	0.0–1.0		
	c/c	C(−)	0.0–0.08		
D	D/D, D/d	D(+)	0.1–0.8	Agglutination	
	d/d	D(−)	0.2–0.9		
I	I/I, I/i	I(+)	0.9–1.0	See text	
	i/i	i(+)	0.0–0.1		
M	M/M, M/m	M	0.0–0.8	Hemolysis	S
	Mx/Mx, Mx/M, Mx/m	Mx	0.0–0.04		
	m/m	M(−)	0.2–1.0		
R	R/R, R/r^o	R	0.2–0.8	Agglutination	
	r^o/r^o	R(−) or O	0.2–0.7		
XZ	X/X	X	0.6–1.0	Hemolysis	J
	X^z/X^z	Z	0.0–0.1		

*The minus sign (−) indicates that no antigen can be detected.

determines the R antigen, whereas r^o determines the O antigen. Both antigens are detectable on the erythrocytes of appropriate animals as well as in their saliva. The antigens are identified either (1) by natural anti-R or anti-O found in the sera of some sheep or (2) by natural anti-J antibodies found in the sera of J(−) cattle (Table 13.6). The expression of R and O antigens depends on the concomitant presence of a dominant I allele at an independent I locus, whereas animals that are homozygous for the recessive i allele at this locus do not express either R or O antigen (Table 13.8). A similar requirement appears to apply to the expression of the C system. To some extent, the I and i alleles of sheep are reminiscent of the Se and se alleles of man (Section 11.11).

The B system of sheep seems to be analogous to the B system of cattle. As many as 52 haplotypes (phenogroups) have been identified and divided into five sets on the basis of serologic cross-reactivity. The five sets possibly correspond to an allelic series at five closely linked loci composing the B complex in sheep. The loci are called E^1 (6 alleles), I (9 alleles), Q (10 alleles), O (19 alleles), and B (8 alleles).

Notably, some sheep antigens are also detectable in goats—species closely related phylogenetically to sheep. However, goats also carry their own species-restricted blood group antigens, which are divided into several distinct systems.

TABLE 13.8. Relationship between the *I* and *R* Genotypes and the R Phenotypes of Sheep

I Genotype	*R* Genotype	R Phenotype	Phenotypic Frequency
I/I or *I/i*	*R/R, R/r⁰*	R	0.21–0.82
	r⁰/r⁰	r	0.17–0.74
i/i	*R/R, R/r⁰, r⁰/r⁰*	i	0.00–0.10

13.9 Rhesus Monkeys (*Macaca mulatta*)

As many as 13 independent systems have been reported in rhesus monkeys (Table 13.9). Two of these systems (G and H) have only codominant alleles with nine and three phenotypes, respectively. The remaining systems have silent alleles in addition to one to three dominant or codominant alleles.

13.10 Chickens (*Gallus gallus*)

Currently, 14 systems are identified in chickens. All except the B system are relatively simple with polymorphism limited to two to three alleles. The highly polymorphic B system, which corresponds to the avian MHC, will be discussed later (Section 17.9). Interestingly, in spite of the intense, intentional inbreeding of chickens in the process of developing breeds with the most desirable commercial features (egg laying, growth, body size, etc.), there is a striking tendency to maintain heterozygosity of the blood group genes. Superficially, this might be construed as evidence that blood group phenotypes are associated with the characteristics for which breeding was carried out. However, it is more likely that the blood group genes are linked to the genes controlling the selected trains and that the preponderance of heterozygosity of blood group genes merely reflect the heterozygosity of other genes.

A peculiar blood group system in chickens is called Hi and consists of an antigen that is expressed in females and not in males. However, the antigen can be induced in males by the administration of estrogens, which suggests that the expression of some blood group antigens is sex hormone dependent.

BLOOD GROUPS IN OTHER SPECIES

Some studies have been done on the blood groups of such species as trouts (*Salmo gardinerii* and *Salmo trutta*), sardines (*Sardinops caerulea*), doves (*Streptopeliae*), and pigeons (*Columbae*). These studies have provided several interesting observations concerning (1) variations in the inheritance of various antigens with the concomitant generation of hybrid antigens and (2) the similarities of blood groups in phylogenetically related species. On the other hand, the blood

TABLE 13.9. Blood Group Systems of the Rhesus Monkeys Maintained in the Regional Primate Center, University of Wisconsin

System	Number of Alleles	Genotype	Phenotype
G	4	G^1/G^2, G^1/G^2	G_1
		G^1/G^3	G_1G_3
		G^1/G^4	G_1G_4
		G^2/G^2	G_2
		G^2/G^3	G_2G_3
		G^2/G^4	G_2G_4
		G^3/G^3	G_3
		G^3/G^4	G_3G_4
		G^4/G^4	G_4
H	2	H^1/H^1	H_1
		H^1/H^2	H_1H_2
		H^2/H^2	H_2
I	3	I^1/I^1, I^1/i	I_1
		I^1/I^2	I_1I_2
		I^2/I^2, I^2/i	I_2
		i/i	i
M	4	M^1/M^1, M^1/m	M_1
		M^1/M^2	M_1M_2
		M^2/M^2, M^2/m	M_2
		M^2/M^3	M_2M_3
		M^3/M^3, M^3/m	M_3
		M^3/M^1	M_3M_1
		m/m	m
N	3	N^1/N^1, N^1/n	N_1
		N^1/N^2	N_1N_2
		N^2/N^2, N^2/n	N_2
		n/n	n
J	2	J^1/J^1, J^1/j	J_1
		j/j	j
K	2	K^1/K^1, K^1/k	K_1
		k/k	k
L	2	L^1/L^1, L^1/l	L_1
		l/l	l
O	2	O^1/O^1, O^1/o	O_1
		o/o	o
P	2	P^1/P^1, P^1/p	P_1
		p/p	p
Q	2	Q^1/Q^1, Q^1/q	Q_1
		q/q	q
R	2	R^1/R^1, R^1/r	R_1
		r/r	r
S	2	S^1/S^1, S^1/s	S_1
		s/s	s

groups of some common laboratory animals such as guinea pigs, hamsters, or gerbils remain true terra incognita.

HUMAN BLOOD GROUP SUBSTANCES DEMONSTRABLE IN ANIMALS

Before closing this chapter, a few words should be spared for the human blood group substances shared by various animal species and animal antibodies reactive with the human antigens. Most information in this area concerns the human A, B, and O substances, which are very common in nature. A wide variety of bacteria, plants, and animals have molecules that react with either the anti-A or anti-B antibodies of man.

All rabbits carry B-like antigen, which is capable of adsorbing human anti-B antibodies. However, the rabbit B-like substance is apparently different from the human B substance since rabbit sera contain natural antibodies that agglutinate human group B cells but not rabbit B erythrocytes. Thus, rabbit anti-B must recognize a human B determinant that is absent from the rabbit B-like substance.

In contrast to B-like substance, which in rabbits is an isoantigen (species specific), a rabbit A-like substance behaves as an alloantigen. Rabbits can be grouped with human anti-A antibodies, as well as the anti-A of some other species, as A-like(+) or A-like(−). Interestingly, the A-like substance of rabbits is present in secretions or on nucleated cells but not on erythrocytes. The substance closely resembles human A_2, and some rabbits have in their sera antibodies reacting with human A_1 cells. In addition, some rabbits have anti-H antibodies in their sera.

Since rabbits are favorite animals for raising antibodies to various human tissue antigens, one should be aware that prior to their use the antisera must be thoroughly absorbed with erythrocytes to remove the anti-A_1, anti-B, and anti-H antibodies.

Horses possess both A-like and B-like substances and can be classified as A, B, or AB. However, these substances are present only in the secretions or secreting tissues, e.g., gastric mucosa, and not on the equine erythrocytes. In human volunteers, antigens of horse gastric mucosa are used to produce strong immune anti-A or anti-B antibodies that are used in clinical blood grouping.

Pigs are either A or O, and the A-like substance, which is called A^p, is present in their secretions and on the erythrocytes. The A^p substance can be detected by natural anti-A^p present in the sera of O pigs as well as by human immune anti-A. Interestingly, anti-A^p also reacts with J(+) cattle erythrocytes and R(+) sheep erythrocytes, indicating that the A^p determinant is shared by these species. One should, however, remember that J, R, and A^p substances, although serologically similar, are quite distinct. For example, the J and R substances are actually serum antigens that are passively adsorbed on erythrocytes, whereas the A substance is an integral component of the cell membrane. Natural anti-J of cattle cross-reacts with cattle J, sheep R, and human A, but the natural anti-R of sheep cross-reacts only with sheep R and human A but not with the cattle J substance.

Finally, as might be expected, primates have human A and O substances (chimpanzee) or

A and B substances (orangutang, gibbon, and gorilla). Notably, the gorilla excretes A and B substances in the urine, but the substance is absent from erythrocytes. Usually, primates have natural anti-A and anti-B in a reciprocal arrangement to the corresponding antigens. In addition to the A and B antigens, primates possess antigens related to the human M, N, Rh, and LW systems.

IV / Suggested Supplementary Reading

The following list of publications has been compiled to provide the reader with a source of specific references. It consists predominantly of the most recent textbooks, monographs, reviews, and some selected original papers. Each publication listed has an extensive list of references that may be useful for the reader who desires to pursue in depth some of the topics discussed in the preceeding section.

Altman, P. L., Katz, D. D. (eds.), *Inbred and Genetically Defined Strains of Laboratory Animals*. Parts I & II. Federation of American Societies for Experimental Biology, Bethesda, Maryland, 1979.

Cohen, C. (ed.), Blood groups in infrahuman species. Ann. N.Y. Acad. Sci. **97**: 1–328, 1962.

Delaney, J. W., Garraty, G., *Handbook of Hematological and Blood Transfusion Techniques*. Appleton-Century-Crofts, New York, 1969.

Fundenberg, H. H., Pink, J. R. L., An-Chuan Wang, Douglas, S. D., *Basic Immunogenetics*. Oxford University Press, New York, 1978.

Galton, D. A. G., Goldsmith, K. L. G. (eds.), *Hematology and Blood Groups*. University of Chicago Press, Chicago, Illinois, 1961.

Giblett, E., *Genetic Markers in Human Blood*. F. A. Davis Co., Philadelphia, Pennsylvania, 1969.

Graham, H. A., Williams, A. N., A genetic model for the inheritance of the P, P_1 and P^k antigens. Immunol. Communic. **9**: 191–201, 1980.

Hildeman, W. H. (ed.), *Frontiers in Immunogenetics*. Elsevier/North-Holland, New York, Amsterdam, Oxford, 1981.

Hildeman, W. H., Clark, E. A., Raison, R. L., *Comprehensive Immunogenetics*. Elsevier/North-Holland, New York, Oxford, 1981.

Huestis, D. W., Bove, J. R., Busch, S. *Practical Blood Transfusion*. Little, Brown, and Co., Boston, 1981.

Issitt, P. D., Issitt, C. H., *Applied Blood Group Serology*. Spectra Biologicals Division of Becton, Dickinson & Co., Oxnard, California, 1975.

Jamieson, G. A., Greenwalt, T. J. (eds.), *Glycoproteins of Blood Cells and Plasma*. Lippincott, Philadelphia, 1971.

Klein, J., *Biology of the Mouse Histocompatibility-2 Complex*. Springer-Verlag, New York, Heidelberg, Berlin, 1975.

Klein, J. Immunology. *The Science of Self-Nonself Discrimination*. A Wiley-Interscience Publication. New York, 1982.

Mohn, J. F., Plunkett, R. W., Cunningham, R. K., Lambert, R. M. (eds.), *Human Blood Groups*. S. Karger, Basel, 1976.

Mollison, P. L., *Blood Transfusion in Clinical Medicine*. F. A. Davis Co., Philadelphia, Pennsylvania, 1979.

Mourant, A. E., *The Distribution of Human Blood Groups*. Blackwell Scientific Publications, London, 1954.

Race, R. R., Sanger, R., *Blood Groups in Man*. Sixth Edition. Blackwell Scientific Publications, London, 1975.

Shifrine, M., Wilson, F. D. (eds.), *The Canine as Biomedical Research Model. Immunological, Hematological and Oncological Aspects*. Technical Information Center, U.S. Department of Energy, Springfield, VA, 1980.

Stansfield, W. D., *Serology and Immunology, A Clinical Approach*. Macmillan Publishing Co., New York, 1981.

Zmijewski, C. M., *Immunohematology*. Meredith Corporation, New York, 1968.

V / Major Histocompatibility Systems

14 / Historical Background

"ANCIENT" HISTORY

Although the expressions histocompatibility antigen and *histocompatibility* gene were introduced in 1948 by George Snell, the idea of histocompatibility has existed much longer. In fact, the concept goes back to the time when the idea of tissue and organ transplantation emerged. Desperate attempts to replace lost organs, not to speak of lost youth, met almost invariably with total failure. Often both the recipient as well as the donor of the graft fell victim to these attempts. Primitive surgical technique alone could not be blamed for the sad and consistent disasters of early transplantation endeavors because, occasionally, autologous grafts of a similar nature brought a remarkable degree of success. Thus, it became readily apparent that an individual receiving a graft from another individual of the same species (allograft) cannot permanently tolerate such a graft even if it becomes temporarily established. The results of grafts between members of different species (xenografts) were even more discouraging. The reason for inability to tolerate allografts and xenografts remained obscure for many years.

An important turn in the work on tissue and organ transplantation came with the advent of studies on tumors. Because these investigations required the constant availability of tumor cells of a given type, attempts were made to propagate these cells in the form of grafts. Initial attempts were also unsuccessful since tumor cells, like normal tissues, were almost invariably and promptly rejected by the recipients. The breakthrough came finally from a most unexpected source—the pet mouse.

To support their colonies and expand their markets, dealers breeding pet mice began supplying animals to research laboratories, unknowingly providing the researchers with a new and powerful tool—partially inbred animals (Section 5.2). The production of fully inbred mice was a long and arduous process that ultimately resulted in an availability of a variety of strains without which our modern immunogenetic studies would be difficult to imagine. This is why one can justifiably say that the pet mouse ushered us into a new era of scientific inquiry.

Probably by sheer chance, Jensen in Copenhagen and Loeb in Philadelphia, both working at the turn of the century on tumor grafting, were supplied with partially inbred mice. Both laboratories demonstrated that in such mice certain tumors could be successfully grafted and, in fact, propagated from one recipient to another for several generations. Successful grafting of tumor cells was obviously a curse to the recipient mouse, since it meant that the tumor grew and ultimately resulted in the death of the animal. The animals did not resist the graft and did not reject the tumor, or, to put it differently, they accepted and succumbed to the tumor graft. Most important, both susceptibility and resistance to the tumor graft were shown to be genetically controlled by dominant alleles of 14 to 15 genes that segregate independently and, conversely, that resistance to a tumor graft is controlled by the recessive alleles of these genes. Subsequent studies showed that the alleles for susceptibility and resistance are codominant and conversely, the resistance to a tumor graft is controlled by the recessive alleles of these genes.

Once the first step on the road to elucidation of the genetic basis for graft rejection was made, three crucial questions emerged. First, what are the products of the alleles that determine susceptibility and resistance? Second, how do the resistance alleles accomplish rejection of the graft? Third, and perhaps the most intriguing, are the resistance alleles that determine tumor graft rejection also responsible for the rejection of normal tissues or organs?

Even before the actual data were available, a hypothesis dealing with all three questions had been advanced by Haldane in 1933. According to this hypothesis, resistance to tumor grafts and probably to grafts of normal cells is due to an immune reaction directed against alloantigens present in the donor but absent from the recipient; susceptibility is the result of the absence of such an immune reaction, i.e., the donor and recipient share relevant antigens. To prove the hypothesis, it was necessary to demonstrate that mice of different strains do indeed carry different alloantigens against which an immune reaction could be elicited. Furthermore, it was essential to demonstrate that graft rejection is in fact mediated by an immune response to an alloantigen(s). It was, unfortunately, easier to say what should be done than it was to accomplish it. Numerous attempts to immunize one mouse against another appeared to fail, according to the serologic tests and criteria used; at that time the armamentarium for detecting an immune response was limited to a few unsophisticated techniques based on agglutination or lytic reactions.

Credit for the unequivocal demonstration of alloantigens in mice belongs undeniably to Peter Gorer who, in 1936, reported the presence of a so-called antigen II, demonstrable by hemagglutination of murine erythrocytes by hetero- as well as alloantisera. Antigen II was present in two strains (A and CBA) but absent in one strain (C57BL). Subsequent studies, clearly demonstrating a correlation between segregation of antigen II and susceptibility to tumor grafts, supported the tenet that the two traits are functionally related. More important, mice that did not carry antigen II and that were resistant to (rejected) tumor grafts from a strain that did carry antigen II produced antibodies to antigen II. Furthermore, these antibodies could be specifically adsorbed by both tumor and normal cells of mice carrying antigen II. With these data at hand, Gorer proposed a hypothesis similar to that of Haldane. The hypothesis stated that isoantigenic factors* present in the grafted tissue but absent from the recipient of this tissue evoked the response that led to rejection of the graft.

The actual demonstration that the reaction responsible for graft rejection is immunologic was accomplished by Sir Peter Medawar and his colleagues in 1943/44. Curiously, Medawar used outbred rabbits rather than the inbred mice quite commonly used in biological research. The choice of animals, however, did not undermine the validity of the results and their interpretations. Medawar demonstrated that skin allografts, but not autografts, are rejected after a period of time in which both types of grafts establish vascular connections with the recipient tissues. The most important observation, however, was the finding that rejection of an allograft sensitizes (immunizes) the recipient only to subsequent grafts from the same, or an alloantigenically related, donor. Such a sensitization results in an accelerated rejection of subsequent grafts often referred to as **second-set grafts**. The specificity and generalized nature of the sensitization is now accepted as prima facie evidence for an immunologic basis of graft rejection.

This early period of work closed when the type of immune reaction against grafts was identified by Mitchison in 1954. Using his, now classic, adoptive transfer system, Mitchison

---

*The original term isoantigen is currently replaced by the term alloantigen.

showed that the reaction could be passively transferred to an unimmunized individual only by lymphoid cells, and not serum, of the graft recipient. Thus, it became clear that the destructive immune reaction toward a **first-set graft** is cell mediated and that antibodies play only a minor or secondary role, if any. Antibodies, however, may significantly contribute to rejection of second-set grafts.

MODERN HISTORY

The next stage of development began with the universal acceptance of the genetic and immunologic theories of graft rejection. The primary objectives of the research in this period were to determine the exact mode of genetic control of the alloantigens responsible for graft rejection, to characterize their chemical structure, and, ultimately, to find a means of manipulating the immune response to such antigens. While some of these objectives have been accomplished at least in part, others continue to be elusive.

Early studies on alloantigens indicated that a great deal of complexity would be involved in defining the immunogenetics of graft rejection. However, only systematic studies have revealed exactly how enormous this complexity is. In fact, the emerging complexity put studies of alloantigens in a sphere often far removed from the mainstream of biologic research. Only recently, attempts have been made to revise the old concepts and construct a simple model to account for the findings accumulated over the years. Historically, the work on the genetic determination of alloantigens has proceeded along two complementary lines.

One line was initiated in 1946 by Snell who undertook the formidable task of attempting to isolate the different alloantigens (histocompatibility antigens) genetically, so that their effect on graft rejection could be studied. As a result of many years of work, Snell, and many other investigators following in his footsteps, produced large numbers of congenic pairs of inbred mouse strains (Section 5.9 and Chapter 21). Members of each pair differed, at least theoretically, by alleles of a single histocompatibility gene, and thus rejection of any graft between the pair was due to an immune reaction to a single antigen. This approach led to the distinction of two groups of histocompatibility genes and their corresponding antigens. The two groups consisted of **major** (strong) and **minor** (weak) antigens distinguished on the basis of the intensity and the speed of the graft rejection caused by the respective incompatibility. The major histocompatibility antigen, identical with the antigen II of Gorer, was found to be controlled by a gene located within the murine genome in the IXth linkage group, and this gene was named the *H-2* gene. Soon after, it became obvious that the *H-2* gene is in reality a cluster of several genes separable by recombination and, therefore, properly should be renamed as the *H-2* complex. The individual genes that comprise the entire complex, now referred to as the **major histocompatibility complex** (MHC), are closely linked and are usually inherited as a block, which is commonly called the *H-2* haplotype. The genes of the *H-2* complex were found to be highly polymorphic, and in early studies using congenic strains, Snell could distinguish as many as a dozen different alleles among laboratory mice.

The second line of investigation, carried out by Gorer and his collaborators, aimed at the serologic characterization of the different allelic products of the *H-2* complex. This line of investigation soon demonstrated that a given antigen consists of several serologically defined determinants or specificities. Some of these specificities were found only in one allelic product, whereas others were shared by several alleles. Serologic studies not only confirmed but also extended the concept of the multigenic structure of the murine MHC.

Both lines of investigation eventually converged in studies of histocompatibility antigens in species other than the mouse. In these studies, the techniques and concepts developed during the work with mice were often employed directly or after appropriate modifications. The major achievement of these studies was the demonstration that virtually all mammalian and probably all vertebrate species have an MHC analogous to that of mice. Perhaps the most enlightening example in this respect are the studies undertaken in the early 1950s by Jean Dausset who reported the first **human leukocyte antigen** (HLA), which he called Mac. This discovery was soon followed by the description of a multitude of human alloantigens by different investigators. In fact, the number of new antigens became so great that it was suspected that some of the antigens were identical and differed only in names given arbitrarily by their discoverer(s). Contrary to the studies in mice, which were carried out on standardized inbred strains and with standardized serologic reagents produced in congenic animals, the studies in man could be done only on random populations and with unstandardized and often multispecific reagents. The First International Workshop, which was organized by Amos in 1965, failed to introduce a semblance of order into available observations, and all its results were deliberately destroyed to avoid even greater controversy. However, the initiative of Amos eventually bore fruit, and subsequent workshops have led to the definition of the *HLA* complex as a cluster of closely linked genes, each with multiple alleles.

The modern era of studies on histocompatibility antigens seemed to have reached an end with seemingly precise definition of the genetics and structure of transplantation antigens. However, during the recent years in which the function of the MHC has become the primary object of studies, so many fascinating vistas have been revealed that it is more than certain that the final chapter has not been written. Surprisingly, the results of studies that originated from problems encountered in tissue and organ transplantation have been only reluctantly accepted by transplantation surgeons, i.e., the individuals who would benefit most significantly from these discoveries. The usefulness of the HLA matching of donor and recipient, to avoid or minimize graft rejection, is still hotly debated although in practice accepted and carried out.

CONTEMPORARY PERIOD

From the onset of studies on histocompatibility antigens, it was suspected that they must play a biologic function other than mediating graft rejection—which, after all, is a man-made phenomenon. Once the *H* genes, and especially the MHC, were defined, their association with a variety of biologic phenomena was looked for and reported. Some 50 or more traits have been found to be associated with the MHC phenotype, making the complex the most pleiotropic of all known mammalian systems. Some of those traits are probably only incidentally associated with the MHC, but at least two phenomena appear to be a reflection of the basic biologic function of the MHC. The discovery of these two phenomena constitutes the basis of most of the current studies in the field.

First, the MHC was found to influence the immune capacity of an individual. The demonstration by Benacerraf and McDevitt (1963–65) that the MHC determines the magnitude of immune responsiveness triggered a flow of studies and speculations on the **Ir phenomenon**, which refers to genetic control of antigen-specific responses (Section 19.2). Second, the already classic work of Zinkernagel and Doherty (1974) provided evidence that the MHC profoundly affects the effectiveness of cell-mediated responses by a phenomenon called **MHC restriction**. There seems to be an emerging consensus that the products of MHC genes serve as primary guides for immunologically competent T cells in their function of distinguishing between self and nonself.

In addition, the MHC was shown to determine susceptibility of an individual to a variety of diseases. The discovery of the first such association resulted in an extensive search still actively going on. It is debatable whether such an association is the direct effect of histocompatibility antigens or just an incidental phenomenon. Still, the implications for genetic counseling, disease prevention, and diagnosis are too great not to pursue all available leads.

With this brief historical overview, one can approach the discussion of our present knowledge of the genetics, structure, and biologic role of the major histocompatibility complexes and their products in various species.

15 / Human Leukocyte Antigen (HLA) System

GENETICS OF THE *HLA* COMPLEX

The *HLA* complex is located on the short arm of chromosome 6, which also carries several other well-defined markers (blood group *P*, enzymes *ME₁*, *PGM₃*, *GLO*, etc.). On the basis of a still limited number of proven recombinants, the size of the complex is estimated to be approximately 2 cM, with the left (centromeric) border being the *HLA-D* locus and the right (telomeric) limit being the *HLA-A* locus. Of the several different loci assigned to the complex, four—*HLA-D, HLA-B, HLA-C* and *HLA-A* (formerly *MLC, Four, AJ,* and *LA,* respectively)—have fairly well established relative positions, which are shown in Fig. 15.1. The positions of other loci known to be linked to the *HLA* complex still remain uncertain. Mapping studies determined that the *HLA-D* locus is oriented toward the centromere, whereas the *HLA-A* locus is toward the telomere of chromosome 6. Population and family studies have provided strong evidence that the genes at the four *HLA* loci form the *HLA* haplotype that is inherited in codominant fashion and behaves in accordance with Mendelian principles. Many basic facts concerning the genetics of the *HLA* complex have become relatively well established during the past decade, whereas other observations are still controversial and the subject of speculation.

Each of the four loci has a series of alleles that determine corresponding products distinguishable from each other by their immunologic properties. The extent of polymorphism varies among different genes, though the full extent of the polymorphism is not yet known for the *HLA-C* and *HLA-D* genes. At present, the *HLA-B* gene appears to be the most polymorphic with at least 32 distinct alleles and is followed by the *HLA-A* gene with at least 17 alleles. For the other two genes, *HLA-C* and *HLA-D*, 8 and 12 alleles, respectively, are currently known (Table 15.1). The precise extent of polymorphism is not yet certain for at least two reasons. First, the frequencies of defined alleles of *HLA-C* and *HLA-D* genes total less than 1.0, being about 0.7 and 0.6, respectively. This indicates that there remain undetected alleles of these genes. Second, alleles of the *HLA-A* and *HLA-B* genes are defined by antisera that are only operationally monospecific. Occasionally, however, some of these antisera detect a determinant

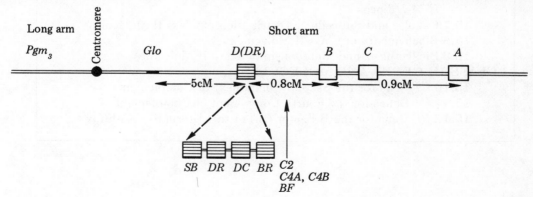

FIG. 15.1. Genetic map of the *HLA* complex and some linked genes of chromosome 6. Distances between loci are indicated in centimorgans: class I genes = white blocks; class II genes = shaded block. Several discrete genes within the *D* are indicated. *Glo* = glyoxylase, *Pgm₃* = phosphoglucomutase 3.

TABLE 15.1. Alleles of the *HLA* Genes

HLA-DR Allele	*HLA-D* Allele	*HLA-B* Allele[a]	Shared Specificity[b] Bw	*HLA-C* Allele[c]	*HLA-A* Allele[a]
DR1	*Dw1*	*B7*	6	*Cw1*	*A1*
DR2	*Dw2*	*B8*	6	*Cw2*	*A2*
DR3	*Dw3*	*B13*	4	*Cw3*	*A3*
DR4	*Dw4*	*B14*	6	*Cw4*	*A11*
DR5	*Dw5*	*B18*	6	*Cw5*	*Aw23* } *A9*
DRw6	*Dw6*	*B27*	4	*Cw6*	*Aw24*
DR7	*Dw7*	*Bw35*	6	*Cw7*	*A25* } *A10*
DRw8	*Dw8*	*B37*	4	*Cw8*	*A26*
DRw9	*Dw9*	*Bw38* } *B16*	4		*A28*
DRw10	*Dw10*	*Bw39*			*A29*
	Dw11	*Bw41*	6		*Aw30* }
	Dw12	*Bw42*	6		*Aw31* } *Aw19*
		Bw44 } *B12*	4		*Aw32*
		Bw45	6		*Aw33*
		Bw46	6		*Aw34*
		Bw47	4		*Aw36*
		Bw48	6		*Aw43*
		Bw49 } *B21*	4		
		Bw50	6		
		Bw51 } *B5*	4		
		Bw52	4		
		Bw53	4		
		Bw54 }	6		
		Bw55 } *Bw22*	6		
		Bw56	6		
		Bw57 } *B17*	4		
		Bw58	4		
		Bw59	4		
		Bw60 } *B40*	6		
		Bw61	6		
		Bw62 } *B15*	6		
		Bw63	4		

[a]"Alleles" on the right side of the brackets indicate the original designation of the alleles on the left side.

[b]Specificities Bw4 and Bw6 are shared by products of different alleles as indicated.

[c]The letter w is retained to avoid confusion with various complement (*C*) genes.

NOTE: The letter *w* after the symbol indicates temporary status of the allele.

shared by two or more distinct allelic products, which, therefore, will appear as a single entity. The allelic products become recognized for what they actually are—i.e., multideterminant molecules or **supertypic** specificities—when antisera specific for the unique determinants of each product are found. This "splitting" of allelic products results in an apparent increase in the number of alleles of the *HLA-A* and *HLA-B* genes for which the sum of frequencies is already close to 1.0.

The frequencies of the *HLA* alleles (f_a) in various racial and ethnic populations are usually calculated from the formula

$$f_a = 1 - \sqrt{1 - f_p}$$

in which phenotypic frequencies (f_p) are utilized. The formula is applicable to a population that is in Hardy-Weinberg equilibrium (Section 1.7). The overall conclusion from all studies is that the HLA frequencies in different populations vary over a broad range from a total absence of certain alleles in some populations (e.g., *HLA-A1* is virtually absent in Japanese) through the restriction of a given allele to a single population (e.g., *HLA-Bw42* is present only in blacks). Furthermore, an extremely high frequency of a given allele can be found in some populations, e.g., 91 percent of Guatemalan Indians have *HLA-Bw35*. The overall polymorphism also varies among populations, with some, e.g., Caucasoids being extremly polymorphic, whereas others (like the Japanese) are relatively less polymorphic. These differences probably reflect, at least in some cases, genetic drift, whereas, in other cases, differential selective pressure may favor certain alleles and eliminate others. The genetic heterogeneity of an individual and of a given population is further increased by the prevalence of *HLA* heterozygosity as observed in most populations studied. It is because of this heterozygosity that in most families both spouses are *HLA* heterozygotes and their children have only a 25 percent probability of being *HLA* identical. Recombination within the *HLA* complex is relatively rare, being approximately 0.02 between the *HLA-D* and *HLA-A* genes. Nevertheless, even seldom recombinations, when given sufficient time to occur, should allow the establishment of a linkage equilibrium between alleles at any two *HLA* loci and thus the generation of all possible combinations of alleles and haplotypes (Section 1.7).

The *HLA* complex deviates from this prediction by displaying striking linkage disequilibrium and certain haplotypes—i.e., particular combinations of alleles at *HLA-A, HLA-B,* and *HLA-D* loci are either more or less frequent than expected from the corresponding allelic frequencies (Table 15.2). The Δ value, measuring the linkage disequilibrium, is positive when the frequency of a given haplotype is greater than expected or negative when the frequency is smaller. Owing to linkage disequilibrium, certain *HLA* haplotypes (e.g., *A1-B8-Dw3, A3-B7-Dw2,* or *A10-B18-Dw2* in Caucasoids) are strikingly common, whereas others are relatively rare.

The mechanism responsible for linkage disequilibrium remains the subject of many speculations. The simplest explanation proposes that one of the two alleles that are in disequilibrium appeared quite recently via mutation and hence has not yet reached equilibrium by random recombinations. This would be especially true if two genes are very strongly linked, since the establishment of equilibrium requires several recombinational events, i.e., events that are extremely rare for strongly linked genes. As much as this explanation might apply for

TABLE 15.2. Some Common *HLA* Alleles Displaying Significant Linkage Disequilibrium

HLA-B Allele	f_a[a]	HLA-DR Allele	f_a[a]	HLA-C Allele	f_a[a]	HLA-A Allele[b]	f_a[a]	Observed Haplotype Frequency	Expected Haplotype Frequency[c]	Δ
B7 ← 0.10		→ DR2	0.11			(A3)		0.046	0.011	0.035
B8 ← 0.09		→ DR3	0.09					0.070	0.008	0.062
← 0.09						A1	0.16	0.064	0.014	0.050
B12 ← 0.17						Aw23	0.02	0.019	0.003	0.015
← 0.17						A29	0.06	0.033	0.010	0.023
B13 ← 0.03		→ DR7	0.16					0.019	0.005	0.014
← 0.03				Cw6	0.13			0.025	0.004	0.021
B14 ← 0.02						Aw33	0.01	0.0066	0.0002	0.0064
B18 ← 0.06				Cw5	0.08	(A25)		0.024	0.005	0.019
B27 ← 0.05				Cw1	0.05	(A2)		0.015	0.003	0.012
← 0.05				Cw2	0.05			0.023	0.003	0.020
Bw35 ← 0.10				Cw4	0.13	(A9)		0.090	0.013	0.077

[a]Allelic frequencies.
[b]Alleles in parentheses are often in weaker disequilibrium.
[c]Calculated as the product of allelic frequencies.
NOTE: All frequencies are rounded off for the sake of simplicity.

disequilibrium between alleles at the *HLA-B* and *HLA-C* loci, it seems less likely for the *HLA-B* and *HLA-A* or *HLA-A* and *HLA-D* loci.

The second explanation invokes a selective suppression of recombination between certain *HLA* genes, a phenomenon described for the murine *H-2* complex (Chapter 16 and Section 24.6). Naturally, such a suppression would prevent separation of alleles at the two loci, and it would maintain a given haplotype once it has been formed. However, at present there is no evidence for the specific suppression of intra-*HLA* recombination in man.

Currently, the third explanation is most preferred, largely on the basis of exclusion of the other two. Specifically, it postulates that certain combinations of alleles at different *HLA* loci are advantageous to the survival of an individual, whereas, by contrast, other combinations might be neutral or clearly disadvantageous. Therefore, individuals with the first type of combination will have better chances of surviving to the age of reproduction and will pass their haplotypes to their offspring. Conversely, the individuals with the other combinations may be eliminated before being able to reproduce. The precise nature of the survival advantage attributed to specific *HLA* haplotypes has not been defined, but it could represent an enhanced resistance to certain infections or diseases, especially those that are prevalent in the environment of a given population. Indeed, it is known that linkage disequilibrium affects different alleles in different racial and geographic populations.

It is increasingly common practice to classify various MHC genes and their products into three categories on the basis of their chemical structures and the biologic properties of the products. The classification, originally introduced for the murine MHC genes, is presently applied to *HLA* genes as well. According to the classification, class I genes comprise *HLA-A*, *HLA-B*, and *HLA-C*; class II consists of *HLA-D* and/or *HLA-DR* genes; and class III encompasses *C2*, *C4*, and *BF* genes of the complement system. Since this classification greatly facilitates discussion of an otherwise extremely complex field, it will be employed from now on whenever feasible.

CLASS I HLA MOLECULES

Although class I consists of *HLA-A, HLA-B,* and *HLA-C* molecules, most of our knowledge is based on the studies of the first two. Thus, if not otherwise stated, the discussion below will concern these two molecules and only by implication will the third one be included.

15.1 Detection of Class I Molecules

Presently, the most common method of detecting class I molecules on the surface of cells is the lymphocytotoxicity test employing a dye exclusion procedure (Section 4.7). Operationally monospecific allosera that contain antibodies to class I molecules are used with complement to induce damage to cells (lymphocytes) carrying the corresponding HLA molecules. Leukoagglutination and complement fixation methods are much less reliable and used only occasionally.

The alloantisera presently used are procured by the screening of sera of multiparous women. About 8 to 30 percent of such women have in their sera IgG antibodies directed against the class I molecules that their children have inherited from their fathers and that are absent from the mothers. The antibodies are elicited in the mother after leakage of her child's cells through the placenta; once induced, these antibodies persist for a long time. No specific correlation was found between the titer of antibodies and the number of pregnancies or the time after the last pregnancy. In most instances, the maternal antiserum is polyspecific since it contains antibodies to several different class I molecules if at each class I locus the father contributed to the child an allele absent from the mother. The antiserum can be rendered operationally monospecific by selective absorption with cells carrying all but one of the paternal molecules.

Even when the difference between a mother and her child is limited to only a single molecule, the antiserum may still be polyspecific. This occurs because, in addition to the antibodies elicited to a unique determinant of the child's allelic product, the mother's serum may also contain antibodies to determinants shared by several other different allelic molecules. Usually, such public determinants (Section 16.3) are shared by some allelic products of the same locus and not by products of different loci although this may also occur. The best examples are determinants Bw4 and Bw6 shared by several HLA-B allelic molecules (Table 15.1). Again, the antiserum may be absorbed by cells carrying public, but not private, determinants to make it specific for the particular allelic product. The most difficult problem to resolve is polyspecificity of an antiserum due to a single antibody that reacts with two genetically different but antigenically similar specificities. Usually, such a true cross-reactivity results in reactions of different affinity, but it still remains a major problem. This cross-reactivity has often been responsible for considering two discrete allelic products as identical until the discovery of a new antiserum that clearly distinguishes them.

Besides polyspecificity, two other phenomena must be considered when using the lymphocytotoxicity test. The **gene dose effect** results in a higher concentration of a given molecule on homozygous cells than on cells heterozygous for a given allele. Differences in concentration may result in different susceptibilities of homozygous and heterozygous cells to a given antiserum. The term **synergism** refers to a phenomenon in which an antiserum containing two distinct antibodies reacts with cells that carry both determinants but is unreactive or reacts only weakly with cells carrying only one of the determinants. It is obvious that synergism may result in false-negative results.

After an early period of chaos when each laboratory arbitrarily named the specificity of its panel of antisera, standardization of antisera was achieved through the international workshops whereby different antisera were tested on a standard panel of cells. Presently, standardized antisera serve as references for defining new antisera procured by a laboratory. Each new

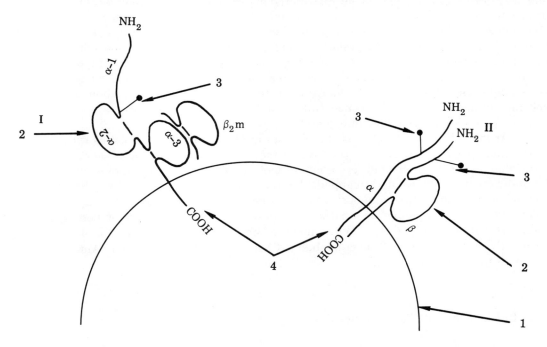

FIG. 15.2. Class I and class II HLA molecules in the cell membrane (**1**). The extracellular portions have disulfide loops (**2**) and sugar side chains (**3**). The short intracellular portion (**4**) corresponding to the C terminus is embedded in cytoplasm. The β_2-microglobulin (β_2m) associated with the α-3 region of the class I molecule is not a transmembrane molecule.

antiserum is defined on the known panel of cells and the pattern of its reactivity compared with the reactivities of the several reference antisera.

Alternative sources of antisera to class I molecules are patients that have received multiple blood transfusions and, only occasionally, individuals consenting to deliberate immunization. So far, xenoantisera, including murine monoclonal antibodies, obtained by immunization of animals with human cells have not gained broad application since they are usually, but not always, species specific and do not detect allelic differences.

15.2 Cellular and Subcellular Distribution of Class I Molecules

On the basis of susceptibility to cytotoxic antibodies, ability to absorb antibodies, and immunofluorescence, it was demonstrated unequivocally that class I molecules are ubiquitously distributed. While class I HLA molecules are present on essentially all cells except erythrocytes and are more or less homogeneously distributed in their membranes, their concentration per cell in various tissues and organs varies considerably. Notably, few class I molecules are present on spermatozoa and virtually none on erythrocytes. There are strong indications that the concentration of class I molecules is relatively higher in immature cells, especially those of the hemopoietic series, and that the amount decreases as the cells differentiate. The biologic significance of this age-dependent change is not fully understood. The highest concentration of class I molecules is believed to be on lymphocytes where they constitute about 1 percent of all cell membrane proteins. The concentration of HLA antigens increases after stimulation of lymphocytes with antigen(s) or mitogen(s).

At the subcellular level, class I molecules are transmembrane moieties with their larger, N terminal portion exposed on the cell surface and only a relatively short portion being intracellular (Fig. 15.2). The different class I molecules are independent of each other and can be individually redistributed (capped) by the corresponding antibodies (Section 4.5). A maximum of six and a minimum of three distinct class I molecules may be found on the cells of a given individual, depending on whether the individual is heterozygous or homozygous at all three, *HLA-A, −B* and *−C*, loci. When anchored on the cell surface, class I molecules are noncovalently associated with β_2-microglobulin (Chapter 18) at a ratio of 1:1. Anti-β_2 serum can cocap all three class I molecules.

15.3 Biochemistry of Class I Molecules

Human class I molecules are glycoproteins consisting of a protein chain and a single carbohydrate side chain. The sugar chain is attached to the asparagine residue at position 86. The molecular weight of the sugar portion is about 3,000. Its exact structure has not been determined, but it seems to be a complex oligosaccharide consisting of a mannose core bearing side chains containing N-glucosamine and sialic acid, as shown below.

```
 SIAL          SIAL              FUC          SIAL
  |             |                 |            |
 GAL           GAL               GAL          GAL
    \         /                     \        /
     GLU-N                           GLU-N
       |                               |
      MAN                             MAN
          \                        /
            MAN
             |
           GLU-N
             |
  FUC ───── GLU-N
             |
            Asp
```

In this scheme, abbreviations are: SIAL = sialic acid; FUC = fucose; GAL = galactose; GLU-N = glucosamine; MAN = mannose; Asp = asparagine.

The protein chain has a molecular weight of about 40,000 and consists of about 339 amino acid residues. The chain can be divided into three distinct portions: intracellular, intramembrane, and extracellular (Fig. 15.3). The intracellular portion consists of 31 amino acids of which 50 percent are chemically polar. Near the inner surface of the membrane is a cluster of arginine residues. This string of basic amino acids probably contributes to the anchoring of the molecule by interacting with negatively charged phospholipids in the membrane. The intracellular portion also contains free cysteine at position 337 and several serines that, presumably by becoming phosphorylated, interact with the cytoskeleton and facilitate anchoring of the molecule in the cytoplasm. The intracellular portion differs most strikingly among various animal species.

The intramembrane portion consists of 24 amino acids, none of which is either polar or charged. This portion is believed to serve solely to anchor the molecule and thus is similar to analogous portions of other transmembrane molecules. Indeed, a striking similarity exists among intracellular portions of class I molecules, cell-surface mIgM (Section 8.3), and glycophorin.

The extracellular portion consists of 271–273 amino acids and can be subdivided into three regions (domains). The α-1 region spans residues 1 to 90, the α-2 region lies between residues 91 and 180, and the α-3 region occupies the stretch between positions 181 and 271 or 273. The α-2 and α-3 regions form loops by disulfide bridges between cysteines at positions 101 and 164 and 203 and 259, respectively. Interestingly, both loops are of the same size as those found in the immunoglobulin domains (Chapter 7). The amino acid sequence of the α-3 region is apparently homologous to the domains of immunoglobulin and to β_2-microglobulin. On the other hand, some level of homology exists between the α-1 and α-2 regions but not between these regions and immunoglobulin domains.

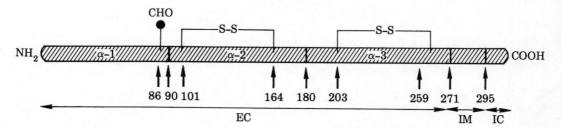

FIG. 15.3. Schematic representation of the class I HLA molecule, which consists of extra-cellular (**EC**), intramembrane (**IM**), and intracellular (**IC**) portions. The extra-cellular portion is divided into regions (α-1, α-2, α-3). The **arrows with numbers** indicate relevant amino acid positions discussed in text. CHO = carbohydrate; S-S = disulfide bond.

Comparison of amino acid sequences of allelic molecules shows a relatively high degree of homology. In fact, the known sequences of cross-reacting allelic molecules HLA-A2 and HLA-A28 differ very little from each other, but it must be kept in mind that sequencing of the latter is not yet complete. A comparison of molecules determined by the alleles of two discrete genes *HLA-A2* and *HLA-B7* shows that approximately 15/100 residues are different. These differences are scattered along the chain with some aggregation of the substitutions localized between positions 65 to 80 and around positions 110 and 175. Still, there is no specific sequence that would identify a given molecule as being determined by either an *HLA-A* or *HLA-B* gene. In fact, there is no sequence typical for human class I molecules as compared with the highly homologous class I molecules of other species. These findings have certain implications for the possible evolution of the *HLA* complex and its relation to speciation.

One of the objectives of amino acid sequencing was to find the relationship between the primary structure and the antigenic properties of the molecules. Thus far, this objective has not been achieved. Although amino acid substitution almost certainly contributes to the formation of an antigenic determinant, such substitution may also bring about conformational changes that are recognized as antigenic determinants per se. It is not possible to decide whether there is a single variable region or multiple antigenic regions. This decision is made difficult by our limited knowledge of the spatial arrangement of the protein chain. Preliminary studies have shown that within the homology region three configurations, characteristic of a polypeptide chain, can be distinguished. The β pleats compose about 75 percent of the molecule; an α helix occupies about 5 percent; and the random arrangements make up the remaining 20 percent. The relative proportion of these configurations changes upon dissociation of the HLA molecule from β_2-microglobulin, suggesting that the latter exerts stabilizing effects upon the spatial structure of the former. Indeed, after dissociation of the class I molecule and β_2-microglobulin, their rejoining in vitro is often only negligible, indicating that dissociation resulted in alteration of spatial structure.

There are two types of class I molecule variants believed to be mutants. One type was found in the HLA-A2 molecule and is considered to be a result of a point mutation involving a single amino acid substitution. The second type (A_2m) represents an HLA-A2 loss mutation that was induced in vitro with a chemical mutagen and then isolated by **immunoselection**, i.e., by growing the clone of cells carrying a particular variant. It is suspected that more extensive changes took place in this type of mutant and resulted in the inability of class I molecules to be anchored in the membrane. Indeed, A_2m cells have an amount of β_2-microglobulin reduced by 25 percent.

15.4 Biosynthesis and Metabolism of Class I Molecules

A great deal of data concerning intracellular synthesis of class I molecules have recently been generated. Each class I molecule is synthesized from a separate mRNA consisting of about 1,600 bases and, thus, has the potential to code for about 500 amino acids. The possibility that different molecules contain an α-3 region determined by a common gene has not found support, especially since apparent amino acid differences within this region were found among allelic molecules. The primary product of translation has an N terminal tail of about 20 amino acids that serves to direct the newly synthesized peptide to the endoplasmic reticulum. This extension is subsequently cleaved off as synthesis continues. After glycosylation takes place the peptide becomes associated with a β_2-microglobulin by the end of synthesis or shortly thereafter. Glycosylation is not required for either the expression or antigenicity of the molecules. If, however, for any reason an association with β_2-microglobulin does not occur, the molecule seems to undergo conformational changes that preclude such an association at a later time. The association between class I molecule and β_2-microglobulin is a condition sine qua non for the transport of the molecule from the reticulum to the cell surface and for the anchoring of the molecule in the membrane. This is well documented by studies of cells of a cell line developed from Burkitt's lymphoma, Daudi cells, which consistently type as class I negative. Although these cells do not synthesize β_2-microglobulin, they are fully capable of synthesizing class I molecules. When such cells are fused with the mouse fibroblast line IT22, which synthesizes β_2-microglobulin, the hybrid cells express class I molecules that are defined as HLA-A10, HLA-A26, HLA-B17, and HLA-Bw38.

During transport of the class I molecule and β_2-microglobulin complex to the cell membrane, a modification of the sugar moiety takes place that converts the high mannose-type to the complex-type carbohydrate. At the same time, some other posttranslational modifications take place including phosphorylation of serine in the intracellular portion and acylation by fatty acids.

The class I molecules in living cells undergo a constant turnover that results in the shedding of old molecules and the synthesis of new ones. There is also an exchange of β_2-microglobulin, but its rate is rather slow, probably because it involves conformational changes. Certain allelic molecules, e.g., HLA-A9, seem to be particularly prone to shedding and are present in abundance in serum. Treatment of living cells with inhibitors of protein synthesis results in a progressive loss of class I molecules. HLA-C molecules are more sensitive to such treatment than HLA-A molecules, which may be indicative of a higher rate of synthesis or of turnover. The old molecules may be either returned to the cell by endopinocytosis and reused, or shed to the surroundings. Free class I molecules found in the serum may play an important role in the prevention of autoimmunity by blocking the receptors of autoreactive lymphocytes.

CLASS II HLA MOLECULES

Class II molecules are the products of the *HLA-D* and *HLA-DR* genes. Our knowledge of these molecules is based primarily on studies of the HLA-DR molecules, which are believed, but not proven, to be identical with the products of the *HLA-D* gene. From a molecular point of view, HLA-DR molecules are analogous to the murine Ia molecules (Section 16.11) and hence are often referred to as human Ia or Ia-like molecules.

15.5 Detection of Class II Molecules

Historically, the putative HLA-D molecules were detected and defined (functionally) earlier than HLA-DR molecules. The detection of HLA-D molecules and their allelic variants is based on their ability to elicit an MLR (Section 4.12) when cells carrying different alleles at the *HLA-D* locus are cocultured in vitro. A difference at the *HLA-D* locus is the only requirement for an MLR. Individuals who carry identical class I molecules, and are therefore serologically identical, still give strong MLR responses when their cells differ by alleles at the *HLA-D* locus. Because of this phenomenon, the concept of **serologically defined** (SD) molecules corresponding to class I and **lymphocyte defined** (LD) molecules corresponding to class II was introduced. This short-lived distinction recently lost most of its validity in the light of the discovery of serologically detectable HLA-DR molecules that appear to be identical with the HLA-D molecules once considered to be lymphocyte defined. We shall return to the question of the relationship between the HLA-D and HLA-DR molecules in the next section of this chapter.

At present, two basic methods, both based on the one-way MLR, are employed in the detection and definition of HLA-D molecules. In the first method, lymphocytes of the individual tested are stimulated with a panel of cells, each of which is homozygous for 1 of the 12 known *HLA-D* alleles. These cells are referred to as **homozygous typing cells** (HTC). The individual carrying either one or both alleles identical with a particular HTC will not react or react only minimally. Such an individual is said to give a **typing reaction** (Fig. 15.4**A**). Thus, if a given individual's lymphocytes fail to react with only one of the HTC employed, he might be considered homozygous for the *D* allele present on the particular HTC. Similarly, if the cells of an individual fail to react with two different HTC, he may be presumed to be heterozygous and to carry alleles identical with the two corresponding HTC that did not elicit the reaction. Finally, an individual whose cells respond to all 12 HTC must carry an *HLA-D* allele that is different from any of the known alleles present in the panel of HTC. However, this method of detection of HLA-D molecules is neither reproducible nor accurate. Equivocal results that are often obtained with this technique are ascribed to possible stimulation by molecules other than HLA-D and possibly the effect of other genes that influence responsiveness itself, e.g., the *MLR-R* gene.

In the second method, a secondary MLR is used. A panel of cells is produced in which each cell of the panel is primed by one of the known HLA-D molecules by being previously cultured with appropriate HTC. These cells are then restimulated by the cells of the individual to be typed, and the magnitude of the response after a relatively short time (24–48 hours) is assessed. This procedure is called **primed lymphocyte typing** (PLT) (Fig. 15.4**B**) and is considered more sensitive and accurate than the HTC method. Its usefulness is further

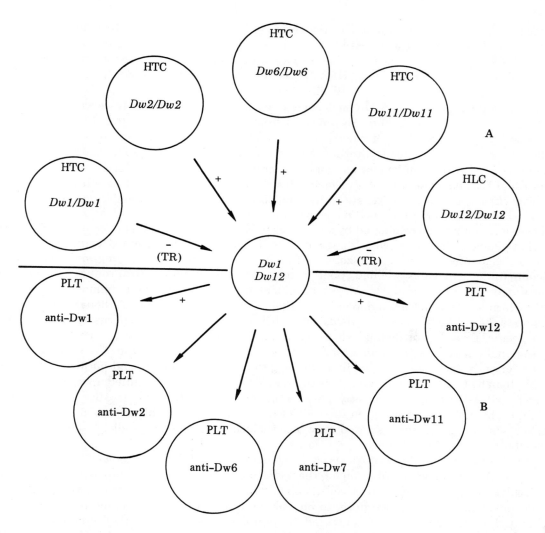

FIG. 15.4. The principle of determination of the HLA-D phenotype of a cell, which is in the center of the scheme. (**A**) The HTC method consists of stimulation (**arrows**) of the tested cell with a panel of known *HLA-D* homozygous cells. Lack of response or typing reaction (**TR**) is indicated by a minus sign (−) and represents the identity of HLA-D of stimulator and tested cell. (**B**) The PLT method consists of stimulation (**arrows**) of a panel of cells, primed to known HLA-D, with tested cells. A secondary response indicated by a plus sign (+) represents the identity of HLA-D of priming and tested cell. For simplicity, only some known HLA-D types are included in the figure.

increased by the recent production of the clones of primed cells that can be maintained in the laboratory. Using PLT, it was possible to demonstrate that an MLR is elicited by both HLA-D and HLA-DR molecules, since positive responses were obtained after restimulation of primed lymphocytes with both HLA-D and HLA-DR as well as with HLA-DR alone. In fact, primed cells seem to recognize primarily HLA-DR differences.

The detection of HLA-DR molecules is based primarily on the dye exclusion lymphocytotoxic test in which alloantisera procured from pregnant women or transfusion recipients are used. Several modifications need to be introduced for the detection of HLA-DR molecules. In most instances, cells after incubation with antiserum must be incubated for a longer period of time with complement at room temperature. In addition, problems similar to those described for alloantisera to class I molecules are encountered (gene dose effect, synergism, polyspecificity, cross-reactivity, etc.) when the alloantisera for class II molecules are used.

The alloantisera for class II molecules are more difficult to select and, as a rule, are weak. They are commonly contaminated by antibodies to class I molecules and must be absorbed with pooled platelets that carry class I, but not class II, molecules. Deliberate attempts to generate specific alloantisera by immunization of volunteers with cells carrying only HLA-DR-incompatible molecules yielded poor results as did attempts to produce alloantisera specific for DR allelic products. Most monoclonal antibodies detect determinants common for DR molecules and which are independent of their allotypic determinants. Although xenoimmunization to the HLA-DR molecules yields antibodies, these antibodies are species specific and not allospecific; they do not distinguish between allelic molecules. Recently, a method to select operationally monospecific antisera has been elaborated. In this method, the specificity of a given serum is determined by its direct binding to chemically isolated and purified molecules, rather than by lymphocytotoxicity. Once the specificity of serum is identified, this serum may be used for HLA-DR typing in an assay in which the binding of antibody to its specific molecule is inhibited by molecules present on the cells of the tested person. This approach, however, has certain limitations because isolated reference molecules of only some allelic specificities are available at this time.

The classic lymphocytotoxic assay for detection of the HLA-DR molecules is limited by the restricted cellular distribution of the molecules. Among blood lymphocytes, HLA-DR molecules are present only on B cells, which constitute 10 to 15 percent of the peripheral blood mononuclear cells. Therefore, to be used as target cells for the assay, B cells must be separated from other cells encountered in peripheral blood. A further limitation of the lymphocytotoxic assay is posed by the fact that individuals undergoing treatment with glucocorticosteroids have a significantly decreased expression of class II molecules, which occasionally makes typing of such individuals virtually impossible.

Cross-reactivity of anti-HLA-DR sera permits the distinction of three supertypic groups of the known HLA-DR allelic molecules: MT1 (DR1, DR2, DRw6, DRw10), MT2 (DR3, DR5, DRw6, DRw8), and MT3 (DR4, DR7, DRw9). Recently, other cross-reactive groups were defined; MB1 (DR1, DR2, DRw6), MB2 (DR3, DR7) and MB3, (DR4, DR5). These findings reopen the question regarding the number of *HLA-DR* loci and their relationship to the *HLA-D* locus, because these cross-reactivities could be attributed to the presence of non-*DR* alleles in multiple linkage disequilibrium with *DR* alleles.

15.6 Number of *HLA-DR* Loci and Question of Their Identity with the *HLA-D* Locus

Since HLA-D and HLA-DR molecules were discovered at different times and by different methods, it was natural to assume that they are distinct moieties. The idea of distinctiveness was supported by reports of putative recombinants between *HLA-D* and *HLA-DR* loci and frequent association of *HLA-DR2* with *HLA-Dw12* in Orientals as opposed to the association with *HLA-Dw2* commonly found in Caucasoids. Also, *HLA-Dw4* was occasionally found to be associated with *HLA-DR1* or *HLA-DR3* instead of being associated with *HLA-DR4*.

A distinction is also suggested by the fact that HLA-D molecules induce a primary MLR (defined with HTC), whereas HLA-DR antigens seem to be detectable only by secondary MLR, i.e., by PLT. However, one could argue that the two reactions are elicited by two sets of determinants present on the same molecules. Presently, many investigators lean toward the idea that HLA-D and HLA-DR molecules are identical and that the two different methods of detection merely reflect two different properties (pleiotropism) of the same molecule. The strongest argument in favor of identity is the finding that anti-HLA-DR sera reacting with the stimulator cells usually abrogate or significantly inhibit the MLR elicited by such stimulators. This contention is further supported by the finding that in mapping studies the *HLA-DR* always follows the *HLA-D* gene in all known recombinants between *Glo* and *HLA*. Finally, a circumstantial argument can be made that the identity of *Lad* genes (murine analogue of HLA-D) and the *Ia* genes (analogue of the *HLA-DR*) is unequivocally established in the analogous murine system.

Equally complicated is the question of the number of *HLA-DR* loci. From biochemical studies, it is obvious that each molecule is determined by at least two genes, each encoding one of the two chains, α and β (see below). Still, it has not been resolved whether the two genes are linked to each other (in tanden) and thereby to the *HLA* complex, or, alternatively, whether the two genes are linked to the *HLA*, whereas the other is on a different chromosome. By analogy to the murine system, it would seem that the former concept is correct. However, some results of experiments with cell hybrids were consistent with the latter. Cell hybrids between human B cells and mouse or hamster fibroblasts, in spite of carrying human chromosome 6 with the *HLA* complex, did not express class II molecules. Although it could be argued that fibroblasts are not permissive for the expression of these molecules, an equally strong case can be made that hybrids have only the one gene linked to *HLA* but lack the other gene and thus cannot produce the molecule. Were this argument correct, it would have to be assumed that the gene determining the more variable chain (β) is linked to *HLA*, whereas the gene for the less variable chain (α) is not.

The question is further complicated by uncertainty as to whether there is only one pair (tandem) of class II genes or, in a fashion similar to mice, whether there are several tandems. On the basis of the experimental data on cross-reactivity, the following concept has been proposed. There could be three closely linked loci for the β chains. One is the *HLA-DR* locus that carries the *HLA-DR* alleles for the β-1 chain of known HLA-DR molecules as defined by the conventional alloantisera. Some of these molecules, in addition to their unique DR determinants, would share public determinants. In the second locus, which is called *DC*, two alleles, *DC1* and *DC3*, each being in linkage disequilibrium with different alleles of the *HLA-DR* locus, have been identified. These alleles encode the β-3 chain of the second human class II molecule. The *DC1* allele is associated with *DR1*, *DR2*, and *DRw6* alleles; *DC3* is in disequilibrium with *DR3* and *DR7* alleles, conforming to the association pattern of *MB1* and *MB2*, respectively. For the third locus, which is called *BR*, one allele has been assigned that shows strong linkage disequilibrium with *DR4* and *DR7* alleles, apparently corresponding to *MT3*. This locus is believed to carry allele for the β-2 chain of still another class II molecule. Each of the three loci for the β chain would have its corresponding locus for the α chain. Molecular mapping of human DNA indicates presence of about 7 β genes and 3–5 α genes. The two tandems would be analogous to the similar murine tandems with *HLA-DR* being similar to the A_e-E_a pair and the *DC* corresponding to the A_a-A_β pair (Section 16.8). This presumptive analogy is supported by the cross-reactivity of alloantisera, similarities in the molecular weights of gene products, and similarities in amino acid sequences of the proposed analogues.

This relatively simple scheme, which emerges from recent immunochemical studies, is complicated by the consistent demonstration of some other polypeptides such as invariable chains (Ii, δ-1, and δ-2) that are not associated with any of the above mentioned β chains. One plausible explanation for the presence of these invariable chains is that they represent metabolic intermediates rather than the integral components of cell-surface molecules. In addition, using the PLT technique a discrete gene called *SB*, that presumably encodes still another class II molecule, has been described. There is no serologic reagent available to detect the molecular product(s) of the *SB* gene(s). The chromosomal positions of the *SB, DR,* and *DC* genes or gene-tandems (Fig. 15.1) are presently determined from the analysis of several cell lines carrying deletion-type mutations within the *HLA* complex.

15.7 Cellular and Subcellular Distribution of Class II Molecules

The cellular distribution of class II molecules apparently is restricted to certain types or subtypes of the cells. Thus far, class II molecules have been convincingly demonstrated in early progeny of myeloid stem cells (myeloblasts and promyelocytes); B cells; monocytes; macrophages; Kupffer cells; Langerhans' cells; endothelium; some, but not all, covering and glandular epithelia; interstitial cells of the ovary; and spermatozoa. Whether class II molecules are expressed on all T cells or only on some of their subsets awaits formal demonstration. The indicative data in this regard are that some investigators have shown that class II molecules are present on PHA-stimulated lymphocytes and that anti-HLA-DR sera block the responses to PHA and to low doses of ConA (Section 4.12). In similarity to class I molecules, the concentration of class II molecules in different cells varies and is usually higher in less differentiated cells.

The class II molecule consists of two transmembrane polypeptides with the larger portions of each being extracellular and only the smaller portion of each chain being intracellular. The two chains are noncovalently bound but are cocapped by the proper antibody. At this time, assuming that there is only a single tandem of *HLA-DR* genes, a maximum of two different class II molecules should be detectable on the cells of an individual if such an individual is an HLA-DR heterozygote. In fact, depending on the antiserum used, multiple molecules can be demonstrated, among which DR molecules constitute 70 percent, while up to six other molecules make up the remaining 30 percent. Apparently, these molecules are not associated with β_2-microglobulin.

15.8 Biochemistry of Class II Molecules

A typical class II molecule consists of two polypeptide chains: the α chain, of molecular weight 34,000 (32,000–36,000), and the β chain, of molecular weight 28,000 (25,000–29,000), that are not covalently linked. There are some indications that the β chain has one or two intrachain disulfide loops. When isolated from the cell by papain digestion, the intramembrane and intracellular portions of both chains are cleaved and only the extracellular portion is released. On the other hand, detergent solubilization results in disruption of the cell membrane and the release of the entire molecule.

Each chain presumably carries a complex-type oligosaccharide. The sugar moieties can be removed from the molecule without an appreciable effect on its antigenic properties. This observation is considered as prima facie evidence that the antigencity of class II molecules resides in the protein component. However, at least one laboratory makes repeated claims that some antigenicity of class II molecules is associated with the sugar moiety (Section 16.11).

Many studies strongly suggest that antigenicity is associated primarily with the smaller chain (β) and, perhaps, with conformational changes resulting from association of the two chains. Most data on the primary structure of class II molecules come from the tryptic peptide mapping of the two chains isolated from B-lymphoid *HLA*-homozygous cell lines carrying different *HLA-DR* alleles. In these studies, the α chains from different allelic molecules were remarkably similar, if not identical. On the other hand, the β chains were strikingly diverse with only 50 percent of tryptic peptides being identical. The structural variability appears to be most pronounced at the N terminal portion of the molecule, whereas the C terminal portion is highly preserved and displays striking homology with the immunoglobulin domains. These structural differences may, at least partially, be related to the antigenic differences. This contention is supported by finding that conventional anti-HLA-DR sera bind preferentially to the variable β chain. However, these same antisera seem to be unable to detect all differences; β chains from two different cell lines that were otherwise considered HLA-DR identical still showed about 30 percent different tryptic peptides. In addition, it was recently shown that from class II molecules isolated by immunoprecipitation with conventional alloantisera one can separate a subpopulation of molecules that reacts and subpopulation that does not react with certain monoclonal antibodies. One subpopulation was shown to contain an α chain that had about 20 percent of its tryptic peptides different from those of the α chain belonging to other subpopulation of the molecules. Similar findings were made for β chains of the two populations, with about 40 percent different tryptic peptides. If these data are confirmed, the two subpopulations of class II molecules may represent two different molecules determined by two different genes in tandem (Section 15.6).

The preliminary data on amino acid sequencing of the N terminal end of class II molecules are consistent with the notion that β chains are more variable than α chains. In two allelic β chains, three of six amino acids were different, whereas in the corresponding α chains only one of five amino acids was different. No homology could be demonstrated, at least for the N terminal part, between class I and class II molecules or between α and β chains. On the other hand, homology was convincingly shown between corresponding chains of human and murine (Ia-5) or rat class II molecules. Recently completed amino acid sequence of 198 N-terminal positions of the DR2 β chain shows presence of two homologous domains and "hypervariable" segment between the positions 60 and 69.

Several cell lines carrying presumed HLA-DR mutations are known. These cell lines either express the class II molecules in a decreased amount or not at all.

15.9 Biosynthesis and Metabolism of Class II Molecules

In contrast to class I molecules, only fragmentary data are available concerning the biosynthesis of class II molecules. It seems that each chain is synthesized on a separate mRNA and glycosylated and assembled in the endoplasmic reticulum. The joining of two chains is a prerequisite for anchoring of the molecule into the membrane. Absence of one chain prevents the expression of the other. The intracellular portion of the α chain is known to be phosphorylated.

The "worn out" molecules are presumably shed from the cell membrane; this shedding is responsible for the presence of free class II molecules in the serum. The serum concentration of the free class II molecules is especially high in patients with chronic lymphocytic leukemia (CLL). Interestingly, the concentration of class II molecules, but not class I, changes significantly during the cell cycle with the lowest amount in the M phase.

CLASS III GENES AND MOLECULES

By convention, complement components C2 and C4 as well as factor B are included in class III molecules.* This is analogous to the mouse in which the gene for C4 is located within the MHC. In man the relationship of the class III genes to those of class I and class II has not been definitely established. It is frequently debated whether class III genes are true members of the *HLA* complex or just incidental "immigrants" by translocation. The argument in favor of the first idea stems from the presumption that all three classes of molecules are involved in some sort of interaction with the cell membrane. On the other hand, striking structural dissimilarities between class III and the other two classes favor the concept that class III is a "stranger." In any case, we shall briefly discuss the genetics of the *HLA*-linked class III genes.

15.10 *C2* Gene for the Second Component of Complement

Polymorphism of C2 was the first one to be demonstrated in association with the HLA. It was originally discovered by finding C2-deficient individuals who were homozygotes for the $C2^-$

---

*The C8 gene originally thought to be linked to the *HLA* was eventually found to segregate independently.

allele (null or silent allele). In the vast majority of such individuals, the $C2^-$ allele was accompanied by, and segregated with, a specific combination of *HLA* alleles, namely, with the haplotype *HLA-A10-HLA-B18-HLA-Dw2*. Thus, not only close linkage but also a pronounced disequilibrium was found. In addition, the $C2^-$ allele appears to be in linkage disequilibrium with certain *BF* alleles (Section 15.12). Subsequent studies revealed several recombinations between the $C2^-$ and *HLA* but never between $C2^-$ and *BF*.

Besides the $C2^-$ allele, there are at least four other alleles that determine structural differences of C2 detectable by isoelectric focusing. The prevalent allele is designated $C2^C$ (frequency 0.9), while the other three are designated $C2^B$ (0.02–0.05), $C2^{A1}$, and $C2^{A2}$ (~0.01). The products of these alleles are expressed codominantly. The $C2^B$ allele was shown to be in linkage disequilibrium with *HLA-Bw15* and *HLA-Cw3*.

15.11 *C4* Genes for the Fourth Component of Complement

Similar to the *C2* gene, the *C4* gene was identified by finding C4-deficient individuals. In the offspring of these individuals, the C4 deficiency segregated with the HLA phenotypes. However, there was no apparent linkage disequilibrium because, in four individuals, the deficiency was associated with different HLA phenotypes (HLA-A2-HLA-B40, HLA-A2-HLA-B12, HLA-A2-HLA-B15, HLA-A2-HLA-B40, HLA-Aw19-HLA-Bw18, and HLA-A26-HLA-B49). Since determination of heterozygosity for the deficiency of C4 poses several technical problems, it was impossible to demonstrate recombinations between the *C4* gene(s) and the *HLA* complex. In addition to the silent or null allele that results in a deficiency of C4, several structural variants were found. To explain their distribution and segregation, it became necessary to postulate that C4 is determined by two closely linked loci, *C4A* and *C4B*, that are closely linked to *C2*, *BF*, and *HLA*, and are positioned between the *HLA-B* and *HLA-D* loci.

The *C4A* gene has at least six alleles (*A1*, *A2*, *A3*, *A4*, *A6*, and *AQO*) determining allelic molecules that carry determinant(s) characteristic for the Rodgers "blood group" (Rg). These molecules form acidic bands that migrate relatively fast toward the anode during electrophoresis. Thus, they were all formerly believed to be a single product of an allele that was designated *F* (for fast). In vivo, the molecules are passively deposited on erythrocytes, conferring upon them the $Rg^a(+)$ phenotype. The *AQO* allele, formerly designated f^o, is silent, and its homozygosity results in a deficiency of Rodgers molecules and produces $Rg^a(-)$ phenotype.

The *C4B* locus carries at least four alleles (*B1*, *B2*, *B3*, and *BQO*) determining molecules bearing determinant(s) characteristic for the Chido "blood group" (Ch). The molecules form basic bands that migrate slowly during electrophoresis and, hence, were originally believed to represent the product of the *S* (for slow) allele. Again, in vivo, they are passively adsorbed on erythrocytes, converting them to $Ch^a(+)$. The *BQO* allele (formerly S^o) is silent, and homozygosity for it is responsible for the $Ch^a(-)$ phenotype.

The alleles at the two C4 loci form several common haplotypes with the frequencies shown in Table 15.3. Obviously, C4-deficient individuals are homozygous for the extremely rare haplotype *AQO-BQO*.

The proposed two-locus model for the determination of C4 best fits the available data, even though there are some discrepancies between the expected and observed frequencies of the haplotypes. These discrepancies may be largely due to difficulties in the detection of half-

TABLE 15.3. Frequencies of *C4* Haplotypes among Caucasoids of the United States

C4A Allele	*C4B* Allele	Haplotype Frequency
A1	*B1*	0.01
A2	*B1*	0.05
A2	*B2*	0.02
A2	*B3*	0.01
A3	*B1*	0.51
A3	*B2*	0.02
A3	*BQO*	0.08
A4	*B2*	0.09
A6	*B1*	0.06
AQO	*B1*	0.10
AQO	*B2*	0.05
AQO	*BQO*	Very rare— homozygotes are C4 deficient

null genotypes in heterozygotes. To some extent, the model resembles the genetics of C4 in mice. However, the resemblance is only partial since of two murine loci only one produces biologically active C4 and, moreover, the expression of the inactive product is testosterone dependent. Recently, it was found that the *AQO* allele is in strong disequilibrium with *HLA-B8*, while the *BQO* allele is in disequilibrium with the *HLA-B12* and *HLA-B5* alleles.

15.12 *BF* Gene for the B Factor (Bf) of the Alternative Pathway

Bf is a single protein chain (molecular weight 93,000) that interacts with C3 and in doing so is cleaved into two fragments—the basic Bb fragment (molecular weight 55,000) and the acidic Ba fragment (molecular weight 40,000). The Bb fragment carries allotypic specificities and the enzymatic activity of a convertase reacting with C3, while the Ba fragment also bears allotypic determinants but is enzymatically inactive. The factor is determined by the *BF* gene with two common alleles—*BF*F* and *BF*S*—and at least nine relatively rare alleles, including *BF*F1*, *BF*S1*, and *BF*0.55*, all of which determine differences in Bb fragments. There are striking racial differences in the frequencies of the *BF* alleles. For example, *BF*F* has a frequency of 0.17 among whites and 0.54 among blacks, whereas *BF*S* frequencies are 0.80 and 0.44, respectively. The names of the alleles are derived from the electrophoretic mobility (F, fast; S, slow) of the second band in a Bf pattern, which consists of at least four bands. There are reports of a certain degree of disequilibrium between *BF*F* and *HLA-B12*, *HLA-Bw35*, and *HLA-B8*, or between *BF*S* and *HLA-B8*, *HLA-Bw40*, and *HLA-B7*. It seems, however, that this disequilibrium reflects the recent development of the alleles rather than a specific selective pressure.

All four genes—*C2, C4A, C4B,* and *BF*—are closely linked, and since no recombination between them has been reported so far, it is impossible to determine their sequence. Although available data suggest that the *BF* and the three other genes are located between the *Glo* and *HLA-B* loci, their relationship to the *HLA-D* locus remains uncertain. It is beyond the scope of this book to discuss the structure and biosynthesis of these complement factors.

16 / The Murine Major Histocompatibility H-2 Complex

GENETICS OF THE *H-2* COMPLEX
CLASS I GENES AND MOLECULES
    16.1 Class I *H-2* Genes
    16.2 Molecular Structure of Class I Genes
    16.3 Detection of Class I Molecules
    16.4 Cellular and Subcellular Distribution of Class I Molecules
    16.5 Biochemistry and Biosynthesis of Class I Molecules
    16.6 Other Class I Molecules
    16.7 Mutations of Class I Genes
CLASS II GENES AND MOLECULES
    16.8 Genetics of Class II Molecules
    16.9 Detection of Class II Molecules
    16.10 Cellular and Subcellular Distribution of Class II Molecules
    16.11 Biochemistry and Biosynthesis of Class II Molecules
    16.12 Mutants of Class II Genes
    16.13 Identity of Different Genes and Products of the *I* region
    16.14 The *I-B* Subregion
    16.15 The *I-C* Subregion
    16.16 The *I-J* Subregion and Its Products
CLASS III GENES AND MOLECULES
    16.17 *C2* Gene
    16.18 *C3* Gene
    16.19 *C4* Gene
    16.20 *BF* Gene

GENETICS OF THE *H-2* COMPLEX

The *H-2** complex of mice was the first MHC to be discovered and, therefore, has been the most extensively studied. In fact, early genetic and serologic studies led to a picture so complicated that a full comprehension of the *H-2* complex became the exclusive domain of a few experts in the area. Only recently has a new trend gained impetus—a trend toward simplification of the structure and possibly the function of the *H-2* complex. In this chapter, an attempt will be made to present the basic facts and some speculations concerning the genes and products of the *H-2* complex.

The *H-2* complex (Fig. 16.1) has been assigned to linkage group IX, which is now known to correspond to the genes on chromosome 17 of the mouse. It is estimated that the complex represents a segment as small as 0.33–0.5 cM, but the segment may actually be larger; the frequency of recombination within the *H-2* apparently is decreased by certain alleles in its close vicinity (Section 24.6). The *H-2* complex traditionally is considered to be comprised of four regions—*K, I, S,* and *D*—each defined by a number of recombinants (Table 16.1). The *I* region is further subdivided into five subregions—*A, B, J, E,* and *C*. Each region or subregion is believed to contain one locus, but probably it contains more. The number of distinct genes assigned to the *H-2* complex once reached well over 50 and seemed to be on a constant rise. This increase in the number of *H-2* genes was partially due to conceptual confusion.

Some investigators assumed that each phenotypic characteristic (phenomenon) must have its corresponding gene. Accordingly, each phenomenon, whether physiologic or actually man-made, was attributed to a specific gene, and if the phenomenon was associated with an H-2 phenotype, the new gene automatically became a member of an ever growing family of *H-2*-linked genes. However, from the point of view of molecular genetics (Section 3.3), the formal proof for the existence of any structural gene rests on the demonstration of its molecular product. Using this criterion, only ten genes within the *H-2* complex currently pass the formal test. The two conceptual approaches to the genetics of the *H-2* complex are easily reconcilable when one accepts that a single product determined by a single gene may be responsible for more than one phenomenon or function. The two concepts are summarized in Table 16.2. It is quite possible that the truth lies somewhere in between the two concepts, but, on the basis of available data, it seems to be closer to a new concept that will constitute the framework of further discussion. It is important to notice that, according to this new concept, the existence of some subregions (*B, J, C*) becomes questionable, as no gene product can be assigned to them, whereas some regions and subregions contain more than one gene (*K, A, S, D*) and thereby determine several products. Taking this into consideration, the new concept calls for total rejection of the traditional division into regions and subregions in favor of a division into discrete genes. Indeed, from a genetic point of view, a gene is the only meaningful structural and functional unit, while the regions and subregions correspond to arbitrary DNA segments defined by the accidental phenomenon of recombination. However, total disregard of traditional

---

*Since it was discovered first, *H-2* should be called *H-1*, but the original designation given by Gorer (antigen II) was kept for sentimental reasons.

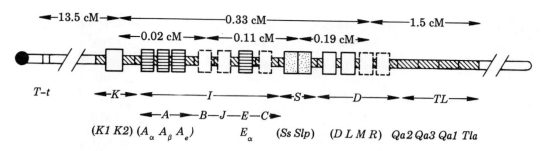

FIG. 16.1. Genetic map of the *H-2* complex. Regions (**K, I, S, D**) and subregions (**A, B, J, E, C**) are indicated: class I genes = **white blocks**; class II genes = **shaded blocks**; Uncertain genes marked with dashed outlines; class III genes = **dotted blocks**. Positions of the *TL* region (Chapt. 22) and the *T-t* complex (Chapt. 24) are also indicated.

terminology poses a problem, viz, some of the genes have not yet been separated from each other by recombination and, thus, cannot be arranged in a sequence. With this in mind, it would appear prudent to preserve, at least temporarily, some of the traditional nomenclature.

The orderly and concise description of *H-2* genes and their products is significantly facilitated by a classification that, based on the structure and function of the products, consists of the three classes—I, II, and III—corresponding to those already proposed for the *HLA* complex of man (Chapter 15). Before discussing individual classes of genes, it would be beneficial to introduce some general concepts and terms concerning the *H-2* complex. Regardless of whether the complex is viewed in the traditional or new perspective, it consists of a cluster of loci, each carrying a gene with multiple alleles. The alleles actually present on a given chromosome are usually, though not always, inherited as a block, and thus the term *H-2 haplotype* has been coined. Obviously, an individual animal carrying a diploid set of chromosomes has two *H-2* haplotypes that comprise its *H-2* genotype. In inbred mice, the two *H-2* haplotypes are, by definition, identical, and, thus, the *H-2* haplotype and the *H-2* genotype are synonymous. Conversely, in outbred mice or F1 hybrids, the two haplotypes may be totally or partially different.

Among the laboratory-maintained inbred mice, well over 100 different *H-2* haplotypes have been distinguished and designated by a lowercase letter(s) and Arabic numeral superscripts (Table 16.3). These haplotypes can be divided into two major categories: unrelated and related. An **unrelated** haplotype carries at each locus a unique allele that was present in the original mice used to develop that particular inbred strain. A **related** haplotype consists of combinations of alleles from two or more unrelated haplotypes. The related haplotypes can be further subdivided into *H-2* recombinant haplotypes and *H-2* mutant haplotypes. Recently, 28 new *H-2* haplotypes derived from wild mice were introduced into laboratory. They consist of both new unrelated haplotypes and 13 related haplotypes. The latter are *H-2* recombinant haplotypes that were carried by the wild mice or occurred after mating wild and laboratory mice.

At the time of the original description of the *H-2* complex, its borders were defined with

TABLE 16.1. Some *H-2* Haplotypes Defining the Regions and Subregions of the *H-2* Complex by Virtue of Crossing-Over Occurring in the Intervals Indicated

Crossing-Over at Interval	Parental Haplotypes	Recombinant Haplotype	Strain(s)
K–I-A	*b–m*	*bq1*	B10.MBR
	s–a1	*t1*	A.TL, B10.TL
	q–a	*y1*	B10.AQR
	Unknown	*ar1*	B10.LG/Ckc
I-A–I-J	*d–b*	*g2*	D2.GD, B10.GD
	a–b	*h4*	B10.A(4R)
	a–b	*i5*	B10.A(5R)
	a–s	*as1*	B10.S(8R)
I-J–I-E	*a–b*	*i3*	B10.A(3R)
	s–t1	*t3*	B10.HTT
	f–t1	*ap5*	A.TFR5
I-E–I-C	Unknown	*a*	A, B10.A, C3H.A
I-C–S	*d–k*	*o1*	C3H.OL, B10.OL
	Unknown	*t5*	BSVS
S–D	*d–k*	*a1*	A.AL, B10.AL
	f–a	*ap1*	B10.M(11R)
	a–f	*aq1*	B10.M(17R)
	a–s	*as2*	B10.ASR
	d–b	*g6*	B6.C-*H-2^{g6}*
	k–q	*h3*	B10.AM
	b–t1	*i8*	A.BTR1
	b–t2	*i21*	B10.S(21R)
	d–k	*o2*	C3H.OH, B10.OH
	t6–b	*sb*	B10.S(26R)
	t2–r	*sr*	B10.RIII(20R)
	s–a	*t6*	B10.S(24R)
	s–a	*t2*	B10.S(7R), A.TH

the *K* region assigned to the left and the *D* region to the right. These borders were established arbitrarily and should not be considered inflexible. The products of the *Tla* genes (Section 22.1) to the right of the *D* region seem to be strikingly similar to the class I molecules. These genes are sometimes considered a part of the *TL* region. They encode products that are also glycoproteins of molecular weight about 45,000. Moreover, the *Tla* products share some functional as well as physicochemical properties with other products of the *H-2* complex (Section 22.2). In fact, it is quite plausible that on both sides of the *H-2* complex there are genes that are homologous and related to those within the complex.

TABLE 16.2. Genes of the *H-2* Complex According to Traditional and New Concepts of the Genetic Structure of the Complex

Region	Subregion	Class	Genes of the Traditional Concept	Genes of the New Concept	Demonstrable Product
K	—	I	*H-2K** *Lad* *Ir* *Hh-3*	*H-2K*	H-2K
I	A	II	*H-2A* *Lad* *Ir-1A* *Ia-1* *CI* *Is*	A_α A_β A_e	Ia-1 (I-A)
	B	II	*Lad(?)* *Ir-1B* *Ia-2*	?	?
	J	II	*Ia-4* *Is(?)*	?	Ia-4 (?)
	E	II	*Lad* *Ia-5*	E_α	Ia-5 (I-E)
	C	II	*H-2C* *Lad* *Ir-1C* *Ia-3* *Is*		Ia-3 (?)
S	—	III	*Ss* *Slp*	*Ss* *Slp*	Ss (C4) Slp
D	—	I	*H-2D** *H-2L* *Lad* *Hh-1*	*H-2D* *H-2L*	H-2D H-2L

*See text for other genes of the *K* and *D* regions.

CLASS I GENES AND MOLECULES

The *H-2K* and *H-2D* genes are the classic members of class I. Recent studies indicate that in the K and D regions, more than a single gene may reside, and they may form a cluster of class I genes. In the *K* region, two genes are reported and have been tentatively named *H-2K1* and *H-2K2*, while in the *D* region four genes are described and are named *H-2D, H-2L, H-2M,* and *H-2R*. These genes may actually represent multiple copies of a single ancestral gene. Since

TABLE 16.3. Partial List of Recombinant *H-2* Haplotypes Derived from Unrelated and Partially Related Haplotypes of Laboratory Inbred Mice

Unrelated *H-2* Haplotype	Prototype Strain(s)	Related *H-2* Haplotype	*H-2* Composition[a]	Recombinant Strain(s)
b	C57BL/10	*bq1*	*b k k k k k k q*	B10.MBR
		i5	*b b b k k d d d*	B10.A(5R)
		i3	*b b b b k d d d*	B10.A(3R)
		bw	*b b b b b b p p*	B10.F(14R)
		bq2	*b b . . . . q q*	BQ2
		i,i7,i8	*b b b b b b b d*	HTI, B10.D2(R107), A.BTR1, A.BTR2,
		i9, i18, i21		B10.A(18R), B10.S(21R)
		i1, i2		B10.BAR-5, B10. RBD
		ak1, oz1	*b b b b b b b k*	B6.AKL, B6-*H-2$^{0az\,1}$*
		ia1	*b b b b b b b dm 1*	B10.D2(R106)
		j^{b}	*j j j j j j b*	B10.WB, I/St
d	DBA/2J	*ar1*	*d f f f f f f q*	LG/Ckc, B10.LG
	BALB/c	*g2*	*d d b b b b b b*	D2.GD, B10.GD
	B10.D2	*o1*	*d d d d d d k k*	C3H.OL
	NZB	*o2*	*d d d d d d d k*	C3H.OH
		g,g1,g3	*d d d d d d d b*	HTI, B10.D2(R107), A. BTR1,
		g4,g5,g6,g7		A.BTR2, B10.A(18R), B10.S(21R),
f	A.CA	*ap3,ap4,*	*f f . q q . s d*	B10.BAR-5, B10.RBD
	RFM	*ap5*	*f f f f k k k d*	B.6AKL, B6-*H-2^{ozl}*
	B10.M	*ap1,ap2*	*f f f f f f f d*	B10.D2(R106)
k	C3H	*m1*	*k . . . . . q q*	B10.QAR
	AKR	*as1*	*k k k s s s s s*	B10.S(8R)
	CBA	*h4*	*k k b b b b b b*	B10.A(4R)
	C57BR	*a,a8*	*k k k k k d d d*	B10.A, A, C3H.A, B10.RKD3
		a7	*k k k k k . q d*	B10.RKD2
		aq1	*k k k k k d d f*	B10.M(17R)
		as2	*k k k k k d d s*	B10.ASR2
		h,h1,h2,h15	*k k k k k d d b*	HTH, B10.A(1R), B10.A(2R), B10.A(15R
		az1	*k k k k k . v v*	B10.SM(22R)
		a3	*k k k k k . d d*	BSVR
		a4	*k k k k k . d d*	B10.RKD1
		h10	*k k . . b b b b*	B10.RKB
		a5	*k k k k k . b d*	A1R1
		a1	*k k k k k k k d*	A.AL, B10.AL
		h3	*k k k k k k k b*	B10.AM
		m	*k k k k k k k q*	B10.AKM, AKR.M
p	B10.P	*bu*	*p p p p p p b b*	B10.F(13R)
	C3H.NB	*td2*	*p p p p p p d d*	B10.RPD2
	P	*td1*	*p p p p p p b d*	B10.RPD1

TABLE 16.3 *(continued)*

Unrelated *H-2* Haplotype	Prototype Strain(s)	Related *H-2* Haplotype	*H-2* Composition[a]	Recombinant Strain(s)
q	DBA/1J	*y1*	q k k k k d d d	B10.AQR
	BUB	*by1*	q k k k k d d b	B10.BYR
	B10.Q	*y2*	q q q q q q q d	B10.T(6R)
	SWR	*qp1*	q q q q q q q s	DA, B10.DA(80NS)
		qb1,qb2	q q q q q q q b	B10.RQB1, B10.RQB2
r	RIII	—	—	
	B10.RIII			
s	SJL	*t1*	s k k k k k k d	A.TL, B10.TL (A_α derived from *H-2^s*)
	B10.S	*an1*	s k k k k k k f	A.TFR1
		at1,at4	s k k k k k k b	A.TBR1, A.TBR4
		at9	s s . q b b b b	B10.RSB1
		at10	s s . k k d d b	B10.RSB2
		at11	s s . q k . k b	B10.RSB3
		t4	s s . k k d d d	B10.S(9R)
		an2	s s . q b b b f	B10.RSF1
		sq2	s s . . . . q q	B10.QSR2
		t3	s s s s k k k d	HTT, B10.HTT
		t5	s s s s s s d d	BSVS
		t2,t6,t11	s s s s s s s d	A.TH, B10.S(7R), B10.S(24R), B10.S(23R)
		sb	s s s s s s s b	B10.S(26R)
		aw1	s s s s s s s r	B10.RIII(20R)
		sq4	s s s s s s s q	NFS/N
		u^b	u u u u u u u d	B10.PL, PL
	NZW	*z^b*	u u u u u u z z	B10.NZW,
w^c	11 unrelated haplotypes	19 related haplotypes		30 strains derived recently from wild mice

[a]Alleles at *K, I-A, I-B, I-J, I-E, I-C, S,* and *D* are given. A dot indicates that the allele is unknown at this time.

[b]Partially related haplotypes carrying unique alleles at the K-side of the complex.

[c]Haplotypes of wild mice (see Table 16.4).

Note: All recombinant haplotypes are related to two or more haplotypes, but for the sake of simplicity they are listed only in connection with haplotypes that share a particular allele in the *K* region.

there are still some doubts surrounding the definition of multiple genes in a given class I region, these genes will be considered separately; here the discussion will primarily concentrate on the two prototype genes and their products.

16.1 Class I *H-2* Genes

The *H-2K* and *H-2D* genes, which are located at two opposite ends of the *H-2* complex, were the first to be defined. Each appears to be extremely polymorphic—e.g., there are 29 *H-2K* and 38 *H-2D* alleles. These figures include the distinct alleles found in laboratory strains and mutants isolated in the laboratory (Section 5.5) as well as alleles of wild mice. The actual numbers allow a theoretical prediction that there may be as many as 100 alleles of each gene in question. This polymorphism exceeds any known genetic system and creates a sui generis paradox. It is conventionally assumed that the term polymorphism, as understood by geneticists, is applicable when a given gene has at least two alleles and both have a frequency of more than 0.01. By the same token, a gene with more than two alleles that are extremely rare (less than 0.01) is for all practical purposes considered nonpolymorphic. With the theoretically predictable 100 class I alleles, all with similar frequencies, class I genes may not fit the definition of polymorphism. In the global population of mice, there seems to be an even distribution of the different alleles with frequencies varying from 0.01 to 0.08. The notably higher frequencies of three alleles (*H-2K^d*, *H-2D^d*, and *H-2K^p*) may reflect a sampling error rather than the true prevalence of these alleles. Finding the same alleles in distant geographic locations suggests that they developed early in evolution or that there has been a convergent evolution. It also argues against the notion that the class I genes are extremely unstable with an unusually high mutation rate.

Inasmuch as the global population of mice has all its class I alleles more or less evenly distributed, any local population can be characterized by two parameters—the spectrum of its alleles and their frequencies. A given local population usually has about 20 to 30 percent of all known alleles with their frequencies distributed on an exponential curve, some being relatively frequent and others being relatively rare. The absence of certain alleles from a local population is the result of various factors such as migration, selective pressure, and/or genetic drift.

Another striking feature of class I genes is their preponderance for heterozygosity. Obviously, this preponderance is demonstrable only in a wild population, since laboratory inbred mice are by definition homozygous. In wild populations, close to 90 percent of individuals are heterozygous for one or both class I genes. Since mice form small populations (demes), there must be a selective pressure maintaining heterozygosity. This finding is analogous to the high degree of heterozygosity of the *HLA* genes in man. The biologic significance of such polymorphism and heterozygosity will be discussed later (Section 19.8).

Some time ago, an alternative concept for the genetics of the class I genes was advanced. In principle, the concept proposes that there are multiple copies of the class I genes in each *H-2* haplotype. The copies are presumed to be the result of several duplications followed by independent mutations of each duplicated copy. This process would ultimately result in a series of related but distinct genes. In a given individual under normal circumstances, only one of these genes is expressed, while all others are suppressed, possibly in a manner similar to the suppression of the genes belonging to the *Ig* family (Section 8.3). However, in some instances, this gene might be repressed and another gene would become expressed. This hypothesis attempts to explain the occasional disappearance of class I molecules from neoplastic cells and the appearance of molecules that are absent in the normal cells of the strain from which the tumor cells were derived (Section 25.1). The new molecules, referred to as **alien antigens**, have not yet been characterized biochemically, and their putative relationship with normal class I molecules is based mostly on serological data. Thus, there are many authors who disagree with the multiple copy concept. A definitive conclusion should be possible when more data are available from recent experiments on *H-2* gene cloning.

16.2 Molecular Structure of Class I Genes

Several cDNA clones that encode either human or murine class I gene products have been isolated and their base sequences determined. The partial amino acid sequences encoded in these cDNA exhibit a high degree of homology with transplantation antigens, even though none of the isolated cDNA clones encodes a known transplantation antigen.

The cDNA clones were used to study the arrangement of their genes by Southern transfer hybridization. Each cDNA hybridized to several restriction endonuclease fragments of DNA, which strongly suggests that each may belong to a multigene family composed of several members. Furthermore, the number of fragments and the intensity of their hybridization were identical for DNA obtained from germ line, embryonic, or adult liver. This fact argues strongly that, unlike the immunoglobulin genes, these genes do not undergo a detectable rearrangement prior to their expression (Section 8.1). Finally, when restriction fragments of DNA from several murine strains carrying different *H-2* haplotypes were compared, there was a high degree of conservation of fragments that hybridized to the cDNA probe, indicating that there is a strong selective pressure to maintain these genes in their conformation. This is consistent with the conservation of the structure of the antigens themselves.

Two of the murine cDNA clones were used to probe a library of mouse genomic DNA. From the 30 to 40 positive phages identified, one was chosen for complete DNA sequence analysis. In this genome-containing phage, designated 27.1, the locations of the coding regions (exons) were identified by Southern transfer with the cDNA probes. Precise exon locations were determined by decoding the possible triplet sequences in three possible reading frames and comparing these potential amino acid sequences with the known amino acid sequence of the murine H-2K^b antigen. The hydrophobic leader exon in 27.1 was identified by its length (21 amino acids), the hydrophobic character of the amino acids, and the presence of an RNA splice site at the 3′ end of the exon (Fig. 16.2).

The gene consists of eight exons that are separated by seven introns. Each exon corresponds to one of the following functional portions of the transplantation antigen: a leader signal peptide, three extracellular regions (Section 16.5), an intramembrane hydrophobic portion, or a hydrophilic intracellular portion. The latter is determined by three small exons. It is interesting to note that a portion of an intron in 27.1 was found in another cDNA clone as an exon for the intracellular portion. This means that the sequence of the intracellular portions may interact with cytoplasmic proteins differently and may play a role in tissue development or the immune response.

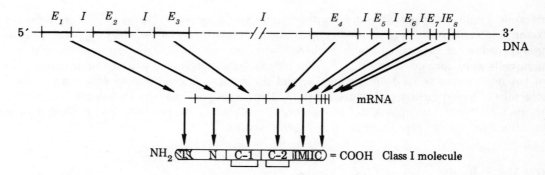

FIG. 16.2. Fine structure of the pseudogene for the product homologous with the class I molecule. The gene is composed of eight exons (**E1-E8**) separated by seven introns (**dotted lines, I**) Single exons code for tail (**T**), each extracellular region (**N, C-1, C-2**), and intramembrane portion (**IM**). Three exons code for the intracellular portion (**IC**).

The gene in 27.1 clone was mapped to the *Qa 2,3* locus (Section 22.24) and thus comes from a gene set that is involved in T lymphocyte differentiation. The sequence of the gene reveals that this is a **pseudogene**, one that cannot be expressed owing to a functional abnormality in its sequence. This gene possesses two translation stop codons (nonsense mutations) at positions 312 and 328 in the transmembrane and intracellular portions, respectively. Pseudogenes are common members of multigene families in eukaryotes. They are thought to be the product of recent gene duplication, which, in the absence of selective pressure, is followed by base sequence changes resulting in the nonsense mutations (Section 3.6). The basic structural arrangement of 27.1 was found in other cloned transplantation antigen genes whose sequences have not yet been reported. It is anticipated that within the next few years most, if not all, of the genes and pseudogenes that determine the class I transplantation antigens will be isolated and their base sequences determined.

Finally, it should be emphasized that the amino acid sequence encoded by 27.1 is highly homologous to the amino acid sequence of the H-2K^b molecule. This means that there must be a high degree of conservation among all class I transplantation antigens, even though the cell types that they are found on and their possible functions in vivo may be strikingly different.

16.3 Detection of Class I Molecules

The detection and definition of the allelic class I molecules are based on their distinct alloantigenic properties, i.e., their ability to elicit an immune response in a member of the same species. Two types of this immune response can be elicited and analyzed—cell-mediated and antibody-mediated (Sections 4.3 and 4.10).

The cell-mediated response to class I molecules is responsible for the rapid rejection of allografts that carry incompatible class I molecules. The ability to reject a skin graft and the segregation of this ability in the progeny constitute the basis of the histogenetic method used to define the unrelated haplotypes of original inbred strains. The in vitro correlate of graft rejection is cell-mediated lymphocytotoxicity (CML) in which the killing of target cells carrying incompatible class I molecules is effected by lymphocytes immunized against these molecules (Section 4.13). The MLR (Section 4.12) that reflects in vitro stimulation of T cells by the histocompatibility antigen(s) can occasionally be used for the detection of class I molecules. However, such a reaction is usually much weaker than that elicited by class II molecules.

The antibody-mediated response is elicited by a series of discrete determinants present in various combinations on the allelic class I molecules. These determinants, often referred to as **specificities**, can be divided into two major groups. One group consists of **private specificities**—each being unique for a given allelic product (Table 16.4). A given molecule carries only one private specificity that identifies it as a product of an allele at either the *H-2K* or *H-2D* locus. A given inbred mouse must have at least two private specificities, one for the H-2K and one for the H-2D molecule with a maximum of four private specificities in a mouse that is heterozygous at both class I loci. Assignment of private specificity to either a K or a D molecule encoded by a given unrelated haplotype is possible only when a crossing-over event separated *H-2K* and *H-2D* genes of such a haplotype. Thus, in some instances, a single specificity (Table 16.4) assigned to the unrelated haplotype in fact represents two specificities that can be "split" when a recombinant haplotype is detected. The second group consists of **public specificities** that are shared by some, but not all, allelic products of either one or both class I genes. The public specificities are sometimes referred to as short, when shared by only a few, or long, when shared by many different allelic products. In addition to more than 80 public and private specificities found in laboratory mice, 42 specificities of wild mice are presently known. The latter consists of both private and public specificities as well.

The lymphocytotoxic test is presently the most common antibody-mediated procedure for the detection and definition of class I molecules. Antibodies elicited by immunization of a mouse with cells or tissues carrying allogeneic specificities are cytotoxic for the immunizing cells in the presence of complement. Antisera for all private and public specificities are available. However, antibodies for private specificities appear to be monospecific, whereas many antibodies for public specificities are not; they tend to cross-react with different specificities to varying degrees. This cross-reactivity formed the basis for several concepts such as **inclusion groups** in which certain public specificities would constitute a component of other public specificities. It should be noted that some alloantisera to mouse class I antigens cross-react with human class I molecules, suggesting a certain degree of interspecies homology. An alternative serologic test for the detection of class I molecules takes advantage of the fact that the class I molecules of mice are expressed on erythrocytes. The hemagglutination test is routinely used to determine the H-2 phenotype in mice.

16.4 Cellular and Subcellular Distribution of Class I Molecules

Murine class I molecules, in similarity to those of man, are ubiquitously distributed. Their concentration per cell varies broadly, depending on the type and degree of differentiation of a

TABLE 16.4. Private Antigenic Specificities of the Class I Molecules Determined by Unrelated and Partially Related *H-2* Haplotypes

Haplotype	Specificities of H-2K Molecules	Specificities Not Assigned	Specificities of H-2D Molecules
b	33		2
d	31		4
f	26		9
j	15		2 (D^b)
k	23		32
p	16		22
q	17		30
r	18		10
s	19		12
u	20		2 (D^b)
v	21		30 (D^q)
z	20 (K^u)		114
w2		102	
w3	103		118
w4	?		104
w5	31 (K^d)		147
w6		143	
w7	132		131
w8	23 (K^k)		110
w9	?		32 (D^k)
w10	21 (K^v)		
w11	26 (K^f)		131
w12	23 (K^k)		112
w13	113		
w14	31 (K^d)		114 (D^z)
w15	115		
w16	116		130
w17	111		118
w18	31 (K^d)		147
w19	19 (K^s)		2 (D^b)
w20	116		110
w21	19 (K^s)		130
w22	116		32 (D^k)
w23		144	
w24	31 (K^d)		114 (D^z)
w25	103		?
w26	17 (K^q)		137
w27	138		
w34	31 (K^d)		118
w35	132 or 145		118
w39	132		2 (D^b)

NOTE: Allelic molecules encoded by unrelated haplotypes of laboratory mice in which the same specificity can also be found are indicated in parentheses.

cell. The richest sources of class I molecules are lymphoid and hemopoietic cells, whereas cells such as muscle fibers and neurons lie on the other end of the spectrum.

At the subcellular level, class I molecules are transmembrane moieties present on the cell membrane. The small C terminal portion is located intracellularly, and the much larger N terminal portion is exposed extracellularly. While anchored in the cell membrane, class I molecules are noncovalently associated with β_2-microglobulin in a 1:1 ratio (Chapter 18). The association between class I and β_2-microglobulin molecules allows cocapping by antibody to either component of the molecular complex (Section 4.5).

16.5 Biochemistry and Biosynthesis of Class I Molecules

There is a striking similarity between the class I molecules of mice and man. In fact, almost all that has been said before in regard to the HLA molecules applies to H-2 molecules (Section 15.3). With this in mind, only the most important points will be reiterated here and some differences emphasized (Fig. 16.3). Class I molecules are glycoproteins of molecular weight about 45,000. The murine molecules have two oligosaccharides attached to asparagines at positions 86 and 176 in contrast to the human counterparts, which have sugar only at position 86. Some investigators reported the presence of three oligosaccharides in some murine molecules. The oligosaccharides appear to be of the complex type with a terminal sialic acid. The protein molecule consists of 344 amino acids divided among intracellular (39 residues), intramembrane (24 residues), and extracellular (281 residues) portions. There are two intrachain disulfide loops that encompass residues 101–164 and 203–259. The extracellular portion is subdivided into three regions: N (residues 1–90), C-1 (residues 91–180), and C-2 (residues 181–281).

Amino acid sequence analysis has revealed homology between allelic products (75 to 87 percent), between two different class I molecules, and between murine and human molecules (67 to 73 percent). Amino acid substitutions between two allelic products do not fall within a definite hypervariable region; they are more or less evenly distributed along the molecule. Still, clusters of substitutions have been distinguished. These clusters are characterized by low homology between alleles (25 to 51 percent) and substitutions that frequently require two-base changes. The clusters are positioned between 61–83 and 95–99 and also between residues 22–24, 30–32, and 41–45. Substitutions are slightly more frequent between two different class I molecules. There is extensive divergence in amino acid sequences of the intramembrane and intracellular portions of murine and human molecules. This divergence may be due to a lack of any selective restriction on these two portions. As in the case of HLA molecules, there is no specific amino acid sequence identifying the products of alleles at a given locus. Nor is there a unique sequence distinguishing class I molecules of mouse and man. Some residues seem to be preserved in all allelic products of a given species; perhaps these residues identify a species.

The biosynthesis of murine class I molecules proceeds along much the same pathway as described earlier for human molecules. The process consists of translation, glycosylation, several posttranslational modifications, and an association with β_2-microglobulin.

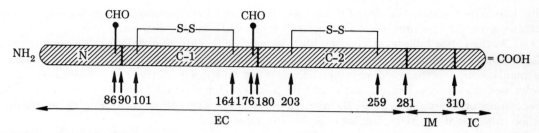

FIG. 16.3. Scheme of the class I H-2 molecule consisting of extracellular (**EC**), intramembrane
(**IM**), and intracellular (**IC**) portions. Within the EC portion, three regions (**N, C-1,
C-2**) are distinguished. **Arrows with numbers** indicate amino acid positions: **CHO**
= carbohydrate residue; **S-S** = disulfide bond. For details, see text.

16.6 Other Class I Molecules

As mentioned earlier, as an alternative to the traditional model of the *H-2* complex, it has been
proposed that class I genes may be present as multiple copies that originated from an ancestral
gene and then mutated independently. This concept, although not yet universally accepted,
finds circumstantial support in the serological demonstration that in some *H-2* haplotypes a
given region may contain more than one class I gene.

Two molecules, tentatively called H-2K1 and H-2K2 were found to be associated with the
K region of the *H-2^d* haplotype. In association with the *D* region of several different haplotypes,
multiple molecules have been described. These molecules, called H-2L, H-2M and H-2R,
apparently are closely related to, but antigentically distinct from, class I molecules determined
by the classic *H-2D* gene. They are distinguishable by the unique combination of public
specificities reactive with both conventional and monoclonal antibodies. The H-2L molecule was
isolated and subjected to extensive biochemical analysis. This analysis indicated that there are
18 to 22 percent amino acid substitutions scattered along the allelic molecules. Different allelic
H-2L molecules strongly cross-react with monoclonal antibodies as well as in the CML assay.
Table 16.5 summarizes the presently known class I molecules determined by the class I genes
and the serological characteristics of these molecules. The functional role of these molecules
remains unclear.

Even more importantly, the genetic determination of different class I molecules assigned
to a single region poses several unresolved problems. The *H-2L* gene that encodes the L
molecule is the only distinct gene that has been firmly established. The existence of other genes
may be only inferred from the DNA cloning studies in which over 30 distinct class I genes have
been identified (Section 16.2). On the other hand, it is possible that some molecules result from
different processing of preRNA transcribed from a single gene. Alternatively, posttranslational
modifications of a single precursor molecule may be responsible for the multiple final products
(Section 3.5). Finally, it cannot be excluded that gene rearrangements or **gene conversions**
(Section 16.7) are not involved in the generation of multiple products of a single or relatively few
genes.

Other unorthodox moieties associated with class I genes are those responsible for the

TABLE 16.5. Antigenic Profiles of Class I Molecules Determined by the Genes in the *D* and *K* Regions of the *H-2* Complex.

Haplotype	Region	Molecule	Antigenic Composition (specificities)										
			[1]	2*	4*	9*	12*	[28]	30*	31*	32*	64	65
b	*D*	D		+				+					
		L						+				+	
d	*D*	D			+			+					
		L						+				+	+
		L2			+			+a					
		M						+a					
		R						+a					
	K	K1						+a		+a	+		
		K2						+a					
f	*D*	D				+							
		L						+					
k	*D*	D1	+							+			
		D2	+a								+		
q	*D*	D						+	+				
		L						+				+	+
		R									+		
s	*D*	D					+	+					
		L						+					

*Private specificities of H-2D and H-2K molecules.
[ ] H-2.1 and H-2.28 are two families, each consisting of several related specificities.
aOnly some specificities of the family are detectable.

phenomenon of **hybrid resistance**. This phenomenon refers to the rejection of parental tissue grafts (hemopoietic or tumor) by the F1 hybrids of two inbred strains. Since, according to the conventional concept, alleles of all histocompatibility genes are codominant, the F1 hybrid should have all the products of parental genes and should not be able to react against them (Section 21.1). To explain the rejection of parental grafts by F1 hybrids, the concept of *Hh* genes (**hybrid** or **hemopoietic histocompatibility**) has been proposed. These genes would carry recessive alleles that result in the full expression of products in homozygotes (inbred parents) but not in heterozygotes (F1 hybrids). Thus, the parent would possess an antigen that is absent in its F1 hybrids and against which an F1 hybrid could react. Three *Hh* genes have been recognized of which two—*Hh-1* and *Hh-3*—were mapped to the *D* and *K* regions, respectively. It is not known whether these genes are identical with either classic or unorthodox class I genes. However, at least in some cases, reactions of F1 hybrids against parent seems to be directed to class I molecules of such a parent. Furthermore, recent experiments with hybrid resistance to some tumors show that mutations of class I genes result in an apparent alteration of hybrid resistance. Interestingly, the immune response to the products of *Hh* genes appears to be mediated by natural killer (NK) cells rather than by the usual cytotoxic T cells (Section 25.12). No obvious hybrid resistance has been observed in the case of skin or other organ grafts.

16.7 Mutations of Class I Genes

Mutants of class I genes were discovered by histogenetic methods before the biochemical structure of the class I molecules was known. By now, a large series of independent mutants has been identified (Table 16.6). The majority of the presently known mutants are of the H-$2K^b$ allele. It is difficult to ascertain whether this reflects an exceptional mutability of this particular allele (2.2×10^{-4}/gamete) or simply biased sampling. However, it should be mentioned that the H-2^d haplotype was actually more extensively screened for mutations than was the H-2^b haplotype and that the H-$2D$ gene of the H-2^b haplotype was tested to the same extent as the H-$2K$ gene. That the mutations affected the class I gene was convincingly demonstrated by serologic isolation and biochemical analysis of the molecules. Besides the specific characteristic of each mutant, there are certain features shared by all, or almost all, known mutants.

With few exceptions, mutants are of the gain-loss type—i.e, mutant class I molecules carry certain determinants that are absent from the original product and, at the same time, lack some determinants of the original product. When private or public specificities are involved, they are changed either quantitatively or qualitatively; in most cases, these changes can be detected serologically. In one of the mutations (H-2^{dm2}), a deletion of the entire gene resulted in lack of expression of the H-2L molecules. Another mutant (H-2^{dm1}) is unusual in that at least two distinct genes—H-$2D$ and H-$2L$—underwent simultaneous mutations. Specifically, it seems that the H-$2D$ gene was duplicated and then both copies were extensively mutated (frame-shift) by mutagenic treatment with diethylsulfate; moreover, the H-$2L$ gene was altered. The mutant molecules are antigenically unique and usually can be distinguished from each other by a variety of immunologic assays. On the other hand, some degree of cross-reaction is commonly observed, as might be expected in the case of a mutation created by a single amino acid substitution. Besides the serologic changes of class I molecules, other functional properties assigned to the genes in the same region are usually altered (graft rejection, GVHR, CML). The simultaneous alteration of several characteristics, after mutation of a single gene, strongly indicates that all these characteristics are the properties of this particular gene or its product.

Biochemical analysis of some mutants clearly showed that the mutations represent one or two amino acid substitutions (Table 16.6). Interestingly, several independent mutants have exactly the same substitutions. It is tempting to speculate that, for enigmatic reasons, certain points in the gene are particularly prone to changes. An alternative possibility, currently under experimental scrutiny, is that the phenomenon of gene conversion may be responsible for some mutants. In this case, within a single gene or between two or more closely linked genes, small fragments of DNA might undergo exchange producing the variants that are detectable as mutants. Biochemical data showing a single amino acid substitution causing multiple serologic and functional changes suggest that some determinants are created by chain conformation rather than by primary amino acid sequences.

CLASS II GENES AND MOLECULES

Murine class II genes are assigned to the *I* region of the *H-2* complex. Functionally, five subregions are distinguished, but only two—*I-A* and *I-E*—have been shown to contain structural genes with detectable molecular products. Summarily, these products are called the *I* region

TABLE 16.6. Mutants of *H-2* Genes and Their Characteristics

Mutant Haplotype (former designation)	Gene Affected	Allele Affected	Strain (synonym)	Type	Amino Acid Substitution		Phenotypic Expression			
					Position	Substitution	Serologic	CM	Ir	Restriction
bm1 (*ba*)	*H-2K*	*b*	B6.6C-*H-2*^*bm1* (Hz1)	GL	155 / 156	Arg→Tyr / Leu→Tyr	+	+	+	+
bm2 (*bb*)	*H-2K*	*b*	B6.C-*H-2*^*bm2* (Hz49)	GL	155 / 156	Arg→Tyr / Leu→Tyr	·	·	·	·
bm3 (*bd*)	*H-2K*	*b*	B6.*H-2*^*bm3* [B6(M505)]	GL	77	Asp→?	+	+	·	−
bm4 (*bf*)	*H-2K*	*b*	B6.C-*H-2*^*bm4* (Hz170)	GL	89	Lys→? / ?	+	+	·	+
bm5 (*bg1*)	*H-2K*	*b*	B6-*H-2*^*bm5*	GL	116	Tyr→Phe	+	+	·	±
bm6 (*bg2*)	*H-2K*	*b*	B6-*H-2*^*bm6*	GL	116 / 121	Tyr→Phe / Cys→Arg	+	+	·	±
bm7 (*bg3*)	*H-2K*	*b*	B6-*H-2*^*bm7*	GL	116 / 121	Tyr→Phe / Cys→Arg	·	·	·	·
bm8 (*bh*)	*H-2K*	*b*	B6-*H-2*^*bm8*	GL	23	Met→?	+	+	·	±
bm9 (*bi*)	*H-2K*	*b*	B6.C-*H-2*^*bm9*	GL	116 / 121	Tyr→Phe / Cys→Arg	−	+	·	·
bm10 (*bj*)	*H-2K*	*b*	B6.C-*H-2*^*bm10*	GL	165	Val→Met	+	+	·	·
bm11 (*bk*)	*H-2K*	*b*	B6.C-*H-2*^*bm11*	GL	77	Asp→?	+	+	·	·
bm12 (*bm*)	*I-A*_β	*b*	B6.C-*H-2*^*bm12*	GL		?	+	+	+	−
bm13 (*bn*)	*H-2D*	*b*	B6.C-*H-2*^*bm13*	GL		?	·	·	·	+
bm14 (*bo*)	*H-2D*	*b*	B6.C-*H-2*^*bm14*	GL		?	+	+	·	+
bm15 (extinct)	?	*b*	B10-*H-2*^*bm15*	L		?	·	·	·	·
bm16	*H-2K*	*b*	B6-*H-2*^*bm16*	GL	116	Try→Phe	·	+	·	·
bm17	*H-2K*	*b*	B6-*H-2*^*bm17* (KH-97)	GL		?	·	+	·	·
bm18	*H-2K*	*b*	B6.C-*H-2*^*bm18* (KH-170)	GL		?	·	+	·	·
bm19	*H-2K*	*b*	B6.C-*H-2*^*bm19* (KH-171)	GL		?	·	+	·	·
bm20	*H-2K*	*b*	B6.C-*H-2*^*bm20*	GL		?	·	+	·	·
bm21	*H-2K*	*b*	B6.C-*H-2*^*bm21*	GL		?	·	+	·	·

(continued)

TABLE 6.6 (continued)

Mutant Haplotype (former designation)	Gene Affected	Allele Affected	Strain(s) (synonym)	Amino Acid Substitution Type	Position	Substitution	Phenotypic Expression Serologic	CM	Ir	Restriction
bm22	H-2K	b	B6-H-2^bm22	GL		?	·	+	·	·
dm1(da)	H-2D	d	B10.D2-H-2^dm1	GL		?	+	+	+	+
	H-2L	d	B10.D2(R106)	GL						
dm2(db)	H-2L	d	BALB-H-2^dm2	L		?	+	+	·	+
dm3(dc)(extinct)	?	d	B6.C-H-2^dm3	L		?	·	·	·	·
dm4(dd)	H-2K	d	C.B6-H-2^dm4	GL		?	−	+	·	·
dm5	H-2K	d	C.B6-H-2^dm5	GL		?	−	·	·	·
fm1(fa)	H-2K	f	A.CA-H-2^fm1 (M506)	GL		?	+	+	·	+
fm2(fb)	H-2D	f	B10.M-H-2^fm2	GL		?	+	+	·	·
km1(ka)	H-2K	k	CBA-H-2^km1 (M523)	GL		?	+	+	+?	+

CM = cell-mediated response (GVHR, HVGR, and/or CML).

Ir = Ir effect.

NOTES: A plus sign (+) indicates an alteration; a minus sign (−) indicates lack of an alteration; a dot (·) indicates lack of data.

*a*ssociated or Ia antigens. Originally, these products were called Lna, Ir-1.1, or β, but now it is generally accepted that they are identical with Ia molecules. The remaining three subregions either have no demonstrable products, viz *I-B*, or the product can only be inferred from a functional assay but has not been isolated in a molecular form, viz *I-J* and *I-C*. The actual product of the gene in the *I-E* subregion was considered to be identical with the putative product of the gene in the *I-C* subregion because the determinants assigned to the two subregions were coprecipitated. However, recently a specific suppressor factor has been associated with the *I-C* subregion, and antiserum specific for the product of this subregion has been produced. The uncertainty about the products of the *I-B*, *I-J*, and *I-C* subregions prompted some investigators to question the existence of these subregions. It seems, however, that passing final judgment at this time would be, to say the least, premature.

16.8 Genetics of Class II Molecules

Until recently, because it was believed that each *I* subregion contains a single gene for a distinct class II molecule, these genes were designated *Ia*. Accordingly, five genes—*Ia-1, Ia-2, Ia-3, Ia-4,* and *Ia-5*—were postulated and assigned to the *I-A, I-B, I-C, I-J,* and *I-E* subregions, respectively. The subsequent finding that each class II molecule consists of two independently synthesized chains—α and β—forced a revision of the original concept of the *Ia* genes. It had to be postulated that a given *Ia* gene represents a set containing not one but two discrete genes—α and β. Furthermore, since no molecular product of the putative *Ia-2, Ia-3,* and *Ia-4* sets could be found and isolated, their nature and even their existence is in doubt (see below). Studies with intra-*H-2* recombinants clearly showed that the two genes forming the *Ia-5* set map into two different subregions—*I-A* and *I-E*. All these findings provide the basis for the current concept of the genetic control of class II molecules in mice (Fig. 16.4).

The Ia-1 molecule, also referred to as the I-A molecule, is determined by a pair of genes designated A_α and A_β, both located in the *I-A* subregion. The two genes appear to be very closely linked, but their order was recently determined to be A_α–A_β and to the right of the *H-2K* locus. The A_α–A_β tandem determines allelic products corresponding to a polymorphism consisting of 21 known alleles. The theoretical estimate calls for as many as 60 alleles of the A_α–A_β tandem. It is believed, on the basis of biochemical studies, that the polymorphism is primarily due to alleles at the A_β locus, but the A_α gene is also polymorphic. Products of both genes must be synthesized in a given cell for the phenotypic expression of the Ia-1 molecule. The presence of only one product results in no expression. Genes A_α and A_β are said to complement each other.

The Ia-5 (I-E) molecule is also determined by a gene tandem designated as A_e (E_β) and E_α. Each member of the tandem, however, maps to a different subregion. While the A_e gene was found to be within the *I-A* subregion to the right of the A_α–A_β tandem, the E_α gene is in the *I-E* subregion. It has been reported that the A_e gene consists of two exons separated by an intervening sequence (intron). The two exons code for the two domains of the A_e (E_β) chain with the border between the domains located at or close to amino acid position 90 of the β chain. Similar to the Ia-1 molecule, several allelic products, mostly due to the A_e alleles, have been defined, but the extent of the polymorphism is much lower and consists of only six known alleles, almost exclusively reflecting polymorphism of the A_e gene. This smaller polymorphism, at least in part,

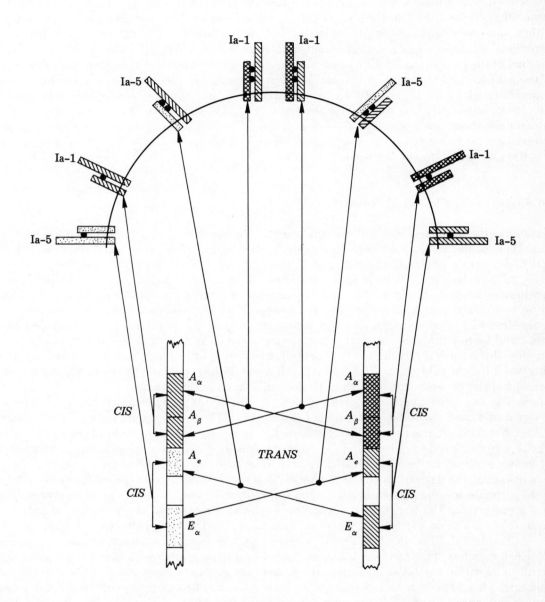

FIG. 16.4. The genetic determination of class II (Ia) molecules in an H-2 heterozygous mouse. **Arrows** indicate intergenic complementation between α and β genes that are in a *cis* or *trans* position. Eight distinct Ia molecules carry either parental combinatorial determinants (●) or hybrid combinatorial (●●) determinants.

may be due to the frequent presence of the silent allele at the E_α locus. Since the expression of the Ia molecule requires the presence of both chains, the silent allele (E_α^o) at one locus prevents the expression of the molecule even though the A_e locus carries a normal allele. At this time, the E_α^o) allele seems to be associated with at least four haplotypes: $H\text{-}2^b$, $H\text{-}2^f$, $H\text{-}2^q$, and $H\text{-}2^s$. Alternatively, rather than being silent, the E_a allele of these haplotypes may be nonantigenic, at least in the allogeneic combination. There are contradictory reports in this regard since some authors were able to raise xenoantisera to the presumptive product of the E_α^o, whereas others failed in such attempts. There are also reports that some A_e alleles are silent (e.g., A_e^f, A_e^q). Some data indicate that at least certain alleles may result in expression of a rather low amount of product rather than a qualitatively distinct molecule. Indeed, molecular analysis by DNA cloning and hybridization revealed that all $H\text{-}2$ haplotypes that do not express the Ia-5 molecule nonetheless carry structural A_e and E_α genes. Authors have suggested that in addition to the E_a gene the $I\text{-}E$ subregion also contains its own E_β gene, but this remains to be confirmed. There are indications that this gene, called $E_{\beta 2}$, lacks one of the exons and, thus, behaves as pseudogene (Section 16.2). The $A_e\text{-}E_a$ tandem consists of complementary genes, since two genes are required for expression of a single molecule.

In either of the two tandems, complementation may occur between genes that are in either the *cis* or the *trans* position. In the first case, products of alleles of the same haplotype form the molecule, whereas in the second case, products of alleles of two different haplotypes are combined (Fig. 16.4). As can be seen, such a complementation phenomenon significantly increases the number of different molecular products without a simultaneous increase in the number of distinct genes. In some F1 heterozygotes, four class II genes may produce eight different molecules. The biologic significance of this will be discussed later (Section 19.6). As mentioned earlier, the Ia-5 molecule appears to be the analogue of the human HLA-DR molecule (Section 15.6). There are speculations that the $A_e\text{-}E_\alpha$ tandem may be ancestral for the $A_\alpha\text{-}A_\beta$ tandem. The latter would develop by duplication of the former and subsequent independent mutation.

16.9 Detection of Class II Molecules

Originally, the *I* subregions were defined by their functional properties, and for some period of time, it was believed that their products were only capable of stimulating a cellular response and were unable to elicit an antibody-mediated response. Class II molecules were considered able to stimulate the proliferation of lymphocytes in vivo or in vitro and thus were called lymphocyte defined (LD) antigens. However, using improved technique, it was unequivocally demonstrated that class II molecules can, and do, induce the production of alloantibodies and, therefore, actually belong to the category of serologically defined (SD) antigens. At present, the most commonly used method to detect and define class II molecules is the lymphocytotoxic assay using alloantibodies and complement. Owing to the restricted distribution of class II molecules, the target cells for the assay must be specially prepared. Most commonly used as target are B cell-enriched preparations of normal cells, B cell tumors, or blast-transformed B cells. The direct cytotoxic assay is complemented by an assay in which cells to be tested for the presence of a given class II molecule are used to absorb a known anti-Ia serum. This approach, however, is limited by the need of sera with a high titer of antibodies and by the nonspecific removal of antibodies during extensive absorption.

Alloantibodies are directed to a spectrum of discrete determinants analogous to those described for class I molecules. As many as 50 different determinants (Table 16.7) are presently defined and assigned to various allelic products on the basis of testing recombinants or sequential immunoprecipitation with appropriate alloantisera. Studies using monoclonal antibodies appear to define additional specificities undetectable with conventional antisera. The determinants can be divided into two categories. In the first category are the true **allotypic determinants**, which correspond to either specific sequences or configurational sites on the α or β chains. These determinants are detectable regardless of whether a given chain is separated from or integrated into the Ia molecule. In the second category are determinants that result from the interaction of the two chains; these determinants cannot be detected on either chain alone. The latter determinants, summarily called **combinatorial**, are probably formed because of conformational changes accompanying the assemblying of the two chains. Whether the combinatorial determinants are actually part of the junction site of the Ia molecule or are physically distant from the site of association has not been determined. Since complementation of corresponding α and β genes may take place in both *cis* and *trans* positions, it follows that, in the latter instances, the combinatorial determinants will be formed in heterozygous F1 hybrids when the products of two parental genes combine into a single Ia molecule. Because such combinatorial determinants are absent from either parent but are present in the F1, they are referred to as **hybrid determinants**. The formation of combinatorial and/or hybrid determinants depends on the properties of the two chains involved, since some combinations of chains are not permissive and cannot combine to form an Ia molecule. In some cases of *trans* complementation, only one of two β chains may form hybrid molecules, while the other contributes only to parental molecules. It should be mentioned that in many instances

TABLE 16.7. Private Antigenic Specificities of Class II Molecules

Haplotype	Specificities of I-A (Ia-1) Molecule	Specificities Not Assigned	Specificities of I-E (Ia-5) Molecule
b	20(w39)*		
d	11		23
f	14		
j		37	
k	2(41)*		22
p		35	21
q	10		
r	34		
s	4		
u		36	
v	38		

*A second specificity so far found to be determined by only this haplotype is shown in parenthesis.

combinatorial determinants become detectable only when the cells have an increased concentration of molecules bearing these determinants, e.g., blast-transformed B cells that have an increased concentration of Ia molecules.

16.10 Cellular and Subcellular Distribution of Class II Molecules

Characteristically, class II molecules have a restricted distribution. They are expressed on virtually all B cells. An extensive search for B cells devoid of class II molecules has not brought convincing evidence that such cells exist. Class II molecules have been demonstrated only on some T cells and in much lower quantities than on B cells. Incidentally, it has been demonstrated that some T cells acquire Ia molecules passively from B cells and/or macrophages with which they interact. It seems that the concentration of class II molecules is inversely related to cell differentiation, with blast forms having more Ia molecules than do more mature cells. Besides lymphoid cells, class II molecules are demonstrated consistently on endothelial cells, macrophages, Kupffer cells, Langerhans cells, dendritic cells, peritoneal neutrophils, and eosinophils. Among macrophages, some appear to express only the Ia-1 molecule, and others both Ia-1 and Ia-5. However, these observations await final confirmation. Recently, Ia molecules were demonstrated in microglial and oligodendroglial cells of the central nervous system. It is worthy of note that all the cells mentioned above are implicated in the process of antigen presentation (Section 4.3). An important observation in this respect is that reticuloepithelial cells of thymic stroma also express class II molecules. No class II molecules have been demonstrated in other cells, suggesting that either they are totally absent or are present in a very low concentration. Contrary to class I, class II molecules are shed easily into the surrounding environment, especially from some tumor cells and also from normal B cells.

At the subcellular level, class II molecules consist of two noncovalent bound transmembrane polypeptides. The two polypeptides are cocapped by antiserum to either of them. During isolation, the two chains of the Ia-1 molecule, but not of the Ia-5, may form a dimer via disulfide bridging, but such a bridge seems not to occur in situ.

16.11 Biochemistry and Biosynthesis of Class II Molecules

Biochemical characterization of class II molecules is still incomplete. The paucity of information is due to the only recent undertaking of systematic studies and the relatively limited source of cellular material from which murine class II molecules can be isolated in quantities sufficient for an extensive analysis.

The class II molecules consist of two glycoprotein chains, α and β. The α chain has a molecular weight of about 33,000, and the β chain has a molecular weight of about 28,000. Some distinct differences in the molecular weights of allelic chains of Ia-5 (I-E) molecules have been reported from various laboratories. Whether these differences represent sampling error or true differences in the size of the chain cannot be decided. Complex sugar moieties are found in both chains, but the number of such moieties in single molecules has not been determined. The β chain of the Ia-5, but not the Ia-1, molecule has an intrachain S-S loop. Tryptic peptide mapping of α and β chains has shown a definitely higher variability of β chains (60 to 85 percent different peptides) than α chains (0 to 53 percent different peptides). However, it should be remembered that tryptic peptide analysis tends to overemphasize the differences. Roughly 50 percent different peptides corresponds to about 10 percent different amino acid residues. There are reports that in addition to α and β chains a third chain of molecular weight 31,000 and called **invariant** (I) is involved in the formation of class II (Ia) molecules. Owing to its invariability, the genetic determination of this chain has not as yet been established. The I chain seems to be associated only with some Ia molecules. It is speculated that those molecules with the I chain are in the process of being synthesized in endoplasmic reticulum, whereas the mature molecules of the cell membrane do not have the I chain. Only limited amino acid sequences of the N terminal portion of the two chains are presently known. These sequences are consistent with serological observations concerning the polymorphism of the two chains. In the β chain, multiple substitutions have been reported in allelic molecules, whereas in the α chain such substitutions are rather infrequent. Because there is a certain degree of homology among corresponding chains found in different species, this homology may be responsible for the cross-reactivity of murine alloantisera with class II molecules of man.

Immunochemical analysis carried out with a panel of monoclonal antibodies (Section 4.9) provided evidence that in a given individual there may be as many as five serologically distinct subsets of Ia-1(I-A) molecules. Among these subsets, one is clearly predominant, whereas others constitute only a minor fraction of the total pool of class II molecules present in the cell. The subsets appear to be formed by combination of four serologically distinct A_β and three A_α chains. The multiplicity of β and α chains may be explained by a multiplicity of the corresponding β and α genes. At least some experimental data seem to support such a contention. A molecular map of murine DNA from the *I* region of the *H-2* complex suggests that it contains several β genes (4–6) but only two α genes. Alternatively, several variants of each chain may be generated by different pathways of preRNA processing or by posttranslational modifications of the product encoded by a single gene. Indeed, electrophoretic analysis revealed that the β chain may occur in two distinct forms that differ from each other by the presence or absence of a disulfide bond but not by differences in amino acid sequence.

There is no appreciable homology between α and β chains, clearly showing that the two chains must be determined by two distinct genes. Even less is known about the biosynthesis of class II molecules. Very preliminary data indicate that the two chains are translated from separate mRNA and combine into a single molecule within the endoplasmic reticulum.

Most investigators agree that the antigenic determinants—and therefore the antigenicity—of class II molecules are associated entirely with the protein part of the molecule. This consensus is supported by the finding that removal of the sugar moiety does not affect the binding of alloantibodies to class II molecules. However, there are persistent reports from one laboratory that a sugar moiety—or to be exact, a monosaccharide—may also be recognized as an alloantigen. It has been suggested that there are two distinct types of class II molecules (Fig. 16.5). One type, roughly corresponding to the molecules presently recognized as class II, would actually represent different glycosyl transferases anchored in the cell membrane and assembling unique sugar moieties. Such sugar moieties then would be transferred to the lipid core. The glycolipids would constitute the second type of class II molecules. These molecules would be shed from cells and possibly play a certain immunoregulatory role. The concept outlined above is far from being universally accepted and requires further systematic experimental studies by independent laboratories.

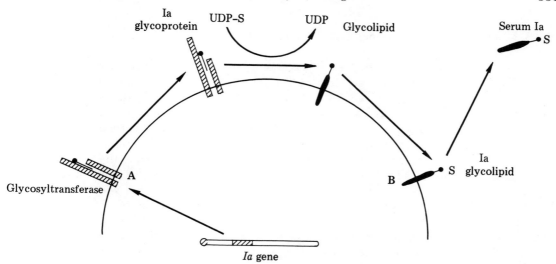

FIG. 16.5. Two proposed kinds of class II molecules involving carbohydrate determinants. (**A**) Glycoproteins that are primary products of the *Ia* genes and have glycosyltransferase activity. (**B**) Glycolipids composed of a sphingosine core to which glycotransferases attach sugars. The glycolipids would be secondary products of the *Ia* genes and are shed from cells.

16.12 Mutants of Class II Genes

There is only one proven and one suspected mutant of class II genes. The proven mutation affects the A_β gene of the H-2^b haplotype. The haplotype carrying the mutant allele has been designated H-2^{bm12} and determines a molecule that is poorly expressed and apparently lacks at least one determinant (Ia.8) present in the nonmutated β chain. It is speculated that this mutation results in structural changes of the molecule and thus not only affects the determinant Ia.8 but also causes deficient anchoring of the molecule. It is also possible that this mutation causes a decreased synthesis of the molecule as indicated by a decreased amount of the I chain that apparently has not been affected by mutational event. The biochemical basis of this particular mutation has been investigated recently. These studies demonstrated that β chains of the mutant molecule differ from the nonmutated chain by at least six tryptic peptides. Three of these peptides are present in mutant but absent from nonmutated molecules, while the other three peptides are absent from the mutant but present in nonmutated molecules. From the functional point of view, the mutation results in the alteration of several different characteristics ascribed to the *I-A* subregion.

The second mutation is suspected to have occurred in the recombinant haplotype called H-2^{g2}, which consists of the *I-A* subregion of the H-2^b haplotype and the *I-E* subregion of the H-2^d haplotype. The Ia-5 (I-E) molecule determined by the H-2^{g2} haplotype apparently lacks a certain determinant (Ia.50). These data are suggestive of an alteration of the A_β gene; in fact recent studies support the concept that this alteration is the result of intragenic recombination and partial deletion of the A_β gene.

16.13 Identity of Different Genes and Products of the *I* Region

According to the traditional concept of the *H-2* complex, each *I* subregion carries at least three genes. The three major genes assigned to the *I* subregions are *Ir*, responsible for controlling specific immune responsiveness; *Ia*, which determines the serologically detectable molecules; and *Lad*, which determines the molecules that stimulate allogeneic lymphocytes and elicit MLR. Extensive search for the molecular products of the *Ir* and *Lad* genes has repeatedly produced negative results. Taking into consideration these negative data, it was postulated some time ago that the products of *Ia* genes may be responsible for the traits attributed to the three genes—*Ir*, *Ia*, and *Lad*—mentioned above. To put it differently, the *Ia* genes would be identical with the remaining two genes—*Ir* and *Lad*. This concept, although originally met with a great deal of skepticism, presently finds strong support owing to recent studies of the $H\text{-}2^{bm12}$ mutant, which showed that all three characteristics—immune responsiveness, Ia molecules, and lymphocyte stimulation ability—are apparently altered. Since a point mutation that affected a single gene changed all three properties, one cannot escape the conclusion that all three properties are determined by a single gene.

16.14 The *I-B* Subregion

Originally, the *I-B* subregion was defined on the basis of its association with immune responsiveness to the IgG allotypic determinant (Section 9.7). Subsequently, responsiveness to some other antigens was mapped to this subregion. However, the Ia-2 molecule, the putative product of the *I-B* subregion, has not been demonstrated serologically despite several attempts. With this in mind, several authors suggested that the *I-B* subregion may not actually exist and that the traits assigned to it may be a reflection of *cis* complementation between the *I-A* and *I-E* subregions. A systematic search for recombinants delineating the limits of the *I-B* subregion should contribute to the resolution of this controversial issue. Interestingly, recent studies on the molecular map of DNA from the *I* region revealed that the *I-A* and *I-E* subregions are separated by a rather small (about 3 Kb) segment of DNA. If these findings are confirmed, it will have to be accepted that the *I-B* subregion does not exist.

16.15 The *I-C* Subregion

The proof of the existence of a distinct *I-C* subregion rests on a single recombinant haplotype (Table 16.1). Since this recombinant ($H\text{-}2^a$) haplotype has been derived from unknown parentage, the reliability of the evidence is often questioned. The doubts are even more justified by demonstration that some Ia specificities originally attributed to the *I-C* subregion product (Ia-3 molecule) are, in fact, borne by the I-E (Ia-5) molecule. Still, at least one specificity (Ia.6) is apparently determined by a gene that maps to the *I-C* subregion. Currently, the presence of the *I-C* subregion is also presumed on the basis of an association between this subregion and certain functional traits. Among these traits are control of immune responsiveness to some antigens (Section 19.3), induction of an MLR by cells differing at the *I-C* subregion, suppression of MLR, and binding of antibodies against receptors for Fc fragments of immunoglobins (Chapter 7).

16.16 The *I-J* Subregion and Its Products

The *I-J* subregion occupies a unique position among the class II genes. The subregion has been defined by several recombinants (Table 16.1) that separated the *I-B* from the *I-E* subregion. The data and arguments concerning the existence of the *I-B* subregion (Section 16.4) apply to some extent to the *I-J* subregion. The animals that differ by the *H-2* segment corresponding to the *I-J* subregion, when reciprocally immunized, produce cytotoxic alloantibodies directed to the product of the *I-J* subregion. These alloantibodies are capable of binding to certain subset(s) of T cells, and, perhaps more important, abrogate the suppressor activity of T cells (Section 22.11). From these observations, it was concluded that the putative product(s)—the I-J or Ia-4 molecule—is expressed selectively on T_s cells and is also detectable in soluble factors produced by these cells (TsF).

In spite of many attempts, the Ia-4 molecule has never been isolated and purified, so that its exact nature remains unknown. Only by inference is such a molecule classified as a member of the class II family. In fact, its exclusive presence on T_s cells makes it an exception to other class II molecules that are found on B cells and macrophages. Recent studies strongly suggest that the Ia-4 molecule(s) is distinctly different from those encoded by other *I* subregions. Characteristically, the Ia-4 molecule does have a two-chain structure and is associated with framework and/or idiotypic determinants of variable regions of the immunoglobin heavy chain (V_H) (Section 19.13). It was found that a given antiserum to I-J products can be absorbed differentially to remove its activity against either antigen-specific or antigen-nonspecific T_s cells. This suggests that there are several discrete products of the *I-J* subregion and thus that the subregion must have several discrete genes. The I-J molecules were also shown to produce weak but significant MLR.

Early reports have not corroborated that I-J products are also expressed on some T_h cells and macrophages. However, these reports did demonstrate that T_h cells express molecules encoded by the *I-A* subregion that are distinct from typical Ia-1 or Ia-5 molecules (see above). These atypical molecules, similar to the I-J (Ia-4) molecules, are frequently associated with V_H structures and are found in the soluble factor (ThF) produced by T_h cells.

CLASS III GENES AND MOLECULES

Three complement factors—C2, C3, and C4—were reported to be associated with H-2 phenotypes, but most attention has been focused on the genetics of C4.

16.17 *C2* Gene

The idea that the *H-2* complex is linked to the putative *C2* gene stems from the observation that *H-2* congenic mice display pronounced variations in the serum concentration of C2. Specifically, mice with the haplotype $H-2^k$ have a high level of C2, whereas mice with the $H-2^d$ haplotype have only about one third as much. Among the *H-2* recombinant strains, those carrying the *S* region derived from the $H\text{-}2^k$ haplotype have a high serum level of C2, whereas those carrying the S region of the $H\text{-}2^d$ haplotype display a low level. These data suggest that the $C2$ gene, or the gene regulating the level of C2 in plasma, might be within the S region. The position of the $C2$ gene in relation to other genes within the S region is unknown.

16.18 $C3$ Gene

Two types of associations between the H-2 phenotype and C3 have been reported. The S region seems to control the level of C3 in plasma. This control is mediated by two alleles associated with the $H\text{-}2^k$ and $H\text{-}2^d$ haplotypes that determine the low and high levels, respectively. The structural gene for C3 has been mapped at a distance of 10–15 cM to the right of the $H\text{-}2$ complex. The codominant alleles of the structural gene determine the electrophoretic variants of C3—one fast (F) and the other slow (S).

16.19 $C4$ Gene

Traditionally, the $C4$ gene of mice is called Ss (for serum substance) and has been unequivocally mapped to the S region. The gene has at least two codominant alleles that determine either a high (Ss^h) or a low (Ss^l) plasma level of Ss protein and, therefore, C4 activity. Recently, it has been suggested that there may be many more alleles, perhaps as many as there are unrelated $H\text{-}2$ haplotypes. Certainly, there are two structural alleles determining the variants of C4 molecule that either carry or do not carry a serological determinant. The determinant, designated H-2.7, is detected on the proteolytic fragment of C4 (C4d), which may be passively adsorbed on erythrocytes in a fashion similar to the C4 of man, which confers on erythrocytes the $Rg^a(+)$ and $Ch^a(+)$ phenotypes (Section 15.11). The Ss gene is accompanied by the closely linked Slp gene (sex limited protein), which determines Slp molecules found in the plasma of males. The two genes, Ss and Slp, have never been separated by recombination and are believed to have developed by duplication of a single ancestral gene. There are at least three Slp alleles: one determining the Slp in males (Slp^a), another determining the absence of Slp (Slp^o) and the third determining the Slp in both males and females (Slp^{w7}). That the Ss and Slp are structural genes for corresponding molecules and that both are located in the S region is supported by several observations. First, apparent differences were found in the molecular weight of the α chain determined by different $H\text{-}2$ haplotypes. Since these differences are expressed codominantly, they must represent structural genes and not posttranslational alterations. Second, tryptic peptide differences of β chains were convincingly mapped to the S region. Third, several electrophoretic variants of the molecules have been associated with different H-2 phenotypes. Fourth, association of the H-2.7 determinant with the specific H-2 phenotype constitutes further evidence that a structural, and not a regulatory, gene resides within the $H\text{-}2$ complex.

Each of the Ss and Slp genes determines a single mRNA for the synthesis of precursor molecules. The precursor molecule (molecular weight 185,000), once synthesized, is cleaved into three peptides: α (molecular weight 100,000), β (molecular weight 75,000), and γ (molecular weight 35,000). Two of these peptides are glycosylated, with the α carrying the complex-type oligosaccharide and the β bearing the mannose-rich sugar. Beginning from the N terminal of the molecule, the linear arrangement of the three peptides within the precursor is β-α-γ. The α chain of the Slp is significantly larger (molecular weight 105,000) than that of the Ss molecule, and it is believed that a mutation occurred in the *Slp* gene that resulted in a shift of the cleavage point of the precursor. The Ss and Slp molecules are quite similar, but tryptic analysis reveals that about 50 percent of the peptides are different, corresponding to about 10 percent amino acid substitution. More important, the Ss, but not the Slp, molecule has complement activity.

The expression of both *Ss* and *Slp* alleles is under complex control, which is more pronounced for Slp. Expression of both genes appears to be influenced by testosterone. This influence results in the absence of Slp in females of most, but not all, strains. In addition, the expression of Slp in some murine strains is specifically regulated by some ill-defined non-*H-2* gene(s).

16.20 *BF* Gene

In the last year, two electrophoretic variants of murine B factor of the alternative complement pathway have been identified. Since the two variants are transmitted in close association with the H-2 phenotype it has been proposed that the *Bf* gene is linked to the murine *H-2* complex just as in the guinea pig it is linked to the *GPLA* complex (Section 17.4). The gene has at least two alleles; *BF*1* and *BF*2* that determine corresponding variants of factor B. During electrophoresis, the B factor is separated into 4–5 distinct bands in males and only 3 bands in females. Therefore, expression of the *BF* gene, in similarity to expression of the *Ss* gene, appears to be influenced by sex hormones.

17 / *Major Histocompatibility Complexes of Various Animal Species*

The interest aroused by studies of the murine, and then the human, MHC prompted systematic studies of various species of laboratory animals in a search for analogues of the MHC. Although in many cases the available data are still fragmentary, the studies unequivocally demonstrate that all species have a gene cluster with features of an MHC. Furthermore, the MHC of various species display remarkable similarities from both the genetic and phenotypic points of view (Table 17.1). This chapter briefly describes the current data concerning the MHC of those species that have been most extensively studied. To facilitate the comparison of different species with each other, and with the mouse as the reference point, the terminology introduced earlier—i.e., class I, class II, and class III genes and molecules—will be used.

THE MAJOR HISTOCOMPATIBILITY COMPLEX OF THE RAT—*RT1*

Second to the mouse, the rat (*Rattus norvegicus*) is the most commonly used laboratory animal. Rats and mice belong to the same family (Muridae) and diverged phylogenetically from a common ancestor. In spite of its frequent use in research, the rat has been investigated less extensively than the mouse from the genetic point of view. One reason, perhaps, is the limited polymorphism of available laboratory strains; most strains currently used (Tables 5.3 and 17.2) were derived from a single stock originally maintained at the Wistar Institute. Second, the MHC of the rat was discovered only two decades ago—hence, its definition and characterization are relatively recent. The MHC of the rat has been assigned to the IXth linkage group, but assignment to a particular chromosome is pending further study. In a very short time, the rat MHC has undergone four name changes with the consecutive designations being *R-1*, *Ag-B*,

TABLE 17.1. Comparison of Characteristics of the Major Histocompatibility Complexes of Various Animal Species

Species	Designation	Number of Regions	Class I		Class II		Class III
			Genes	Alleles	Genes*	Alleles	Genes**
Mouse (*Mus musculus*)	*H-2*	4	2	29–38	2	6–21	+
Rat (*Rattus norvegicus*)	*RT1*	2–4	2	13	2	12	−
Rabbit (*Oryctolagus cuniculus*)	*RLA*	3	2	~10	1	5	−
Hamster (*Mesocricetus auratus*)	*Hm-1*	1	?	?	1	5	−
Guinea pig (*Cavia porcellis*)	*GPLA*	3	2	2–4	3	2–3	+
Dog (*Canis familiaris*)	*DLA*	4	3	3–7	2	2–3	−
Pig (*Sus scrofa*)	*SLA*	2	1	4	1–2	?	−
Cow (*Bos bovis*)	*BoLA*	2–3	1–2	11	4	?	?
Sheep (*Ovis aries*)	*OLA*	1	2	>5	?	?	?
Rhesus monkey (*Macaca mulatta*)	*RhLA*	3	2	13–14	1–2	8–10	+
Chimpanzee (*Pan troglodytes*)	*ChLA*	3	2	>7	1–2	~10	+
Man (*Homo sapiens*)	*HLA*	4	3	17–32	1–3	>12	+

*Tandem α-β genes are considered a single gene.

**Plus sign (+) indicates that gene(s) was identified, minus (−) indicates that gene has not been identified, question mark (?) indicates no studies were done.

RtH-1 (or *H-1*), and finally *RT1*. The last designation is now universally accepted and will be used in this and subsequent chapters.

17.1 Genetics of the *RT1* Complex

Fig. 17.1 schematically depicts the *RT1* complex. The complex probably consists of four regions; however, only two (*A* and *B*) have been firmly documented.* The latter two regions,

---

*The genes at the two regions were in the past designated by the presently obsolete terms (*H-A, Aa-1, MLR-A, H-B, Ba-1, MLR-B,* etc.). These terms should not be used and are mentioned here only to enable the reader to understand the old literature.

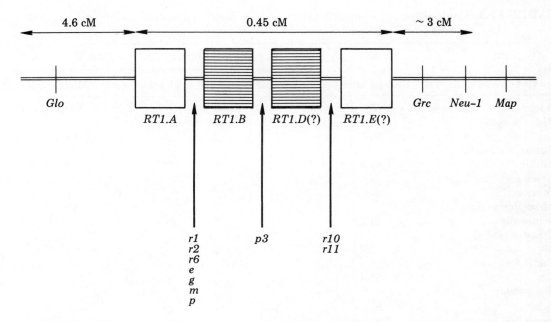

FIG. 17.1. Genetic organization of the rat major histocompatibility complex, *RT1*, and its genes: **white blocks** = class I regions (***RT1.A*** and ***RT1.E***); **shaded blocks** = class II regions (***RT1.B*** and ***RT1.D***); **arrows** = position of crossing-over that occurred in haplotypes listed; ***Glo-1*** = glyoxylase; ***Grc*** = growth and reproduction complex; ***Neu-1*** = neuraminidase; ***Map*** = mannosidase processing enzyme. The relationship of the RT1 complex to the centromere has not been established. Neither the position of the *RT1.C* nor the *CT* locus (see text) has been determined.

called *RT1.A* and *RT1.B*, carry class I and class II genes, respectively. Close (~4.5 cM) to the *RT1* complex is the gene determining glyoxylase (*Glo-1*). Interestingly, the *Glo* gene has also been demonstrated in a similar location in both mice and man.

The *RT1.A* region carries at least one gene that determines a class I molecule. At the moment, on the basis of serologic studies using hemagglutination by alloantibodies, at least 13 alleles have been characterized and assigned symbols represented by lowercase letter(s) and an Arabic numeral used as superscript for the *RT1* designation. The number of class I alleles found among laboratory rats is not significantly different from the number found among standard strains of mice. However, when rats captured from wild populations in various geographical locations are tested, most animals will be found to carry at least one, and often two, well-defined allele(s). This observation suggests that the polymorphism of the MHC of rats is significantly less extensive than that of mice. Such a limited polymorphism may be a true phenomenon or merely a reflection of certain selective forces acting on wild rat populations. Rats are the subject of periodic extermination attempts that could conceivably reduce polymorphism by randomly removing individuals carrying less frequent alleles. However, further studies are needed to elucidate this phenomenon. The existence of an additional class I region, tentatively designated *RT1.E*, was postulated on the basis of biochemical studies that suggested that during amino acid sequencing of RT1.A molecules two different molecular species were actually analyzed. Presently, more direct evidence of the *RT1.E* is available since a recombinant between the putative region has been reported. The polymorphism of the *RT1.E* gene has not been fully determined.

Recently, the presence of a region, tentatively called *RT1.C*, has been reported. However, it has been claimed that the *RT1.C* is not another class I region but a locus or cluster of loci with genes determining T cell alloantigens homologous with murine Qa antigens (Section 22.23–25).

The *RT1.B* region presumably carries four class II genes arranged in two tandems. Each pair of genes determines a single class II molecule that consists of two polypeptide chains. There are at least nine different pairs of *RT1.B* "alleles," each pair determining one class II allelic product. The discrepancy between the number of unique *RT1.A* "alleles" and *RT1.B* "alleles" reflects the fact that a given *RT1.B* "allele" is sometimes associated with two distinct *RT1.A* alleles. In the light of data concerning the murine MHC (Section 16.13), it is plausible to consider that rat class II genes display significant pleiotropism that may well account for the three biologic functions—lymphocyte antigens, immune responsiveness, and histocompatibility antigens—originally attributed to the three discrete genes within the *RT1.B* region. Recently, another class II region, tentatively called *RT1.D*, was proposed on the basis of a recombination demonstrated in an *RT1* complex derived from wild rats. This region is believed to contain another pair of genes determining another class II molecule.

The alleles at different regions form 37 *RT1* haplotypes, which can be divided into distinct categories—11 unrelated haplotypes designated by a small letter superscript (e.g., $RT1^a$), 16 recombinant haplotypes, and 10 variant haplotypes (Table 17.2). The nature of the variant haplotypes is not clear at this time; they may represent variability of known genes, or, alternatively, they may correspond to differences of still unidentified genes. Thus far, no mutant haplotypes have been defined. The order of the regions in the *RT1* appears to be similar to that of mouse, i.e., class I regions being peripheral and class II regions being centrally located.

Finally, it should be mentioned that in the close vicinity of the *RT1* complex at least two genes called *CT* have been identified. There is no information whether these genes are related to the *RT1* complex. The genes encode cell surface alloantigens detectable as targets for the T_c cells, but, thus far, no antibodies directed to these antigens have been experimentally produced.

17.2 Products of the *RT1* Complex

The class I molecules of rats are glycoproteins (molecular weight 45,000) that are associated noncovalently with β_2-microglobulin (molecular weight 11,000). They can be detected by hemagglutination or, still better, by the lymphocytotoxic test. Both tests utilize alloantisera produced by immunization of appropriate *RT1*-congenic strains. The antisera recognize a series of discrete specificities that can be divided into private and public categories. The distinction is based on the same principle as in mice: i.e., private specificities are unique for a given class I allelic product of the *RT1*, whereas public specificities are shared by different allelic products. Thus far, two of the known allelic products do not have an identified private specificity. Assignment of a single private specificity to each RT1 phenotype may incorrectly suggest the

TABLE 17.2. *RT1* Haplotypes and Their Composition

RT1 Haplotype		Alleles at Regions		Prototype Strain	Number of Strains	Strains Congenic with		
Unrelated	Related	*A*	*B*			LEW	BN	Others*
a		a	a	AVN	6	+	+	F344
	r1	a	c	PVG-*H-1*^*ac1*	1			
	r2	a	u	LEW.1AR1	1	+		
	r3	a	a	LEW.1AR2	2	+		
	e	a	c	BDVII	1			
	av1	a	a	DA	1		+	
b		b	b	BUF	9	+	+	
c		c	c	PVG	11	+	+	
d		d	d	BDV	7	+		
	o	d	a	MR	1			
	p1	d	a	WRA	1			
	dv1	d	d	BDIX	1			
f		f	f	AS2	2	+		AS
	g	g	l	KGH	1		+	PVG
	p2	g	l	WRB	1			
h		h	h	HW	2	+		
k		k	k	WKA	3		+	PVG,LOU
l		l	l	LEW	15		+	AS2,AUG
	r5	l	l	LEW.B3	1	+		
	lv1	l	l	F344	1			
	lv2	l	l	BS	1			
	lv3	l	l	BH	1			
	lv4	l	l	A990	1			
	m	m	c	MNR	1			PVG
n		n	n	BN	4	+	+	DA,AUG,F344
	i	a	n	BI(B3)	1			
	p3	n	n	—	1			
	r10	n	l	—	1			
	nv1	n	n	LEW.B3	1	+		
t		t	t	TO	1			
u		u	u	WF	25	+	+	
	r4	u	u	LEW.1WR1	1	+		
	r6	u	a	LEW.1WR2	1	+		
	p	u	l	RP	1			
	uv1	u	u	LEP	1			
	uv2	u	u	LE	1			
	uv3	u	u	OM	1			

*Background strain indicated.

NOTE: Related haplotypes designated with a second letter of *v* (for variant) are similar but not identical to haplotypes designated by the same first letter.

presence of a single class I molecule; more likely, a single private specificity represents a combination of two private specificities—one for each class I product. The detectability of some specificities may pose a serious problem owing to cross-reactivity. Class I molecules are found on essentially all cells; however, their concentration, especially on erythrocytes, varies depending on the *RT1* haplotype. Preliminary amino acid sequencing of the N terminus of RT1.A molecules reveals remarkable homology with analogous molecules of other species.

Class II molecules were originally defined in the rat by their ability to elicit an MLR. As judged from MLR patterns, there are nine distinct alleles, each associated with a unique *RT1.A* allele. In most instances, an MLR is induced between RT1.A-incompatible, and only occasionally between RT1.A-compatible animals. There are rather infrequent exceptions to this rule. For example, some RT1.A-incompatible strains—KGH (*RT1.A^g*) and LEW (*RT1.A^l*)—do not stimulate each other. Conversely, RT1-compatible animals such as LEW and F344, both *RT1.A^l*, may stimulate each other. These exceptions are interpreted as evidence of recombination between the *RT1.A* and *RT1.B* loci. The KGH and LEW strains probably share the *RT1.B^l* allele, whereas LEW and F344 carry the standard and variant *RT1* haplotypes, respectively.

Serologic detection of the rat class II molecules has been greatly facilitated by the finding that some murine alloantisera cross-react with rat molecules. Using these antisera, as well as antisera produced in mice against the rat, two distinct class II molecules can be demonstrated. These two class II molecules appear to correspond to the Ia-1 and Ia-5 molecules of the mouse. Each molecule consists of two chains, α (molecular weight 30,000) and β (molecular weight 26,000–31,000). Biochemical analysis of the α chains that correspond to the Ia-5 molecule revealed that those determined by the different *RT1* haplotypes are almost identical. Surprisingly, the α chains that correspond to the murine Ia-1 molecule could not be sequenced, probably owing to blockade of its N terminus. On the other hand, sequencing of the β chains derived from the different haplotypes revealed pronounced heterogeneity involving several amino acid substitutions. Both chains show significant homology with the corresponding chains of other species. There are about 17 discrete specificities (determinants) assigned to class II molecules, but only two of them can be assigned to specific molecules.

THE MAJOR HISTOCOMPATIBILITY COMPLEX OF THE RABBIT—*RLA*

The rabbit (*Oryctolagus cuniculus*) has been used in immunologic studies from the inception of the discipline. However, knowledge of the rabbit MHC, although it was discovered about 10 years ago, is still very fragmentary. The main reason for this is the difficulty in raising and maintaining inbred strains. Inbreeding depression (Section 5.2) in the rabbit is difficult to overcome and eventually results in the loss of many strains. Most of the initial studies were done either on outbred populations or on only partially inbred lines. These studies permitted a preliminary definition of the MHC of the rabbit, termed the *RLA* (formerly *RLC* or *RbH-1*), as depicted in Fig. 17.2. According to the presently available data, the complex consists of three loci (regions)—two class I (*RLA-A* and *RLA-B*) and one class II (*RLA-D*). The three loci form the *RLA* haplotype; as of now, 13 different haplotypes have been defined. An additional six haplotypes are postulated, but further studies are required to decide whether all of them differ

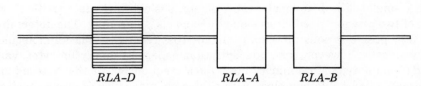

FIG. 17.2. Genetic organization of the rabbit major histocompatibility complex, *RLA*: **white blocks** = class I regions (**RLA-A** and **RLA-B**); **shaded block** = class II region (***RLA-D***). The order of regions and relationship to the centromere have not been established.

from those already defined. Since no proven recombination has been found, the sequence of the three regions cannot be determined. Furthermore, it should be mentioned that the product of the *RLA-B* region has been demonstrated serologically for only one of the several known *RLA* haplotypes.

Class I genes determine molecules present on all cells in the rabbit. Allelic molecules are distinguishable by alloantisera that recognize multiple determinants on each molecule. Each allelic molecule has a unique combination of specificities. Recently, using *RLA* homozygous cell lines, the partial amino acid sequence of the *RLA-A11* allele product was determined. The limited data demonstrate a significant degree of homology between the corresponding molecules of the rabbit and other species.

The genes at the class II region appear to be less polymorphic. Moreover, they determine a glycoprotein molecule that is found predominantly on B cells. So far, two distinct molecules— Ia-1 and Ia-2—are known. Each consists of two chains—the larger has a molecular weight of 30,000 to 32,000, the smaller has a molecular weight of 28,000. Presumably, the two chains correspond to the α and β chains of other species.

THE MAJOR HISTOCOMPATIBILITY COMPLEX OF THE SYRIAN HAMSTER—*Hm-1*

The Syrian hamster (*Mesocricetus auratus*)* was introduced to the laboratory in 1930, when three litter mates were captured near Aleppo, Syria. Until recently, all hamsters used in the laboratory were direct descendants of these three individuals. Because of the limited gene pool from which all presently available strains were derived (Table 5.5), there seemed to be a relatively small number of polymorphic histocompatibility genes. It appeared that only two or three histocompatibility genes could be demonstrated by the histogenetic method. In studies on recently captured wild hamsters, the presence of as many as 12 genes has been demonstrated. Among these proven histocompatibility genes, one appears to be the major histocompatibility gene and has been designated *Hm-1*.

---

*The Syrian hamster belongs to the family Cricetidae, which contains the genera *Causumys*, *Cricetulus*, *Cricetus*, *Mesocricetus*, and *Phodopus*.

There is very little information on the genetics and products of *Hm-1*. Originally, only two alleles (haplotypes), designated $Hm-1^a$ and $Hm-1^b$, were defined; they appear to differ only by class II genes. Alloantisera precipitate products from cell homogenates that appear analogous to the class II products of other species, i.e., two chains of molecular weights 39,000 and 29,000, but do not reveal the presence of a product of molecular weight 45,000 that would be analogous to a class I molecule. Thus, either *Hm-1* contains only class II genes or the class I gene carried by laboratory hamsters is nonpolymorphic. More recently, using alloantisera and newly captured wild hamsters, investigators have identified four additional *Hm-1* haplotypes designated $Hm-1^c$, $Hm-1^d$, $Hm-1^e$, and $Hm-1^f$. It remains unresolved whether these new haplotypes contain polymorphic gene(s) for class I molecules or also differ only by class II alleles.

THE MAJOR HISTOCOMPATIBILITY COMPLEX OF THE GUINEA PIG—*GPLA*

The guinea pig (*Cavia porcellis*) was introduced to Europe and then to the United States by Spaniards who acquired the animals from Peruvian Indians in the sixteenth century. Controlled breeding of these animals was initiated in 1906 within a colony maintained by the U.S. Department of Agriculture. These efforts resulted in the production of the first two inbred strains, which were designated strain 2 and strain 13. Inbreeding of other strains was begun in 1926 and resulted in the production of several additional strains (Table 5.4). In recent years, the breeding of several new lines was initiated. Perhaps because the guinea pig is an animal in which the Ir phenomenon (Section 19.2) was demonstrated, its major histocompatibility complex, which is called *GPLA*, has been studied relatively well.

17.3 Genetics of the *GPLA* Complex

The *GPLA* complex consists of four regions—two class I (*GPLA-B* and *GPLA-S*), one class II (*GPLA-Ia*), and one class III (Fig. 17.3).

Each of the class I regions contains at least one class I locus. The *GPLA-B* locus carries a gene with four recognized alleles (*GPLA-B1, GPLA-B2, GPLA-B3*, and *GPLA-B4*), whereas the *GPLA-S* locus carries a gene with at least two alleles ($S1$ and S^o). The S^o represents either a silent allele or a series of alleles undetectable by available methods. The limited polymorphism of class I genes in the guinea pig may be due to the limited gene pool from which the laboratory strains were originally derived. To confirm this supposition, systematic studies must include wild animals from Peru. Preliminary results have revealed that about half of the wild animals possess haplotypes absent in laboratory animals. This suggests that the actual polymorphism may prove to be greater than presently ascertained although it is unlikely to be as great as that documented for mice.

The class II region has been divided into three subregions. Each of the subregions presumably carries two tandem genes that determine one class II molecule. The extent of polymorphism of class II genes is not known presently, but it seems to be rather limited among both laboratory and wild animals.

The class III region contains at least three distinct structural genes with limited

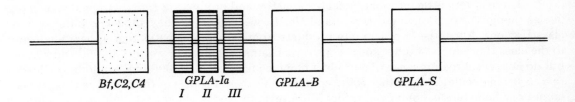

FIG. 17.3. Genetic organization of the guinea pig major histocompatibility complex, *GPLA*: **white blocks** = class I regions (**GPLA-B** and **GPLA-S**); **shaded blocks** = class II region (**GPLA-Ia**) subdivided into three subregions; **dotted block** = class III region containing *Bf, C2,* and *C4* loci. The order and distances between the regions are still tentative.

polymorphism. The *C4* locus carries the gene for the C4 factor of complement with four alleles designated *F, S, S1,* and *C4°*. The first three alleles determine electrophoretic variants (fast, slow, and very slow) of C4. The fourth, *C4°*, allele is silent and, if homozygous, results in total C4 deficiency. The *C2* gene has three alleles—*A, A1,* and *B*—that determine either acidic or basic electrophoretic variants of C2. The *Bf* gene determines the B factor of the alternative pathway. Alleles *F* and *S* have been distinguished electrophoretically; they determine differences associated with the Bb fragment of the Bf molecule (Section 15.12).

17.4 Products of the *GPLA* Complex

The class I genes (*GPLA-B* and *GPLA-S*) determine glycoprotein molecules (molecular weight ~45,000), which are ubiquitously distributed. In the cell membrane, these molecules are noncovalently associated with β_2-microglobulin. Four allelic molecules have been defined by available alloantisera. Partial amino acid sequencing of the N terminus of GPLA-B molecules has revealed extensive homology with analogous molecules of other species. Thus far, evidence for the GPLA-S1 molecule has been found only in the haplotype that carries the *GPLA-B1* allele, whereas haplotypes carrying the *GPLA-B2* or *GPLA-B3* alleles seem to be associated with the *GPLA-S°* allele.

Genes at class II loci determine three distinct molecules, each consisting of two chains, α (molecular weight 33,000) and β (molecular weight 25,000–26,000). The three molecules and their allelic variants are distinguished by the distribution of eight serologically defined determinants (Ia.1-Ia.8). On the basis of this distribution, two or three alleles can be distinguished in each subregion (Table 17.3). The two chains determined by the genes in subregion I are noncovalently bound, whereas the two chains determined by the genes in subregion II are joined by a disulfide bridge. The specificities of the product of subregion III appear to be associated with only one chain (β). The amino acid sequence of the β chains shows a great deal of homology with human, but surprisingly little with murine, chains. Nothing is known about the α chain(s) sequence.

TABLE 17.3. Allelic Ia Molecules Determined by
Three Class II Subregions of the *GPLA*
Complex

| Strain | Subregions of *GPLA-Ia* | | |
	I	II*	III
2	Ia.2	Ia.4, Ia.5	Ia.6
13	Ia.3, Ia.5	Ia.7	Ia.1, Ia.6
	Ia.8		

*Two chains form a dimer bound by a disulfide bridge.

Class III genes determine C2, C4, and Bf molecules and their structural variants. The chemistry of C4 is quite similar to that of the mouse. It consists of three peptides—α (molecular weight 95,000), β (molecular weight 78,000), and γ (molecular weight 31,000)—derived by proteolytic cleavage of the pro-C4 molecule (molecular weight ~200,000).

THE MAJOR HISTOCOMPATIBILITY COMPLEX OF THE DOG—*DLA*

Studies on the histocompatibility systems of larger animals were prompted by an obvious need for an experimental model that could be used prior to undertaking transplantation studies with human subjects (preclinical studies). These studies, initiated about two decades ago, have provided us with a relatively extensive knowledge of the MHC of four species: dog (*Canis familiaris*), pig (*Sus scrofa*), rhesus monkey (*Macaca mulatta*), and chimpanzee (*Pan troglodytes*).

17.5 Genetics of the *DLA* Complex

The postulated arrangement of the *DLA* complex is schematically depicted in Fig. 17.4. The model bears striking resemblance to that of the *HLA* complex of man (Chapter 15).

Three class I genes—*DLA-A, DLA-B,* and *DLA-C*—are separated by an estimated distance of 0.7 cM. These genes are quite polymorphic, each having three to seven defined alleles in addition to a significant fraction of alleles that cannot be identified by available alloantisera. Alleles of the three genes form the *DLA* haplotype. The frequency of particular haplotypes is strongly influenced by linkage disequilibrium. Interestingly, the linkage disequilibrium appears to affect different alleles in various breeds and in mongrels. The Δ values, reflecting the extent of linkage disequilibrium, are exceptionally high for many haplotypes, reaching 0.185, as compared with values for various haplotypes in man or primates, which are at the range of 0.02–0.03. To some extent, this may reflect the founder effect (Section 1.8) since, in many canine populations, a limited group of individuals constituted a nucleus of the future breed or population. It is expected that the haplotypes of these founding individuals will become

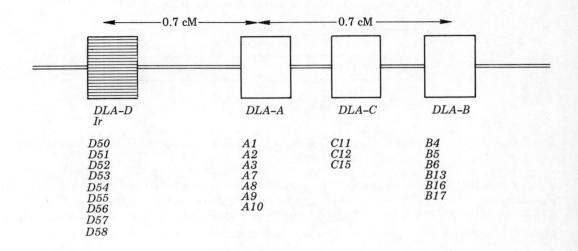

FIG. 17.4. Genetic organization of the dog histocompatibility complex, *DLA*, and some alleles assigned to different regions: **white blocks** = class I regions (***DLA-A***, ***DLA-B***, and ***DLA-C***); **shaded block** = class II region (***DLA-D***). The relative position of the *DLA-C* and another class II region (*DLA-E*) (not shown) are still tentative.

exceptionally frequent in subsequent quasi-inbred populations that are prevented from mating with individuals of other breeds.

Currently, two class II loci are proposed—*DLA-D* and *DLA-E*. Only the former has been formally documented to be about 0.7 cM to the left of the *DLA-A* gene. The *DLA-E* gene, proposed on the basis of serologic characteristics, seems to be on the right side of the *DLA-B* because it has stronger linkage disequilibrium with *DLA-B* than with *DLA-A*. The polymorphism of class II genes is not fully known, though it is believed that the *DLA-D* gene has at least 5 alleles, whereas the *DLA-E* gene carries four alleles (*D54, D55, D57,* and *D58*).

Some authors distinguish the *Ir* gene as a separate entity located to the left of the *DLA-D*. However, most likely the *Ir* gene is identical with *DLA-D* (Section 19.3). In addition, an *R* gene located to the right of the *DLA* complex has been described. This polymorphic gene (3 or more alleles) is believed to control the resistance of lethally irradiated animals to allogeneic bone marrow grafts. In some respects the gene is similar to the *Hh* genes of mice (Section 16.6). Neither its exact location nor its product have been identified.

No class III genes have been identified in the dog at the present time.

17.6 Products of the *DLA* Complex

Class I genes determine molecules that are present on lymphocytes and thrombocytes but absent from erythrocytes. There are also indications that class I molecules are present on the cells of the skin, intestines, and heart since allogeneic grafts of these organs result in the production of strong alloantibodies reactive with class I molecules. In fact, by analogy with other species, it might be expected that class I molecules are present on virtually all cells. These molecules can be detected by the lymphocytotox test with monospecific antisera. Such antisera detect different allelic products of the three class I genes (Fig. 17.4). However, there are several other specificities that cannot be assigned to any of the known series. Antisera, though believed to be monospecific, often display significant cross-reactivity, especially in cases of certain allelic products. This cross-reactivity might be due to the presence of public specificities or to a reaction with products of two discrete genes that are in strong linkage disequilibrium. Essentially nothing is known about the chemistry of the DLA molecules.

Class II genes determine moieties responsible for the MLR between DLA-D- and/or DLA-E-incompatible individuals. Using HTC (Section 15.5), it is possible to define and divide several allelic products into two allelic series (*D* and *E*). Nothing is known about the chemical structure of the latter moieties, and only by inference can it be assumed that these moieties are analogous to the class II molecules of other species.

THE MAJOR HISTOCOMPATIBILITY COMPLEX OF THE PIG—*SLA* (*PLA*)

The pig (*Sus scrofa*) has been used only occasionally in immunologic studies. Nevertheless, studies on the blood groups of pigs led to the discovery of alloantigens present on the cell membrane of their nucleated cells. One of these antigens turned out to be a member of the MHC that was named the *SLA* or *PLA*. Cytotoxic antibodies induced by allografts were instrumental in the detection of at least four allelic products presumably representing class I molecules (SLA-A1, SLA-A2, SLA-A3, and SLA-A4). The MLR is essential in the detection of class II molecules. Further studies resulted in the concept that the SLA consists of at least two regions or loci—*SLA-A* and *SLA-D*—the latter corresponding to class II. Apparent recombinants between the two loci made possible their recognition as two distinct entities. It seems that the polymorphism of class I genes is more extensive than that of class II, since different individuals frequently share *SLA-D* alleles. This notion is further supported by the finding of an *SLA-D* allele of domesticated pigs in a wild boar.

The SLA class I molecule is a typical glycoprotein with a molecular weight of about 45,000 and is associated with β_2-microglobulin. The class II molecules, in turn, are found on B cells and have the characteristics of the Ia molecules.

More extensive genetic and structural studies of the swine MHC became possible with the selection of a special breed of miniature pigs. In contrast to conventional pigs, the MHC of miniature swine is called *MSLA* (M for miniature), though it seems to be structurally identical with *SLA*. At the moment, four herds are maintained, each homozygous for a different *MSLA* haplotype. Recently, an intra-*MSLA-D* recombination was reported, indicating that this region contains more than one locus.

THE MAJOR HISTOCOMPATIBILITY COMPLEX OF THE COW—*BoLA*

Studies of the MHC of the cow (*Bos bovis*) were initiated about a decade ago. These studies were carried out using alloimmune sera obtained from multiparous dams or from animals intentionally immunized with allogeneic skin grafts. Serologic studies resulted in a definition of at least 11 codominant alleles determining the class I molecules BoLA-A. Inasmuch as the presence of one class I gene, *BoLA-A*, is firmly established, evidence for a second gene is still only circumstantial.

Employing the MLR test, the presence of a class II region, *BoLA-D*, was established. Family studies indicate that this region contains more than one locus; there are possibly four class II loci. The extent of the polymorphism of the class II gene(s) in the cow has not been fully established.

THE MAJOR HISTOCOMPATIBILITY COMPLEX OF SHEEP—*OLA*

Serologic testing of "Préalpe" breed of sheep (*Ovis aries*) led to demonstration of the two series of class I products determined by alleles at two closely linked loci; *OLA-A* and *OLA-B*. These two loci separated by a distance of 0.6 cM form the MHC of sheep. There are 5 alleles at the *OLA-A* locus (*A1, A2, A4, A8,* and *A10*) and 4 alleles at the *OLA-B* locus (*B3, B6, B7,* and *B9*). The alleles occur with frequencies of 0.05 to 0.23. Since in the numerous individuals tested no known allele at one or both loci can be detected with presently available antisera, there must be still unidentified alleles. The alleles at two loci form the *OLA* haplotype with apparent linkage disequilibrium (Δ varies from -0.004 to 0.047). So far no data on class II and class III genes of the *OLA* complex are available.

THE MAJOR HISTOCOMPATIBILITY COMPLEX OF THE RHESUS MONKEY—*RhLA*

The rhesus monkey (*Macaca mulatta*) has attracted the special interest of biologists for a variety of reasons. One very obvious reason is the monkey's close relation to humans, making it a desirable model for various preclinical studies. At this time, the MHC of the rhesus monkey and its structure are firmly established (Fig. 17.5).

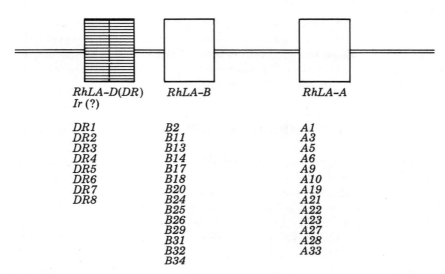

| RhLA-D(DR) | RhLA-B | RhLA-A |
| Ir (?) | | |

DR1	B2	A1
DR2	B11	A3
DR3	B13	A5
DR4	B14	A6
DR5	B17	A9
DR6	B18	A10
DR7	B20	A19
DR8	B24	A21
	B25	A22
	B26	A23
	B29	A27
	B31	A28
	B32	A33
	B34	

FIG. 17.5. Genetic organization of the rhesus monkey major histocompatibility complex, *RhLA*, and some known alleles: **white blocks** = class I regions (***RhLA-A*** and ***RhLA-B***); **shaded block** = class II region [***RhLA-D(DR)***].

17.7 Genetics of the *RhLA* Complex

The *RhLA* contains three loci (regions). Two of them, called *RhLA-A* and *RhLA-B*, carry highly polymorphic genes belonging to class I. The *RhLA-A* gene has 13 known alleles, and the *RhLA-B* gene has 14, but both of them in all likelihood have other still unidentified alleles. The frequencies of certain haplotypes differ significantly from the frequencies expected on the basis of individual allele frequencies. Apparently, in this monkey species the extent of linkage disequilibrium is similar to that in man. Interestingly, no evidence for a third class I locus has been reported.

The *RhLA-D* region was originally defined on the basis of the MLR. With the development of the HTC procedure (Section 15.5), 10 alleles of the *RhLA-D* gene have been identified. These alleles appear to correspond to the eight alleles of the *RhLA-DR* (originally called the Ia_1 gene). Since no recombination between *RhLA-D* and *RhLA-DR* genes has been observed thus far, it is tempting to assume that the two genes are in fact identical. There are still doubts concerning the mapping position of the *Ir* gene(s) and its possible identity with the *RhLA-D(DR)* gene. In addition to the three histocompatibility genes, the *RhLA* complex is linked to the class III genes, *BF* and *C2*, but their positions with respect to the other genes have not been determined.

17.8 Products of the *RhLA* Complex

The class I genes determine allelic molecules distinguishable by alloantisera in the lymphocytotoxic assay. Class I molecules are glycoproteins of molecular weight 44,000 and are associated with β_2-microglobulin. Class II molecules (RhLA-DR) are similar to those of the Ia-like molecules of man and other species. The latter similarity is further increased by the finding that class II molecules can be arranged into cross-reacting sets, possibly analogous to the MT1 sets of man (Section 15.5). In addition, it was recently proposed that there are actually two pairs of genes in tandem within the *RhLA-DR* segment.

THE MAJOR HISTOCOMPATIBILITY COMPLEX OF THE CHIMPANZEE—*ChLA*

Although studies of the chimpanzee (*Pan troglodytes*) began much later than studies of man or the rhesus monkey, a defined MHC (Fig. 17.6) was soon discovered and found to be remarkably similar to that of the two other species. Two class I loci (*ChLA-A* and *ChLA-B*) carry apparently polymorphic genes. However, only a fraction of all possible alleles have been identified, mostly because of the limited availability of animals. The sum of *ChLA-A* frequencies is 0.58 and *ChLA-B* is 0.69, indicating the presence of possibly 30 to 50 percent more alleles than presently identified. The allelic products of either class I gene of the chimpanzee are very similar to those of man. This structural similarity is probably responsible for the extensive cross-reactivity of human anti-HLA sera with certain chimpanzee antigens. The class II (*ChLA-D*) locus is well established on the basis of the MLR and presumably carries gene(s) with at least 10 alleles. On the other hand, the existence of the *ChLA-DR* gene is only suggested by the cross-reactivity of human antisera with chimpanzee B cells. Linkage of the *BF* and *C2* genes to *ChLA* was recently reported; they appear to be on the left side of the complex.

THE MAJOR HISTOCOMPATIBILITY COMPLEX OF THE CHICKEN—THE *B* COMPLEX

Studies of the chicken (*Gallus gallus*) were initiated over 30 years ago. Besides their purely theoretical significance, such studies have a practical aspect. It was hoped that these studies would provide useful information for commerical breeding of animals with the most desirable traits, such as meat quantity and quality, egg-laying capacity, disease resistance, etc. Inasmuch as there are strong indications that the selection for certain genetic markers does permit the production of superior animals, only the theoretical aspects of these studies will be addressed in this section.

17.9 Genetics of the *B* Complex

The name *B* locus, or strictly speaking, *B* complex, was initially proposed for one of the several blood groups of the chicken (Section 13.10). Later, it was demonstrated that the B blood group is associated with graft rejection and several other features typical of histocompatibility antigens. More recent studies have revealed that the *B* complex consists of a cluster of closely linked loci (regions). The present model for the *B* complex is depicted in Figure 17.7. The complex consists of three distinct regions—*B-G*, *B-F*, and *B-L*—but their sequence cannot be determined at

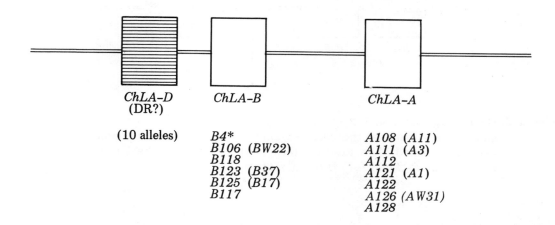

FIG. 17.6. Genetic organization of the chimpanzee major histocompatibility complex, *ChLA*, and some of its known alleles: **white blocks** = class I regions (***ChLA-A*** and ***ChLA-B***); **shaded block** = class II region (***ChLA-D***). Alleles of the *HLA* complex encoding the molecules that cross-react with antibodies to *ChLA* products are indicated in parentheses.

this time since all seven known recombinants separate only *B-G* from the *B-F* and *B-L* segments but not *B-F* from the *B-L* region. Clearly, the *B-G* and *B-L* regions contain more than one locus each, but neither the number nor the sequence of such loci can be established because the recombination frequency within the *B* complex is extremely low (10^{-4}), i.e., corresponding to a size of 0.01 cM. In any case, genes at the three regions form the *B* haplotype; as many as 30 different *B* haplotypes are known and designated by Arabic numeral superscripts. However, since these haplotypes were defined by different investigators employing nonstandardized sera, there is the possibility that some reported haplotypes may be identical. The production of monoclonal antibodies to several allelic products of the *B* complex should ultimately alleviate this problem and permit standardization of the typing procedure.

17.10 The *B-F* Region and Its Products

The *B-F* region of the chicken MHC is analogous to the class I region of mammals. The question that still awaits a definitive answer is whether this region contains a single locus or several closely linked loci. While some investigators claim that there is no indication of multiple loci,

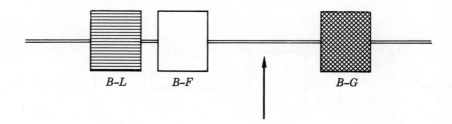

FIG. 17.7. Genetic organization of the chicken major histocompatibility complex, *B*. The order and distances between the class I region (***B-F***) and the class II region (***B-L***) have not been established. The **arrow** indicates the postion of the known crossing-over between the *B-G* and *B-F–B-L* segments.

others report data suggesting that there are as many as three loci. Whichever claim is correct, the *B-F* region appears to be highly polymorphic with many alleles determining products that are distinguishable both serologically and electrophoretically.

The products of the *B-F* region are glycoproteins of molecular weight 40,000–45,000 found in the membranes of both lymphocytes and erythrocytes, and are associated with β_2-microglobulin. The amino acid sequence of the B-F molecules shows several amino acid substitutions between allelic products. There is extensive homology in the amino acid sequence of B-F molecules and class I molecules of other species, which supports the notion that, indeed, the B-F molecules are avian analogues of mammalian class I molecules. When the B-F molecules isolated from the cells of a given B phenotype are separated by two-dimensional electrophoresis, three discrete molecular species can be demonstrated. This is construed as evidence that a given *B-F* region carries three distinct class I genes. However, one should keep in mind that the different electrophoretic mobilities may be due to a difference in composition or content of carbohydrate moieties associated with otherwise identical protein molecules. More convincing evidence has been provided by sequencing data in which two different amino acids appear to be assignable simultaneously to the same position. The final answer requires further evidence, such as the finding of recombination between putative genes, or more sophisticated studies with monoclonal antibodies. Such antibodies have been raised for several B phenotypes, but their exact specificities have not yet been defined.

17.11 The *B-L* Region and Its Products

The *B-L* region appears to be analogous to the class II regions in other species. Its genes determine glycoproteins of molecular weight ~30,000 that are found on lymphocytes and macrophages but not on erythrocytes. These cell-membrane molecules are not associated with β_2-microglobulin. However, lymphocytes bearing the B-L molecule(s) usually bear immunoglobulin molecules, suggesting that such cells are B lymphocytes (bursacytes). As in the case of the *B-F* region, the question of the number of distinct loci in the *B-L* region remains unanswered Electrophoretic analysis of B-L molecules suggests the presence of two molecular species, a finding consistent with the idea that a given *B-L* region contains two genes. The two genes could well represent analogues of the α and β genes that determine a single Ia-like molecule. This idea is further strengthened by the finding that the allelic differences appear to be associated with only one of the two molecules. On the other hand, sequential precipitation by two different antibodies suggests that both molecules must be antigenically different.

The B-L molecules are defined by alloantisera that are rather difficult to produce. Antisera to B-L molecules determined by a given *B* haplotype are usually cross-reactive with the B-L molecules of other haplotypes. This cross-reactivity, however, can be removed by proper absorption, indicating that B-L molecules carry both private and public determinants. Interestingly, the B-L molecules also react with human anti-HLA-DR antigens, suggesting that there is a significant homology between the two species.

17.12 Class III Genes in the Chicken

Although no specific complement genes have been mapped to the *B* complex, the level of total serum complement has been shown to be associated with the B phenotype. It has not been determined which specific component(s) is responsible for variability of the complement level or whether the gene is homologous to the complement genes in other species.

17.13 The *B-G* Region and Its Products

The *B-G* region seems to be unique for the chicken and has no analogue in other species. It has been proposed that this region belongs to a separate class of its own—class IV. The region contains a highly polymorphic gene that determines products found on erythrocytes and their progenitors. This specific and restricted expression makes it plausible to consider the *B-G* gene products as differentiation antigens of hemopoietic cells. Chemically, the product is a glycoprotein with a molecular weight of 42,000 that forms in situ trimers or tetramers and is not associated with β_2-microglobulin. There is strong linkage disequilibrium between alleles at the *B-F* and *B-G* regions. This disequilibrium is exemplified by the almost invariable copresence of the $B\text{-}F^{13}$ and $B\text{-}G^{13}$ or $B\text{-}F^6$ and $B\text{-}G^6$ alleles and, rarely, dissociation of $B\text{-}F^{12}$ from $B\text{-}G^{12}$. Even when the $B\text{-}G^{12}$ allele is associated with an allele other than $B\text{-}F^{12}$, the product of the other allele is strongly cross-reactive with the B-F$_{12}$ molecule. It has been speculated that the B-F and B-G molecules somehow interact at the level of the cell membrane; this interaction may require some degree of structural similarity of the two molecules.

18 / β_2-Microglobulin

GENETIC DETERMINATION OF β_2-MICROGLOBULIN
MOLECULAR STRUCTURE OF β_2-MICROGLOBULIN
DISTRIBUTION OF β_2-MICROGLOBULIN
β_2-MICROGLOBULIN-LIKE MOLECULES

A common feature of class I molecules in all species studied so far is their association with a small and mostly invariant polypeptide chain. This polypeptide chain is called β_2-microglobulin even though in some species its electrophoretic mobility does not correspond to that of a β_2-globulin. Since β_2-microglobulin is required for the expression and stabilization of class I molecules, it deserves a certain amount of attention. Such attention is even more warranted by the recent suggestion that β_2-microglobulin may influence not only the expression but also the synthesis of class I molecules.

GENETIC DETERMINATION OF β_2-MICROGLOBULIN

The β_2-*microglobulin* gene ($\beta_2 m$) is physically separated from the MHC as well as from the immunoglobulin genes. In man, the $\beta_2 m$ gene has been assigned to chromosome 15 and in mice to chromosome 2, whereas in other species the chromosomal position of the gene remains unknown. It was generally believed that the gene is nonpolymorphic and that no structural variants were demonstrable in any given species. However, a recent report on the heterogeneity of murine β_2-microglobulin has been published. Two electrophoretic variants were found in two mouse strains and designated as β_2M-A and β_2M-B. The alleles determining these two variants appear to be codominant and are equally expressed in F1 hybrids. Biochemical studies strongly indicate that the two variants differ from each other by a single amino acid substitution at position 85. The polymorphism of β_2-microglobulin will permit classic genetic studies of this molecule in the future.

MOLECULAR STRUCTURE OF β_2-MICROGLOBULIN

β_2-microglobulin is a polypeptide of molecular weight ~11,600 and consists of 100 amino acid residues in man and 99 in several other species. The amino acid sequence of the entire molecule in different species has been determined. The sequence shows a high degree of homology among these species with amino acid substitutions involving 30 to 40 percent of the residues which are distributed more or less uniformly along the chain, albeit with greater aggregation at the C and possibly N termini. In addition, β_2-microglobulin shows a significant degree of homology with one of the domains of the immunoglobulin heavy chain. In fact, it has been postulated that β_2-microglobulin may be the product of a gene determining a free domain—perhaps an ancestral gene for the immunoglobulins (Section 8.3). A similarity to the Ig domain is further emphasized by the presence of an intrachain loop formed by a disulfide bridge between cysteines at positions 25 and 80. The β pleat secondary structure of the molecule also resembles the structure of immunoglobulin. On the basis of homologies among the immunoglobulin domains, β_2-microglobulin, and the third region, α-3 in man or C2 in mice, of class I molecules, it is speculated that β_2-microglobulin is bound to the third region of class I molecules. However, there are no documented data to support this speculation. The tertiary structure of β_2-microglobulin is not fully known, but recent crystallization of the bovine homologue (lactolline) should facilitate a more detailed study.

DISTRIBUTION OF β_2-MICROGLOBULIN

β_2-microglobulin is noncovalently bound to class I molecules at a ratio of 1:1 with a ubiquitous distribution. Binding to class I molecules does not utilize all β_2-microglobulin present in cell membranes as there is a significant number of molecules that are either free or bound to the other cell membrane components. The latter include such molecules as H-Y antigens (Section 21.8), TL antigens (Section 22.3), tumor-associated antigens (Section 25.2), and Qa antigens (Sections 22.23–25). Interestingly, it seems that most of the cell membrane components that are associated with β_2-microglobulin are determined by genes within the MHC or closely linked to it. This association may be purely incidental, or it may reflect a specific functional aspect of these components.

Originally, β_2-microglobulin was found in the urine of people with a certain renal tubular dysfunction, but it is also present in normal sera either as a free molecule or associated with some other plasma molecules. One such molecule seems to resemble, both structurally and antigenically, class I molecules released from the cell membrane. These molecules lack certain antigenic features of the native class I molecules and at the same time acquire new determinants. It is speculated that these molecules may be the metabolic products of shed class I molecules or products of other genes related to the MHC. Interestingly, serum β_2-microglobulin was also found to associate with fragments of the heavy chains of immunoglobulins.

β_2-MICROGLOBULIN-LIKE MOLECULES

Molecules similar to β_2-microglobulin are associated with C4 and putative products of the *T-t* complex (Section 24.8). In contrast to the classic β_2-microglobulin, these molecules do not react with specific antibodies raised against β_2-microglobulin. Lack of reaction could be due to structural differences or to conformational changes conferred by binding to other molecules. This question still requires study.

19 / Biologic Function and Significance of the MHC

THE FUNDAMENTAL BIOLOGIC FUNCTION OF THE MHC

It was suspected from the very beginning that the MHC and its products must serve a function other than to participate in the man-made process of graft rejection or to help in deciding (also man-made) cases of disputed paternity. In retrospect, the first hint of a more basic function for the MHC came in the 1920s and 1930s from studies on resistance and susceptibility of various animals (mostly mice) to a variety of bacteria and viruses. However, since at that time the MHC had not yet been defined, these studies could not link the phenomenon of immunne responsiveness with the MHC. Nevertheless, these studies laid a groundwork for future investigations of the genetic control of immune responsiveness. These investigations, culminating in the discovery of the *Ir* genes, assigned the first "dignified" role to the, by then firmly defined MHC. Indeed, from the sphere of interest of a narrow circle of specialists and transplantation surgeons, the MHC sprang into the center of basic immunology.

This chapter will present briefly the major facts and current speculations concerning the biologic role of the MHC. One must, however, keep in mind that in these days of active investigation, in which each day brings new data, a comprehensive synthesis is extremely difficult, if at all possible. It must be remembered also that, at least for the more speculative aspects of the topic, the authors' views may bias the presentation, and, therefore, should not be taken as dogma. Rather, the content of this chapter should be considered as a sui generis conceptual framework that must be adjusted and expanded constantly as new data become available.

Experimental data generated in numerous studies employing various animal species led to a unifying concept of the biologic function of the MHC. This concept, which currently has gained almost universal acceptance, proposes that the primary function, and common denominator, of the various products of MHC genes is to provide guidance for the various T cell subsets (Sections 4.2 and 22.11). The data are consistent with the idea that class I molecules guide T_c cells, whereas class II molecules guide T_h and T_s cells. This role of MHC molecules is reflected in the requirement for presentation of an antigen in the context of, or in association with, one of the MHC molecules. It is well established that different T cells of an individual become activated and functionally effective only when an antigen is recognized in conjunction with the MHC molecules of this particular individual, i.e., self-MHC. Indeed, the two basic phenomena associated with the MHC, Ir effect and MHC restriction, are presently considered to be a prime expression of the T cell guiding properties of the MHC products.

THE Ir PHENOMENON

19.1 Resistance and Susceptibility

In the early studies employing mostly outbred mice, it was discovered that some individuals are highly resistant, whereas others are highly susceptible to a given bacterium. By selective breeding, it was possible to produce lines of resistant and susceptible mice presumably homozygous for alleles determining the resistance or susceptibility trait. It was always suspected, though not formally demonstrated, that such resistance reflects a high and/or effective immune response to the microorganism, whereas susceptibility represents a low and/or ineffective response. More important was the demonstration that resistance preexists in an animal before it actually encounters the bacterium—hence, it is the capability to mount a good response that is inherited and not the response itself. Other studies demonstrated that a similar phenomenon also applies to certain viruses and parasites. In many of these earlier studies, no association of resistance or susceptibility to a specific gene or gene complex could be made beyond the demonstration that the phenomenon was often inherited as a single dominant and autosomal trait. More recent studies, however, clearly show that many, but not all, genes for resistance and susceptibility are either linked to the MHC or actually map within it. At the same time, other genes that influence resistance have been found to be totally independent of the MHC, with many of them subsequently mapped to different chromosomes.

Selective breeding from an outbred population has been employed in a series of studies in which immune responsiveness to a variety of bacterial and nonbacterial antigens was investigated. In principle, selective breeding entailed repeated mating for several generations (usually 15–20) and selection in each generation of the animals expressing a given trait. The process ultimately resulted in lines homozygous for the alleles that influence the given trait—in this particular case, either high or low responsiveness to a given antigen. At the end of the selection process, the magnitude of the response in the two lines differed by a factor of from 10^2 to 10^3. The data obtained from testing the two lines permitted the determination of the number of independent genes involved in responsiveness. For each of five different antigens such as heterologous erythrocytes, heterologous proteins, or several bacterial antigens, such studies showed that 2 to 11 independently segregating genes are involved. Since these genes are inherited independently, only one could be linked to the MHC. Indeed, such a linkage has been found in some but not all instances. MHC-linked genes(s) contributed between 10 and 25 percent of the total differences between the two lines. Apparently, an immune response to a given antigen is under polygenic control with each gene contributing to the overall responsiveness.

Selection for a specific response often resulted in a nonspecific effect—i.e., the selection affected not only the response to a specific antigen but also responses to other unrelated antigens. This nonspecific effect is most likely due to the simultaneous selection for certain basic immunologic features that affect in a similar way the responses to a variety of antigens.

An interesting observation reported from selective breeding was that humoral responses (antibody formation) are influenced by a set of genes different from those influencing cell-mediated reactions (HVGR or GVHR). Furthermore, because the phagocytic activity of macrophages appears to be regulated by still another set of genes, selective breeding can be used as a means of raising animals with high or low macrophage activity.

19.2 The Ir Control of Antigen-Specific Responses

The phenomenon described above pointed toward the genetic control of immune functions such as antibody or cell-mediated responses, but it still did not clearly demonstrate a crucial role for the MHC. In fact, even the first case of antigen-specific control was shown to be MHC associated only in retrospect. It has been known for a long time that immunization with certain antigens results in a high titer of antibodies in some outbred animals, whereas in other animals a low, if any, titer of antibodies is produced. Originally, this was considered more of a nuisance than a biologically important phenomenon. The antigen-specific control of the immune response has since been shown to be a basic immunologic phenomenon of immense theoretical and practical importance. The concept of **Ir (immune response) control** has been introduced, and the related terms—*Ir* genes and Ir phenomenon—added to the vocabulary of the immunologist. According to the current operational definition, Ir control represents the dominant and heritable ability of some individuals (or inbred strains) to recognize a specific antigen and mount a humoral immune response to that antigen, whereas other individuals or strains do not recognize and do not respond to the same antigen. The most crucial part of this definition is the specificity clause, as it eliminates from the concept all cases of general immunodeficiencies, e.g., lack of immunoglobulins. It also puts the specificity of the Ir phenomenon on the same level of importance as that attributed to the specificity of the immunoglobulins. Still, the two types of specificities—Ir control and immunoglobulins—are clearly different, as are the two sets of genes that determine them. Although at this time Ir control encompasses several variations, the basic principles appear to be common for different situations.

Ir control has been demonstrated in mice for more than 40 different antigens. These antigens fall into the following three broad categories: synthetic polypeptides, heterologous proteins, and alloantigens; Ir control concerns the response to specific antigenic determinants borne on these antigens. Thus, in the case of a multideterminant entity (e.g., heterologous protein), the response to each determinant is often controlled independently of responses to the other determinants. Since the response to a multideterminant entity may be viewed as the sum of responses to its individual determinants, it might be difficult to demonstrate Ir control of responses to a particular multideterminant antigen. It is precisely for this reason that Ir control was first clearly demonstrated for responses to synthetic polypeptides that bear a limited number of determinants. Subsequently, Ir control was shown for responses to native proteins, provided that relatively low doses were used, thus limiting the number of determinants that are presented in a quantity sufficient to induce a response. Recently, the specific determinants of some proteins have been isolated and even synthesized artificially. As a result, it became possible to carry out a detailed analysis of the effect that Ir control has on the response to complex native antigens.

Ir control appears to be exquisitely specific. An animal that is a low responder to a given antigen (determinant) may be a good responder to other antigens (determinants). Studies with synthetic polypeptides show that an animal is capable of discriminating among determinants that differ by a single amino acid substitution.

All responses that are under Ir control are T-dependent, i.e., they require the participation of T cells. It is generally accepted that the T cells affected by the Ir phenomenon belong to the category of T helper (T_h) cells. In most, but not all, such responses, it appears that *Ir* genes control the switch from a primary (IgM) to a secondary (IgG) response. As a result, the distinction between a high and low responder usually can be made only during a secondary response. The Ir effect can be demonstrated and measured by two basic methods. One method ascertains qualitatively and quantitatively the production of specific antibodies by either serologic (serum titration, antigen binding) or cellular (determination of plaque-forming cells [PFC]) assays. The second method determines qualitatively the ability of specific primed T cells to proliferate in vitro upon contact with the antigen. With rare exceptions, the results obtained with these two methods correlate closely, which is understandable if one remembers that both methods presumably probe either directly or indirectly the function of the same subset of T cells, i.e., T_h. The crucial role of T cells in the Ir phenomenon was demonstrated further by numerous experiments in which the function of T cells was replaced by soluble factors derived from them.

In most systems, the Ir effect is quantitative, with some animals being good (or high) responders and others being poor (or low) responders. However, in certain cases the effect may be qualitative, with animals being either responders or nonresponders. Regardless of the type of effect, the responsiveness in the progeny of good and poor responders, with few exceptions, behaves as a dominant or codominant autosomal trait.

19.3 *Ir* Genes

An obvious consequence of the discovery of Ir control was a search for the specific genes responsible for this control. Studies with inbred mice were instrumental in demonstrating that the large number of genes, referred to as the *Ir* genes, map within the murine MHC, i.e., the *H-2* complex (Section 16.13). Since these *Ir* genes were the first to be described and mapped, the MHC-linked *Ir* genes were named *Ir-1*. Subsequently, the *Ir* genes that controlled the responses to different antigens were mapped into different subregions of the *H-2* complex, and the nomenclature was extended to *Ir-1A, Ir-1B,* and *Ir-1C* genes. For those *Ir* genes that could not be assigned to a specific subregion, the term *Ir-x* was accepted, *x* standing for an arbitrary designation of the antigen in question. The early studies seemed to be compatible with the idea that the response to each antigen is controlled by a distinct *Ir* gene with two alleles—one for a good and one for a poor response. Accordingly, it was presumed that the *I* subregions contain an array of antigen-specific *Ir* genes, each controlling the response to a different antigen (Table 19.1). Although the *I* region theoretically could accommodate several hundred structural genes, the search for the corresponding number of molecular products did not bring the expected results. The only molecular products that could be assigned to genes at the *I* subregions that were thought to contain the putative *Ir* genes were class II (Ia) molecules (Section 16.8). Only one, or at most three, such molecules were found in any given individual inbred mouse and, thus, were definitely too few to fulfill the role of products of the multiple *Ir* genes. With this in mind, it had to be concluded that either the Ia molecules are not the actual products of the *Ir* genes or, conversely, that there are very few *Ir* genes. The second case, if correct, would mean that the specificity of *Ir* genes for different antigens is not determined by the principle of "one antigen-one *Ir* gene." To choose between the two possibilities, several experiments were carried out among which the most important was the finding that treatment of cells with antiserum against Ia molecules of a good responder abrogated the ability of such cells to produce a good response. This finding is the strongest argument in favor of the identity of the Ia (A_α, A_β, A_e, E_α) and the *Ir* genes. Another crucial piece of evidence was provided by the discovery of a single gene mutation that alters both Ia and Ir characteristics. Accepting these data means that there are only a few MHC-linked *Ir* genes and that the specificity for different antigens must reside in a relatively limited set of molecular products.

TABLE 19.1. Positions of Murine *Ir* Genes within the *H-2* Complex

Antigen[a]	*Ir* Gene	Map Position[b]			Other Genes Influencing Response[c]	Hapten Conjugated
		I-A	*I-B*	*I-E/I-C*		
Synthetic polypeptides						
(T,G)-A-L	*Ir-1A*	+			+(*Ig*)	
(H,G)-A-L	*Ir-(H,G)-A-L*	+				
(Phe,G)-A-L	*Ir-(Phe,G)-A-L*	+				
(T-A-G-Gly)	*Ir-(T-A-G-Gly)*	+			+	
GLPro	*Ir-GLPro*	+				
GAT[10]	*Ir-GAT*	+			+(*I-J*)	
GLLeu	*Ir-GLLeu*	+(β)		+(α)		
GLPhe	*Ir-GLPhe*	+(β)		+(α)		
GLT[5-15]	*Ir-GLT(Ir-1C)*	+(β)		+(α)		
Soluble Alloantigens						
IgA (allotype)	*Ir-IgA*	+				
IgG (allotype)	*Ir-1B*		+			
Liver F antigen	*Ir-F*	+			+	
Slp	*Ir-Slp*	+				
Thyroglobulin	*Ir-Tg*	+			+	
Thy-1	*Ir-Thy-1*	+(A,B)			+(*Ir-5*)	
Cell surface alloantigens						
H-2.2	*Ir-H-2.2*	?			+	
H-4	*Ir-H-4*		+			
H-Y	*Ir-H-Y*		+			
Ea-2.1	*Ir-Ea-2.1*	?				
Ea-1.2	*Ir-Ea-1*	?			+(*Ir-2*)	
Ly-6.2	*Ir-Ly-6.2*	?			+	
Native Proteins						
Bovine gamma globulin	*Ir-BGG*	+				DNP,BPO
Bovine ribonuclease	*Ir-RNase*	+?				BPO
Bovine insulin	*Ir-BI*	+?				
Porcine lactate dehydrogenase-A	*Ir-LDH$_A$*	+?				
Porcine lactate dehydrogenase-B	*Ir-LDH$_B$*			+		
Human hemoglobin						
α chain	*Ir-$_α$Hb*	+(A$_β$)				
β chain	*Ir-$_β$Hb*	+			+	
Whale myoglobin						
Determinant 1	*Ir-Mb-1,2(A)*	+			+(*H-2D*)	
Determinant 2	*Ir-Mb-1,2(C)*			+		
Determinant 4	*Ir-Mb-4*	+				
Determinant 5	*Ir-Mb-5*	+				
Ovalbumin	*Ir-1-OA*	+			+	

(continued)

TABLE 19.1 (continued)

Antigen[a]	Ir Gene	Map Position[b]			Other Genes Influencing Response[c]	Hapten Conjugated
		I-A	I-B	I-E/I-C		
Ovomucoid	Ir-OM	+?				DNP
Hen albumin lysozyme	Ir-HEL	+			+	
Calf collagen I	Ir-Col-I	+			+	
Calf procollagen I	Ir-Procol-I	+				
Staphylococcal nuclease	Ir-Nase		+		+	
Bacteriophage fd	Ir-fd	+(β)		+(α)		
Ragweed pollen extract	Ir-RE	+				
TNP-self-H-2[d]	?	+(?)				
TNP-mouse serum albumin	Ir-6	+	+(?)		+	

[a]Amino acid symbols: T = tyrosine; G = glutamine; A = alanine; L = lysine; H = histidine; Phe = phenylalanine; Gly = glycine; Pro = proline; Leu = leucine.

[b]In parenthesis is the symbol of the Ir gene assigned to the subregion.

[c]+ indicates involvement of Ir genes other than those assigned to the I region of the H-2. If the name and/or position of such a gene are known, they are shown in parentheses.

The postulate that class II molecules are the actual products of Ir genes found further support in the discovery of complementation between Ir genes. Complementation, which has been described for the Ir control of responses to several different antigens, reflects the requirement for the expression of two distinct Ir genes for a good response to a given antigen. Two types of complementation may be distinguished: **pseudocomplementation** and **true complementation**. The former refers to a situation in which different Ir genes are required for a response to two determinants on the same molecule; these two Ir genes may be expressed on two different cells because they affect two independent responses. However, owing to their being directed against determinants present on the same molecule, these two responses are additive in the overall response to this molecule. True complementation, in contrast, encompasses a situation in which two different Ir genes are needed for a response to a single determinant; in this case, the two genes and their products must be expressed on the same cell and must operate in concert to determine a single response. True complementation of Ir genes remarkably parallels the cis and trans complementation of the α and β genes that determine the two chains of class II molecule and the resulting combinatorial specificities (Section 16.9).

19.4 Ir Genes Not Linked to the MHC

Most, but not all, Ir genes are linked to the MHC. The Ir genes that are not linked to the MHC (Table 19.2) fall into the following three categories: Ir genes linked to the genes determining the heavy chains of immunoglobulins (Igh), Ir genes located on the chromosome X, and Ir genes linked to various other autosomal markers.

TABLE 19.2. Murine *Ir* Genes Not Linked to the *H-2* Complex

Class	*Ir* Gene	Antigen	Involvement of the *H-2*	Low Responder
Allotype-linked	V_H-*DEX*	α-1,3 dextran	−	C57BL/6
	Ir-GAC (*Ir-ASA*)	Streptococcal group A polysaccharide	+	?
	?	(T, G)-A-L	+	?
X-linked	*Ir-X*(?)	Various thymus-independent antigens: pneumococcal SSSIII polysaccharide, poly I: poly C RNA		CBA/N
	?	DNA-methylated BSA		DBA/2
Non-H-2	*Ir-2*	Ea-1.2	+	BALB, CBA/J
	Ir-3	(T,G)-Pro-L		DBA/1
	Ir-4	LPS		C3H/HeJ
	Ir-5	Thy-1.1	+	C57BL/6,
	Ir-7	A-CHO*		C57BL/6, C3H

*Polysaccharide of streptococcus group A.

The genes linked to the *Igh* genes are associated with a particular allele of the heavy chain (allotype). Since these genes are very closely linked to the V_H genes that encode the variable portion of the immunoglobulin, it is possible that the low response "allele" merely represents lack of the gene for the variable segment (idiotype) that determines a binding site for a particular antigen (Section 10.5). Conversely, a good response "allele" would correspond to a V_H gene encoding the idiotype associated with an antigen-binding site of specific antibodies. If this is the case, this category contradicts the original concept (Section 19.2) that the *Ir* genes do not code for immunoglobulin (Chapter 8), and, accordingly, the term Ir is a misnomer.

The *Ir* genes on the *X* chromosome can be further subdivided into two types. One type is associated with poor responsiveness to a wide spectrum of antigens rather than with a poor response to a single antigen. Furthermore, these genes affect T-independent responses. Both these characteristics are inconsistent with the definition of true *Ir* genes. Another type of *X*-linked *Ir* genes appears to be antigen specific, but this specificity requires confirmation.

The third category contains *Ir* genes scattered throughout the genome. Most of these appear to be antigen specific and are probably true *Ir* genes that happen not to be associated with the MHC. In mice, these *Ir* genes are designated *Ir-2* through *Ir-5* and *Ir-7*.* Although *Ir* genes that are not linked to the MHC must be considered as important in the overall immunoregulatory mechanism, in most instances the information available is insufficient for a reasonable hypothesis of their mode of action. In addition to the genes listed in Table 19.2, there are indications that strains with the C57BL/10 background produce responses to various

---

*The *Ir-6* gene has been assigned to the *H-2* complex in defiance of the convention that only *Ir-1* genes should be associated to this complex.

antigens (polypeptide GAT, staphylococcal nuclease, sperm whale myoglobin, and sheep erythrocytes) that are lower than responses elicited by the same antigens in the H-2-identical strains with the A strain background. Whether this effect is due to a single gene or to several discrete genes remains unknown.

19.5 *Ir* Genes and the Ir Phenomenon in Various Species

The original discovery of Ir control was made in the guinea pig, but the most extensive studies have been carried out in inbred mice. These studies provided the theoretical basis and experimental models to be applied to various other species. The results of experiments in different species clearly corroborate the general idea that the Ir phenomenon is one of the basic functions of the MHC in all species. Table 19.3 briefly summarizes the available data concerning the Ir phenomenon in the species so far studied.

In guinea pigs, linkage between *Ir* genes and *GPLA* has been established by segregation analysis. However, since no recombination between *I* subregions has been found, the specific *Ir* genes cannot be assigned to particular subregions. Responses to some antigens seem to be under polygenic control exerted by genes that are *GPLA*-linked and genes independent of *GPLA*. Responses to haptens applied topically were studied extensively in the guinea pig. Although responses to such compounds as dinitrophenyl, aspirin anhydride, beryllium fluoride, dinitrochlorobenzene, mercuric chloride, phenetidin, and potassium dichromate are under Ir control exerted by *GPLA*-linked genes, non-*GPLA* gene(s) occasionally appeared to be involved.

The immune response of rats to various synthetic and natural antigens is under the control of genes linked to the *RT1* complex. The genes have been mapped to the class II region (*RT1.B*) and display properties similar to those of the murine *Ir* genes. These common properties include a high degree of specificity, dominance of the alleles that determine a good response, and complementation.

The least amount of information is available concerning the *Ir* genes of primates and man. Nevertheless, there is strong evidence for control exerted by genes in the class II regions, i.e., *RhLA-D* and *HLA-D(DR)*, respectively. This is in contrast to some early reports of associations of putative *Ir* genes with class I rather than class II genes.

Without going into excessive detail, a single important conclusion can be drawn. In most instances so far studied, the Ir effect—and, thus, the *Ir* genes—were associated with the class II genes of the MHC in various species. Therefore, the Ir phenomenon appears to reflect a genuine and common biologic function of the MHC.

19.6 Cellular and Molecular Mechanism of the Ir Phenomenon

Although most of the experimentally established facts about Ir phenomenon are beyond serious challenge and are commonly accepted, the possible mechanism of the Ir phenomenon still remains the subject of continuous debate; ideas about the Ir phenomenon change almost incessantly as new facts become available. Some concepts have been discarded as untenable, whereas others have been modified to accommodate the new observations. One must become familiar with two basic concepts to arrive at an overall understanding of the phenomenon.

TABLE 19.3. The *Ir* Genes in Animal Species Other Than the Mouse

Species	Antigen	*Ir* Gene	MHC Association*	Other *Ir* Genes	Hapten**
Rat	(T,G)-A-L	*Ir-(T,G)-A-L*	+		
	(H,G)-A-L	*Ir-(H,G)-A-L*	+		
	(Phe,G)-A-L	*Ir-(Phe,G)-A-L*	+		
	(T-G-A-Gly)	*Ir-(T-G-A-Gly)*	+	+	
	(GAT)	*Ir-GAT*	?		
	(GA)	*Ir-GA*	+		
	(GLT)	*Ir-GLT*	+	+	
	(GT)	*Ir-GT*	+		
	TAL	*Ir-TAL*	+		
	Bovine serum albumin	*Ir-BSA*	?		
	Bovine gamma globulin	*Ir-BGG*		+(Ig?)	
	Porcine lactate dehydrogenase-A4	*Ir-LDH*$_{A4}$	+		
	Ovomucoid	*Ir-OM*		+	
	Streptococcal group A vaccine			+(*Ig*)	
	Sheep erythrocytes			+	
Guinea pig	(T,G)-A-L	*Ir-(T,G)-A-L*	+	+	
	(T-G-A-Gly)	*Ir-(T-G-A-Gly)*	+		DNP
	GL	*Ir-GL*	+		
	GA	*Ir-GA*	+		
	GT	*Ir-GT*	+		
	Poly-L-lysine	*Ir-PLL*	+		DNP
	Poly-L-arginine	*Ir-PLA*	+		DNP
	Poly-L-ornithine	*Ir-PLO*	+		DNP
	Bovine serum albumin	*Ir-BSA*	+		
	Bovine gamma globulin	*Ir-BGG*	+	+	BPO
	Human serum albumin	*Ir-HSA*	+		
	Rabbit serum albumin	*Ir-RSA*	+		
	Insulin				
	A chain	*Ir-InA*	+		
	B chain	*Ir-InB*	+		
	Protamine	*Ir-Pro*	+		DNP
	DNP-GPA	*Ir-DNP-GPA*	+		
Rhesus monkey	(T,G)-A-L	*Ir-(TG)AL*	+		
	GA	*Ir-GA*	+		
	GL	*Ir-GL*	+		DNP
Man*	(T,G)-A-L	*Ir-(T,G)AL*	+(*B*)	possibly two genes	DNP
	Ragweed antigen	*Ir-RA*	+	+	
	Rye grass	*Ir-Rye*	+		
	Gluten	*Ir-Glu*	+(*DW3, B8*)		
	Mycobacterium leprae	?	+(*BW21, B14, A19*)		
	Rubella		+(*BW17, A28*)		

(continued)

TABLE 19.3 *(continued)*

Species	Antigen	*Ir* Gene	MHC Association*	Other *Ir* Genes	Hapten**
	Influenza		+		
	Measles		+		
	Streptococci		+(*B5*)		
	Diphtheria toxoid		+(*B5*)		+

*Specific *HLA* alleles associated with good responsiveness are indicated in parentheses.

**Hapten indicated was conjugated with a given antigen; anti-hapten response serves as an indicator of a response to the antigen.

NOTE: For an explanation of symbols, see Table 19.1.

In its most basic form, the **receptor hypothesis** (Fig. 19.1) postulates that the *Ir* gene determines an antigen-specific receptor that is expressed predominantly, if not exclusively, on T cells. According to this hypothesis, a good or high responder, within its T cell repertoire, has a clone of T cells bearing the receptor for a given antigen. Conversely, a poor or low responder lacks such a clone. In this hypothesis, there are several predictions that have been extensively tested, some of which were not borne out by the actual data.

True *Ir* genes would have to be expressed on T cells, and low responsiveness would thus represent a clonal deficiency of T cells. To support this contention, the following observations have been cited: (1) all Ir-controlled responses are T-dependent; (2) thymectomy converts a good responder into a poor responder; (3) low responders produce specific antibodies to the antigen, provided their cells receive help from T cells taken from good responders or from soluble factors produced by such T cells; (4) a poor responder can be converted into a good responder when the antigen is presented in association with a carrier moiety that is immunogenic for this poor responder; and (5) the T cell proliferative assay parallels the Ir effect. Even with this array of supportive data, one cannot exclude the possibility that the defect in a low responder is, at least partially, associated with B cells that must interact with the T cells. In fact, some data pointed to the Ir defect as being expressed in bone marrow derived cells, since an occasional low response appeared to be associated with either a quantitative or qualitative deficiency of B cells. These observations led to the conclusion that either the receptor hypothesis is totally incorrect or there must be several different mechanisms to account for the Ir effect observed in different experimental systems.

The second basic assumption of the receptor hypothesis was that, if *Ir* genes code for actual T cell receptors, there should be as many distinct structural *Ir* genes as there are antigens to which a response is genetically controlled. This prediction has still not been experimentally proved. On the contrary, several observations speak against this concept. The issue of the number of molecular products of the *I* region has already been discussed (Section 16.11). Class II molecules, multiple as they are, cannot account for the specificity of all postulated *Ir* genes, at least in a manner known to operate for the specificity of antibodies. Moreover, in none of the known recombinants within the *I* region has separation of the two or more putative *Ir* genes mapping within a given subregion been demonstrated. Certainly, if each subregion carries several *Ir* genes, independent crossing-over events should occasionally separate these genes and

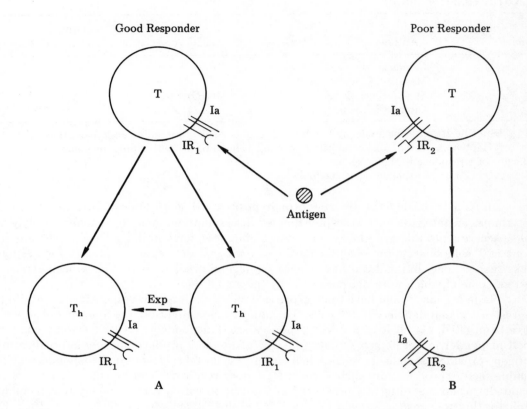

FIG. 19.1. Receptor hypothesis of the Ir phenomenon. **(A)** Good responder has a T cell clone with Ir-encoded receptor (**IR₁**) for the antigen. Upon exposure to the antigen, the clone expands (**Exp**), producing specific T helper (Tₕ) cells. **(B)** Poor responder has a T cell clone with a different receptor (**IR₂**), which does not combine with the antigen, so that there is no expansion. In either case, the receptors are distinct from Ia molecules (**Ia**).

also separate them from the *Ia* genes, assuming that *Ia* genes are distinct from *Ir* genes. Thus, the evidence for multiple *Ir* genes as predicted by the receptor hypothesis is still lacking.

Perhaps the most important and most controversial prediction of the receptor hypothesis is that there should be a broad spectrum of receptors, each carried by a distinct clone of T cells of an individual. Early searches for such receptors were fruitless. Recently, however, with the acquisition of new data, the issue has returned to a center of controversy. The question of the origin and nature of the putative T cell receptors will be discussed separately (Section 19.13), since this topic is much broader than the issue of the Ir phenomenon.

In summary, the receptor hypothesis, initially quite attractive and accompanied by circumstantial support, cannot account for all the findings and predictions. Therefore, many investigators have advanced an alternative concept.

The **associative recognition hypothesis** (Fig. 19.2) proposes that the Ir effect is mediated through presentation of the antigen. According to this concept, it would be conditio sine qua non that the antigen, in order to be recognized and to trigger a good immune response, must be presented by a macrophage or any other antigen-presenting cell in the context of, or in association with, class II molecules. It follows that the antigen and the class II molecule(s) must be capable of forming some sort of physical or functional association. Class II molecules of the good responder would be capable of association with a given antigen, whereas a poor responder would have molecules that cannot form an association with this particular antigen. The associative recognition hypothesis accounts for the specificity of *Ir* genes by assuming that a given antigen can associate with some allelic class II molecules but not with others. Conversely, a given allelic molecule can associate with some but not with other antigens. Thus, several different alleles for class II molecules may serve as a good response *Ir* allele for a given antigen, while a given class II allele may serve as a good response allele for several antigens. The association by itself would not be specific because neither the given class II molecule nor the antigen has a unique preference for each other. However, the complex formed between the antigen and a given class II molecule would be a unique entity. There are several predictions that the associative recognition hypothesis must make—predictions that must be checked experimentally.

The Ir effect would have to be mediated by Ia molecules, and, therefore, the blocking of Ia molecules should result in the abrogation of the Ir effect. Indeed, as mentioned earlier, pretreatment of the responder cells with sera directed against the responder Ia molecules did result in conversion of a good responder to a poor responder. On the other hand, similar treatment of the poor responder cells had no appreciable effect on the response.

If Ia molecules are intimately involved in the presentation of the antigen, these molecules would have to be expressed on antigen-presenting cells. Furthermore, in the case of heterozygosity of the responder, only the Ia molecules determined by the *H-2* haplotype contributed by the good responder parent should be able to accomplish an effective presentation of the antigen. The actual cellular distribution of Ia molecules is fully compatible with the above prediction; the Ia molecules have been demonstrated on macrophages, dendritic cells, Langerhans' cells, Kupffer cells, and oligo- or microglial cells (Section 16.10). Even more important, T cells of an F1 hybrid between good and poor responder parents could be stimulated to antigen-specific proliferation only when the antigen was presented by macrophages of the F1 or the good responding parent. The same T cells could not be stimulated by the antigen presented by macrophages of the poor responding parent. It must be emphasized that the macrophages of both parents are equally efficient in the presentation of an antigen that is not under Ir control. Thus, it is the class II molecules on antigen-presenting cells that actually determine, at least partially, the Ir phenotype.

A third prediction of the associative recognition hypothesis is that if Ia molecules serve as the presenters of a wide spectrum of antigens they would have to be highly polymorphic. The role of class II molecules, as products of the *Ir* gene, hinges to a great extent on the heterogeneity of class II molecules. This requirement for heterogeneity stems from the idea that the

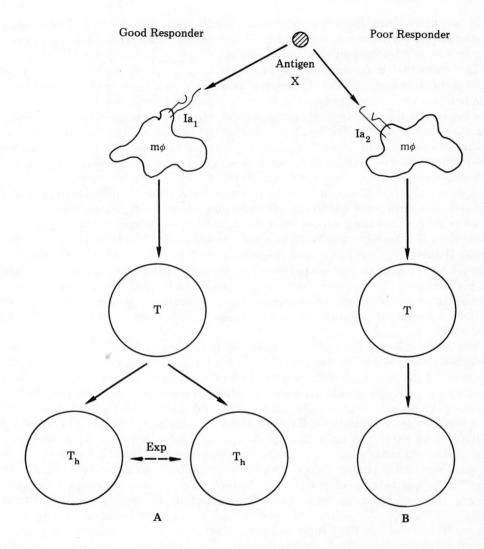

FIG. 19.2. Associative recognition hypothesis of the Ir phenomenon. (**A**) Good responder has macrophages (**mϕ**) bearing Ia molecules (**Ia$_1$**) capable of associating with the **antigen X.** Complex (Ia$_1$ + X) is recognized by T cells, which expand (**Exp**), generating T helper cells (T$_h$). (**B**) Poor responder has **mϕ** bearing different Ia molecules (**Ia$_2$**), which do not associate with the **antigen X.** Lack of (Ia$_2$ + X) complex precludes both recognition of X and clonal expansion of T cells.

class II molecules present in an individual and in the population must be capable of associating with the broad array of antigens that may be encountered by the individual and/or population. A single and nonpolymorphic class II molecule would have a grossly limited capability to associate and therefore would lead to low responsiveness against many potential antigens. Should such an antigen happen to belong to highly pathogenic bacteria or viruses, low responsiveness of an entire population could have a disastrous effect that could eventually lead to the elimination of that population. The potential to form an association with various antigens is significantly increased by the presence of multiple class II molecules in an individual and by the preponderance for heterozygosity in a random population. The heterogeneity of class II molecules is also increased by the formation of combinatorial specificities due to *cis* or *trans* complementation (Section 16.9). Although complementation produces eight distinct molecules in any heterozygote, this is still too few to account for the number of putative *Ir* genes. However, if each individual allotypic and/or combinatorial determinant acts as a unique antigen-binding site, then the extent of variability becomes compatible with the proposed function. In addition to the easily detectable standard class II molecules, other equivalent, but less readily demonstrable, molecules may also exist (Sections 15.6 and 16.11).

Finally, according to the associative recognition hypothesis, the structural change of the Ia molecules should result in altered capability of association with some antigens. Such an alteration would, in turn, affect the responsiveness to some antigens. Indeed, studies employing a mutant of the A_β gene (Section 16.12) revealed that the mutation has apparently changed, positively or negatively, the Ir control of the responses to some antigens.

One may recast the associative recognition hypothesis in slightly different words and say that the response to a given antigen is restricted by the class II molecules of the responder, since a specific allelic variant of the class II molecules determines whether the association with a given antigen is possible and, thereby, whether a good response can ensue. With this in mind, the hypothesis may alternatively be called the **restrictive recognition hypothesis**. The hypothesis presupposes that low responsiveness reflects the failure of antigen-presenting cells to form a complex between an antigen and self-MHC molecule(s). Recently, reported data suggest that under experimental conditions the low responsiveness may also be associated with the lack of the T cell clone capable of recognizing a complex involving a particular MHC molecule. The associative or restrictive recognition hypothesis permits one to account for a broad range of immunoregulatory phenomena being associated with class II molecules. As much as a prevalent T_s rather than T_h cells. This would account for the occasional reports mapping **Is (immune** preferentially bind to I-E molecules. Since the α and β genes for these molecules are in different subregions, a response to such antigens appears to be restricted or controlled by two complementary *Ir* genes. *Trans* complementation between A_α and A_β may produce a similar effect for *Ir* genes encoded within a single subregion. Finally, the preferential association of an antigen with an I-J molecule may yield a complex that selectively triggers T suppressor (T_s) cells. In fact, one can envision a situation in which even an association with I-A or I-E molecules could induce T_s rather than T_h cells. This would account for the occasional reports mapping **Is (immune suppression) genes** into the *I-A* and *I-E* subregions. Since some of these *Is* genes follow the classic interregion complementation pattern it is probable that in fact the *Is, Ir,* and *Ia* genes are identical.

THE MHC RESTRICTION PHENOMENON

The Ir phenomenon discussed in the preceding section ascribed a central role to class II molecules, but it still left class I molecules without a function other than to elicit an artificial phenomenon of HVGR (and possibly a GVHR). This static situation did not last long, however, since in the 1970s several laboratories almost simultaneously reported a phenomenon called **MHC restriction**.

19.7 MHC-Restricted Responses

In contrast to the humoral responses affected by Ir control, MHC-restricted responses belong to the cell-mediated type of immunity. By definition, these responses involve T cells and, therefore, are T dependent. The antigens that elicit restricted responses may be certain cell-surface alloantigens, viruses, or simple chemical compounds (haptens*). All these antigens have one basic characteristic in common—they are associated with the surface of certain cells and they elicit a response aimed at the destruction of these cells. The response is mediated by T_c cells which are similar to those involved in some HVGR and/or GVHR (Sections 4.10, 4.11, 20.2 and 20.3).

MHC restriction was clearly demonstrated in mice studied for cytotoxic responses to virus-infected cells, cells expressing incompatible non-MHC alloantigens, and autologous cells altered by simple chemicals, e.g., trinitrophenol (TNP). Subsequently, restriction was also shown in man for the male histocompatibility antigen, i.e., a non-MHC alloantigen.

In its most basic form, MHC restriction can be defined as the requirement for identity of the class I molecule(s) borne by responder cells and cells that present the antigen. The latter consist of (1) the stimulator cells that originally present the antigen at the time of initiation of the response and (2) the target cells that are ultimately attacked and damaged by responder T_c cells. Specifically, responder cells appear to recognize the restricted antigens only when they are presented by stimulator cells carrying at least one class I molecule that is identical with that carried by the responder. The T_c cells that are induced under such conditions can lyse the target cells only if such cells carry the antigen and a class I molecule identical with those of the stimulator cells. However, it has been shown that in some instances removal of cells reactive against non-identical (allogenic) class I molecules alone before stimulation with antigen does not preclude restriction of subsequently generated T_c cells that now may be restricted by the non-identical class I molecules. Therefore, it may be speculated that class I matching of responder and stimulator may not be absolutely necessary. The restriction is highly specific for both the antigen and the class I molecule—hence, alteration of either of them on target cells results in inability of a given T_c cells to lyse the target cells. The specificity applies to the major allelic variants of class I molecules as well as to class I point mutants (Section 16.7). In the latter case, however, some degree of cross-reactivity between the mutant and the wild-type molecule, or between different mutants of a given allele, occasionally is observed. Another important aspect of

---

*Haptens actually modify self cell surface molecules, conferring immunogenicity on such molecules.

MHC restriction is its clonality. In an F1 hybrid that carries at least four different class I molecules, i.e., two H-2K and two H-2D in the mouse, there are four distinct clones of T cells, each recognizing the antigen in association with one of the four different class I molecules. To put it differently, a given *H-2* heterozygous responder may recognize a given antigen in the context of each class I molecule; such recognition is executed by the cell clone that is specific for both the antigen and a given class I molecule.

19.8 Cellular and Molecular Mechanism of MHC Restriction

After excluding some trivial explanations for the MHC restriction phenomenon, two alternative concepts remained to be examined.

The first concept, termed the **altered-self hypothesis**, proposes that an antigen and a class I molecule interact in such a way that a new moiety is created (Fig. 19.3). This new moiety, sometimes referred to as a **neoantigen**, consists of the antigen and class I molecule either one, or both of them in an altered form. It is this altered-self (class I molecule) or neoantigen that is recognized by responder cells, presumably via a single receptor for the neoantigen; the recognition generates a single signal for the development of specific T_c cells. The cells are incapable of recognizing either the antigen or the class I molecule alone. The drawback of this concept is that only in some instances can a true physical and permanent association between an antigen and a class I molecule be demonstrated unequivocally. In the vast majority of cases, the actual association of the two entities is presumed, but not proven.

The second concept, called the **dual recognition hypothesis**, postulates, in its extreme form, that the antigen and the class I molecule are recognized independently and generate two signals for the development of the T_c cells. However, both moieties must be recognized simultaneously to stimulate the cells to differentiate into effector T_c cells. The requirement for simultaneous recognition could reflect an additive effect of the two ligands, antigen and class I molecule, whereas each ligand separately and the single signal it generates might be insufficient to initiate the recognition and subsequent generation of specific T cells.

Between the two hypotheses mentioned above lies a spectrum of intermediate concepts to be considered. The spectrum ranges from a loose association of the two moieties, which would preserve their native characteristics, to their total independence; and from a single receptor with two binding sites, one for each moiety, to two receptors, each binding one of the moieties in question (Fig. 19.4). At this time, experiments have not been designed that can discriminate between these two hypotheses; therefore, both must be considered as equally viable alternatives. In fact, one might speculate that either one or the other may be operative, depending on the antigen involved. Whichever concept is correct, the phenomenon of MHC restriction has profound biologic implications. Upon cursory inspection of the facts, class II molecules ("*Ir* gene" products) appear to restrict the humoral responses to certain antigens, whereas class I molecules (restriction gene products) seem to restrict cellular responses to another set of antigens. In fact, it is the restriction of the T cells that represents a common denominator in the biologic function of both classes of MHC molecules. More detailed analysis clearly shows that the two types of restriction have a great deal in common (Table 19.4 and Fig. 19.4). The most striking similarity is a presumed interaction of the antigen with the self-molecule (MHC

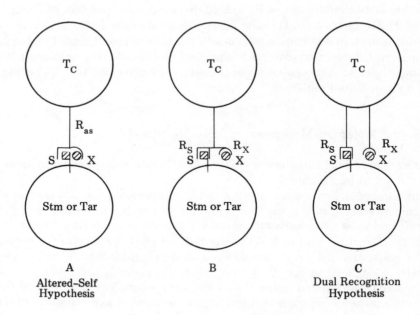

FIG. 19.3. Concepts of MHC restriction of cytotoxic T cells (**T**$_c$). (**A**) The altered-self hypothesis proposes that T$_c$ and its precursor have a receptor (**R**$_{as}$) that binds to a complex of self class I molecule (**S**) and antigen (**X**) on the surface of a stimulator (**Stm**) or target (**Tar**) cell and generates a single signal. (**B**) The alternative hypothesis suggests that **T**$_c$ and its precursor have a single receptor with two discrete binding sites: **R**$_s$ for the self class I molecule (**S**) and **R**$_x$ for the antigen (**X**). Simultaneous binding at two sites generates a single signal for the **T**$_c$ cell. (**C**) The dual recognition hypothesis postulates that **T**$_c$ and its precursor have two receptors: one (**R**$_s$) for the self class I molecule (**S**) and the other (**R**$_x$) for the antigen (**X**). Simultaneous binding of two receptors with corresponding molecules on stimulator (**Stm**) or target (**Tar**) cell generates two signals and permits activity of **T**$_c$.

product) and the requirement for the simultaneous recognition of both interacting moieties. Along the lines of the concept of associative recognition, it has been speculated that MHC molecules may represent a form of "primitive antibodies" with a broad, albeit limited, spectrum of combining abilities. Such binding of an individual determinant is relatively weak, but when it is amplified by numerous determinants and numerous MHC molecules, it may result in a complex sufficiently strong and stable to elicit the response. Since in all instances the interaction in itself is nonspecific and depends on the capability of a given antigen and a given MHC molecule to associate, it follows that MHC molecules must be as heterogeneous as possible to enable the recognition of a large spectrum of nominal antigens by an outbred population. Indeed, both class I and class II molecules are extremely polymorphic, and in a

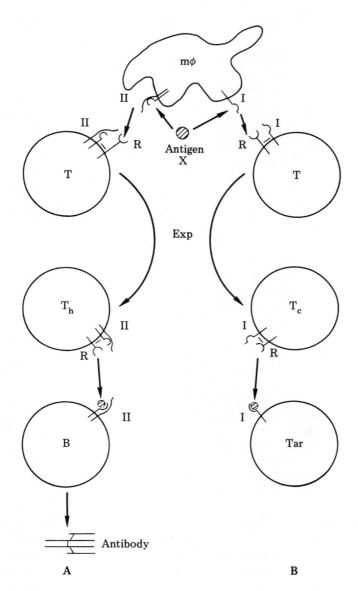

FIG. 19.4. Comparison of the cellular mechanisms of the Ir phenomenon and MHC restriction. (A) The Ir phenomenon involves presentation of **antigen X** by macrophage (**mφ**) via a class II molecule (**II**) and recognition of the (II + X) complex by a T cell, which expands (**Exp**), generating specific T_h cells that interact with B cells, stimulating them to production of antibodies. All interactions are class II restricted. (B) MHC restriction involves presentation of **antigen X** by stimulator cells (**mφ**, grafted cells, virus-infected cells) via class I molecule (**I**) and recognition of the (I + X) complex by a T cell, which expands (**Exp**) and generates specific T_c cells that recognize the (I + X) complex on the target cell (**Tar**). All interactions are class I restricted.

TABLE 19.4. Comparison of the Ir Phenomenon and MHC Restriction

Feature	Ir Phenomenon	MHC Restriction
Genes	$Ir = Ia$ (class II)	*H-2K, H-2D,* and *H-2L* (class I)
Antigens	Synthetic polypeptides	Haptens
	Heterologous proteins	Viruses
	Alloantigens	Alloantigens
Response	Antibody-mediated	Cell-mediated
Cells affected	T_h	T_c
	Macrophages	
Postulated mechanism	Associative recognition of antigen + class II molecules	Associative recognition of antigen + class I molecules

random population, there is a strong preponderance of heterozygosity. Still, to accept fully the proposed concepts, one must reconcile them with the relatively limited polymorphism in some species (rat, hamster, guinea pig) (Chapt. 17).

19.9 *Ir*-Like Genes Controlling MHC-Restricted Responses

The magnitude of the cytotoxic response in the presence of restrictive class I molecules is further influenced by certain allelic forms of class I molecules. Thus, an Ir-like effect might be postulated, with *Ir*-like genes mapping to class I rather than to class II regions. Most *Ir*-like genes are dominant. The mechanism of the Ir-like effect could be explained simply by assuming that a given allelic variant, which is capable of associating with a given antigen, acts as a good response allele, whereas those that do not form an association, or that form it to a limited extent, represent low response alleles. In some instances, however, low responsiveness appears to be dominant. In these cases, it is necessary to consider that the response to the class I molecule preempts the response to the nominal antigen associated with this molecule. Alternatively, it is possible that certain allelic class I molecules not only are unable to associate with the antigen but, at the same time, reduce the expression of other class I molecules. Such a reduction could be mediated by a specific suppression of synthesis of other class I molecules. In addition, it is possible that some complexes of the class I molecules and the antigen induce development of the T_s rather than T_c cells.

Finally, it was shown that in some instances MHC-restricted responses are influenced additionally by class II genes—e.g., the response of mice to an H-Y antigen, while being restricted by class I molecules, also requires the presence of certain class II molecules. It has been proposed that such class II molecules permit the generation of T_h cells that, in turn, amplify the T_c responses. An important implication of this observation is that there is a very close link between the two phenomena—Ir control and MHC restriction. It seems that both phenomena represent two forms of the same basic process, perhaps even applicable to the same antigen depending on the form of its presentation (Table 19.4).

19.10 "Learning" the Restriction

If it is accepted that associative recognition is the common denominator of both the Ir phenomenon and MHC restriction, the following question must be posed: When and how is the recognition of self (restriction) acquired? There is still no definitive answer to this question, but a large body of data is compatible with the idea that both forms of restriction—i.e., those mediated by class I or class II molecules—are acquired by T cells independently of the particular H-2 phenotype of the T cells affected by restriction and independently of exposure to the antigen. The restriction or definition of self appears to be imposed by the genotype of thymuses in which the maturation of T cells takes place (Fig. 19.5). Having in mind that "learning" results in sui generis adaptation of T cells to the environment in which they mature, the term **adaptive differentiation** has been coined. In reality, such a differentiation seems to result from the selection of some clones and deletion of others rather than the modification of preexisting clones.

The strongest evidence in favor of "learning" the restriction—i.e., for the Ir effect to be under the influence of the thymic environment—comes from elegant experiments employing irradiation chimeras. The basic design of such experiments consists of grafting T cell precursors with the MHC genotype and phenotype of a poor responder into a heavily irradiated host with the MHC genotype and phenotype of a good responder. The grafted cells that repopulate the host retain their MHC genotype and phenotype but become capable of good responsiveness. This conversion from poor to good responder phenotype depends on the H-2 phenotype of the radioresistant reticuloepithelial stroma or thymic macrophages of the host thymus. In thymectomized animals grafted with thymus, the responsiveness of grafted cells agrees with the responsiveness of the donor of a simultaneous thymic graft. Such a correlation exists even in the case of an Ir effect involving true complementary genes. This suggests that hybrid combinatorial determinants are actually responsible for the Ir effect.

Similarly, in the case of MHC-restricted responses, the T cell precursors of F1 animals, when grafted into an irradiated parental host, generate cells that recognize the antigen in the context of that parent's class I molecules but not in the context of the other parent's molecules. Again, the selection of a restrictive molecule is directed by the thymus environment, since grafted cells become restricted by the molecules of the reticuloepithelial stroma of the parental host thymus. The selection of the restrictive element is essentially independent of the antigen, but introduction of the antigen in the early period of chimeric development may influence the selection of the restrictive element. The antigenic challenge occurring during selection may cause simultaneously the expansion of the clone restricted by molecules with which the challenging antigen is associated and the contraction of clones restricted by molecules with which the antigen is not associated.

Although most experiments are consistent with the above concept, several distinct exceptions have been observed. To what extent such exceptions reflect experimental artifacts or true differences in various systems remains unknown. There is an important implication of the data obtained in experiments with chimeras. Since the restriction for either class I or class II molecules essentially is developed before a specific antigenic challenge takes place, it is tempting to conclude that subsequent recognition must involve dual recognition (self and

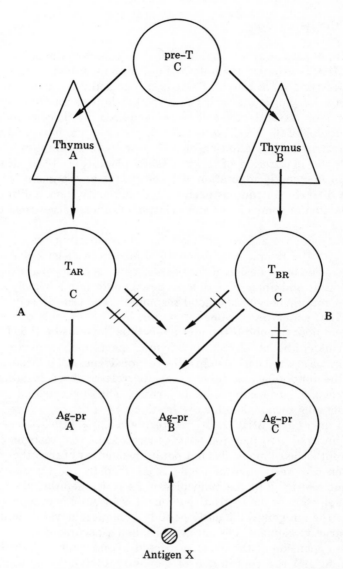

FIG. 19.5. "Learning" the restriction by prethymic (**pre-T**) cells of phenotype C. (**A**) The pre-T cells, after passing through thymus A, retain their phenotype C but become restricted by molecules A (**T$_{AR}$**) and recognize **antigen X** in the context of A ($\rightarrow$) but do not recognize ($\nrightarrow$) antigen X presented by antigen-presenting (**Ag-pr**) cells of phenotype B or C. (**B**) The same cells passing through thymus B retain phenotype C but become restricted by molecules B (**T$_{BR}$**) and recognize ($\rightarrow$) **antigen X** presented by cells B but not ($\nrightarrow$) by cells A or C.

antigen) rather than an altered-self mechanism. This conclusion is based on the assumption that the recognition of altered-self cannot be "learned" without actually encountering the antigen generating the alteration (neoantigen).

19.11 Restrictions of Cell-Cell Collaboration

The restriction imposed by MHC molecules affects not only antigen presentation by macrophages to T cells or their precursors but also cell-cell collaboration or interaction. Such an interaction constitutes an essential event in most humoral and cell-mediated immune responses. Three specific cell-cell interactions are commonly distinguished: macrophage-T cell (mϕ-T), T cell-B cell (T-B), and T cell-T cell (T-T). The first two types were extensively studied, but there is still a paucity of data concerning the third.

The importance of the mϕ-T interaction was ascertained when it was demonstrated that so-called glass- or plastic-adherent cells (mϕ) are indispensible for an in vitro primary response. Subsequently, it was shown that the mϕ during antigen presentation interact with T cell, stimulating the proliferation of the latter only if both T and mϕ are histocompatible for class II genes. Apparently, the interaction, and thus the ensuing response, is restricted by class II molecules. Subsequently, this conclusion was confirmed by the demonstration that antibodies to the class II molecules shared by the two interacting cells can inhibit the interaction. Interestingly, the antibodies were shown to react invariably with the mϕ but not necessarily with the T cells. The prevalent idea accounting for this restriction is, in essence, identical with that described for the Ir phenomenon. It proposes that the macrophage presents the antigen in the context of, or in association with, class II molecules. Attempts to demonstrate the complex of antigen and class II molecules on mϕ have so far failed. Significantly, antibodies to the antigen do not block the interaction between mϕ and T cells, suggesting that the antigen associated with mϕ either has been sequestered or is present in a form that cannot bind the antibodies directed to the entire native molecule. At this time one must conclude that although mϕ and their class II molecules are clearly involved in antigen presentation, the molecular mode of such presentation remains a mystery. Subsequent studies have demonstrated that discrete clones of T cells interact with each of the allelic self class II molecules (Fig. 19.6). Furthermore, among the interacting T cells, there are clones that recognize complexes between different allelic class II molecules and antigen. Such clones, however, are different from those recognizing allogeneic class II molecules alone. The restriction of mϕ-T collaboration is imposed upon T cells during their maturation in the thymus. How absolute this restriction is remains the subject of debate.

T-B interaction was the first example of MHC restriction to be described and probably has been the most extensively studied. Restriction of the T-B interaction was originally ascribed to the entire MHC, but it was soon shown that the products of genes at the *I-A* subregion are primarily, if not exclusively, involved in the phenomenon. Initially, no link between the *Ia* and *Ir* genes was established, and the putative genes affecting cellular interaction were called *CI* (cell interaction). Subsequent studies unequivocally equated the *CI* genes with *Ia* genes and, thereby, with *Ir* genes. Interestingly, several experiments strongly indicated that the restriction of T-B collaboration is imposed upon T cells by class II restrictive molecules of the macrophages originally presenting the antigen to these T cells. Thus, T-B restriction seems to be essentially

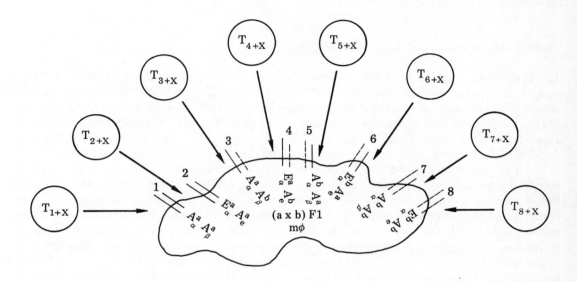

FIG. 19.6. Clonality of T cells. Macrophage (**mɸ**) of (a × b)F1 hybrid heterozygous for MHC may express eight class II (Ia) molecules (**1–8**) generated by *cis* and *trans* complementation of *α* and *β* genes. An antigen (**X**) may be associated with any one molecule, and the complex [II(Ia) + X] is recognized by the clone specific for a particular class II (Ia) molecule and antigen (X).

identical to mɸ-T restriction; macrophages that present an antigen associated with Ia molecules select a T cell clone that is restricted by these particular Ia molecules in the subsequent interaction of T cell with B cell. Experiments show that the restriction of T-B interaction is "learned" by T cells during their ontogeny; this "learning" takes place in the thymus by the selection and deletion of appropriate clones. It is still unresolved whether the T-B restriction is a true restriction or only reflects the restriction of the mɸ-T interaction that precedes T-B collaboration. Still, many results presently available strongly support the notion that both interactions are specifically and independently restricted.

19.12 Unrestricted Responses

The recognition of and responses to allogeneic MHC molecules and some alloantigens closely related to them, such as Qa and TL (Sections 22.2 and 22.3), are the exceptions to what has been said so far. The recognition of and response to these antigens do not require the identity of class I or class II molecules of the responder and stimulator or target cells. The apparent lack of restriction is interpreted differently by the two concepts that account for the mechanism of the MHC restriction.

According to the altered-self hypothesis, allogeneic MHC molecules and some MHC-related alloantigens may themselves be considered as altered-self. This consideration is based on the notion that both self-MHC and allogeneic MHC molecules are allelic variants and apparently variants of each other or to put it another way, each molecule is an altered form of the other. Still, the molecules have a significant identical portion, and this identical portion, in fact, serves as a restrictive element. The same reasoning is applicable to the closely related Qa and TL molecules, which are believed to be the products of the genes that arose by duplication and mutation of a common ancestral gene.

Accepting the concept of allelic molecules as sui generis, altered-self is consistent with the assumption that among T cells bearing receptors for various alterations of self there will be T cells with receptors for allogeneic MHC and MHC-related molecules. Furthermore, it has been speculated that the receptors develop progressively, beginning from the receptors to non-altered-self, and proceeding to receptors for subtle alterations, and finally, leading to receptors for drastic alterations. In this scheme, allogeneic molecules would represent relatively subtle alterations; cells with corresponding receptors would develop early in the process and would be relatively numerous. This is consistent with the well-established fact that there is a high frequency of alloreactive T cells.

The dual recognition hypothesis postulates that unrestricted alloreactivity reflects the presence of a unique set of T cells that bears only a single receptor. Alternatively, it could be speculated that allogeneic molecules, being related to self, cross-react with some of the self-receptors. This would account for the high frequency of alloreactive cells, since essentially all cells would have the self-receptor and, therefore, would be potentially capable of recognizing alloantigens. However, it must be assumed that the interaction between self-receptor and alloantigen results in blocking the receptor for the nominal antigen, since the alloantigen should otherwise be able to act as a restricting element.

There are no experimental data to support either of the two concepts outlined above. Until such data are generated, the two concepts must remain in the sphere of speculation.

T CELL RECEPTORS

Perhaps the most controversial of all issues discussed so far is the nature and origin of T cell receptors. The existence of receptors was accepted as a matter of fact even before any experimental proof was available. Even today, after literally hundreds of studies, the issue has not been resolved and remains clouded by controversy. Still, this chapter would not be complete without a brief summary of the present state of the art.

19.13 Nature of the T Cell Receptors

Although it is plausible to consider that there is a single general type of receptor, for didactic reasons it may be helpful to discuss the putative receptors for alloantigens and receptors for heterologous antigens separately.

The evidence for receptors for alloantigens rests heavily on experiments in which F1 hybrids are immunized with lymphocytes from one of the parents. The lymphocytes of this parent are believed to carry receptors specific for a variety of alloantigens including those of the other parent. On the other hand, the F1 hybrid is believed not to have receptors for alloantigens of either parent. Therefore, immunization is presumed to lead to the production of antibodies directed to the receptors that are carried by lymphocytes of the immunizing parent and are specific for alloantigens of the other parent. Indeed, the resulting antibodies were able to react with the T cells and alloantibodies of the immunizing parent. Significantly, the antibodies elicited in the F1 hybrid reacted only with the T cells and alloantibodies of the immunizing parent that were directed to the second parent of the F1. The parental determinant that induced the antibodies in the F1 hybrid is associated with the heavy chain of immunoglobulin and not with the product(s) of the MHC. This association constitutes a central argument for the concept that the heavy chain, or some part of it, contributes to the molecular structure of the T cell receptor for alloantigens and that T cells have membrane-bound immunoglobulins. As convincing as these results are, one must remember that several observations suggest that the F1 animals do have T cells reactive against certain parental antigens (Chapt. 16). Therefore, it is conceivable that, contrary to the original assumption, the F1 individuals do have receptors for some of the parental alloantigens.

To demonstrate receptors for heterologous antigens, a similar approach has been used. Animals were immunized with antibodies specific for a given heterologous antigen. The antibodies elicited by such an immunization were shown to react with the specific T cells of the donor of antibodies used for immunization. The results support the tenet that antibodies and T cells capable of reacting with a given antigen share a common structure.

A general conclusion from both approaches is that a putative T cell receptor includes a portion of the immunoglobulin heavy chain and that this portion probably corresponds to, or contains, the variable portion of the heavy chain (V_H). To be more specific, the portion carries the idiotypic determinant of V_H (Section 10.1). Further support for this conclusion came from studies in which presumably "free" receptors shed by T cells were studied. Again, such free receptors were shown to contain the V_H idiotype but no other markers of immunoglobulin, e.g., allotype. These data are consistent with the results of studies in which animals immunized with purified V regions or with (Fab') produced antibodies that were shown to react with specific T cells as indicated by inhibition or stimulation of the functions of these T cells. The next question put forth was: What is the actual structure of the putative receptor? In this regard, the studies of soluble factors that can substitute for the function of either helper or suppressor T cells are of crucial importance. There is a long list of such factors, each somehow different from the others, but all sharing certain basic structural characteristics. While it is tempting to speculate that many of the differences may be due to the method used to isolate the various factors, it is still possible that various factors represent the products of distinct cell populations that form immunoregulatory circuits (Chapter 10). The most striking features of the soluble factors are the antigen specificity and the presence in them of class II determinants. Antigen specificity seems to be associated with the V_H component of the factors. Interestingly, no constant portion of any known immunoglobulin chain could be detected in the factors studied. Comparison of the specificity of T cells carrying the putative receptor and the factor derived from these T cells shows that the factor is usually less specific than the intact cells. It is still too early to conclude whether the differences in specificity are real or merely artifactual.

The class II component, in factors isolated from murine cells, corresponds to either an Ia-1 (I-A) molecule in helper factors or an Ia-4 (I-J) molecule in the suppressor factors. It should be emphasized that in studies of these receptors no genetic association with the MHC has been found. It is, however, conceivable that because the V_H studied in receptors can associate itself with all allelic class II molecules, there is phenotypic but not genotypic association between the two components.

Considering all the available data, the structure of the factor or receptor has been proposed (Fig. 19.7). According to this model, the antigen-binding segment of V_H is bound, perhaps by means of disulfide bridges, to a class II molecule. This otherwise very attractive model has one serious drawback. As discussed earlier, the Ir effect seems to depend on class II molecules, especially those expressed on macrophages. So far, no evidence for the presence of a V_H portion in macrophages, or factors derived from them, has been obtained. The apparent discrepancy between concept and facts could be explained by postulating that macrophages present the antigen through direct association with class II molecules, whereas T cells superimpose a higher level of specificity by possessing receptors that contain the V_H segment in addition to class II molecules. Alternatively, one could speculate that the class II molecule of T cells is actually derived from macrophages and not internally synthesized by T cells. If this were true, then the actual T receptor could consist of just V_H with specificity for both the class II molecule and the antigen. Currently, there is no evidence to support the above concept.

To close this topic, it is necessary to mention briefly the so-called macrophage factors. Factors demonstrated in several systems consist of a class II molecule and the immunogenic fragment of the antigen. The class II molecule is encoded by the subregion that determines the *Ir* gene(s) controlling the response to the antigen in question. Macrophage factors do not contain a detectable component of the immunoglobulin chain. The antigen fragment appears to be avidly associated with the factor and cannot be displaced from it by affinity columns. This finding bears heavily on the earlier described concept of associative recognition by either a single or double receptor.

19.14 Origin of the T Cell Receptors

In spite of numerous experimental data directly related to the possible nature of the receptors, the issue of the origin of such receptors, especially their diversity, is totally speculative.

Accepting the idea that the receptor, or at least its antigen-combining portion, is encoded

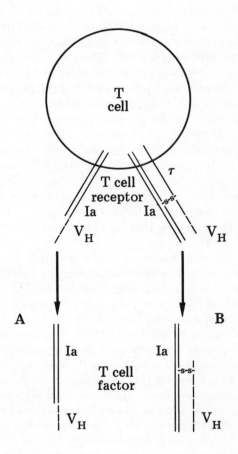

FIG. 19.7. T cell receptors and T cell factors. (**A**) Ia molecule (molecular weight 25,000–33,000) serves as the constant portion for V_H (molecular weight 10,000), and the entire complex is released as factor (molecular weight 30,000–50,000). (**B**) Ia molecule is attached by S-S band(s) to putative IgT consisting of V_H and a constant portion (τ). The molecular weight of the complex is about 200,000. The factor is produced by cleavage of the τ portion of the receptor.

by V_H genes, one may speculate how different V_H segments are generated. Essentially, two alternative concepts have been proposed. According to one concept, the single germ line V_H gene undergoes somatic mutations or recombinations (Section 8.8). When such a process eventually produces a receptor specific for both self-MHC and nominal antigen, further mutations become precluded. Generation of a receptor specific only for antigen leads to low responsiveness, while cells that generated a receptor only for self are promptly eliminated. The other concept proposes that two germ line V_H genes are initially involved. One of the genes, encoding the receptor for self-MHC, is precluded from mutation, whereas the second gene does either concept. However, considering that the same self molecule or even a portion of this molecule *frequently* restricts response to a variety of unrelated antigens, it might be speculated that receptors for self and for antigens are derived from the same self germ line gene.

20 / Clinical Significance of the HLA

Initial interest in the MHC was almost exclusively stimulated by its putative role in the rejection of tissue and organ grafts. It was believed that by defining the genetic determination and molecular nature of the MHC products, a major stepping stone on the way to matching donors and recipients would be reached. It was also hoped that, ultimately, manipulation of the immune response of recipients would become possible, thereby precluding a specific response against MHC products and subsequent rejection of the graft. Neither of these hopes has been fulfilled so far. Nevertheless, studies of the MHC have led to discoveries that have placed the MHC in the limelight of modern immunology. Two of these discoveries, the Ir phenomenon and MHC restriction (Chapter 19), may be considered as turning points in the conceptual and practical approaches to the study of the MHC. In this chapter, the clinical role of the MHC will be discussed briefly.

MHC AND GRAFT REJECTION

20.1 Nomenclature

The major classification of grafts is based on the relationship between the donor and recipient. There are three main types of grafts.

A graft taken from one location in an individual and returned to the same individual at any site is called an **autograft** (autogeneic graft).

An **allograft** (allogeneic graft) is taken from one individual of a given species and placed in another individual of the same species. Within this major category, several subcategories can be distinguished. Graft between two genetically identical individuals (identical twins, members of an inbred strain) is called **isograft** (**syngeneic** or isogeneic graft). Graft from either inbred parent donor to its F1 hybrid is referred to as **semisyngeneic** graft, whereas graft from the F1 hybrid to either of its parents is called **hemiallogeneic**. Finally, graft between two genetically unrelated individuals of the same species represents a true allograft.

A **xenograft** (xenogeneic graft) is taken from an individual of one species and placed in an individual of a different species.*

Depending on its composition, a graft may be a cellular, tissue, or organ graft. This distinction, however, is not clear-cut, since by definition any organ contains tissues and cells, whereas any tissue contains cells. Still, for practical purposes, one distinguishes between grafting a piece of bone (tissue graft) and grafting an entire kidney (organ graft).

Grafted cells, tissues, or organs may be placed in their normal location or in an atypical location. In the first case, the graft is called **orthotopic**, and in the second case, it is called **heterotopic**.

Finally, grafts can be divided into **allostatic** and **allovital**. This division is based on the relationship between survival of the cellular components of the graft and its eventual function. In the case of allostatic grafts, as long as their anatomic structure is preserved, the survival of

---

*In the older literature, the term homologous (homogeneous) and heterologous (heterogeneous) grafts were used for allogeneic and xenogeneic grafts, respectively.

the cells is neither achievable nor often desirable. The best example of an allostatic graft is transplantation of bone tissue in which the graft provides the framework for the proliferation and differentiation of the recipient's own cells. In an allovital graft, the survival of cells and/or preservation of the anatomic structure are required for the normal function of the graft. A kidney graft is an example of an allovital graft.

Although at one time or another each type of graft has been attempted and subjected to analysis, allografts (being the most commonly employed) have always attracted the most attention. With this in mind, the following section will deal predominantly with allografts, whereas other types of grafts will be only occasionally mentioned.

20.2 Host versus Graft Reaction

While autogeneic and syngeneic or semisyngeneic grafts are, as a rule, accepted, true allogeneic and xenogeneic grafts are invariably rejected. Rejection is the result of an immune response of the recipient against molecules present on the surface of the grafted cells but absent from the recipient. These molecules are recognized by the recipient as foreign and, therefore, are commonly referred to as **transplantation antigens** or **histocompatibility antigens**. The antigens determined by the MHC elicit an exceptionally rapid and strong response that usually overshadows a response elicited by any other transplantation antigen that might be recognized in a given donor-recipient combination. In this section, the response to MHC antigens will be considered; the response to other histocompatibility antigens, called minor antigens will be the subject of another chapter (Chapter 21). The response to histocompatibility antigens, generally referred to as the **host versus graft reaction** (HVGR), is the single major cause of allograft failure. The mechanism of the HVGR has been the subject of numerous extensive studies outside the scope of this book and will not be discussed in great detail. Still, a brief description of the basic facts seems to be in order.

It has been established beyond reasonable doubt that the histocompatibility antigens elicit a predominantly cell-mediated response in a recipient who previously has not been challenged with these antigens. The antigens of a first-set graft trigger precursor T cells, which subsequently proliferate and differentiate into specific effector T (T_{ef}) cells (Section 4.10). These effector T cells act in concert with macrophages to infiltrate the graft and either directly or via soluble factors (lymphokines) inflict damage on the graft. The infiltration itself and the subsequent damage ultimately lead to graft rejection (Section 4.10). In reality, the process is much more complex that this. It seems that class II antigens preferentially stimulate the generation of T_h cells, which, in turn, amplify the triggering and generation of either T_{ef} cells or B cells. The former are primarily responsible for first-set graft rejection, whereas the latter produce so-called **transplantation antibodies** that are only marginally, if at all, involved in rejection of the first-set graft. The magnitude of HVGR stimulation varies widely, depending on the following factors: the size and type of graft, the allelic variants of histocompatibility antigens involved, the immune and general state of the recipient, etc. Ordinarily, the HVGR elicited by MHC antigens results in the rejection of allogeneic skin grafts in mice within 10 to 12 days. In fact, such a rapid rejection occurs when the donor and recipient differ for the entire MHC haplotype. On the other hand, when the difference is limited to some segments of the MHC rejection may be delayed to about 20 days. The rejection of the first-set grafts is followed by the development of immunologic memory, which is mediated by a specific subset of long-lived T cells. Immunologic memory is responsible for an accelerated rejection of a subsequent allograft from the same donor. Such a graft, called a second-set graft, is often rejected in mice within five to seven days. The accelerated rejection of a second-set graft is exquisitely specific and can be transferred by lymphoid cells but not by the serum of the recipient. The latter finding has been accepted as irrefutable proof that allograft rejection is primarily a cell-mediated phenomenon. Although rejection of a first-set graft is cell mediated, grafts can and do elicit production of specific antibodies. These transplantation antibodies directed to various products of the MHC may, to a varying extent, participate in rejection of a second-set graft. In extreme cases, when the recipient of a second-set graft has a high titer of specific transplantation antibodies, these antibodies may inflict severe damage and prevent establishing blood circulation (**white graft**) or cause a **hyperacute rejection** of the graft. An antibody-mediated hyperacute rejection occurs within hours, or even minutes, after grafting, especially with such highly vascularized organs as the kidneys or the heart.

It should be obvious by now that the HVGR requires fulfillment of two conditions: the donor must have some histocompatibility antigens that are absent from the recipient, and the recipient must be capable of recognizing and responding to these antigens. These two conditions form the basis of five basic rules or **laws of transplantation**. These laws, which were formulated for and are applicable to highly inbred animals, ignore the effect of sex-linked histocompatibility genes (Section 21.8) and *Hh* genes (Section 16.6). They may be stated as follows:

I. All animals accept syngeneic grafts.
II. All recipients eventually reject true allogeneic grafts.
III. All F1 hybrids accept semisyngeneic grafts, i.e., grafts from either of the parental strains.
IV. The vast majority of F2 or backcross hybrids reject both parental grafts (in the case of backcross hybrids, the rule applies to the graft from the parent that has not been used for backcrossing).
V. All F1 hybrids accept grafts from any F2 or backcross hybrid.

It should be apparent that in all instances when the grafts are accepted, the donor does not have antigens that are absent from the recipient, whereas the grafts are rejected when the donor has some antigens that are lacking in the recipient. The few F2 or backcross hybrids that accept parental grafts correspond to individuals that happen to have all parental antigens. The fraction of such individuals is inversely related to the number (n) of antigens involved in the HVGR and can be calculated for F2 individuals from the formula $(3/4)^n$ and for backcross individuals from the formula $(1/2)^n$.

20.3 Graft versus Host Reaction

What has been said above is fully applicable to a nonlymphoid tissue allograft that has been placed in an immunologically competent recipient. Under such circumstances, the grafted cells have no capacity to recognize and react against the recipient's antigens, whereas the recipient's lymphoid cells can recognize a foreign donor's antigens. In the case of lymphoid tissue grafted to an immunologically competent recipient, both the graft's and recipient's cells are potentially capable of recognizing each other's antigens. In the long run, the reaction of the recipient, since it draws on a practically unlimited pool of cells, overtakes the reaction of the graft, and ultimately the graft is rejected. However, when lymphoid tissue capable of recognizing the recipient's antigens is grafted into an allogeneic recipient that is unable to recognize the donor's antigens, the grafted cells are unopposed in their reaction against the host. An example of such a situation is grafting lymphoid cells from either of inbred parents into their F1 hybrid. The parental cells are capable of recognizing the antigens of the other parent present in the F1, but the F1 possesses all antigens of the donor parent and, hence, cannot recognize these antigens on the grafted cells. As a result, the grafted cells are triggered to proliferate and differentiate into effector T cells, which ultimately inflict damage on the recipient. Such a **graft versus host reaction** (GVHR) in its extreme form may result in the death of the recipient. While the genetic situation described above for inbred strains does not occur in man, the acute GVHR is an important cause of failure of about 30 percent of cases of human allogeneic bone marrow grafts. In this case, bone marrow contains a significant number of immunologically competent cells, and the recipient usually has a compromised (diminished) immunologic competency resulting from either the disease itself (bone marrow aplasia, leukemia, inherited immunodeficiency) or the treatment for the disease (antimetabolites, irradiation, etc.). Though in principle the HVGR and GVHR are mediated by the same cellular process, the specific events and the ultimate outcome of the two reactions are often quite different. More specific information concerning the two reactions may be found easily in any textbook of immunology.

20.4 Effect of the MHC on Allograft Survival

The finding that among the multiple histocompatibility antigens those determined by genes of the MHC cause exceptionally acute and rapid rejection led to the presumption that matching a donor and recipient for these antigens should have a profound effect on the fate of the graft. Accordingly, it was believed that elimination of the HVGR against MHC-determined antigens would significantly delay graft rejection. To this end, numerous studies were undertaken in various animal species to prove this assumption, and some results are given in Table 20.1.

Two conclusions can be drawn from these data. First, the effect of MHC matching is somewhat more pronounced in related than in unrelated donor-recipient combinations. Second, although statistically significant, the effect of matching is not as impressive as one would expect on the basis of the severity of a HVGR elicited in nonmatched combinations. An additional conclusion is that the overall effect of the MHC on graft survival varies among species and among different tissues or organs. While the data do not refute the contention that MHC antigens have an effect on the fate of allografts, they clearly indicate that such an effect is not an exclusive one and that a pronounced HVGR can be elicited by antigens other than those determined by the MHC. In spite of the relatively unimpressive effect of MHC matching on overall graft survival, the procedure of matching has been introduced and is widely used in

TABLE 20.1. Effect of Matching for MHC Antigens on Survival of Allografts of Skin and Kidney in Various Species

Species	Donor-Recipient Relationship[a]	MHC Match[b]	Median Survival Time of Allografts (days)[c]	
			Skin	Kidney
Man	Related	−	10	} See text
		+	15	
	Unrelated	−	—	Short
		+	—	Slightly longer
Chimpanzee	Unrelated	−	11	—
		+	17	—
Rhesus monkey	Related	−	9	—
		+	14	—
	Unrelated	−	10	Short
		+	12	Slightly longer
Dog	Related	−	12	20
		+	18	43
	Unrelated	−	—	Short
		+	—	Slightly longer
Swine	Related	−	6	20
		+	16	76–490
Rat	Unrelated	−	14	15
		+	Slightly longer	121–664
Mouse	Unrelated	−	10–16	—
		+	25–200	—

[a]Related—donor and recipient are members of the same family.
[b]Matching for known MHC determinants regardless of other histocompatibility differences.
[c]Values from various sources are rounded off for simplicity.

clinical transplantation. However, the benefits of the matching procedure are influenced by several factors that will be discussed later.

20.5 Clinical Transplantation of Kidneys

Although transplantation of almost every tissue or organ has been attempted, only the following two situations have gained the status of an approved therapeutic method that offers an acceptable chance for long-term success: the kidney (with well over 25,000 grafts in the last two decades) and bone marrow (estimated over 2,500 grafts). At this time, 50 percent or more of renal grafts survive for a period of time that can be measured in years. The grafting of other organs such as heart, liver, lung, or pancreas is still a highly experimental procedure, and only a small fraction (2 to 20 percent) of these grafts have survived for any significant length of time.

Allostatic grafts of bone tissue, fascias, blood vessels, tendons, etc., although accompanied by a higher rate of success, will not be discussed here because the MHC antigens and the HVGR appear to play only a marginal role in their outcome.

Predictably, the success of clinical renal transplantation depends on solution of two basic problems: perfection of the surgical technique and circumvention of graft rejection. For all practical purposes, the technical and logistic difficulties encountered in the early period have been largely resolved. International cooperation among various centers and the implementation of computers have permitted quick selection of potential donors and recipients. Also, significant advancement in the short-term preservation of kidneys has made possible the transportation of organs, even between distant centers.

On the other hand, in spite of a great deal of progress, a solution to reliable circumvention of graft rejection remains elusive. At present there are two major means of combating rejection. Immunosuppression by drugs such as 6-mercaptopurine, cyclophosphamide, azathioprine, methotrexate, or prednisone significantly improves the prognosis for graft acceptance. Immuno-suppression, although it has many drawbacks, is responsible for much of the success of renal grafting. Identification of the MHC and defining its role in determining the outcome of renal grafting prompted extensive efforts to elaborate a quick and reliable method of HLA matching of prospective donors and recipients. It was once believed that such matching, combined with immunosuppressive therapy, should ensure almost unhindered long-term survival of renal allo-grafts. However, after some enthusiastic initial reports, the truth began to emerge that HLA matching, at least at the present state of the art, does not constitute the ultimate means of avoiding the HVGR. In fact, at one point the value of HLA matching as a routine procedure was seriously questioned. Such doubts stemmed from contradictory reports from different trans-plantation centers—some claiming a beneficial effect and others denying any effect of HLA matching on the outcome of renal grafts. Interestingly, extensive analysis revealed that the beneficial effects of matching were most demonstrable in those centers that had a relatively low rate of overall success. Conversely, in centers with a high rate of overall success, matching had little, if any, effect on the final outcome. One may think of a variety of reasons for such dis-crepancies in the data and opinions: differences in the number of matched antigens, patient population, clinical status of the patients, or immunosuppressive regimens employed are only a few possible reasons for the different results. Even accepting the differences in the effect of HLA matching as real, certain general conclusions may be drawn from past experience with HLA matching.

Overall, it seems that HLA matching has a definite effect on the survival of renal grafts. This effect clearly emerges when the percentages of renal grafts surviving at different times after transplantion are compared among sufficiently large groups of recipients who received grafts from a HLA-identical sibling (fully compatible), a parent (haplocompatible), or a cadaver (incompatible). It is obvious that the effect of HLA matching differs depending on the relationship between the donor and recipient (Table 20.1). The matching of related (sibling) donor-recipient combinations for both classes of antigens (class I and class II) significantly improves survival of the grafts. On the other hand, matching only for class I antigens appears to have a significant but definitely smaller effect. It seems that mismatching class II antigens is more deleterious than mismatching class I antigens. This conclusion seems to be further supported by the finding that the production of antibodies to class II, but not to class I, antigens correlates with the onset and progress of usually an irreversible process of rejection. It should be mentioned that some reports claim comparable effectiveness of matching for class I antigens (HLA-B) and for class II antigens (HLA-D). However, it is plausible to speculate that owing to linkage disequilibrium between these two genes, matching for one of them results in coincidental matching for the other.

Even more controversial are data concerning the matching of unrelated donor-recipient combinations. Since in this combination donors usually are deceased accident victims, the graft is referred to as cadaveric. While some claim that a complete matching has at least some beneficial effect, others do not find this to be true. In the case of matching only for class I antigens, the effect, although statistically significant, is not large enough to have clinical impact. There seems to be an additive effect of matching for an increasing number of class I antigens. Thus, a graft that shares no antigens or only one antigen with the recipient has a poorer survival potential than a graft that shares two to three antigens with the recipient. The latter has still poorer survival than one sharing all four class I antigens. Matching for class II seems to have a definite effect on graft survival. In fact, there is an inverse relation between the intensity of MLR that indicates class II mismatching and the rate of kidney graft survival. In donor-recipient combinations with low MLR, i.e., presumably matched for class II antigens, long-term survival is about 70 percent, whereas in combinations with high MLR, the survival is about 25 percent. The effect of matching for HLA-C antigens (class I) has not been established because of difficulties in typing and unavailability of a complete battery of sera detecting all possible allelic variants.

Many factors other than HLA matching must be taken into consideration when renal graft outcome is predicted. These factors, their relative importance, and their effect are summarized briefly in Table 20.2. Early observations strongly indicated that preimmunization to histo-compatibility antigens usually led to an accelerated rejection of the graft. Indeed, hyperacute rejection has been observed often when the recipient had a high titer of antibodies to class I

TABLE 20.2. Some Factors Influencing the Outcome of Renal Allografts in Man

Factor	Relative Importance	Specific Effect on Graft Survival
Clinical center	Very important	High success rate obliterates effect of HLA matching
Blood transfusion	Very important	Multiple transfusions improve survival in unrelated donor-recipient combination
HLA matching	Important	Matching, especially for class II antigens, improves survival in related donor-recipient combinations
Delayed hypersensitivity	Important	Responsiveness to certain haptens reduces survival in unrelated donor-recipient combinations
ABO matching	Important	ABO mismatch decreases survival
ABO phenotype	Marginally important	Mismatch in non-O males reduces survival
Sex	Marginally important	See above
Age	Marginally important	Old age reduces graft survival

and/or class II antigens of the donor at the time of placing the graft. Based on these observations, three rules were incorporated into the scheme of clinical transplantation.

First, the serum of the prospective recipient is always tested for the presence of antibodies against cells of the prospective donor. Prospective recipients having such antibodies are deemed to be unsuitable candidates for a graft of the kidney from the particular donor. However, it was reported recently that, in many instances, no deleterious effect on the kidney graft was ascertained despite a positive crossmatch test. Apparently, the serum antibodies detected in the crossmatch are not always directed to MHC antigens. Thus, the results of any crossmatch should always be interpreted cautiously before they are accepted as contraindication for grafting in a particular donor-recipient combination.

Second, when grafting a second kidney because the first was rejected, the mismatch in the two grafts should not involve the same antigens. Clearly, the identical mismatch of two consecutive grafts will considerably increase chances of an acute or hyperacute rejection of the second graft.

Third, blood transfusions were once held to be strongly contraindicated for a prospective recipient because of the potential anti-HLA immunization by the nucleated cells of blood. However, retrospective analysis of a large number of cases revealed a rather unexpected phenomenon. The multiple blood transfusions performed prior to transplantation turned out to have a beneficial, rather than a deleterious, effect on the survival of a subsequent graft. This beneficial effect seems to be especially pronounced in cases involving unrelated donor and recipient mismatched for class II antigens. Some preliminary data suggest that, in fact, matching for class II antigens and pretransplantation transfusions may have an additive advantageous effect. The mechanism of the beneficial effect of blood transfusion is presently the subject of extensive studies in numerous laboratories. Two possibilities are being considered: the induction of specific suppressor cells or the induction of antibodies that block graft antigens, preventing the recognition of these antigens and thus abrogating the HVGR and graft rejection. Indeed, antibodies to either class of HLA antigens of the stimulator seem to inhibit MLR.

One of the areas to be explored in search of further improvement of the outcome of renal grafts is immunologic monitoring of the prospective and actual recipients. Availability of methods to test T cell functions should allow determination of the probability of an unusually strong HVGR as well as detection of the imminent onset of graft rejection.

HLA AS A GENETIC MARKER

20.6 Determination of Disputed Paternity

The legal and medical professions are often faced with a fundamental question: Is a given man the father of a given child? This question can be rephrased to read: What is the probability that a given man is the biologic father of a particular child by a particular mother? The question can also be broken down into the following two interrelated parts: Can the paternity of the man be excluded? And, if not, what is the probability that he is actually the father? Usually, maternity is assumed, that is, the woman who claims to be the mother is accepted to be truthful. In the search for an answer to either of these questions one may choose any polymorphic trait (i.e., having at least two allelic variants) and test the child for the presence of an allele that could be contributed by the man in question. If the child has such an allele, the paternity of the man cannot be excluded, whereas if the child does not have either of the alleles of the accused man, paternity can be positively excluded. The fewer the allelic variants in a chosen system, the more frequently at least one of them will occur in a population and, thereby, the higher the chance that two individuals will share a given allele, even if these two individuals are unrelated. Several inheritable markers (blood groups, isoenzymes, blood proteins) are used in attempts to determine paternity, but because of their limited polymorphism, an exclusion of paternity can be made only in a limited portion of cases (Sections 11.17 and 12.3). Among the 22 traits commonly examined, the highest a priori chances of exclusion are about 30 percent for the MNS blood group system (Section 12.3). These chances can be increased up to about 90 percent by simultaneous testing for all 22 traits, but such a testing is cumbersome and possible only in highly specialized laboratories that have all the necessary reagents and equipment to test for the specific markers. This problem may be circumvented by testing for a single but extremely polymorphic trait where the chances of sharing a particular allele by two unrelated individuals are very low. The HLA system seems to suit this purpose ideally, and its usefulness for the exclusion and/or proving of paternity has already been demonstrated in several thousand cases.

All the cases can be divided into two major categories. In about 24 percent of cases, an **absolute exclusion** of paternity can be made by the demonstration that the child does not have either of the two *HLA* haplotypes of the putative father. Obviously, in such an instance, the probability of the man being the biologic father of this particular child equals zero. In a small fraction of cases (about 3 percent), only **probable exclusion** can be made, e.g., when the child has one antigen that is also present in the putative father, say HLA-B, but the second antigen, HLA-A in the child is blank (undeterminable). Although the putative father has two demonstrable HLA-A antigens, there is a small possibility that one paternal antigen became converted in the child to a blank. Because of such an (admittedly remote) possibility, absolute exclusion cannot be made. In the remaining 73 percent of cases, no exclusion can be made since the child has one haplotype identical to the putative father. In those instances, one must determine the probability that the child's antigens were contributed by the putative father and not by some other male. This is done by calculating the probability on the basis of the haplotype frequency in a given population (considering race, ethnic origin, etc.). In most instances of **nonexclusion**, the probability of paternity is over 90 percent and occasionally as high as 99 percent. The range of probabilities reflects differences in the haplotype frequencies and rare cases when determination of the antigens of the mother, child, or putative father is questionable. The available data strongly indicate that HLA typing is the most reliable basis for exclusion or determination of the probability of paternity. One should, however, remember that because nonexclusion does not constitute proof of paternity, it is advisable to test for other markers in all cases of nonexclusion.

20.7 HLA Typing as a Tool in Anthropologic Studies

The extreme polymorphism and pronounced linkage disequilibrium of the *HLA* alleles make HLA an ideal marker for various population studies. Indeed, HLA frequencies were studied in both general and selected human populations. These studies revealed unique alleles in some populations (Chapter 15) and permitted speculations concerning the migration of various human groups and races. Finally, cross-reactions of MHC molecules of various species provides an insight into events underlying the evolution of the animal kingdom.

20.8 The HLA and Disease Predisposition

An important but still poorly understood aspect of the biology of the MHC is its association with certain diseases. Studies of such an association were initiated almost at the same time that the *HLA* complex was discovered. The first reports that people carrying certain *HLA* haplotypes or alleles have a greater incidence of various diseases—psoriasis, coeliac disease, and ankylosing spondylitis—met with understandable reservations. Perhaps this lack of enthusiasm was partially due to the memories that speculative associations between disease and blood groups proved to have little clinical significance. As the list of the diseases associated with HLA grew, the initial reservations were replaced by overenthusiasm. At present no one questions the reality of the association, but its meaning and mechanism remain enigmatic.

There are numerous pitfalls in establishing a specific association. Such pitfalls must be considered in each individual case before the results are accepted. The most important considerations can be summarized briefly. There is never an absolute association—i.e., not all patients with a given disease carry the same *HLA* allele, and, conversely, not all people carrying a given allele suffer from a particular disease. Thus, the association must be, in each case, based on a statistical analysis with all its limitations. At the moment, the most common approach consists of an estimation of the significance of association by a 2 × 2 contingency table.

HLA Allele

		+	−
Disease	+	a	b
	−	c	d

In this table, a, b, c, and d are the number of individuals in four classes. The plus sign (+) signifies the presence and the minus sign (−) the absence of overt disease and/or a given allele. If the χ^2 value calculated from the standard formula indicates a statistically significant association, the relative risk (Rr) is then estimated according to the formula

$$Rr = \frac{ad}{cb}.$$

It is important to keep in mind that since each race and even local populations have their own characteristic frequencies of *HLA* alleles, the patients (disease +) and normal (disease −) subjects must be drawn from the same population.

An alternative method of assessing the association between two traits, i.e., HLA phenotype and the disease, is linkage analysis. This method consists of determining the recombination frequency between HLA and a putative gene determining the disease. This method is more difficult since it requires studying large families consisting of several individuals with overt disease. Presently, the International Disease Registry for all diseases found to be associated with HLA is kept in Copenhagen, Denmark. The registry is constantly revised and updated as new observations are made.

The strength of an association depends on the component of the HLA system used in the determination of association. Early observations were made almost exclusively using class I molecules, since typing for class II molecules was cumbersome and not available to all centers interested in this type of study. With the discovery of the HLA-DR molecules and development of a serological method for their detection, it was demonstrated that many of the diseases that appeared to be associated with one of the class I molecules are even more strongly associated with class II molecules HLA-D(DR). In fact, it is very likely that, in many instances, what appeared to be association with class I molecules simply reflected linkage disequilibrium between the alleles composing the *HLA* haplotypes.

The association between any two factors can be unequivocally established if both factors are strictly defined. Although typing for HLA phenotypes is at this time relatively precise, the same precision does not always apply to the diagnosis of various diseases. Because the reliability of a specific diagnosis does vary over a rather broad range, the final conclusion about association must also vary. Besides the obvious errors in diagnosis, one must realize that certain diseases actually represent a collection of different syndromes or clinical forms that are difficult to distinguish. An association may apply only to one of the syndromes or forms but not to the other, but as long as they are not precisely distinguished, an association may be obscured. The best example in this regard is psoriasis: two forms called **psoriasis vulgaris** and **psoriasis pustularis** can be distinguished, but only the former is associated with HLA. Furthermore, detailed studies show that among patients suffering from psoriasis vulgaris, only those who developed the disease at an early age show association with HLA. Similar findings apply to **diabetes mellitus**, where only the juvenile-onset form is associated with HLA, or to **myasthenia gravis** in which the early-onset form without thymoma shows significant association.

20.9 Specific Associations

The list of diseases found to be associated with HLA is too long to be cited here in its entirety; some of the more striking examples are given in Table 20.3. A brief examination of the table shows several interesting features of the HLA-associated diseases. The diseases do not have a common etiology. Moreover, although some of the diseases do, or may, have an immunologic basis, others clearly do not. A second striking characteristic is that many of the diseases listed are rather rare in comparison with the spectrum of diseases commonly encountered. Whether the latter characteristic reflects a true phenomenon or is simply a bias in selection of material for study is too early to decide.

Special attention should be directed to the association between HLA and malignancies.

TABLE 20.3. Selected Examples of the Association between Disease and the *HLA* Allele in Caucasoids

Disease	HLA Allele	Frequency Ratio Patients/Controls	Relative Risk	Comment
Ankylosing spondylitis	B27	9.6	87.4	
Acute anterior uveitis	B27	5.5	10.4	
Behcet's disease	B5	4.1	6.3	
Celiac disease	Dw3(DR3)	3.0	10.8	
Chronic hepatitis	Dw3(DR3)	4.1	13.9	
(autoimmune)	B8	3.0	9.0	
Congenital adrenal	B47	1.5	15.4	
hyperplasia	B5	2.9	3.6	
(21:OH deficiency)				
Dermatitis herpetiformis	Dw3(DR3)	3.2	15.4	
Graves' disease	Dw3(DR3)	2.2	3.7	
Herpes labialis	A1	1.8	2.7	
Hemochromatosis	A3	2.7	8.2	
(idiopathic)	B14	4.2	4.7	
Hashimoto's thyroiditis	Dw5(DR5)	2.8	3.2	
Idiopathic Addison's disease	Dw3(DR3)	2.6	6.3	
Juvenile arthritis	B27	3.4	4.5	
	Dw8(DRw8)	3.1	3.6	Also Dw5(DR5)
Juvenile-onset diabetes	Dw4(DR4)	2.3	6.4	Dw2 less frequent in patients
mellitus	Dw3(DR3)	2.0	3.3	
Manic-depressive psychosis	B16	2.2	2.3	
Myasthenia gravis	B8	2.3	4.1	
	Dw3(DR3)	1.8	2.5	
Multiple sclerosis	Dw2(DR2)	2.3	4.1	
Optic neuritis	Dw2(DR2)	1.8	2.4	
Pemphigus	Dw4(DR4)	2.7	14.4	in Jews
	Cw6	2.6	13.3	
Psoriasis vulgaris	B13	4.1	4.8	
	B17	3.6	4.8	
	B37	4.2	4.4	
Psoriatic arthritis	B27	3.1	4.0	
	B16	2.5	2.8	
Pernicious anemia	Dw5(DR5)	4.3	5.4	
Reiter's syndrome	B27	8.4	37.0	
Rheumatoid arthritis	Dw4(DR4)	2.5	4.2	
Systemic lupus	Dw3(DR3)	2.5	5.8	
Derythematusus	B8	1.7	2.1	
Subacute thyroiditis	B35	4.8	13.7	
Tuberculosis	B8	2.9	5.1	

Table 20.4 shows a general summary of many studies done in this area. A clear-cut association has been found between HLA and various neoplastic diseases. Notably, since these studies were done before HLA-DR typing was introduced or widely used, the association seems to be mostly with class I genes. Moreover, it appears that certain HLA molecules are selectively associated with malignancies, e.g., B5, B12, B18, or A2. It is not clear whether this reflects linkage disequilibrium of the corresponding alleles with some other genes that influence susceptibility to malignancy or whether the products of these particular alleles predispose to the neoplasia. The prognostic value of associations, although strongly indicated, has not been firmly established. Still, in the future, HLA typing in early childhood may provide an important clue to susceptibility of an individual to certain etiologic agents or carcinogens. Obviously, such information could be utilized in designing specific prophylactic measures.

20.10 Possible Mechanisms of the HLA-Disease Association

Assuming that in most of the instances studied so far, the ascribed association is both statistically and biologically significant, one must pose a crucial question: What is the mechanism(s) underlying such an association? An extension of this question is whether single or multiple mechanisms are involved. There is no simple answer to either of these questions. It is precisely because of this that speculations in the area are so abundant.

The most extensively deliberated mechanism is the one that proposes that the *HLA-D(DR)* gene determines immune responsiveness in much the same way as do the *Ir* genes in mice. Poor or good responsiveness to certain exogenous or endogenous antigens would play a decisive role in predicting the clinical significance of the etiologic agent for the disease under consideration. It follows that the disease would have to be immunologic in nature. This

TABLE 20.4. Association between Some Common Malignancies and Certain *HLA* Alleles

Malignancy	*HLA* Alleles*	Relative Risk
Acute lymphoblastic leukemia (ALL)	*A2, (Bw44, Bw45)*	1.24–1.39
Chronic lymphocytic leukemia (CLL)	*B18, Bw35, (Bw51, Bw52)*	5.24
Chronic myelocytic leukemia (CML)	*A2, (Aw23, Aw24)*	39.42
Hodgkin's disease (all forms combined)	*A1, A11, B8, B18, Bw35, B37, (Bw51, Bw52)*	1.23–8.0
Multiple myeloma	*(Bw51, Bw52)*	1.93
Lymphoma	*(Bw44, Bw45)*	2.75–3.51
Carcinomas (all localizations combined)	*A2, B8, B18, Bw35, Bw46, Bw52*	1.35–6.45
Sarcomas	*(Bw51, Bw52)*	4.00
Retinoblastoma	*Bw35*	2.75

*In parentheses are given the designations of alleles that were previously recognized as a single allele (see Table 15.1).

explanation could conceivably be applied to such diseases as juvenile-onset diabetes mellitus, coeliac disease, or various malignancies. Credibility is lent to this explanation by the finding that in these diseases antibodies to the affected organ are commonly found and that the immune responses in mice to some organ-specific antigens are known to be influenced by *Ir* genes (Section 19.3). However, accepting immune control as the major involvement of the MHC in the disease necessitates some additional considerations. Assuming that a given allele at the *HLA-D(DR)* locus represents a high response allele, one would expect that all homozygotes would suffer from a given disease. This is rarely true. To explain the lack of an absolute association, it is necessary to consider either heterogeneity of the disease or a significant influence of environmental factors.

Although the above factors do not rule out an immunologic mechanism for association, they make it more complex. It is worth mentioning that in juvenile-onset diabetes, association with products of two different alleles (*HLA-DR3* and *HLA-DR4*) has been found, but heterozygotes carrying both alleles seem to be at higher risk than homozygotes. This phenomenon resembles the effect of complementary *Ir* genes (Section 19.3). The role of environmental factors appears well demonstrated by the finding that, in some instances, an association established for one ethnic or racial population apparently is invalid for another population. It remains to be demonstrated that the *HLA-D(DR)* alleles and their products are directly responsible for the disease and not simply markers for still undefined genes that are in strong disequilibrium with the *HLA-DR(DR)*. Obviously, the most likely condition for the HLA effect via an immune response is an infectious disease. Though in several cases the effect of HLA on the immune response to pathogens was demonstrated, a significant association was found only in **tuberculoid leprosy** (DR2/DR2). Interestingly, in this case an immune response is present as opposed to the lepromatosus form that is not associated with HLA.

An alternative, but not mutually exclusive, concept is that the MHC and its products may influence a variety of nonimmunologic functions. Such nonimmunologic traits have been described in mice and range from smell perception or mating preference to the receptors for glucagon. Thus, *HLA* itself or genes closely associated with it could influence a variety of phenomena such as hormone binding, receptors for oncogenic viruses, bacteria, or toxins. This mechanism could underlie the association with such diseases as **hemochromatosis, 21-hydroxylase deficiency** (congenital virilizing adrenal hypertrophy), or **ataxia telangectasia**.

Because it seems that no definitive conclusion can be reached presently, the safest approach is to wait for more specific data as well as further refinement in clinical diagnosis and HLA typing before passing final judgment.

However, it must be emphasized that the association between HLA and various diseases reflects a more general phenomenon of MHC and disease relationships. Such a relationship was clearly demonstrated in all species (mice, rats, chickens) studied in this respect.

20.11 Clinical Significance

Even though the mechanism of HLA-disease association remains poorly understood, the phenomenon itself should not be disregarded. Its discovery and subsequent study have contributed enormously to the progress of medical science.

First, in some instances, e.g., hemochromatosis, studies of association with HLA were instrumental in proving that the disease is inherited. Second, in this particular case, the association is so obvious that HLA typing of siblings constitutes a valuable basis for the detection of individuals at risk and the institution of prophylactic measures. Third, it was demonstrated that many endocrine diseases encompass several distinct forms with different etiologies and, even more important, with different prognoses.

Although the diagnostic and prognostic value of HLA typing, in many instances, is minimal, it is unwise to abandon the studies entirely. Rather, one is tempted to agree with the proposition that particular emphasis should be put on in-depth studies of known associations rather than on the search for still other specific associations.

V / *Suggested Supplementary Reading*

The following list of publications has been compiled to provide the reader with a source of specific references. It consists predominantly of most recent textbooks, monographs, reviews, and some selected original papers. Each publication listed has an extensive list of references that may be useful for the reader who desires to pursue in depth some of the topics discussed in the preceding section.

Altman, P. L. Katz, D. D. (eds.), *Inbred and Genetically Defined Strains of Laboratory Animals*, Federation of American Societies for Experimental Biology, Bethesda, 1979.

Benacerraf, B., *Immunogenetics and Immunodeficiency*. University Park Press, Baltimore, 1975.

Benacerraf, B., Role of MHC gene products in immune regulation. Science **212**: 1229–1238, 1981.

Benacerraf, B., Katz, D. H., The histocompatibility linked immune response genes. Adv. Cancer Res. **21**: 121–173, 1975.

Blanden, R. V., How do immune genes work? Immunol. Today **1**:33–36, 1981.

Braun, W. E., *HLA and Disease*. CRC Press, Boca Raton, 1979.

Briles, W. E., Briles, R. W., Identification of haplotypes of the chicken major histocompatibility complex (B). Immunogenetics **15**: 449–459, 1982.

Caldwell, J., Cumberland, P. A., Cattle lymphocyte antigens. Transpl. Proc. **10**: 889–892, 1978.

Cramer, D. V., Kunz, H. W., Gill III, T. J., Immunogenetics, in *The Laboratory Rat*. Volume 2. Academic Press, New York, 1980.

Démant, P., Ivanyi, D., Oudshoorn-Snoek, M., Calafat, J., Roos, M. H., Molecular heterogeneity of H-2 antigens. Immunol. Rev. **60**: 5–22, 1981.

Dick, H., HLA-DR: more than three loci? Immunol. Today **3**: 199–203, 1982.

Dorf, M. E. (ed.), *The Role of the Major Histocompatibility Complex in Immunobiology.* Garland STPM Press, New York, London, 1981.

Ferrone, S., David, C.S. (eds.), *Ia Antigens.* CRC Press, Boca Raton, 1982.

Ferrone, S., Solheim, B.G (eds.), *HLA Typing: Methodology and Clinical Aspects.* CRC Press, Boca Raton, 1982.

Festenstein, H., Démant, P. *HLA and H-2 Basic Immuno Genetics; Biology and Clinical Relavance.* E. Arnold (Publisher) Ltd. London 1978.

Fougereau, M., Dausset, J., *Immunology 80*, Progress in Immunology IV (3 volumes). Academic Press, London, New York, 1980.

Fudenberg, H. H., Pink, J. R. L., Wang, An-Chuan, Douglas, S. D., *Basic Immunogenetics.* Oxford University Press, New York, 1978.

Gill III, T. J., Günther, E., Štark. O., Alloantigenic systems in the rat. Transplant. Proc. **11**: 1549–1664, 1979.

Gill III, T. J., Kunz, H. W. (eds.), Alloantigenic systems in the rat. Transplant. Proc. **13**: 1307–1497, 1981.

Goldberger, R. F. (ed.), *Biological Regulation and Development.* Volume 2. Plenum Publishing Company, 1980.

Götze, D. (ed.), *The Major Histocompatibility System in Man and Animals.* Springer-Verlag, Berlin, Heidelberg, New York, 1977.

Guy, K., van Heyningen, V., Further intricacy of HLA-DR antigens. Immunol. Today **3**: 236–237, 1982.

Hildeman, W. H. (ed.), *Frontiers in Immunogenetics.* Elsevier/North-Holland, New York, Amsterdam, Oxford, 1981.

Hildeman, W. H., Clark, E. A., Raison, R. L., *Comprehensive Immunogenetics.* Elsevier/North-Holland, New York, 1981.

Janeway, C., Jones, B., Binz, H., Frischknecht, H., Wigzell, H. T-cell receptor idiotypes. Scand. J. Immunol. **12**: 83–92, 1980.

Jerne, N. K., The somatic generation of immune recognition. Eur. J. Immunol. **1**: 1–9, 1971.

Katz, D. H., Genetic control of cell-cell interaction. Pharm Rev. **34**: 51–62, 1982.

Katz, D. H., Benacerraf, B. (eds.), *The Role of Products of the Histocompatibility Gene Complex in Immune Response.* Academic Press, New York, San Francisco, London, 1976.

Kaufman, J. F., Strominger, J. L., HLA-DR light chain has a polymorphic N-terminal region and a conserved immunoglobulin-like C-terminal region. Nature **297**: 694–697, 1982.

Klein, J. *Immunology: the Science of Self-Nonself Discrimination.* John Wiley & Sons, New York, 1982.

Klein, J., *Biology of the Mouse Histocompatibility-2 Complex.* Springer-Verlag, Berlin, Heidelberg, New York, 1975.

Klein, J., Figueroa, F., Polymorphism of the mouse *H-2* loci. Immunol. Rev. **60**: 23–57, 1981.

Klein, J., Flaherty, L., Vandeberg, J. L., Shreffler, D. C., *H-2* haplotypes, genes, regions, and antigens: First listing. Immunogenetics **6**: 489–512, 1978.

Klein, J., Juretić, A., Baxevanis, C. N., Nagy, Z. A., The traditional and a new version of the mouse H-2 complex. Nature **291**: 455–460, 1981.

Krco, C. J., David, C. S., Genetics of immune response: a survey. CRC Critical Review in Immunology **1**: 211–257, 1981.

Kvist, S., Bregegere, F., Rask, L., Cami, B., Garoff, H., Daniel, F., Wiman, K., Larhammar, D., Abastado, J. P., Gachelin, G., Peterson, P. A., Dobberstein, B., Kourilsky, P., cDNA clone coding for part of a mouse H-2^{d} major histocompatibility antigen. Proc. Natl. Acad. Sci. USA, **78**: 2772–2776, 1981.

Loor, F., Roelants, G. E. (eds.), *B and T Cells in Immune Recognition*. John Wiley & Sons, London, New York, Sydney, Toronto, 1977.

McDevitt, H. O. (ed.), *Ir Genes and Ia Antigens*. Academic Press, New York, 1978.

Michaelson, J., Genetic polymorphism of β_2-microglobulin (β2m) maps to the *H-3* region of chromosome 2. Immunogenetics **13**: 167–171, 1981.

Millot, P., Genetic control of lymphocyte antigens in sheep. The *OLA* complex and two minor loci. Immunogenetics **9**: 509–534, 1979.

Murphy, G. P., Cohen, E., Fitzpatrick, J. E., Pressman, D. (eds.), *HLA and Malignancy*. Alan R. Liss, New York, 1977.

Nairn, R., Yamaga, K., Nathenson, S. G., Biochemistry of the gene products from murine MHC mutants. Ann. Rev. Genet. **14**: 241–277, 1980.

Nagy, Z., Baxevanis, C. N., Ishii, N., Klein, J., Ia antigens as restrictive molecules in *Ir*-gene controlled T cell proliferation. Immunol. Rev. **60**: 59–83, 1981.

Ogra, P. L. Jacobs, D. M. (eds.), *Regulation of the immune response*. S. Kerger, Basel, 1982.

van Oss, C. J., Atassi, Z., Absalon, D., *Molecular Immunology*. M. Dekker, New York, Basel, in press.

Parnes, J. R., Seidman, J. G., Structure of wild-type and mutant β_2-microglobulin genes. Cell **29**: 661–669, 1982.

Pierce, C. W., Cullen, S. E., Kapp, J. A., Schwartz, B. D., Shreffler, D. C. (eds.), *Ir Genes: Past, Present, and Future*. Humana Press, Clifton, N.J., 1983.

Ploegh, H. L., Orr, H. T., Strominger, J. L., Major histocompatibility antigens: The human (HLA-A,-B,-C)) and murine (H-2K,H-2D) class I molecules. Cell **24**: 287–299, 1981.

Poulik, M. D., Reisfeld, R. A., β_2-microglobulins. Contemp. Top. Med. Immunol. **4**: 157–204, 1975.

Reisfeld, R. A., Ferrone, S. (eds.), *Current Trends in Histocompatibility*. Plenum Press, New York, London, 1981.

Roos, M. H., Démant, P., Murine complement factor B (BF): sexual dimorphism and *H-2*-linked polymorphism. Immunogenetics **15**: 23–30, 1982.

Rose, N. R., Friedman, H., *Manual of Clinical Immunology*. American Society of Microbiology, Washington, D.C., 1976.

Rose, N. R., Milgrom, F., van Oss, C. J. (eds.), *Principles of Immunology*. Macmillian Publishing Co., New York, 1979.

Rosenthal, A. S., Determinant selection and macrophage function in genetic control of the immune response. Immunol. Rev. **40**: 136–152, 1978.

Ryder, L. P. Svejgaard, A. Dausset, J., Genetics of HLA disease association. Ann. Rev. Genet. **15**: 169–187, 1981.

Schwartz, R. H., Yano, A., Paul, W. E., Interaction between antigen-presenting cells and primed T lymphocytes. Immunol. Rev. **40**: 153–180, 1978.

Seligman, M., Preud'homme, J. L., Kourlisky, F. M. (eds.), *Membrane Receptors of Lymphocytes*. Elsevier/North-Holland, Amsterdam, Oxford, New York, 1975.

Snell, G. D., Dausset, J., Nathenson, S. *Histocompatibility*. Academic Press, New York, San Francisco, London, 1976.

Steinmetz, M., Minard, K., Horvath, S., McNicholas, J., Frelinger, J., Wake, C., Long, E., Mach, B., Hood, L., A molecular map of the immune response region from the major histocompatibility complex of the mouse. Nature **300**: 35–42, 1982.

Steinmetz, M., Winoto, A., Minard, K., Hood, L., Clusters of genes encoding mouse transplantation antigens. Cell **28**: 489–498, 1982.

Steinmetz, M., Moore, K. W., Frelinger, J. G., Sher, B. T., Shen, F., Boyse, E. A., Hood, L., A pseudogene homologous to mouse transplantation antigens: Transplantation antigens are encoded by eight exons that correlate with proteion domains. Cell **25**: 683–692, 1981.

Stone, W. H., Bovine lymphocyte antigen (BoLA) system. Adv. Exp. Med. Biol. **137**: 433–450, 1981.

Svejgaard, A., Hauge, M., Jerslid, C., Platz, P., Ryder, L. P., Staub Nielson, L., Thomsen, M., *The HLA System*. Second Edition. S. Karger, Basel, 1981.

Terasaki, P. I. (ed.), *Blood Transfusion and Transplantation*. Grune & Stratton, New York, London, Paris, San Diego, San Francisco, Sao Paulo, Sydney, Tokyo, Toronto, 1982.

Zaleski, M. B., Abeyounis, C. J., Kano, K. (eds.), *Immunobiology of the Major Histocompatibility Complex*. S. Karger, Basel, 1981.

Zinkernagel, R. M., Doherty, P. C., MHC-restricted cytotoxic T cells. Studies on the biological role of polymorphic major transplantation antigens determining T-cell restricted-specificity, function and responsiveness. Adv. Immunol. **27**: 51–177, 1979.

VI / Cell Surface Alloantigens of Nucleated Cells

21 / Minor Histocompatibility Genes and Antigens

The terms histocompatibility (*H*) gene and histocompatibility (H) antigen designate allogeneic moieties that (1) can be recognized by the recipient of an allograft and (2) can elicit an immune response, which results in rejection of that graft. These seemingly simple definitions, however, require certain qualifications. To cause graft rejection, the antigen must be expressed on the grafted cells. Hence, an antigen that is present exclusively on, for example, thymocytes will cause their rejection and, thus, is classified as an H antigen; however, the same antigen will not cause kidney graft rejection and, in this case, should not be classified as an H antigen. With this in mind, one must consider the term H antigen as a relative one, depending on the specific situation under consideration. The *H* genes are traditionally divided into two categories, major and minor. The distinction is based on the intensity of graft rejection caused by incompatibility involving either one or the other category of *H* genes. Specifically, the incompatibility for major *H* gene(s) leads to the rejection of a skin graft within 21 days,* whereas the incompatibility for minor *H* genes results in rejection usually after more than 21 days (see below). In this chapter, only minor histocompatibility genes will be discussed. It should be kept in mind that most likely it is only a chance occurrence that the product of a given gene acts as an H antigen. Thus, the designation *H* gene or H antigen is useful only for the transplantation biologist and says nothing about the actual biologic function of the gene or its product.

THE NUMBER OF MINOR HISTOCOMPATIBILITY GENES

Initially, the minimal number of *H* genes in mice was estimated to be about 15. The estimate was made using the formula

$$S = (3/4)^n,$$

where S is the fraction of F2 animals that accept parental allografts and n is the number of *H* genes segregating independently. This figure was definitely an underestimate; today, over 50 distinct *H* genes have been defined, and some of them have been the subject of extensive genetic analysis. The initial underestimation was due to several factors that were well known to the early investigators.

First, it is presently known that many minor *H* genes, as well as those comprising the MHC, are linked to various extents. Given only a single chance of crossing-over in the F2 generation, most of such linked genes will not cross over but will behave as a single gene. Obviously, the closer the linkage, the greater is the probability that crossing-over will not occur and, subsequently, the greater is the probability of an underestimate. This shortcoming has been eliminated in subsequent studies that examined multiple backcross generations instead of a single F2 generation. Employing the formula

$$n = 2^{(g-1)},$$

where n is the number of segregating *H* genes and g is the number of the generation in which all grafts from a backcross to a parent used for backcrossing are accepted, the estimate of *H* genes

---

*In fact, in most instances, the graft is rejected after about 12 days.

has been raised to about 28. Alternatively, the number of genes was estimated to be about 34 by using mice from the nth generation (F_n) of intercrossing and the formula

$$S = (3/4)^{rL}(5/8)^{vL},$$

where S is the fraction of surviving grafts, L is the number of *H* genes segregating, and r and v are constants for each generation tested.

A second cause of *H* gene number underestimation is that a gene will be detected only if its product is expressed on the grafted tissue and if it evokes a strong enough reaction to cause graft rejection within the period of observation, usually 100 days. In the early studies, either tumor cells or skin grafts were used for grafting. As shall be seen later, some H antigens elicit a relatively weak reaction that is unable to cause graft rejection even after 400 days, and in some instances, there is a permanent survival of the graft. Some of these drawbacks can be eliminated by extending the time of observation and enhancing the weak reaction by preimmunization of the recipients. The total estimate should also take into consideration that some antigens may not be expressed on skin or tumor cells and, therefore, may escape detection by means of skin or tumor graft rejection.

Third, it must be remembered that any two strains may differ by alleles of some *H* genes while sharing alleles of other *H* genes. Obviously, any test will detect the former but not the latter. Usually, the number of *H* genes detectable in any particular strain combination corresponds to about 11 percent of all *H* genes of a species. Thus, the estimate of the number (x) of *H* genes in any particular combination of strains reflects the number of genes detectable in such a combination and not the total number (n) of genes in the species. All studies using various strain combinations produce estimates close to 30 *H* genes, suggesting that this the true number of genes by which two mouse strains can actually differ. This number would correspond to about 273 *H* genes in the species according to the formula

$$n = x/0.11.$$

However, using the rate of mutation, which is independent of segregation, certain investigators have estimated the number of *H* genes to be in the range of 430 to 720. In this method of estimating the number of *H* genes, the number of mutants detected by graft rejection, i.e., mutants of *H* genes, is compared with the number of mutants of other genes whose number is known. Assuming that the mutation rate is similar for different genes (about 5×10^{-3}/gamete/generation for all *H* genes and about 7.5×10^{-6}/gamete for a single *H* gene), the number of detected mutants permits the calculation of the total number of *H* genes. The extremely large numbers of *H* genes obtained by this method are, at least in part, due to the facts that (1) the method also detects nonpolymorphic genes and (2) a given gene can undergo several independent mutations, each being attributed to a discrete gene.

THE GENETICS OF THE MINOR HISTOCOMPATIBILITY GENES IN MICE

The minor *H* genes are scattered throughout the murine genome as illustrated in Fig. 21.1. The figure shows only 32 genes with chromosomal assignments. In addition, there are 13 *H* genes not assigned to any particular chromosome; these genes are listed in Table 21.1.

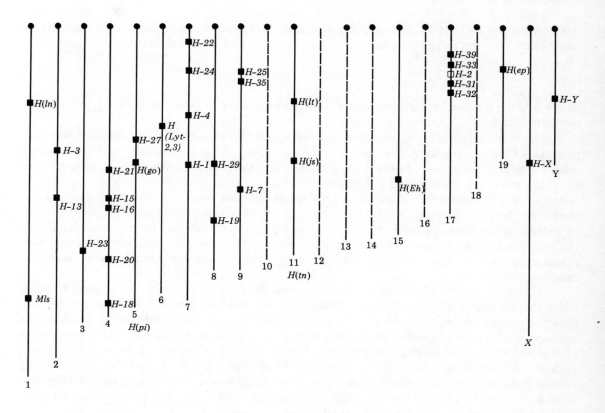

FIG. 21.1. Chromosome positions of murine minor histocompatibility genes. Chromosomes with minor *H* genes are represented as **solid lines** and chromosomes without genes as **dashed lines**. Positions of centromeres are indicated by **solid circles**. Relative positions are based on available recombination data. Positions of **H-X** and **H-Y** are assigned arbitrarily. The positions of **H(pi)** and **H(tn)** genes have not been established.

Both assigned and unassigned genes are designated by the capital letter *H* for histocompatibility and a sequential Arabic number. Unfortunately, some numbers had to be omitted (5,6,14) because they were used previously to designate murine blood groups (Section 13.1). Additionally, there are at least eight *H* genes (Table 21.2) with temporary designations that consist of the letter *H* and an abbreviation of the genes to which they are closely linked. Once the histocompatibility nature of these genes and their separate identities are firmly established, the temporary designations will be replaced by standard ones. Most of the minor *H* genes have only two alleles, but in a few instances several alleles have been distinguished. Specifically, *H-8* and

TABLE 21.1. Murine Minor Histocompatibility Genes without Chromosome Assignment

Locus	Number of Alleles	Alleles Carried by the Strains*			
		a	b	c	?
H-8	3	B6, B10	D2	C	
H-9	2	B6, B10	C		
H-10	2	B10	129		
H-11	3	B10	129		D2
H-12	2	B10	129		
H-17	2		B6	C	
H-26	2		B6	C	
H-28	2		B6	C	
H-30	2		B6	C	
H-34	2		B6	C	
H-36	2		B6	C	
H-37	2		B6	C	
H-38	2		B6	C	

*For abbreviations of strains, see Table 5.2.

H-11 genes have three alleles each, *H-1* and *H-13* have four alleles each, and *H-3* has six alleles. The alleles are designated by small letter superscripts e.g., $H-1^a$, with the letter usually corresponding to the standard abbreviation of the name of the strain in which the allele was identified, i.e., *a* corresponds to the A strain, *b* corresponds to B6 or B10 strains, *c* to BALB/c, and *l* to the LG/Ckc strain. Alleles of any minor *H* gene usually have a unique strain distribution, but in many instances this distribution has not been extensively studied.

IDENTIFICATION OF THE MINOR *H* GENES

The following three basic methods are employed in the identification of *H* genes.

21.1 The F1 or Complementation Test

In this test, a pair of congenic strains differing by alleles of the gene *x* and designated $A.x^a$ and $A.x^b$ are used to find out whether a given strain, e.g., T, carries the x^a or x^b allele or still another allele, x^z. This is done by producing two hybrids $(T \times A.x^a)F1$ and $(T \times A.x^b)F1$ and grafting them with $A.x^a$ and $A.x^b$ skin. If the strain T carries the x^a allele, the $A.x^a$ graft will be accepted by both hybrids, whereas the $A.x^b$ graft will be rejected by the $(T \times A.x^a)F1$ but accepted by the $(T \times A.x^b)F1$ recipient. Conversely, if the strain T has the x^b allele, an $A.x^b$ graft will be accepted by both hybrids, whereas the $A.x^a$ graft will be accepted by the first but rejected by the second F1 hybrid. However, when T carries neither the x^a nor x^b allele, an $A.x^a$ graft will

TABLE 21.2. Murine Minor Histocompatibility Genes Identified by Association with Mutant Alleles of Nonhistocompatibility Genes

Histocompatibility Locus	Chromosome Position	Mutant Designation	Phenotype of Mutant
$H(ln)$	1	Leaden	Bluish-gray coat color
$H(go)$	5	Angora	Angora type of coat
$H(pi)$	5	Pirouette	Circling movement, head shaking, deafness
$H(js)$	11	Jackson shaker	Circling movement, head shaking, deafness
$H(lt)$	11	Lustrous	Shining coat
$H(tn)$	11	Teetering	Progressive hypertonia
$H(Eh)$	15	Hairy ears	Hair growth on ears
$H(ep)$	19	Pale ears	Deficient vascularization of ears

be rejected by the $(T \times A.x^b)F1$ and $A.x^b$ graft will be rejected by the $(T \times A/x^b)F1$ recipient. The outcome of the F1 test in different situations is summarized in Fig. 21.2. Using the F1 test, six known H genes (H-7 through H-12) have been identified.

The complementation test is also used to determine whether the two alleles (a and b) are variants of the same gene or of two different genes. In this case, congenic strains A.a and A.b and their F1 hybrids (A.a × A.b) are produced and grafted with tissue obtained from the donor strain A carrying the c allele at either one or both loci. If the a and b alleles are variants of the same gene, both congenic strains and their F1 hybrids will reject the graft of A. If the a and b alleles are variants of two genes, the congenic strains will reject but F1 hybrids will accept the graft from A, since the two parental haplotypes complement each other (Fig. 21.3) and all genes of the strain A are present in the hybrid.

21.2 The Strain Distribution Pattern (SDP) in Recombinant Inbred Strains

In this test, recombinant inbred strains (RI) are derived by strict sister-brother breeding for 20 consecutive generations of the progeny of F2 hybrids of two inbred strains (Section 5.3). The resulting strains represent a fixed random assortment of all the alleles derived from the original parental strains. Each RI strain is then subjected to F1 tests using a congenic pair differing by an allele at a given differential locus. In this way, the strain distribution pattern (SDP) of parental alleles in various RI strains can be determined. Using this approach, investigators have identified 21 distinct H genes (H-15 through H-38 except for H-31, H-32, and H-33).

21.3 Linkage Analysis

For this test, a visible or easily detectable marker—e.g., coat color, eye color, enzyme variant, etc.—is introduced from one strain into the other during the production of congenic pairs

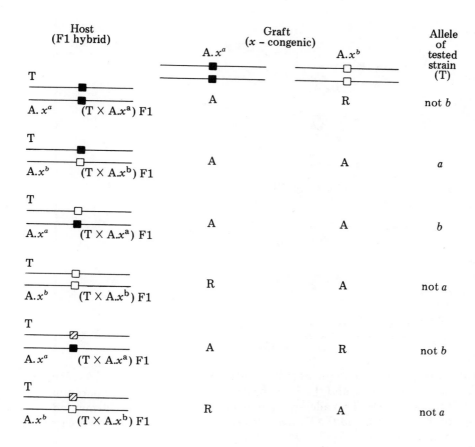

FIG. 21.2. Principle of the F1 test. The allele of gene x carried by tested strain (**T**) is determined by the pattern of rejection (**R**) and acceptance (**A**) of the graft from x-congenic strains by F1 hybrids between these strains and strain T.

(Section 5.4). If a congenic pair that differs by the marker in question rejects reciprocal skin grafts, either the marker itself is an H gene or it is closely linked to an H gene. By this method, about 15 H genes have been identified. In most instances, the products of these genes elicit relatively weak reactions, and often the histocompatibility character of the genes remains questionable. Unfortunately, only in some instances has the putative H gene been separated from the differential gene by crossing-over, thus indicating independence of the two genes.

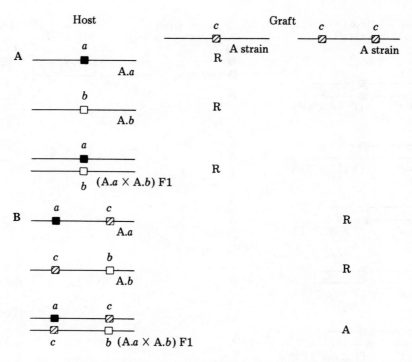

FIG. 21.3. Principle of the complementation test. (**A**) Two alleles, *a* and *b*, of the same gene do not complement, and the F1 hybrids reject a graft from the parental donor carrying the *c* allele. (**B**) Two alleles, *a* and *b*, of two genes are complemented by the *c* alleles of these genes, and the F1 hybrids accept a graft from the donor carrying *c* alleles of both genes.

PHENOTYPIC EXPRESSION OF THE MINOR *H* GENES

As said at the beginning of this chapter, graft rejection due to donor-recipient incompatibility for alleles at a given locus constitutes the primary criterion to classify the locus as carrying an *H* gene. Rejection of a first-set graft is almost exclusively mediated by a cellular mechanism, although antibody production to minor H antigens has been demonstrated in a few instances. The cell-mediated responses against H antigens can be demonstrated and measured in several different systems, which will be discussed briefly.

21.4 Graft Rejection

Rejection of either tumor cells or skin grafts is used extensively to demonstrate minor H antigens and their properties. The rejection is caused by a mononuclear infiltration of the graft,

TABLE 21.3. Immunogenicity of Some Histocompatibility Antigens Measured by MST of Skin Graft

Donor	Recipient	Response to the Antigen	Median Survival Time (days)
B10.AKM	B10.MBR	H-2K^k	∼12
B6-H-2^d	B6-H-2^{g6}	H-2D^d	∼15
B10	B10.LP-H-3^b	H-3^a	21–30
B10-H-3^b	B10	H-3^b	50
B10	B10.129-H-4^b	H-4^a	120
B10.129-H-4^b	B10	H-4^b	25
B10	B10.C-H-7^b	H-7^a	24
B10.C-H-7^b	B10	H-7^b	33–47
B10	B10.129-H-11^b	H-11^a	78
B10.129-H-11^b	B10	H-11^b	164

which leads to its necrosis and ultimately to its replacement by a scar. The intensity of the HVGR customarily is measured by the time that is required for complete rejection of the graft. The median survival time (MST) of a graft is considered an indicator of the immunogenicity of the antigen involved and the capability of the recipient to mount a specific response. The MST is influenced by several factors.

The immunogenicity of different minor H antigens varies broadly, as illustrated in Table 21.3. The H-4 and H-7 antigens cause the rejection of all grafts within four to five weeks, whereas the H-1 and H-13 antigens elicit rejection of only some grafts, and usually after several months. In addition, two allelic products of a given H gene often differ in their immunogenicity. For example, the antigen determined by the H-4^a allele elicits rejection after about three months, whereas the product of the H-4^b allele causes rejection in less than one month. These differences in immunogenicity of the different minor H antigens are also reflected in the number of lymphoid cells needed to preimmunize a recipient for rejection of a second-set graft. The required number of priming cells is relatively small for strong antigens and relatively large for weaker antigens or the weaker of two allelic products.

The dose effect of the minor antigen on the immune response elicited by such an antigen is clearly reflected by slower rejection of hemiallogeneic H-13^a/H-13^b than allogeneic H-13^a/H-13^a grafts by H-13^b/H-13^b homozygous recipients. The rejection of skin grafts across the minor histocompatibility barrier is also influenced by the size of the graft with large grafts being rejected more slowly.

In some instances, the effect of several minor H antigens expressed simultaneously on the grafted cells is cumulative—i.e., the MST of a graft bearing two or more antigens may be shorter than the MST of grafts carrying each antigen alone. In an extreme case, the MST of a graft expressing multiple minor H antigens may be as short as the MST of a graft carrying incompatible MHC antigens. The cumulative effect of minor H antigens may be responsible for the relatively unimpressive effect of MHC matching, as discussed earlier (Section 20.4). It has been speculated that the exceptionally rapid rejection of grafts that carry allogeneic MHC antigens may represent the cumulative effect of antigens determined by the different genes constituting the MHC and that each MHC antigen alone may not be significantly different in its immunogenicity from some of the stronger minor H antigens. The cumulative effect is limited by the immunogenicity (strength) of two or more minor antigens and is usually pronounced when the individual antigens involved have rather similar immunogenicity. Conversely, the effect is obliterated when one of the antigens is significantly stronger than the other. The mechanism of the cumulative effect remains unknown except that the activation of several different antigen-specific clones most likely plays an important role.

Recently, an interesting phenomenon of gene interaction that underlies the expression of some minor H genes was reported. A mutant of a minor H gene called $H(KH-11)$ requires that the H-$2D^b$ allele be phenotypically expressed. The interaction is highly specific since other H-$2D$ alleles, or even a mutant of the H-$2D^b$ allele (H-$2D^{bm14}$), do not permit the expression of this specific minor antigen. The mechanism of this interaction is a total enigma.

The immunogenicity of minor H antigens and the MST of grafts bearing them are affected in some instances by the MHC of the recipient and/or donor. Such an effect, reminiscent of Ir control and/or MHC restriction, has been demonstrated for several minor antigens (H-3, H-4, H-7, H-Y) and even for the mutant called H(KH-29A). Interestingly, the effect has been mapped to various segments of the H-2 complex. In addition it has often been observed that female hosts reject allografts incompatible for minor H antigens more rapidly than do male hosts. This higher reactivity of females appears to be mediated by sex hormones rather than by an immune mechanism per se.

21.5 Graft versus Host Reaction

Since the GVHR (Sections 4.13 and 20.3) is mediated by cellular processes essentially similar, if not identical, to those involved in the HVGR, it should come as no surprise that minor H antigens can and do elicit a GVHR. Because the standard methods suitable for detection and measurement of the GVHR in vivo are less sensitive than the method used to detect the HVGR, it was originally believed that minor H antigens do not elicit a GVHR. However, systematic studies have shown beyond reasonable doubt that minor H antigens can elicit a serious and even lethal GVHR. Such a reaction may not be detectable by ordinary methods—e.g., splenomegaly assay (Section 4.13))—and often has a chronic character, but in some instances, the reaction is strongly pronounced and may lead to a high mortality rate in animals. As in the case of the HVGR, the minor antigens involved in the GVHR often display a cumulative effect but occasionally may counteract each other and inhibit the GVHR by a rather mysterious mechanism.

21.6 Responses to Minor H Antigens in Vitro

The early phase of the response to alloantigens, as represented by the MLR, is often difficult to demonstrate in vitro. Both positive and negative results have been reported involving a difference of a single minor H antigen. On the other hand, differences for more than a single H antigen usually produce a definite primary MLR. It should be mentioned that one of the systems —Mls antigens (Section 21.13)—has been identified exclusively on the basis of the MLR. The magnitude of the MLR elicited by minor H antigens may be influenced by the MHC genes of the responder. The genes affecting the MLR induced by a minor H antigen have been mapped to the *I-A* and *I-C* subregions. The last phase of the response to alloantigens is represented by the CML assay, which has been positive for several different minor antigens (H-3, H-4, H-7, H-8, H-13, and H-Y). The inductive and effectoral phases of the CML are MHC restricted—i.e., the lysis of target cells carrying minor H antigens requires identity of the class I antigens of the stimulator and target (Section 19.7). Whether the identity of the MHC antigens of the effector cells is also required remains the subject of speculation.

21.7 Antibody Responses to Minor H Antigens

Although under normal circumstances a single challenge with minor H antigens does not result in appreciable antibody production, the titers of such antibodies can be boosted by repeated challenges. Once induced, the antibodies have specificity for several distinct determinants and are often cross-reactive with other minor H antigens. Production of antibodies in a conditio sine qua non for the isolation and chemical analysis of the antigenic molecules from cell homogenates. So far, antibodies against H-3, H-4, and H-Y antigens have been successfully produced. At least one such antigen (H-4) has been isolated and characterized as a glycoprotein of molecular weight 45,000.

SOME MINOR H ANTIGENS OF MICE

There is little specific information concerning most of the minor H antigens in mice. Some antigens, however, have attracted special attention and have become the subject of more extensive studies.

21.8 The Male Histocompatibility (H-Y) Antigen

At least one minor H antigen is located on the male Y chromosome since within highly inbred strains grafts from males to females are rejected, while female grafts with few exceptions are accepted by males. Originally, it has been postulated that at least two alleles—$H\text{-}Y^a$ and $H\text{-}Y^b$— are identifiable. However, these early reports could not be confirmed in subsequent studies; currently, the prevalent view is that the $H\text{-}Y$ gene is nonpolymorphic, unless there are some allelic variants in wild mice. The expression of the $H\text{-}Y$ gene appears to be influenced by male hormones, but this influence is not solely responsible for the expression; a male castrated at birth still expresses the antigen. It seems that the H-Y antigen is expressed on most cells of an individual. Interestingly, H-Y seems to be expressed on the acrosomal part of more than 50 percent of spermatozoa. Whether the spermatozoa that express H-Y correspond to those that carry a Y chromosome is a matter of conjecture. Specific total removal of such spermatozoa has not been accomplished; however, treatment of sperm with antibodies to H-Y does reduce the proportion of males in subsequent litters. The H-Y antigen, besides eliciting graft rejection, is also able to induce an MHC-restricted CML both in mice and in man. Furthermore, antibodies to the H-Y antigen have been produced by the immunization of females with multiple male skin grafts. However, some authors believe that the molecules responsible for male graft rejection (H-Y) and those responsible for induction of antibodies (serologically detectable male [SDM] antigen) are two distinct moieties. The distinction is based on findings that tissues of a mutant lacking the H-Y antigen by skin grafting criteria and lacking the entire Y chromosome still carried SDM antigen detectable by antibody formation. However, the two antigens may be related since antibodies to the SDM antigen block cytotoxic cells directed against the H-Y antigen. The rejection of a skin graft bearing the H-Y antigen is influenced by several genes, including genes in the MHC. In fact, it was reported that responses to H-Y and SDM are controlled by different MHC genes. These genes, or at least some of them, may act as either Ir genes or as restrictive elements. Some strains—e.g., carrying the $H\text{-}2^b$ haplotype—invariably reject an H-Y-incompatible graft within about 30 days, while other strains—e.g., carrying the $H\text{-}2^k$ haplotype—reject only some grafts or do not reject at all. Factorial analysis indicates that several genes with complementary properties may be involved in this effect.

The physiologic role of either H-Y or SDM remains the subject of dispute. Although available data are still fragmentary, they permit a conclusion that neither antigen is a primary factor responsible for sexual differentiation of an individual.

21.9 The Female Histocompatibility (H-X) Antigen

Using the reciprocal hybrids (A × B)F1 and (B × A)F1, one obtains males that differ according to the source of their sex chromosomes: X^aY^b or X^bY^a, respectively. F1 females in both instances are identical, being X^aX^b. In such a situation, a skin graft from a female F1 may be rejected by a male F1 recipient. This rejection has been accepted as support for the idea of a polymorphic $H\text{-}X$ gene. At least three alleles—$H\text{-}X^b$, $H\text{-}X^c$, and $H\text{-}X^l$—are known at present. Virtually nothing is known about the nature of the antigen and its tissue distribution, although the antigen must be expressed on skin cells since skin grafts are rejected.

21.10 Skin-Specific (Skn) Histocompatibility Antigen

The Skn antigen was postulated to explain skin graft rejection occurring in lymphoid and hemopoietic chimeras, which, by definition, must be tolerant of lymphoid cells. Rejection of skin grafts, while simultaneously tolerating lymphoid cell grafts, suggested that skin must have an antigen that is absent in lymphoid tissue. Such an antigen was named Skn and its gene $Skn\text{-}1$ (formerly Sk). The $Skn\text{-}1$ gene has at least two alleles, $Skn\text{-}1^a$ and $Skn\text{-}1^b$, that determine corresponding allelic products, Skn-1.1 and Skn-1.2, found in prototype strains A and C57BL, respectively. The products elicit immune responses that result in skin graft rejection with an MST of about 26 days. However, the immunogenicity of allelic products of the $Skn\text{-}1$ gene varies broadly. For example, the Skn-1.2 antigen causes rejection of only 50 percent of grafts and then in a chronic manner. This difference may also reflect an Ir effect on the recipient's response to Skn antigens (Section 19.2). Also, the presence of specific cytotoxic T (T$_c$) cells directed to Skn antigens has been demonstrated in vitro. The skin graft rejection is accompanied by the production of specific antibodies. The availability of antibodies made it possible to demonstrate that the Skn antigen is expressed only on epidermal, normal brain, and neuroblastoma cells but not on lymphoid cells. Although at this time the *Skn* gene is considered to be an independent entity, further studies are needed to rule out the possibility that it is identical with one of the known minor *H* genes. In addition, some recently conducted progeny studies suggest that there may be at least two *Skn* genes (*Skn-1* and *Skn-2*) that segregate independently and affect graft rejection.

21.11 Epidermal Alloantigens (Epa)

In a series of experiments, it was demonstrated that immunization of mice with isolated allogeneic epidermal cells results in the generation of cytotoxic T (T$_c$) cells that are exquisitely specific for epidermal cells. The activity of these T$_c$ cells was found to be restricted by the *K* region of the *H-2* complex. Most significantly, the survival of skin allografts was clearly correlated with the induction of the T$_c$ cells. On the basis of these data, it was postulated that both T$_c$ cells and graft rejection are elicited by the molecules determined by the *Epa-1* gene that is expressed selectively on epidermal cells. The *Epa-1* gene is believed to have two alleles that determine two phenotypes characterized by the presence (Epa-1$^+$) or absence (Epa-1$^-$) of the antigenic molecule. Preliminary data indicate that there may be another gene, *Epa-2*, with alleles determining the presence (Epa-2$^+$) or absence (Epa-2$^-$) of still another molecule expressed selectively on epidermal cells. The relationship between *Skn* and *Epa* genes remains so far unresolved.

21.12 *H* Genes Associated with Allogenic Markers

In some instances, when congenic lines differing by certain allogenic markers are produced, members of the congenic pairs reject reciprocal skin grafts. Two explanations can be invoked for this. On the one hand, the allogenic marker itself may be expressed on skin cells and act as a histocompatibility antigen; on the other hand, a histocompatibility gene may be closely linked to the marker gene for which these congenic lines were selected. While in some instances the first explanation cannot be ruled out, in other cases the existence of distinct *H* gene(s) has been experimentally demonstrated.

The *H-Thy-1* gene associated with the *Thy-1* gene (Section 22.4) has been proposed because *Thy-1*-congenic strains A and A-*Thy-1^a* or B6 and B.PL(74NS) (Table 5.7) reject, at least in some instances, reciprocal skin grafts. The rejection is unrelated to production of anti-Thy-1 antibodies. Since the Thy-1 antigen may be present on some epithelial cells, it is possible that this antigen could be responsible for skin graft rejection. Alternatively, it may be that the rejection is due to the closely linked *H-25* and/or *H-35* genes that are on the same chromosome as the *Thy-1* gene.

Originally, two histocompatibility genes—*H(Tla-1)* and *H(Tla-2)*—associated with the

Tla complex (Section 22.1) were proposed. Incompatibility for alleles of these genes would account for the rejection of an A skin graft by the (A-*Tla^b* × B6-*Tla^a*)F1 hybrids and the rejection of an A-*Tla^b* skin graft by (A × B6-*Tla^a*)F1 hybrids. Such a rejection could not be caused by an incompatibility of the *Tla* complex because TL antigens are not expressed on skin cells. The two loci were subsequently renamed *H-31* and *H-32*, respectively, and mapped between the *H-2D* gene and the *Tla* complex.

Similarly, the *H* genes were postulated to be located in close vicinity to the *Lyt-1* and *Lyt-2-Lyt-3* genes (Sections 22.9 and 22.10), since *Lyt*-congenic mice reject reciprocal skin grafts. The *H(Ly-1)* gene, which is presumably associated with the *Lyt-1* gene, appears to be a separate gene, since two independently derived congenic pairs differed with respect to graft rejection. The difference in rejection suggests that in one pair the *H(Ly-1)* and *Lyt-1* genes were still connected, while in the other pair the two loci had been separated by crossing-over at some stage in the production of the congenic strains. The skin graft rejection observed between Lyt-2,3-congenic mice suggested an *H* gene closely linked to the *Lyt-2* and *Lyt-3* genes. In fact, two or even three genes had to be postulated to account for the different patterns of rejection in various backcross generations. Genes called *H(Ly-2,3)*, *H(Ly-2-N8)*, and *H(Ly-2-N16)* are believed to be distinct from the *Lyt-2* and *Lyt-3* genes, but formal proof is still lacking.

To this same category belong other minor *H* genes that have been identified on the basis of an association with some other morphological and behavioral markers; these still bear provisional names (Table 21.2). Among these genes, those assigned to the same chromosome have not been formally separated; they may turn out to be identical.

21.13 Minor Lymphocyte-Stimulating (*Mls*) Gene

At least some cases of MLR attributed to stimulation by minor H antigens could be due to differences at the *Mls* locus. This locus is assigned to murine chromosome 1; the gene at this locus has four alleles—*Mls^a*, *Mls^b*, *Mls^c*, and *Mls^d*. The products of the *Mls^a* or *Mls^d* allele elicit the strongest MLR reaction and are sometimes designated Mls^{++} to distinguish them from the others designated Mls$^+$ or Mls$^-$. The Mls antigens, while invariably eliciting an MLR, may also elicit graft rejection, but the pattern of rejection is often inconsistent. Interestingly, the MLR elicited by Mls antigens is restricted by class II molecules, is mediated by T_h cells, and does not lead to the generation of T_c cells (Section 22.11). Recently, it has been reported that there is active recruitment of the T cells during an ongoing reaction; this recruitment may be responsible for the apparent lack of restriction during a secondary MLR elicited by Mls.

MINOR HISTOCOMPATIBILITY ANTIGENS IN OTHER SPECIES

There is a great deal of evidence that multiple minor histocompatibility antigens exist in various species other than mice. Unfortunately, only some of these species have been investigated to an extent that permits even partial comparison with the murine model.

In the rat, at least six antigens have been distinguished (Table 21.4). The antigens are present in skin and some are also found on erythrocytes, but analysis of their tissue distribution

TABLE 21.4. Minor Histocompatibility Genes in Rats

Histocompatibility Locus	Former Nomenclature	Genomic Position (linkage group)	Number of Alleles*	Tissue Distribution
RT2	AgC, H-3	V	2	Skin, erythrocytes
RT3	AgD	?	2	Erythrocytes
RT4	H-4	I	2	Skin, lymphocytes
RT5	H-5	VII	2	Skin
H-Y	—	Y	?	Skin
H-X	—	X	?	Skin

*Designated by lowercase a or b superscripts.
NOTE: T cell alloantigens are excluded.

is incomplete at present. As in mice, the minor H genes of the rat seem to have a rather limited polymorphism, since usually only two allelic products are distinguishable by the histogenetic method. Thus far, only one antigen, RT2, has been chemically isolated and found to be a glycoprotein of molecular weight 36,000. Among the isolated molecules, two types are distinguishable on the basis of chemical and immunologic properties. The RT2 antigen may be a homologue of the murine blood group antigen, Ea-1 (Section 13.1). Skin-reactive transplantation antibodies (SRTA) found in rats seem to detect the antigen analogous to the Skn antigen of mice. However, in contrast to mice, the SRTA antigen was shown to be present in low concentration on lymphoidal cells, and there is no evidence that this antigen is responsible for skin graft rejection. In the dog, at least two minor histocompatibility antigens have been reported. One antigen seems to be determined by a gene linked to the *Pgm-2* gene that encodes phosphoglucomutase. The antigen was shown to cause GVHR. The second gene is located on the Y chromosome and has properties similar to the murine *H-Y* gene. Two alloantigens—OL-X and OL-Z—were described in sheep, but their role in graft rejection remains to be established.

Even less is known about human minor H antigens, though neither their existence nor their role in graft rejection has ever been in doubt. Evidence for such antigens stems from observations of renal graft rejection that occurs even in cases of a complete HLA match and the finding of antibodies unabsorbable with either HLA or blood group antigens. The antibodies react with either T or B cells or both; some of these antibodies may define lymphoid cell antigens (Chapters 22 and 23). Recently, it was shown that CML reaction not directed to the HLA antigens could be induced in vitro. The target antigen of this reaction has been named effector (Ef) and may represent the product of one or several minor histocompatibility antigens. Some of these antigens may be analogous to Skn and Epa of mice.

It should be noted that apparently two distinct antigens, H-Y and SDM, were described in man. Their biologic properties seem to be analogous to those of the murine antigens. The H-Y induces a cell-mediated response, resulting in rejection of male graft, whereas the SDM elicits production of antibodies.

22 / Cell Surface Alloantigens of T Cells

Considering the functional diversity of immunologically competent cells, it is not at all surprising that they carry a large number of various cell surface markers. Furthermore, different functional subsets within both the T and B cell populations are distinguishable by specific alloantigens and/or their combinations. In this chapter the genetics, biochemistry, and biologic properties of the alloantigens expressed by T cells will be discussed in some detail. From the anatomical point of view, thymus-derived (T) cells can be subdivided into two broad classes: **extrathymic** or peripheral (T cells) and **intrathymic** (thymocytes). The T cell population can be further subdivided into **prethymic** and **postthymic**. Although no specific markers have yet been identified on prethymic T cells, intrathymic and extrathymic cells can be more or less clearly distinguished. Table 22.1 lists the different subsets of T cells and their most important markers.

THE *Tla* COMPLEX

The thymus leukemia antigen complex (*Tla*) determines a set of so-called TL alloantigens, which, under normal conditions, are expressed only on intrathymic T cells. Because of this restricted expression, products of the *Tla* complex can be considered as differentiation antigens. This notion is further supported by the fact that TL antigens, normally absent from the extrathymic T cells, may reappear when such cells undergo neoplastic transformation.

22.1 Genetics of the *Tla* Complex

The *Tla* complex is located on the right (telomeric) side of the *H-2* complex at a distance of about 1.5 cM from the complex. Its fine structure still remains the subject of speculation. To

TABLE 22.1. Major Subsets of Murine T Cells and Their Alloantigenic Profiles

Class	Subset (synonym)	Frequency in Periphery (percent)	Restricting Class of MHC Molecules	TL	Thy-1	Lyt-1	Lyt-2,3	Qa-1	Ia
Intrathymic (thymocytes)	(T_0)	0	?	+ (80–90 percent)	+ (90–100 percent)	+ (95 percent)	+ (95 percent)	?	?
Postthymic (T cells)	Precursors (T_1, T_E)	50–55	?	–	+	+	+	?	?
	Helper $(T_2, T_h$ or $T_{DTH})$	30–35	II	–	+	+	–	?	+ (I-A,I-E)
	Suppressor $(T_2$ or $T_s)$	5–10	I	–	+	–*	+	+	+ (I-J)
	Cytotoxic $(T_2$ or $T_c)$	5–10	I	–	+	–*	+	–	–

*In fact, a certain amount of Lyt-1 can be detected with high affinity antibodies.

account for the presently available data, a model consisting of three closely linked loci, each carrying a gene with a limited number of alleles, has been proposed.

The *Tla.1* gene presumably has a single allele that determines a molecule that carries TL-1 antigenic specificity. This allele is present in all laboratory strains even though in some of these strains it may not be expressed on normal thymocytes. The *Tla.2* gene also has a single allele that determines a molecule with TL-2 specificity. This allele is also present in all laboratory mice, but occasionally it may not be expressed on normal thymocytes. The *Tla.3* gene probably has several alleles, each determining a molecule bearing a combination of four specificities, TL-3, TL-4, TL-5, and TL-6. According to this concept, at least five different alleles of the *Tla.3* gene can be identified. The three genes form a complex, and the alleles actually present in a given genome form the *Tla* haplotype that is inherited as a unit. No intra-*Tla* crossing-over has been reported. There are five distinct *Tla* haplotypes designated Tla^a, Tla^b, Tla^c, Tla^d, and Tla^e.

To determine the haplotype of a given strain, one must test not only normal thymocytes but also leukemic cells that arise in this strain. This is because normal thymocytes often do not express alleles of certain loci even though the alleles are actually present in the genome. Table 22.2 shows the phenotypes of normal thymocytes and the corresponding leukemic cells that allow the determination of the five haplotypes. As can be seen, leukemic cells of all tested strains except those carrying the Tla^a haplotype express one or more specificities that are not detectable on normal thymocytes. One can explain this phenomenon by postulating that the expression of the structural *Tla* genes is under the control of regulatory genes that selectively suppress or derepress *Tla* genes during both normal and neoplastic differentiation of T cells. A particular TL phenotype is found to be associated with a corresponding H-2 phenotype—an arrangement that implies that the regulatory, but not necessarily the structural, genes must be linked to the *H-2* complex. The exact position of the structural *Tla* genes has not been established, but it seems likely that they are on chromosome 17, because established cell lines that have lost chromosome 17 lack both TL and H-2 antigens. Activation and deactivation of the regulatory genes require a thymic environment. Bone marrow-derived prethymic T cells, which are TL$^-$, repopulate the host thymus and become TL$^+$ when grafted into an irradiated host. The TL phenotype of repopulating cells corresponds to that of the donor and not of the host. However, when the same cells are grafted into irradiated and thymectomized animals, no expression of the TL antigens can be demonstrated.

22.2 Phenotypic Expression of the TL Antigens

TL molecules are detected by the standard cytotoxic assay in which cells are first treated with alloantibodies to a given TL specificity and then with complement (Section 4.7). The allo-antisera are produced in selected mouse strains that lack a given antigen (specificity) by immunization with thymocytes or leukemic cells that possess or express that antigen. Curiously, although postthymic cells (lymph node or splenic peripheral lymphocytes) do not express detectable TL antigens, immunization with such TL$^-$ cells occasionally may induce a specific anti-TL response. This can be explained by assuming that some of the cells used for immunization reach the responder's thymus and, under the influence of the thymic environment,

TABLE 22.2. *Tla* Genotypes and TL Phenotypes of Normal Thymocytes and Leukemic Cells

Tla Haplotype	*Tla* Genotype[a]			TL Phenotype of Normal Thymocytes (leukemic cells)[b]					
	Locus 1	Locus 2	Locus "3"	TL-1	TL-2	TL-3	TL-4	TL-5	TL-6
a	*Tla.1*	*Tla.2*	*Tla.3,5,6*	+	+	+	−	+	+
				(+	+	+	−	+	?)
b	*Tla.1*	*Tla.2*	*Tla.4*	−	−	−	−	−	−
				(+	+	−	+	−	?)
c	*Tla.1*	*Tla.2*	*Tla.4,5*	−	+	−	−	−	−
				(+	+	−	+	+	?)
d	*Tla.1*	*Tla.2*	*Tla.3*	+	+	+	−	−	−
				(		none known			)
e	*Tla.1*	*Tla.2*	*Tla.3,5*	+	+	+	−	+	−
				(		none known			)

[a]Three-locus model assumed.
[b]Some leukemias of the same genotype may have different phenotypes.

become TL$^+$. This assumption is based on the fact that no anti-TL response appears in thymectomized mice immunized with TL$^-$ cells, although these mice do respond to immunization with TL$^+$ cells.

TL antigens are present almost exclusively on thymocytes, of which 80 to 90 percent react with specific anti-TL antibodies. Only the most mature, cortisone-resistant thymocytes seem to lack TL antigens. TL antigens cannot be detected in any other lymphoid organ; hence they are either totally absent or present only on an extremely small fraction of cells. TL antigens are present on the cell membrane of thymocytes and on the mitochondrial membrane. The most interesting property of the TL antigens is their expression on cells of some leukemias, even when the strain of origin of a given leukemia does not express any (the *Tla^b* haplotype) or expresses only some (the *Tla^c* haplotype) specificities. In fact, the TL-4 specificity encoded by *Tla^b* and *Tla^c* haplotypes is expressed on leukemic cells but never on normal thymocytes. The mechanism of derepression of *Tla* genes during neoplastic transformation remains unknown. Moreover, the role of TL antigens in such a transformation is not clear, since some mutants of leukemic cells that have lost *Tla* genes still remain highly malignant.

The expression of the TL antigens is influenced by two phenomena—**interaction** and **modulation**. The interaction phenomenon refers to the reduced amount of a given TL antigen in heterozygous animals, depending on the two *Tla* haplotypes. Reduction, however, cannot be explained by a simple gene dose effect since it also occurs in some homozygous animals that carry two identical alleles. An alternative explanation is based on the observation that the quantities of the TL and H-2D antigens expressed in a given cell are inversely related. Thus, TL$^+$ thymocytes (*Tla^a*, *Tla^c*, *Tla^d*, and *Tla^e* haplotypes) have fewer H-2D molecules as compared with TL$^-$ thymocytes (*Tla^b* haplotype). Reduction does not depend on the particular *H-2D* allele nor on the relative position of the *Tla* and *H-2D* loci involved. Three explanations are possible:

the two antigens may interact in such a manner that the TL antigen masks the H-2D molecules; or the two antigens may physically compete for space on the cell surface; or each antigen may compete for the same common precursor. There is no direct evidence to favor any one of these mechanisms over the others.

The modulation phenomenon refers to a decrease in the quantity of TL molecules on cells exposed to antibodies specific for the TL antigen expressed on these cells. An exception is the TL-2 antigen, which not only does not modulate but it elicits antibodies that inhibit modulation of other TL antigens on the same cells. The process of modulation requires metabolic activity and is temperature dependent but does not require complement or bivalency of antibodies. The monovalent F(ab) fragment is as efficient in modulation as is the divalent $F(ab')_2$ fragment or intact IgG. Modulation can be elicited in vitro by incubation of thymocytes or leukemic cells with appropriate anti-TL serum. In vivo modulation can be evoked by injecting anti-TL antibodies into TL^+ animals or by injecting TL^+ leukemic cells into animals that have anti-TL antibodies. Modulation does not cause redistribution of TL molecules (capping), though some patching does appear (Section 4.5).

Modulated cells become resistant to the lytic action of anti-TL and complement. Resistance induced by modulation explains why preimmunization of a TL^- animal does not result in accelerated rejection of TL^+ leukemia grafts. Although it would be appealing to assume that resistance to lysis is the direct result of the loss of TL molecules during modulation, there are certain data that contradict this supposition; modulated cells that resist lysis by guinea pig complement are nevertheless lysed by rabbit complement. It is, therefore, possible that modulation represents, rather than the simple loss of TL antigen, an alteration of the antigen on the membrane in such a way that guinea pig complement cannot be activated, whereas rabbit complement can be. The mechanism of modulation is still unresolved. Both blocking of antigenic sites and selection of TL^- cells appear unlikely explanations. The possibility remains that modulation per se reflects enhanced degradation of TL molecules. This concept is supported by the finding of dependency of modulation on metabolic activity, reversibility of modulation, and an increase in the quantity of H-2D molecules with concomitant decrease of TL molecule concentration.

22.3 Biochemistry of TL Molecules

TL molecules isolated from thymocytes or leukemic cells are tetramers (molecular weight $\sim$ 120,000) bound by disulfide bridges. Each tetramer consists of two identical or similar heavy chains (molecular weight 44,000–50,000) and two light chains (molecular weight 12,000). The heavy chains are glycoproteins, whereas the light chains are β_2-microglobulin. The structure of the TL molecules is remarkably similar to that of the class I MHC molecules, and it is widely speculated that TL antigens both phylogenetically and functionally are related to the H-2 antigens.

THE MURINE THYMUS ANTIGEN—Thy-1

An alloantigen specific for both extra- and intrathymic T cells is the Thy-1 antigen, formerly called theta (θ). Since its discovery, the Thy-1 system has been a powerful tool in the analysis of the cellular components of the murine lymphoid system. Treatment of cell suspensions with anti-Thy-1 antibodies and complement specifically eliminates the T cells from a mixed population and, thus, permits the study of the properties and functions of B cells and/or macrophages.

22.4 Genetics of the Thy-1 System

The Thy-1 system appears to be one of the simplest; it consists of a single locus on chromosome 9 with a gene that has two alleles—*Thy-1*^{a} and *Thy-1*^{b}. The two alleles determine two antigenic molecules, Thy-1.1 and Thy-1.2, formerly called θ-AKR and θ-C3H, respectively. The alleles are codominant and equally expressed in heterozygotes. Although Thy-1 antigens are expressed on all T cells, their concentration varies from low in prothymocytes to intermediate in mature thymocytes and peripheral T cells and high in immature thymocytes. Whether these differences depend on regulatory genes or on the effect of the thymic environment has not been determined. Recently, monoclonal antibodies to the Thy-1 antigens were shown to distinguish between long-lived and short-lived T cells on the basis of their expression of the Thy-1 antigen. Short-lived T cells appear to be more susceptible to lysis by high dilutions of these antibodies.

22.5 Thy-1 Phenotypes

The Thy-1 phenotypes of various inbred strains can be determined using specific anti-Thy-1.1 or anti-Thy-1.2 sera raised in *Thy-1*-congenic strains by reciprocal immunization. Presently, the following four *Thy-1*-congenic pairs are available: A and A-*Thy-1*^{a}, B6 and B6.PL(74NS), B10.S(7R) and B10.S(7R)-*Thy-1*^{a}, and B6.C-H-*2*^{d} and B6.C-*Thy-1*^{a}. Using specific alloimmune sera or monoclonal antibodies, one can determine both the strain and tissue distribution of the Thy-1 alloantigens.

Among the hundreds of inbred strains presently maintained in laboratories, only 15 carry the *Thy-1*^{a} allele that determines the Thy-1.1 antigen. All other strains carry the *Thy-1*^{b} allele and express the Thy-1.2 antigen. As Thy-1 antigens are present on thymocytes as well as on virtually all T cells, the number of Thy-1$^+$ cells in various lymphoid organs reflects the T cell content. Thus, 95 percent of thymus cells, 55 to 60 percent of lymph node cells, 30 percent of spleen cells, and about 1 percent or less of bone marrow cells are Thy-1$^+$. Interestingly, about 20 percent of all spleen cells in athymic mice express a low amount of the Thy-1 antigen. These cells probably represent prethymic T cells, but this conjecture requires experimental confirmation. In this connection it seems relevant to note that recently, it was reported that under conditions of in vitro cultures many bone marrow cells may express a significant amount of the Thy-1 antigen. The subcellular location of Thy-1 antigen is not known except for its presence on the cell surface. If it is a transmembrane molecule, it is shed extremely easily. Thymocytes incubated for about 24 hours lose almost all of their Thy-1 molecules, which then can be found free in the culture medium.

A most interesting finding concerning the phenotypic expression of the Thy-1 antigen is its presence on cells of the central nervous system. The concentration of Thy-1 antigen in brain tissue increases significantly during the first three weeks of postnatal life, and this increase parallels the process of **synaptogenesis**. The concentration of Thy-1 antigen in various parts of the nervous system is proportional to the number of synapses in these parts.

The Thy-1 antigen is not subject to modulation, since the immunization of a pregnant female with the Thy-1 antigen of her fetus has no appreciable effect on the Thy-1 phenotype of the fetus. The Thy-1 antigen elicits a specific humoral immune response, which has been extensively studied in several laboratories from both the practical and theoretical points of view. There are extremely complex genetic and cellular requirements for eliciting a good anti-Thy-1 response in vivo. Such a response, when elicited by the injection of Thy-1 disparate thymocytes, is restricted by both class I and class II molecules. This restriction suggests that the Thy-1 antigen may be recognized as cell bound and/or cell free, depending on the genetic makeup of the responder and donor animals. Responsiveness to cell free antigen seems to be under the control of complementary *Ir* genes, and combinatorial class II determinants probably play an important role in determining the magnitude of the response. Interestingly, although the cell-mediated response to the Thy-1 antigen has been studied only superficially, preliminary data suggest that the antigen does not elicit this type of response.

22.6 Biochemistry of Thy-1 Antigens

The chemical structure of Thy-1 is still the subject of debate. Some workers consider that the Thy-1 molecule is a glycoprotein of molecular weight 19,000–25,000; others suggest that Thy-1 antigenicity is associated with a glycolipid (ganglioside GM1), a finding so far not confirmed adequately. The molecule is almost certainly glycoprotein since both allo- and xenoantisera reproducibly precipitate a glycoprotein of molecular weight 19,000. It has been estimated that there may be as many as 600,000 molecules of Thy-1 per cell. After solubilization, the single molecules may form large aggregates (molecular weight 250,000). Antigenic specificity of the molecule seems to reside in the protein rather than the carbohydrate portion, even though the latter constitutes as much as 30 percent of the molecule. Amino acid sequence analysis revealed that murine brain Thy-1 antigen is remarkably similar to that of rat (Section 22.8). The two allelic Thy-1 molecules differ by a single amino acid at position 89, at which Thy-1.1 has arginine and Thy-1.2 has glutamine.

22.7 Biologic Properties of Thy-1 Antigens

Since the Thy-1 antigen is found on T cells as well as in nonlymphoid (brain) tissue, it is rather doubtful that its primary function is immunologic. Nevertheless, there are reports that Thy-1 molecules may participate in cell-cell interaction between T and B cells. This supposition is based on the finding that anti-Thy-1 serum influences humoral responses by decreasing the effect exerted on such a response by the T suppressor factor(s). Furthermore, the role of Thy-1 in cell-cell interaction does not have to be limited to lymphoid cells; the Thy-1 antigen present in the synapses may well participate in neuronal interaction. It has been proposed that the protein segment serves to anchor the molecule to the cell membrane, whereas the carbohydrate residue actually mediates the cell-cell interaction.

22.8 Thy-1 Analogues in Other Species

All laboratory strains of rats have on their cells a molecule analogous, if not identical, to the murine Thy-1.1. The similarity is especially striking when the chemical composition and reactivity with anti-Thy-1.1 sera are compared. However, there are striking differences in the tissue distribution of the rat molecule. The rat antigen is present on 95 percent of thymocytes but only on 5 to 15 percent of peripheral T cells. On the other hand, as many as 40 percent of rat bone marrow cells are lysed by anti-Thy-1.1 serum. This cellular distribution indicates that the rat antigen cannot be considered as a bona fide T cell marker. Rather, it may be that the rat Thy-1 antigen represents a marker of prethymic and intrathymic cells, a marker that disappears from most of the mature T cells. In similarity to the mouse, the rat Thy-1 antigen is also found in the brain in decreasing concentrations in cortex, cerebellum, brain stem, spinal cord, and olfactory areas. Interestingly, a high concentration of Thy-1 antigen is present in an established cell line of neurinoma cells. Serologic studies suggest that whereas both allelic molecules of the murine Thy-1 share some determinants with the rat antigen, the rat and mouse share only the Thy-1.1, not the Thy-1.2, determinant.

The amino acid sequence of the Thy-1 molecule from rat brain was reported; this molecule consists of 111 amino acid residues that form two overlapping disulfide loops. One loop is between cysteines at positions 9 and 111, while the other is between cysteines at positions 19 and 85. The molecule seems to be similar to immunoglobulin domains (V, C and β-m) both by amino acid sequence and secondary structure (extensive β pleats). This homology may be only incidental, but it warrants further studies. The molecule has three sugar chains attached to asparagines at positions 23, 74, and 98. Although the C terminus has hydrophobic properties, it does not have an apparent sequence of hydrophobic amino acids. Perhaps this unusual situation is responsible for the ease with which Thy-1 is shed from the cell membrane.

So far, no clear-cut evidence for a Thy-1 analogue has been found in man. However, an antigen that can be detected on 70 percent of thymocytes but not on the peripheral lymphocytes has been given the designation THY (T6). This antigen can be detected with a commercially available monoclonal reagent. Its genetic determination and polymorphism are not yet established. It should be mentioned that structurally similar glycoproteins were isolated from brains of various species (man, dog, chicken and squid).

LYMPHOCYTE (Ly) ANTIGENS

At this time, there are over two dozen of distinct antigens that are expressed on murine lymphocytes. Originally, they were given the designation Ly followed by a number, but subsequent studies suggested that some are expressed exclusively on T cells, while others are found only on B cells, and still others are on both T and B cells. This prompted the classification of Ly antigens into three groups: Lyt, Lyb, and Ly. This renaming was intended to introduce some order into the steadily growing number of lymphocyte markers, but, unfortunately, it led to more confusion. Follow-up studies carried out with better reagents and by more sensitive methods revealed that some antigens classified as Lyt are present on some B cells and, thus, should be called Ly. With this in mind, both nomenclatures will be given to help the reader in following current and earlier publications. Since it has been demonstrated that in many instances conventional and monoclonal antibodies may detect different determinants, it has been proposed that for the markers defined with monoclonal antibodies the assigned number should be preceded by a lower-case letter m. In this chapter, discussion will be limited to those Ly antigens that are expressed exclusively on T cells (Lyt) or on both T and B cells (Ly) (Tables 22.3 and 22.4), whereas antigens expressed exclusively or predominantly on B cells (Lyb) will be described in the next chapter.

22.9 The *Lyt-1* Gene and its Products

Lyt-1 (formerly called Ly-A, Ly-1, or μ) was the first lymphocyte antigen system described in mice. Its presence is determined by the *Lyt-1* gene on chromosome 19. This gene has two alleles—*Lyt-1^a* and *Lyt-1^b*—that determine two allelic molecules—Lyt-1.1 and Lyt-1.2, respectively. Among laboratory mice, the *Lyt-1^a* allele is relatively rare and found only in four strains (CBA, C3H, DBA/1, and DBA/2). Both allelic products are detectable by appropriate antisera raised by reciprocal immunization of either *Lyt-1*-congenic mice or by immunization of noncongenic mice. In the second case, appropriate absorption makes the antisera monospecific for Lyt-1 antigen. Monospecific or monoclonal antibodies can be used to demonstrate that Lyt-1 antigens are present on most T cells (thymocytes and peripheral T cells). Only 5 to 10 percent of Thy-1$^+$ cells do not express Lyt-1 antigen. Even this small fraction of T cells that seem to lack Lyt-1 antigen may actually express it, but in very low concentration. During ontogenesis, the Lyt-1 antigen first appears by the end of the second week of embryogenesis, and thereafter the percentage of T cells that express this antigen rapidly increases to the adult level by the time of birth. Chemical analysis of Lyt-1 antigen isolated from T cells has revealed a single chain glycoprotein of molecular weight $\sim$67,000.

22.10 The *Lyt-2* and *Lyt-3* Genes and Their Products

These two antigens were described separately, and there are convincing data that they are two distinct entities. However, the two genes—*Lyt-2* (formerly *Ly-2* or *Ly-B*) and *Lyt-3* (formerly *Ly-3* or *Ly-C*)—reside on chromosome 6 and are so closely linked that, thus far, they have not been separated by crossing-over. Each gene has two alleles that determine two allelic products. According to convention, the alleles are designated *Lyt-2^a*, *Lyt-2^b*, *Lyt-3^a*, and *Lyt-3^b*, while the corresponding molecules are called Lyt-2.1, Lyt-2.2, Lyt-3.1, and Lyt-3.2. The two alleles of the *Lyt-2* gene are equally common among laboratory mice, but the *Lyt-3^a* allele is rather rare, being found in only four strains (AKR, RF, C58, and PL).

The allelic products can be detected and identified by appropriate antisera or monoclonal antibodies. Both antigens together are present on 95 percent of thymocytes and on about 30 percent of lymph node and spleen cells. The percentage corresponds to about half of the T cell population of a lymph node but almost the entire T cell population of the spleen. Interestingly, the concentration per cell seems to be higher for thymocytes than for the peripheral T cells. Normal cells either express both or neither of the two antigens, but some neoplastic cells express only one or the other antigen. Lyt-2 and Lyt-3 molecules appear to be glycoproteins composed of two chains of molecular weight 30,000 and 45,000. The chains are linked by disulfide bridge. Since they can be sequentially precipitated by corresponding antibodies, they must be distinct molecular species. This is further indicated by different susceptibility of the two antigens to trypsin digestion; Lyt-2 is resistant, whereas Lyt-3 is susceptible. Expression of the Lyt antigens during ontogenesis resembles that of Lyt-1, although the first appearance of Lyt-3 seems to be slightly delayed in time.

22.11 Functional Considerations

Because the expression of the three Lyt antigens seems to be closely related, their possible functional significance will be discussed together. With the discovery and serologic characterization of the first three Lyt antigens, it became apparent that these antigens distinguish unique subsets of T cells (Table 22.1). The function of such subsets is a topic of immunology rather than immunogenetics. However, as a preamble, a brief summary of the available data will be made here. The Lyt antigens described above permit the distinction of at least three subsets of lymphocytes characterized by the presence of the antigens in various combinations. The subsets are referred to as Lyt-1$^+$2,3$^+$, Lyt-1$^+$, and Lyt-2,3$^+$. It is believed that the three subsets have a common precursor, a thymocyte that is TL$^+$, Lyt-1$^+$2,3$^+$. Upon maturation, these precursor cells become TL$^-$ and reach the peripheral lymphoid organs where the subset Lyt-1$^+$2,3$^+$ constitutes about 50 percent of all peripheral T cells. This subset is sometimes referred to as "early" T cells (T$_E$) or T$_1$ cells and presumably constitutes the source of two additional, more differentiated subsets jointly referred to as T$_2$ cells. One subset has the phenotype Lyt-1$^+$, corresponds to helper (T$_h$) and delayed-type hypersensitivity (T$_{DTH}$) cells, and constitutes about 30 percent of peripheral T cells. The other subset has the phenotype Lyt-2,3$^+$ (with a very low concentration of Lyt-1) and corresponds to cytotoxic (T$_c$) and suppressor (T$_s$) cells that make up about 5 to 10 percent of murine peripheral T cells. The subsets differ not only by Lyt phenotypes but also by other markers, e.g., I-J molecules, which are present on T$_s$ cells but not on T$_h$ cells. In addition, the different subsets perform different functions and are restricted by different MHC molecules (Section 19.9). Fig. 22.1 shows the postulated relationship between Lyt phenotypes and cell function. One should, however, remember that this scheme is both largely speculative and grossly oversimplified.

For example, the T$_h$ cells involved in responses to allogeneic class I molecules (Section 16.3) have the phenotype Lyt-1$^+$ 2,3$^+$, whereas the T$_c$ cells directed against aloogeneic class II molecules may have the Lyt-1$^+$ phenotype. In addition, there are subsets of augmenting (T$_a$) cells that are involved in the generation of other T cell subsets. Specific Lyt molecules, although associated with functional subsets of T cells, do not appear to be directly responsible for the ultimate function of such subsets. To appreciate fully the complexity of the relationship between Lyt phenotypes and the function of various T cell subsets, more details must be obtained from modern textbooks of immunology. Analogous markers and subsets of human T cells will be described later in this chapter.

TABLE 22.3. Alloantigen Markers of Murine T Cells

Gene	Previous or Synonymous Designation	Chromosome Position	Alleles	Products	Chemical Nature[a] and Molecular Weight	Cellular Expression (percent)[b]			Functional Subset
						Thymus	Spleen	Lymph Nodes	
Tla	—	17	Tla^a Tla^b Tla^c Tla^d Tla^e	TL-1,2,3,5,6 none TL-2 TL-1,2,3 TL-1,2,3,5	gp45,000–50,000	90–95	—	—	—
Thy-1	θ	9	$Thy\text{-}1^a$ $Thy\text{-}1^b$	Thy-1.1 Thy-1.2	gp19,000–25,000	90–100	30	60	All T cells
Lyt-1	Ly-A,Ly-1,μ	19	$Lyt\text{-}1^a$ $Lyt\text{-}1^b$	Lyt-1.1 Lyt-1.2	gp67,000	95	35	60	T_h, T_{DTH}
Lyt-2	Ly-B,Ly-2	6	$Lyt\text{-}2^a$ $Lyt\text{-}2^b$	Lyt-2.1 Lyt-2.2	gp35,000	90	13	20	T_c, T_s
Lyt-3	Ly-C,Ly-3	6	$Lyt\text{-}3^a$ $Lyt\text{-}3^b$	Lyt-3.1 Lyt-3.2	gp35,000	90	11	35–45	T_c, T_s
Lyt-4	Ly-5	1	$Lyt\text{-}4^a$ $Lyt\text{-}4^b$	Lyt-4.1 Lyt-4.2	gp15,000	95	30	60	T cells, pro-T
Ly-6	Lyt-5 ALA-1 Ren-1	9	$Ly\text{-}6^a$ $Ly\text{-}6^b$	Ly-6.1 Ly-6.2	?	5–10	25–70	70	T_c, B cells (PFC)
Ly-7	—	?	$Ly\text{-}7^a$ $Ly\text{-}7^b$	— Ly-7.2	?	+	70–80	70–80	T and B cells
Ly-8	Lyt-5(?)	?	$Ly\text{-}8^a$ $Ly\text{-}8^b$	Ly-8.1 Ly-8.2	?	15	65	40–50	T and B cells

440

Antigen	Alternative	Chromosome	Alleles	Specificities	Molecular nature[a]				Cell distribution[b]
Ly-9	—	1	Ly-9^a, Ly-9^b	Ly-9.1 (Lgp100, T100), Ly-9.2	gp100,000	+	+	+	T and B cells
Ly-10	—	19	Ly-10^a, Ly-10^b	Ly-10.1, —	?	+	+	+	—
Ly-11	—	?	Ly-11^a, Ly-11^b	Ly-11.2, —	?	−	22	22	pro-T, NK
Asialo-GM1	—	?	Asialo-GM1^a, Asialo-GM1^b	—, —	Ganglio-N tetraosylceramide	−	?	?	NK
NK-1	—		NK-1^a, NK-1^b	NK-1.2, —	?	?	?	?	NK
Qa-1	—	17	Qa-1^a, Qa-1^b	Qa-1.1, —	?	+	+	+	T_s, T_a
Qa-2	—	17	Qa-2^a, Qa-2^b	Qa-2.1, —	gp43,000	15–35	40	60	T_h(?)
Qa-3	−	17	Qa-3^a, Qa-3^b	Qa-3.1, —	gp43,000	−	20	30–50	T_h(?)
Qa-4	Qat-4	?	Qa-4^a, Qa-4^b, Qa-4^c	Qa-4.1, Qa-4.2, Qa-4.3	?	?	?	?	T cells
Qa-5	Qat-5	?	Qa-5^a, Qa-5^b	Qa-5.1, Qa-5.2	?	?	+	?	T and B cells
Ia-1	I-A	17	21 alleles	Ia	gp28,000 and 33,000	?	?	?	T_h, T_{DTH}
Ia-4	I-J	17	?	Ia	?	?	?	?	T_s
Ia-5	I-E	17	6 alleles	Ia	gp 28,000 and 33,000	?	?	?	T_h

[a] gp = glycoprotein.
[b] A plus sign (+) = presence, a minus sign (−) = absence, and question mark (?) = lack of precise data.

TABLE 22.4 Recently Reported New Alloantigen Markers of Murine Lymphoid Cells

Gene	Chromosome position	Allele	Detectable Product	Cellular Expression (percent)[a]					Functional Subset
				Bone Marrow	Thymus	Spleen	Lymph Nodes	Non-lymphoid Cells[b]	
Ly-12	?	Ly-12a	Ly-12.1	?	+	+	+	?	
Ly-13	?	Ly-13a	Ly-13.1	?	+	+	+	L,K,B,E	
Ly-14	7	Ly-14b	Ly-14.2	?	?	+	+	L,K,B	
Ly-15	9	Ly-15a	Ly-15.1	?	>95	>95	>95	L	
		Ly-15b	Ly-m15.2	?	>95	>95	>95		
Ly-17	?	Ly-17a	Ly-17.1	21	2	39	32	L	B cells
Ly-18	12	Ly-18	Ly-18	−	−	+	+		T$_c$
Ly-m18	?	Ly-m18b	Ly-m18.2	45	90	55	45	L,KB	early B, some
Ly-m19	4	Ly-m19b	Ly-m19.2	35	15	75	75		T cells
Ly-m20	1	Ly-m20b	Ly-m20.2	50	5	60	40	L,K	B cells (PFC)
Ly-21	7	Ly-21b	Ly-21.2	70	83	80	74	L	B and T, dividing cells

[a] A plus sigh (+) = presence, a minus sign (−) = absence, and question mark (?) = lack of precise data.

[b] L = liver, K = kidney, B = brain and E = erythrocytes.

442

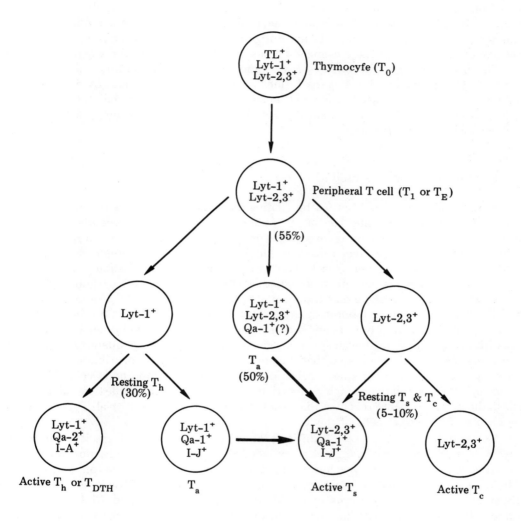

FIG. 22.1. Differentiation and relationship between subsets of murine T cells: T_h = helper; T_a = augmenting; T_s = suppressor; T_c = cytotoxic cells. **Thin arrows** indicate conversion and **bold arrows** represent interaction. The phenotypes indicated include only major markers. Percentages in parentheses correspond to the frequency of corresponding cells in the peripheral lymphatic tissue.

22.12 The *Lyt-4* Gene and Its Products

The Lyt-4 antigen (formerly Ly-5) is found predominantly on T cells, but recent data suggest that a variety of other cells may also express this antigen. Included among these cells are some myeloma cells, spleen cells of athymic mice, macrophages, neutrophils, and kidney cells. It is not yet known whether the presence of this antigen on these various cells reflects an actual expression of the antigen or the presence of cross-reactive antibodies in the sera used to define Lyt-4. The *Lyt-4* gene has two alleles—*Lyt-4^a* and *Lyt-4^b*—that determine the corresponding molecules, Lyt-4.1 and Lyt-4.2, but the former nomenclature—*Ly-5^a* and *Ly-5^b* or Ly-5.1 and Ly-5.2—is still occasionally used. The *Lyt-4^b* allele is carried by only four laboratory strains (DA, RIII, SJL, and STS). The Lyt-4 molecule is a glycoprotein of molecular weight 150,000; its biologic properties are unknown.

22.13 The *Ly-6* Gene and Its Products

The Ly-6 antigen was renamed Lyt-5 after finding that it is expressed predominantly on mature T cells. However, the renaming has been premature, because more recently several laboratories have reported that Ly-6 antigens are also present on cells other than mature T cells, i.e., B cells, mast cells, brain cells, liver cells, and kidney cells; the renal antigen was described independently and initially named Ren-1. Thus, the original name Ly-6 should be retained.

The *Ly-6* gene has not been assigned a chromosomal position though it has been suggested that the gene may be on chromosome 2. It has two alleles, *Ly-6^a* and *Ly-6^b*, of which *Ly-6^a* is less common among laboratory mice. Two corresponding allelic products, Ly-6.1 and Ly-6.2, are detected by appropriate antisera. Determination of the Ly-6 phenotype occasionally meets with some difficulties because some strains express a very low quantity of the antigen. Nevertheless, early studies revealed that the antigen is present on approximately 10 percent of thymocytes, 25–70 percent of spleen cells, and 70 percent of lymph node cells. This distribution, except for the relatively high proportion of thymocytes, resembles the distribution of T cells in these organs. More recent studies show that Ly-6 is expressed on all T_c cells regardless of the nature of the target cells of the T_c.

A clear definition of the Ly-6 is difficult for a number of reasons. First, it was noticed that the strain distribution of the Ly-6.2 antigen was for all practical reasons identical with the strain distribution of the activated lymphocyte antigen—ALA-1; ALA-1 is the antigen present on lymphoid blast cells, regardless of whether the blast cells belong to a T or B cell lineage but not on thymoblasts. Two allelic forms of the ALA antigen, ALA-1.1 and ALA-1.2, have been described. It was also shown that the strain distribution of these forms corresponds to the distribution of the Ly-6.1 and Ly-6.2 allelic molecules. With this information available, it seems justified to propose that the *Ly-6* and *ALA-1* genes are identical.

A second difficulty in defining the Ly-6 system was the finding that anti-Ly-6.2 sera could be almost completely absorbed by purified preparations of murine leukemia virus (MuLV). This finding raised the question of whether the Ly-6 antigen is a true alloantigen or merely a viral antigen similar to that determined by the G_{IX} (Section 25.7).

The alloimmune response against Ly-6.2 antigen appears to be under complex genetic control that involves complementary *Ir* genes linked to the H-2 complex as well as non-*H-2 Ir* genes. In simularity to the response to Thy-1 antigens (Section 22.5) the response to Ly-6 seems to be augmented by simultaneously occurring response to some other cell-surface alloantigens.

22.14 The *Ly-7* Gene and Its Product

Of two putative alleles Ly-7^a and Ly-7^b, the molecular product of the latter, Ly-7.2, can be detected serologically in most mouse strains. Only two strains (C57BL and C58) seem to carry the Ly-7^a allele, which appears to be silent. Since Ly-7.2 molecules have been demonstrated on 70 to 80 percent of spleen and lymph node cells that contain 30 and 60 percent T cells, respectively, it must be presumed that the antigen is expressed on both T and B cells. This presumption is supported by the finding that only 50 percent of T cells in the spleen and 80 percent of T cells in lymph nodes express the Ly-7 molecules. Thymocytes, although not directly reactive with anti-Ly-7 sera, are capable of absorbing such sera, suggesting that thymocytes do in fact express antigen, albeit in small quantity.

22.15 The *Ly-8* Gene and Its Products

The Ly-8 gene and its two alleles, Ly-8^a and Ly-8^b, determine two allelic molecules, Ly-8.1 and Ly-8.2. Analysis of the strain distribution of these two molecules shows striking similarity with the distribution of the Ly-6 antigens. Since, in addition, both Ly-6 and Ly-8 antigens are coexpressed on similar cells, the question arises whether the two genes and the two antigens are distinct or actually the same. In the first case, the two genes would have to be very strongly linked to each other.

22.16 The *Ly-9* Gene and Its Products

The Ly-9 gene and its two alleles, Ly-9^a and Ly-9^b, have been assigned to chromosome 1 where it is closely linked to the *Mls* gene (Section 21.13). The Ly-9^a is carried by many strains, whereas the Ly-9^b is found in relatively few strains (C57BL/6, C57L, C57BR, C58). The two alleles determine corresponding molecules, Ly-9.1 (formerly called Lgp100 or T100) and Ly-9.2 (or Ly-m9.2) both detectable with monoclonal antibodies. The molecules are found on 90 percent of T and B cells and on about 40 percent of bone marrow cells. The antigen is also present on liver and brain cells. Chemically the Ly-9 antigen is a glycoprotein of molecular weight 100,000.

22.17 The *Ly-10* Gene and Its Product

The Ly-10 gene was assigned to chromosome 19 since the expression of the Ly-10^a and Lyt-1^a alleles in congenic strains coincided. The gene must have two alleles—Ly-10^a and Ly-10^b—but only the product of the former, i.e., the Ly-10.1 molecule, is identifiable by monoclonal antibodies. The antigen is expressed on both T cells (thymocytes and T cells) and B cells and also on the stem cell lines. Its concentration on peripheral T cells is twice that of thymocytes. Ly-10.1 is also expressed on kidney and brain cells.

22.18 The *Ly-11* Gene and Its Product

The *Ly-11* gene is closely linked to the *Ly-6* and *H-30* genes but is definitely distinct from either of them. By convention, it has two alleles: $Ly-11^a$, which determines a putative molecule Ly-11.1, and $Ly-11^b$, which determines the allelic Ly-11.2 molecule to which cytotoxic antibodies have been produced. The Ly-11.2 molecule is expressed on a subset of the peripheral T cells (22 percent in spleen, 22 percent in lymph node, but very few thymocytes) and on 28 percent of bone marrow cells. There is no evidence that the molecule is expressed on any other cells, but further studies are required before the formal designation Lyt-11 can be accepted. Functional studies show that Ly-11 is primarily expressed on prothymocytes and natural killer cells (NK) (Section 25.12). In addition, the antigen is expressed on cells that are selectively susceptible to infection with certain oncogenic viruses. Consistent with this concept is the observation that the number of cells expressing Ly-11 is greater in virus-susceptible than in virus-resistant animals.

22.19 Some Other *Ly* Genes and Their Products

In the past two years a number of new markers of murine lymphoid cells were reported. For the sake of comprehensiveness of this chapter a brief description of these new markers will be given even though in most instances the available data are still preliminary and require further independent confirmation. Particularly, in some instances it cannot be ruled out that a given marker is not identical with some already known markers or that it is not an allelic variant of the known markers. While some of these markers were identified with conventional antibodies others were defined with monoclonal antibodies (Section 4.9).

Table 22.4 summarizes briefly the information available on these newly described markers. For most markers only one allelic variant can be serologically identified, whereas the antithetical product is only presumed and remains undetectable. Most of the markers are apparently expressed on both T and B cells and notably in a number of cases also on a significant fraction of bone marrow cells. The latter observation suggests that some of the markers may be useful for future characterization of the lymphoid precursor cells. Conversely, some markers appear to be expressed preferentially or even exclusively on certain types of cells—Ly-17, Ly-m19, and Ly-m20 on B cells and Ly-18 on Tc cells. At the other end of the spectrum are those markers that are demonstrable not only on lymphoid cells but also on cells of other tissues (liver, kidney, brain, or erythrocytes).

At least in three instances it cannot be excluded that the markers are either antithetical or identical with markers of other systems. Specifically, the Ly-17 and Ly-m20.2 markers appear to have reciprocal strain distribution and similar cellular expression. However, to determine whether these two markers are indeed allelic products of the same gene, formal genetic analysis is required. Such an analysis should also provide evidence in favor or against the notion that Ly-m20.2 marker may be identical to one of the LyM-1 markers of the B cells (Section 23.8). The Ly-m19.2 is found in strains that carry Lyb-2.1, Lyb-2.2, or Lyb-2.4 markers (Section 23.2) but never in those that carry Lyb-2.3 marker. This might be construed as an argument that Ly-m19.2 represents a determinant on some Lyb-2 molecules, whereas other Lyb-2 molecules do not have this determinant and correspond to unidentifiable Ly-m19.1. However, it must be emphasized that Ly-m19.2 antigen has been demonstrated on both B and T cells while Lyb-2 antigen only on B cells.

Further genetic and biochemical studies are needed to resolve all these and many other speculations that certainly will evolve in the near future as the result of increasing use of monoclonal antibodies. These studies should be complemented by experiments aimed at elucidation of the functional significance of the markers.

22.20 The *Asialo-GM1* Gene and Its Product

This marker is present on natural killer (NK) cells (Section 25.12) and probably some other mature T cells but evidently not on thymocytes or T_c cells. The antigenic determinant is associated with the glycolipid (ganglio-N-tetraosylceramide)—hence the putative *Asialo-GM1* gene must determine an enzyme responsible for synthesis of the antigen and not the antigen itself.

22.21 The *NK-1* Gene

The *NK-1* gene and its two alleles, *NK-1^a* and *NK-1^b*, determine alloantigens selectively expressed on natural killer cells. Available antiserum has defined one (NK-1.2) product of the *NK-1* gene present in the CE strain of mice. The allelic product—NK-1.1—is believed to be expressed in the C3H strain, but no antibody to this product has been raised.

22.22 The *LyX* Genes and Their Products

Purportedly, there are three distinct *Ly* genes located on the sex chromosome X and named *LyX-1*, *LyX-2*, and *LyX-3*. The *LyX-1* and *LyX-3* genes have two alleles each—one structural *LyX-1^a* and *LyX-3^a* determining the corresponding molecules, LyX-1.1 and LyX-3.1, and the other silent *LyX-1°* and *LyX-3°* with no detectable products. The *LyX-2* gene probably has two structural alleles, *LyX-2^a* and *LyX-2^b*, that determine the allelic molecules, LyX-2.1 and LyX-2.2, and one silent *LyX-2°* allele. Serologically detectable LyX molecules were demonstrated on about 10 percent of thymus, spleen, and lymph node cells. It has been speculated that the LyX molecules confer, upon the cells that express them, sensitivity to stimulation by some thymus-independent antigens (pneumococcal polysaccharide, DNA, etc.). If this speculation is correct, the LyX molecules would not only represent the products of the X-linked *Ir* genes (Section 19.4), but their presence would indicate good responsiveness, whereas their absence

TABLE 22.5. Organ Distribution of Qa Antigens

Antigen	Bone Marrow	Thymus	Spleen	Lymph Node
Qa-1	?	+	+	+
Qa-2	+	+	+	+
Qa-3	−	−	+	+

would determine a low responsiveness to a given antigen. Many more studies are needed to elucidate fully the nature and biologic function of LyX molecules.

THE *Qa* GENES AND THEIR PRODUCTS

Five *Qa* genes have been identified. These represent another family of genetic markers of T cells (Table 22.5). Their biologic significance remains to be unraveled.

22.23 The *Qa-1* Gene and Its Product

The Qa-1 antigen was discovered in studies that employed anti-TL sera. Since such sera should react solely with thymocytes and not with normal peripheral cells, which are TL⁻, the positive reactions observed suggested that the anti-TL serum contained antibodies to an antigen or antigens other than TL. Subsequently, the *Qa-1* gene has been identified and mapped on the basis of recombinants to chromosome 17 between the *H-2* and *Tla* complexes or to the right of the *Tla* complex. Presumably, it has two alleles—*Qa-1ᵃ* and *Qa-1ᵇ*—that are present in a similar frequency among laboratory mice. Of the two alleles, only *Qa-1ᵃ* seems to determine a serologically detectable product; the other appears to be silent. There is a striking correlation between the *Qa-1* and *Tla* alleles, since the *Qa-1ᵃ* allele is present in strains that carry the *Tlaᵃ*, *Tlaᵈ*, or *Tlaᵉ* haplotypes, whereas *Qa-1ᵇ* appears to be associated with the *Tlaᵇ* or *Tlaᶜ* haplotypes. In the strains that carry the *Qa-1ᵃ* allele, the molecular product of this allele is present on about 66 percent of peripheral T cells found in lymph nodes and in the spleen and also on thymocytes. Among the T cells that express Qa-1.1 molecules are cells with the Lyt-1⁺ and Lyt-1⁺2,3⁺ phenotypes. Thus, the two subsets defined by the Lyt antigens are further subdivided into still smaller subsets—one expressing and another not expressing the Qa-1.1 molecules. It appears that the subset that expresses Qa-1 is involved in inhibitory feedback circuits. Elimination of Qa-1 bearing cells from a cell population in vitro results in increased antibody production, suggesting that the removed cells belonged to the category of T$_s$. Interestingly, the Qa-1-positive T$_s$ cells are activated by the Qa-1-positive helper cells.

22.24 The *Qa-2* Gene and Its Products

The *Qa-2* gene has been mapped between the *H-2* and *Tla* complexes and is probably located to the left of the *Qa-1* gene. It has two alleles, *Qa-2^a* and *Qa-2^b*, that determine the presence and absence of the Qa-2.1. Although the *Qa-2^b* allele appears to be silent, recent immunochemical studies revealed in the *Qa-2^b*-bearing mice the presence of a molecule with characteristics of the Qa antigen. This molecule, designated provisionally Lq, and the Qa-2.1 molecule have certain antigenic properties in common with class I antigens encoded by the *H-2* complex (Section 16.5). The strain distribution of the *Qa-2* alleles does not correlate with either the *Tla* haplotypes or *H-2D* alleles. In strains that carry the *Qa-2^a* allele, Qa-2.1 molecules are present on 15 to 35 percent of thymocytes, 65 percent of lymph node cells, and about 40 percent of spleen cells. These figures correspond approximately to the distribution of T cells in lymph node and spleen, but in the spleen some B cells may also express the Qa-2.1 antigen. Removal of the cells that express Qa-2.1 molecules decreases proliferation induced by a mitogen that selectively activates T cells. More detailed studies are greatly hindered by the difficulty encountered in distinguishing the Qa-2-positive from Qa-3-positive cells.

22.25 The *Qa-3* Gene and Its Product

An antiserum that originally detected the Qa-2 antigen was still reactive after extensive absorption with EL4 lymphoma cells that are Qa-2 positive. Such an absorbed antiserum reacted with 30 to 50 percent of lymph node cells and about 20 percent of spleen cells but did not react with thymocytes, thereby distinguishing it from anti-Qa-2 serum. Hence, it was postulated that the molecule that reacted with such an antiserum represents still another antigen, Qa-3.1. This antigen is presumably determined by a structural allele, *Qa-3^a*, at the *Qa-3* locus, which maps close to the other two *Qa* loci. Although the *Qa-2* and *Qa-3* genes have not been separated by crossing-over, the distinct strain distribution of *Qa-2^a* and *Qa-3^a* alleles strongly suggests that the latter are true alleles of two distinct genes and not simply alleles of the same gene. Perhaps the most convincing evidence for this concept is that strains SWR and DBA/1, as well as some wild mice, have the genotypes *Qa-2^a/Qa-2^a* and *Qa-3^b/Qa-3^b*, while other strains have genotypes *Qa-2^a/Qa-2^a* and *Qa-3^a/Qa-3^a* or *Qa-2^b/Qa-2^b* and *Qa-3^b/Qa-3^b*. Preliminary studies on the biochemistry of the Qa-2 and Qa-3 antigens showed that they are glycoproteins, each consisting of two chains—one heavy (molecular weight 43,000) and one light (molecular weight 12,000); the light chain is β_2-microglobulin. In addition, 21 to 43 percent identity was found among peptides in tryptic peptide analysis of Qa and H-2 class I antigens. These findings prompted speculations that the genes for these antigens might have a common origin (Section 16.2).

22.26 The *Qa-4* and *Qa-5* Genes

These two genes were recently proposed on the basis of reactions of two monoclonal antibodies with murine lymphoid cells. Originally, the putative molecules appeared to be expressed exclusively on T cells. This prompted the names Qat-4 and Qat-5. Further studies, however, suggested that those molecules may also be on other lymphoid cells; therefore, the less committal term Qa seems to be more appropriate. Each of the two genes has at least two alleles, and in the case of *Qa-4*, the presence of a third allele cannot be ruled out. Interestingly, the third allele (*Qa-4ᶜ*) appears to be associated with specific alleles at the *H-2D* locus—*H-2Dᵈ* and *H-2Dᵍ*. Qa-4 products are present on 75 percent of T cells, whereas Qa-5 appears on 35 percent of T cells and also on the spleen cells of athymic mice and on some B cell blasts.

OTHER T CELL MARKERS

The Ia antigens, especially those determined by the gene(s) in the *I-J* region, may be considered as markers of T cells or their subsets. Because these antigens were described earlier (Section 16.16), there is no need to repeat the discussion here. Tables 22.3 and 22.4 list the basic information available for all markers of murine T cells.

CELL SURFACE ANTIGENS OF RAT T CELLS

T cell markers are also known for rats. Since these markers were identified in several independent laboratories using different panels of antisera, the different names that were introduced for the same marker initially caused a great deal of confusion. Only recently have collaborative efforts involving the exchange of antisera brought a semblance of uniformity and subsequent agreement on the definitions of the two distinct systems (Table 22.6).

The *RT-Ly1* (formerly *ART-1*) gene has two alleles—*RT-Ly1ᵃ* and *RT-Ly1ᵇ*; the first appears to be more frequent among laboratory strains. The corresponding allelic products—RT-Ly1.1 and RT-Ly-1.2—are present on 96 percent of thymocytes, about 50 percent of lymph node cells, and about 33 percent of spleen cells, as well as 15 percent of peripheral blood nucleated cells. Judging from its tissue distribution, the RT-Ly1 marker seems to be expressed on most of the peripheral T cells, but this conclusion still requires confirmation by functional tests of the RT-Ly1⁺ cells.

The *RT-Ly2* (formerly *ART-2*, *Pta*, or *Ag-F*) gene also has two alleles—*RT-Ly2ᵃ* and

TABLE 22.6. Alloantigen Markers of Rat T Cells

Gene	Synonyms	Number of Alleles	Chromosome Assignment	Expression (percent)	
RT-Ly1	*ART-1*	2	?	Thymocytes	(96)
				Lymph node	(50)
				Spleen	(33)
RT-Ly2	*ART-2, AgF, Pta*	2	LG I	Thymocytes	(0)
				Lymph node	(42)
				Spleen	(20)
Thy-1	—	1	?	Thymocytes	(95)
				Lymph node	(5–15)
				Spleen	(5–15)
				Bone marrow	(40)

RT-Ly2^b—that determine RT-Ly2.1 and RT-Ly2.2 products, respectively. The two alleles appear to be equally frequent in laboratory rats. The gene has been assigned to linkage group I and is linked to the minor histocompatibility gene *RT4*. The products are virtually absent from thymocytes but present on 42 percent of lymph node cells, 20 percent of spleen cells, and 20 percent of peripheral blood lymphocytes. If this determination of tissue distribution is confirmed, *RT-Ly2* must be expressed on a distinct subset of T cells. Preliminary studies have shown that such a subset does not include T_c cells. Biochemical analysis indicates that RT-Ly2 is a single protein chain of molecular weight ~25,000. The molecule has an intrachain disulfide loop.

Although the existence of the two T cell alloantigens in the rat is firmly established, their strain and tissue distribution require further investigation. Different antisera, presumably specific for a given antigen, often show quite different activity. This suggests either that the density of the antigen in various strains is different or, more likely, that the sera contain antibodies to still another unidentified system(s). This problem will be resolved when *RT-Ly*-congenic strains are available.

Recently, it has been proposed that the *RT1.C* region of the rat major histocompatibility complex (Section 17.1) represents an analogue of the murine *Qa* gene(s).

CELL SURFACE ANTIGENS OF HUMAN T CELLS

The existence of subsets of murine and rat T cells and their definition, according to antigenic and functional points of view, prompted the search for similar subsets in other species. The major thrust of such a search, for obvious reasons, was directed toward the characterization of human T cells. Although it was quite a difficult task, considering the outbred nature of the human population, a formidable achievement surfaced in a relatively short time. Ten distinct antigens designated T1, T2, T3, T4, T5, T6, T8, T9, T10, T11, and T12 have been described and partially characterized from the chemical standpoint. There is some degree of confusion concerning the nomenclature of human T cell antigens, since they have been detected and named by several independent laboratories employing different monoclonal antibodies. The specific hybridoma lines, used to produce the antibodies that were instrumental in detecting and characterizing T cell antigens, subsequently were patented; some of the original names have become commercial trademarks. Until an international agreement on the scientific terminology is reached, use of the noncommittal terms listed above is most prudent. As mentioned above, monoclonal reagents are instrumental if not essential for the work on human T cell markers. Previously, attempts to produce monospecific reagents by absorption of polyvalent antisera were difficult to interpret because in responding to xenogeneic immunization with human cells, animals are capable of recognizing many different antigens. The resulting antisera are usually too polyspecific to be of practical use. However, the monoclonal technique (Section 4.9), when applied to studies of human alloantigens, does have a serious limitation since mouse antihuman heteroantibodies do not detect allelic differences within any antigen system studied. Thus, virtually nothing is known about the genetic determination of human T cell antigens. There are several reports of alloantibodies presumably directed to human T cells, but their definite characterization is still remote.

22.27 Ontogenesis of Human T Cells

Nearly 95 percent of human thymocytes (intrathymic T cells) express the T10 antigen, the earliest detectable ontogenic marker of human T cells. About 10 percent of such cells simultaneously express another antigen called T9. Neither marker is truly specific for T cells since T10 is associated with various dividing cells and T9 corresponds to the transferrin receptor found on a variety of cells including those of nonlymphoid origin. Following further maturation of the thymic cells, the T9 marker disappears and a new marker, T6, appears on about 70 percent of thymocytes. The T6 (Leu-6) marker is a glycoprotein, of molecular weight 49,000, and is associated with β_2-microglobulin. Since T6 is present only on thymocytes, one is tempted to speculate that it might represent the human analogue of the murine TL antigens (Section 22.2). Almost simultaneously with the appearance of T6, about 70 to 80 percent of the cells begin to express three additional markers—T4, T5, and T8—which, to some extent, are similar to the murine Lyt-1, Lyt-2, and Lyt-3 markers, respectively. T4 antigen appears to be identical with the antigen previously identified by two other sets of monoclonal antibodies, and the antigen was named Leu-3a or Leu-3b, An argument was made by some investigators that Leu-3 or T4 has the following features in common with Lyt-1 of mice: it is present on all thymocytes and a majority, if not all, of peripheral T cells and consists of a single chain (molecular weight 65,000–71,000). However, other authors suggest that another marker called T1 (Leu-1) is the true homologue of the murine Lyt-1 antigen (Table 22.7).

TABLE 22.7 Summary of the Human T Cell Markers

Marker	Synonym	Molecular weight	Expression	Murine homologue
T1	Leu-1	69,000	Immature and mature thymocytes, All T cells (variable concentration)	Lyt-1 (?)
T3	Leu-4	20,000	Mature thymocytes, All T cells	Thy-1 (?)
T4	Leu-3a,b	62,000	Immature and mature thymocytes, About 60% of T cells (T_h)	Lyt-1 (?)
T5 & T8	Leu-2a,b; TH$_2$	30,000 and 32,000	Intermediate and mature thymocytes, About 30% of T cells (T_s and T_c)	Lyt-2
T6	Leu-6	49,000	Immature and intermediate thymocytes	TL
T9	Transferrin receptor	?	Intermediate thymocytes	
T10	—	37,000 or 45,000	Immature and mature thymocytes	
T11	Leu-5 HuLyt-3	55,000	All thymocytes, All T cells	
T12	—	120,000	Intermediate and mature thymocytes, All T cells	
TQ1	—	?	About 50% of T cells (T_h and/or T_a)	Qa-1
JRA	—	?	About 60% of T cells (T_a)	

The T5 and T8 are apparently identical with TH_2 or Leu-2a, 2b antigens detected by other monoclonal antibodies. The similarity of these molecules and murine Lyt-2,3 is evidenced by the following observations. The antigens are present on most of thymocytes but only on about 30 percent of peripheral T cells, and the molecules are composed of two chains (molecular weight 30,000 and 32,000–45,000) bound by a disulfide bridge.

Interestingly, while preserving the pattern of expression and molecular characteristics, T4, T5, and T8 diverged antigenically from their presumptive murine homologues—Lyt-1, Lyt-2, and Lyt-3; the anti-T and anti-Lyt sera do not show cross-reactivity.

During the last stage of intrathymic differentiation, the T6 and T10 markers are lost and two other markers, T1 (Leu-1) and T3 (Leu-4), appear on a small (10 percent) fraction of thymocytes. In fact, T1 appears much earlier but in a low concentration that gradually increases, making a maximum level in the mature thymocytes. Thus, the ontogenically mature thymocyte has a phenotype of T1, T3, T4, T5, and T8 and, at this stage, is released from the thymus into the periphery as a postthymic T cell. The sequential phenotypic conversions are depicted in Fig. 22.2, which also shows further differentiation taking place in the periphery.

22.28 Subsets of Human Peripheral T Cells

During their life-span, the majority of T cells retain the T1 and T3 markers, which are molecules of molecular weight 69,000 and 19,000, respectively. The T3 marker may represent the human analogue of the murine Thy-1 antigen. However, the remaining three markers—T4, T5, and T8—become distributed in a specific manner since 55 to 60 percent of T cells express a significant amount of the T4 marker but not the T5 and T8 markers, whereas 20 to 30 percent of T cells express the T5 and T8 markers but only a negligible amount of the T4 marker.

The subset that bears T1, T3, and a significant amount of T4 antigens (for convenience, referred to as $T4^+$ cells) has been identified as T helper (T_h) or inducer cells as well as T_{DTH} cells and, thus, corresponds closely to murine Lyt-1^+ cells. The nature of this subset has been revealed in experiments in which the proliferation of $T4^+$ cells was stimulated by exposure to either mitogens (PHA or ConA) or soluble antigens, as well as cell-bound alloantigens. Functionally, this subset is required for the generation of antibodies, for delayed-type hypersensitivity reactions, and for generation of antigen-specific T suppressor (T_s) cells. In addition to the T1, T3, and T4 markers, $T4^+$ cells carry several other cell surface molecules. All cells have a receptor for the Fc portion of IgM molecules and a receptor for sheep erythrocytes that is involved in the formation of so-called E rosettes. The erythrocyte receptor is present on all thymocytes and peripheral T cells and is detected by the specific monoclonal antibodies that define T11 marker occasionally referred to as HuLyt-3 or Leu-5. Resting $T4^+$ cells do not express class II molecules of the HLA system. However, 20 percent of $T4^+$ cells upon activation with mitogen and 40 percent of cells after challenge with soluble antigen begin to express class II (Ia-like) molecules. The $T4^+$ subset may be further dissected into two discrete subpopulations. The T-T interaction, required for the generation of T_s cells, involves those $T4^+$ cells that also express an antigen called JRA* and, hence, are designated as $T4^+JRA^+$. These cells are probably analogous to murine T_a cells. They constitute about 60 percent of peripheral T cells and express the TQ1 marker, which is homologous with the murine Qa-1 antigen (Section 22.23).

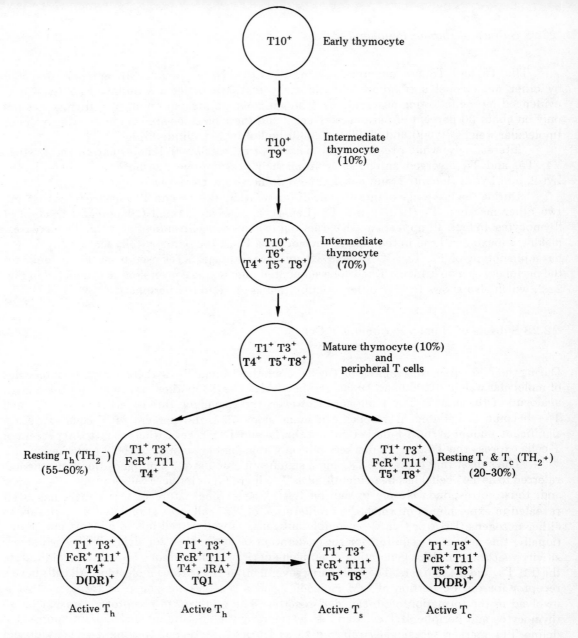

FIG. 22.2. Differentiation and relationship between subsets of human T cells: $T_h(TH_2^-$ or $T4^+)$ = helper; T_s and $T_c(TH_2^+, T5^+,$ or $T8^+)$ = suppressor and cytotoxic cells, respectively; FcR = receptor for Fc portion of immunoglobulin; HuLyt-3 = receptor for sheep erythrocytes; JRA = antigen detected on cells by serum from patients suffering from juvenile rheumatoid arthritis. **Thin arrows** indicate conversion and **bold arrow** represents interaction. Percentages in parentheses correspond to the frequency of corresponding cells in the peripheral lymphatic tissue.

454

The subset that bears the T1, T3, T5, and T8 markers is for simplicity called T8$^+$, since the expression of T5 is always accompanied by the expression of T8, which is found on a slightly larger proportion of T cells than cells expressing T5. It should be kept in mind that these cells also express T4 but in distinctly low concentration. Previously, this subset was identified by xenogeneic antiserum and was called TH$_2^+$, as opposed to T4$^+$ cells that were called TH$_2^-$ These cells have cytotoxic (T$_c$) and suppressor (T$_s$) activity and, therefore, may be analogous to murine Lyt-2,3$^+$ lymphocytes. T8$^+$ cells proliferate in the presence of mitogens ConA and PHA, though admittedly less intensively in presence of the latter. The T8$^+$ cells also respond to cell-bound alloantigens but not to soluble antigens. In a fashion similar to T4$^+$ cells, T8$^+$ cells carry T11 marker, i.e., a receptor for sheep erythrocytes, and a minor fraction bears receptor for the Fc portion of IgG molecules. Resting T8$^+$ cells do not express class II molecules, but they become Ia$^+$ upon stimulation with alloantigens. There are no data available about further heterogeneity of the T8$^+$ subset. The analogy to murine Lyt-2,3$^+$ cells is obvious, not only from a functional point of view, or because T5 and T8, like Lyt-2 and Lyt-3, are always expressed simultaneously, but also from preliminary structural studies. T5 and T8 molecules each has two glycoprotein chains of molecular weight 30,000 and 32,000–45,000 that are linked with each other, probably by disulfide bridge(s).

22.29 Implications of Human T Cell Subsets

There is still a long way to go for final definition and characterization of the human T cell alloantigens. Still, the available data appear to be of great importance not only from a theoretical but also from a practical point of view. For example, different immunodeficiencies may represent the arrest of T cell ontogenesis at a certain stage of differentiation. In the peripheral blood of patients with **severe combined immunodeficiencies** (SCID), T cells expressing only T9 and T10 markers may be found, whereas patients with **acquired agammaglobulinemia** lack T$_h$ cells belonging to the T4$^+$ subset. Analysis of **acute lymphocytic leukemias** (ALL) shows that those that are less well differentiated, and potentially more malignant, may express T9 and T10 alone; only in 20 percent of cases do blast cells also have the T6 marker. On the other hand, **chronic lymphocytic leukemia** (CLL), which is thought to develop from a more mature T cell precursor, displays a prevalence of either the T4$^+$ or the T8$^+$ antigen in the malignant population. From a practical point of view, the selective expression of human T markers and the availability of highly specific monoclonal antibodies ultimately may open an avenue for the selective elimination of an abnormal subset without affecting other subsets. In fact, anti-T3 antibodies have already been used successfully to abrogate the T-cell proliferative responses elicited by renal allografts.

*JRA antigen is found on a subset of normal T cells and is serologically defined by reaction with sera from patients suffering from *juvenile rheumatoid arthritis*.

23 / Cell Surface Alloantigens of B Cells

T cells, by virtue of their regulatory function in immune responses, understandably have attracted the lion's share of efforts aimed at identification of cell surface markers. Nonetheless, both B cells and macrophages perform sufficiently complex and divergent functions to envision the subdivision of these cell types into subsets identifiable by unique cell surface determinants. Although no clear-cut subdivision of these cell populations is presently known, several molecules have been described to be predominantly, if not exclusively, associated with B cells. This chapter contains a brief description of the B cell markers of the mouse, the species in which they have been most extensively studied (Table 23.1).

MURINE ANTIGENS DETECTABLE BY ALLOANTIBODIES

23.1 The *Lyb-1* Gene and Its Products

The *Lyb-1* gene has been mapped to chromosome 2 in the close vicinity of the *H-3* locus. Formerly, the *Lyb-1* gene was referred to as *Ly-4*, and it seems that this name better reflects the true distribution of its product. The Lyb-1 molecules are found predominantly, but not exclusively, on B cells. The gene has two alleles—*Lyb-1^a* and *Lyb-1^b*—determining the allelic molecules Lyb-1.1 and Lyb-1.2. The degree of expression of the Lyb-1 molecules, at least in some instances, appears to be strongly influenced by the *H-2* genotype. In mice carrying the *H-2D^k* allele, the B cells express an exceptionally low quantity of Lyb-1 molecules, making their detection quite difficult. Originally, it was believed that Lyb-1 molecules are expressed exclusively on B cells, but recent data have shown that anti-Lyb-1 sera react not only with B cells but also with purified T cells. Moreover, purified T cells were shown to adsorb anti-Lyb-1 antibodies or reduce their concentration in some antisera. Predominant among B cells that express the Lyb-1 molecules are those in the early stages of development, but some fully mature antibody-producing cells also express a small amount of the antigen. Whether Lyb-1 molecules are present on all early B cells or only on some subsets has not been determined. Also unknown are the biologic role and chemical structure of the molecules.

23.2 The *Lyb-2* Gene and Its Products

The *Lyb-2* gene is located on chromosomes 4 and has four alleles—*Lyb-2^a*, *Lyb-2^b*, *Lyb-2^c*, and *Lyb-2^d*—that determine the corresponding molecules Lyb-2.1, Lyb-2.2, Lyb-2.3, and presumably Lyb-2.4. The alleles are more or less evenly distributed among laboratory strains of mice. The *lyb-2* gene is linked with two other *Lyb* genes, *Lyb-4* and *Lyb-6* (Fig. 23.1) as well as with the *Ly-m19* gene (Section 22.19). In fact, the possibility that the Ly-m19 determinant is located on the same molecule as the Lyb-2 determinant has not been formally ruled out. The Lyb-2 molecules are expressed on antibody-producing cells. However, only those cells producing IgG antibodies express Lyb-2 molecules; IgM-producing cells do not. The Lyb-2 molecule is a polypeptide of molecular weight 40,000–45,000.

TABLE 23.1. Alloantigen Markers of Murine B Cells

Gene	Chromosome Position	Alleles	Products	Chemical Nature	Cellular Expression (percent)				Functional Subset
					Th	Sp	Ln	Bm	
Lyb-1 (Ly-4)	2	Lyb-1^a Lyb-1^b	Lyb-1.1 Lyb-1.2	?	10	60	30	35	Early B cells, some T cells
Lyb-2	4	Lyb-2^a Lyb-2^b Lyb-2^c Lyb-2^d	Lyb-2.1 Lyb-2.2 Lyb-2.3 Lyb-2.4	Protein 40,000–45,000	5	60	30–40	40	IgG antibody-forming cells
Lyb-3	?	Lyb-3^a	Lyb-3.1	Protein 68,000	nt	30	?	nt	B cells (differentiation signal)
Lyb-4	4	Lyb-4^a Lyb-4^b	Lyb-4.1 —	Protein 44,000	5	45	35	5	B cells (signal for alloreactive T cells)
Lyb-5	?	Lyb-5^a Lyb-5^b	Lyb-5.1 Lyb-5.2	?	nt	nt	nt	nt	50–60 percent of B cells
Lyb-6	4	Lyb-6^a Lyb-6^b	Lyb-6.1 Lyb-6.2	Protein 45,000	?	+	+	?	Lyb-4$^+$ B cells
Lyb-7	12	Lyb-7^a Lyb-7^b	Lyb-7.1 Lyb-7.2	?	nt	nt	nt	nt	B cells
LyM-1	1	LyM-1^a LyM-1^b LyM-1^c	LyM-1.1 LyM-1.2 LyM-1.3	?	nt	75	30	75	B cells with FcR
Pca-1	?	Pca-1$^+$ Pca-1$^-$	Pca-1 —	Protein 115,000	nt	nt	nt	nt	Antibody-forming cells, plasmacytomas, nonlymphoid tissues
Pc.2	?	Pc.2$^+$	Pc.2	?	nt	nt	nt	nt	Antibody-forming cells, plasmacytomas

Th = Thymus.
Sp = Spleen.
Ln = Lymph nodes.
Bm = Bone marrow.
nt = not tested

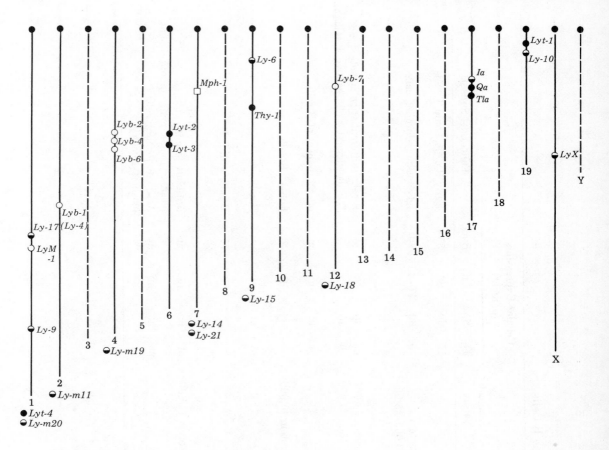

FIG. 23.1. Chromosome positions of genes encoding alloantigens of T cells (**black circles**), B cells (**open circles**), T and B cells (**half-black circles**), and macrophages (**square**). The chromosomes to which no antigen has been assigned are indicated by **dashed lines**. Except for the position of *LyX*, which is arbitrarily assigned, the relative positions of genes on the chromosomes are based on available recombination data. The genes indicated below the chromosome have been mapped to this chromosome but their exact positions are unknown.

23.3 The *Lyb-3* Gene and Its Product

The *Lyb-3* gene appears to be nonpolymorphic, since all strains studied so far are Lyb-3 positive, i.e., presumably they carry the *Lyb-3ᵃ* allele that determines the Lyb-3.1 molecule. In light of the lack of polymorphism of the *Lyb-3* gene, its product should not be detected by alloimmunization. However, demonstration of the Lyb-3 and two other molecules, Lyb-5 and Lyb-7, became possible when a mutant strain of mice (CBA/N) was found in which, owing to mutation of a regulating gene, all three Lyb molecules cannot be expressed. The mutant strain has a general immunodeficiency and is called CBA/N-xid (X-linked immunodeficiency) (Table 23.2). The mutation in CBA/N is sex-linked and recessive, and thus males (X/Y) of F1 hybrids between CBA/N females (which contribute an X chromosome with the mutated gene) and males of the other strain (which contribute the Y chromosome) lack the Lyb molecules. Such F1 males, upon immunization with lymphoid cells from a normal donor, produce the anti-Lyb-3 antibodies. Using antibodies produced in F1 crosses, investigators have demonstrated that the Lyb-3 molecule is expressed on 30 percent of splenic B cells. The molecule detected by anti-Lyb-3 serum is a single chain polypeptide of molecular weight 68,000. It seems that the molecule participates in the generation and/or transmission of a signal for B cell differentiation. This conclusion is based on the observation that the treatment of normal B cells with anti-Lyb-3 serum results in a significantly enhanced antibody response to antigenic challenge. Apparently, antibodies against Lyb-3 bind to the Lyb-3 molecules, and as a result, the signal for B cell differentiation is generated and followed by enhanced antibody production.

23.4 The *Lyb-4* Gene and Its Product

The *Lyb-4* gene has been mapped to chromosome 4 where it is linked with the *Lyb-2* and *Lyb-6* genes. However, in one mouse strain (C3H/He), an apparent translocation of the *Lyb-4* gene has occurred. Of the two alleles—*Lyb-4*[a] and *Lyb-4*[b]—only the former determines a detectable product, Lyb-4.1. This molecule is found on many B cells but only on a few bone marrow cells, T cells, or thymocytes. Since anti-Lyb-4.1 serum abrogates an MLR elicited by either Mls or H-2 molecules, it has been speculated that the Lyb-4 molecules provide the augmenting signal to the T cells responsible for the MLR, i.e., cells responding to alloantigens. The molecule has been tentatively characterized as a polypeptide of molecular weight 40,000–44,000.

23.5 The *Lyb-5* Gene and Its Products

The *Lyb-5* gene has been identified in a manner similar to that used for the *Lyb-3* gene, i.e., via the CBA/N-xid mutant. Two alleles, *Lyb-5*[a] and *Lyb-5*[b], code for the structural products Lyb-5.1 and Lyb-5.2. The products are expressed on 50 to 60 percent of immature B cells; the removal of these cells results in an enhanced antibody response. Since the Lyb-3 and Lyb-5 molecules appear to be phenotypically associated, though they have different strain distributions, further genetic studies are required to determine whether the two genes are separate entities.

23.6 The *Lyb-6* Gene and Its Product

The Lyb-6 product was discovered before the gene was identified. Antibodies to what is now known to be the Lyb-6 molecule precipitated from cell homogenates a polypeptide of molecular

TABLE 23.2. Comparison of Characteristics Distinguishing CBA Mice from
CBA/N-xid Mutant

Characteristic	CBA	CBA/N-xid
Predominant mIg	mIgM	mIgD
Lyb-3,5, and 7	+	−
Concentration of Mls molecules	High	Low
B cell colony formation	+	−
Responses to		
Thymus independent antigens type 1	+	+
Thymus independent antigens type 2	+	−
Thymus dependent antigens	High	High or low

weight 45,000. Retrospectively, the *Lyb-6* gene was postulated and mapped to chromosome 4 in linkage with the *Lyb-2* and *Lyb-4* genes. The Lyb-6 molecules were found on the B cells of the spleen and lymph nodes but not on the cells of the bone marrow or on thymocytes. All cells that are Lyb-6 positive are also Lyb-4 positive; 50 percent of these cells are also Lyb-5 positive.

23.7 The *Lyb-7* Gene and Its Products

The *Lyb-7* gene is the last in the Lyb series, as it is currently known. It has been proposed that the *Lyb-7* gene is located on chromosome 12. The gene has two alleles—*Lyb-7^a* and *Lyb-7^b*— determining the allelic molecules Lyb-7.1 and Lyb-7.2. Antisera to these molecules inhibit the response to TNP-ficoll. Since Lyb-7 molecules are absent in the mutant CBA-xid, which also lacks the Lyb-3 and Lyb-5 molecules, it has been speculated that the three molecules are complexed into a single entity. In such an entity, the Lyb-3 molecule would constitute the common constant portion associated with the sui generis variable portion composed of the Lyb-5 and/or Lyb-7 molecules.

23.8 The *LyM-1* Gene and Its Products

The *LyM-1* gene and its products are defined by an antiserum that is cytotoxic for 75 percent of bone marrow cells, 75 percent of spleen cells, and 30 percent of lymph node cells—a distribution consistent with that of B cells. Indeed, treatment of cells with anti-LyM-1 serum eliminated all functions commonly assigned to B cells. The *LyM-1* gene is located on chromosome 1 and seems to be closely linked, but not identical, to the Mls gene (Section 21.13). There are speculations that the *LyM-1* gene may be closely linked to, or identical with, the recently described *Ly-m20* gene (Section 22.19). Three alleles determine three allelic products— LyM-1.1, LyM-1.2, and LyM-1.3. These products presently are identified on the basis of the percentage of spleen cells killed by anti-LyM serum. Particular *LyM-1* alleles appear to be associated with particular *Mls* alleles. Specifically, *LyM-1^a* is usually present with *Mls^c*, but the presence of its product, LyM-1.1, does not cause lysis of lymphocytes. The *LyM-1^b* allele accompanies Mls^a, Mls^b, or Mls^d and renders 50 to 70 percent of splenic cells susceptible to lysis by anti-LyM serum. $LyM-1^c$, when accompanying Mls^a and Mls^d, is responsible for lysis of almost 70 percent of cells. Although there is no reported crossing-over between the *LyM-1* and *Mls* genes, the two genes seem to be distinct because serologically different (LyM-incompatible) individuals do not produce an MLR. This observation suggests that LyM-incompatible animals may be Mls identical. The reverse situation, in which serologically identical individuals produce a strong MLR, has also been observed. Some authors speculate that the two loci are closely linked and, reminiscent of the MHC, form a complex determining LyM-1 molecules that induce a serologic reaction and Mls molecule(s) that produce a cellular response (MLR). Antibodies to LyM molecules were shown to interfere with the ability of B cells to bind the immunoglobulins via Fc receptors (FcR).

23.9 The *Pca* Genes and Their Products

The *Pca-1* (*PC.1*) gene has been postulated to account for the expression of an antigen present on plasma cells (plasma cell antigen) but absent from less mature B cells. The antigen is found on myeloma cells and normal antibody-producing cells but, surprisingly, also on kidney, liver, and brain cells. This unusual cellular distribution led to the introduction of the term **PKLB antigen**, where the letters represent the organ localization of the antigen. Interestingly, a similar, if not identical, antigen has been identified by rabbit-anti-mouse myeloma xenoantisera and has been named **mouse-specific plasma cell antigen** (MSPCA). There are speculations that the antigen may actually represent the expression of latent virus. Of two presumptive alleles, only $Pca-1^+$ determines a structural product, a protein of molecular weight 115,000, whereas the $Pca-1^-$ allele appears to be silent. The PC.1 molecule is a dimer composed of two identical chains joined by disulfide bond. The latter is much less common among laboratory animals and is found in only six strains (C57BL/6, C57BR, C57L, C58, DBA/2, and 129). Recently, a second gene was proposed and tentatively designated *PC.2*. The gene appears to be nonpolymorphic since all mouse strains express the same product that is detectable by a monoclonal antibody. The PC.2 molecule is expressed on all murine plasmacytomas and antibody-forming cells (PFC). In contrast to Pca-1 it is absent from kidney, liver and brain cells.

MURINE ANTIGENS DETECTABLE BY XENOANTISERA

Many antigens expressed on various murine lymphoid cells have been detected and partially characterized as a by-product of attempts to produce antilymphocyte serum. It was hoped that such a serum would be a potent immunosuppressant. To be of any clinical use, the antiserum would have to be produced by heteroimmunization. However, the heteroantiserum, even if produced by immunization with a highly purified cell population, is usually polyspecific. Still, upon extensive absorption, such an antiserum can be made relatively monospecific. The achieved monospecificity is for a given type of cells in a given species, but these antisera do not discriminate between allelic variants within that species. Three broad groups of antigens can be distinguished with xenoantisera.

Mouse-specific lymphocyte antigen (MSLA) is present on all lymphocytes (thymocytes, T cells, B cells, and cells of various leukemias). Proper absorption of an antiserum that detects the MSLA converts the antiserum into a reagent that detects the **mouse peripheral lymphocyte antigen** (MPLA), an antigen present on the T and B cells but not on thymocytes.

Further absorption of anti-MPLA serum or immunization with purified T cells permits the detection of **mouse T lymphocyte antigen** (MTLA) which is present on all T cells. In the same group, an antigen present exclusively on the killer cells and called **mouse killer T cell antigen** (MKTCA) can be detected.

The third group of antigens consists not only of **mouse-specific B lymphocyte antigen** (MBLA), detectable on B cells, but also the antigen mentioned earlier that is present on plasma cells, kidney, liver, and brain (PKLB).

THE *Mph-1* GENE AND ITS PRODUCT

A macrophage antigen determined by the *Mph-1* gene has been identified in two strains (I and F). The gene maps to chromosome 7 and has two alleles of which only one codes for a structural product, Mph-1.1. The product seems to be expressed predominantly on macrophages, but a small quantity of antigen can be detected on neutrophils and monocytes. Neither the effect of anti-Mph-1 serum nor the biologic function of Mph-1.1 molecules is known at this time.

24 / *The Genetic Determination of Morphogenesis*

Differentiation antigens appear only at a certain stage of the development of a given cell type and disappear when the cell reaches a later stage of differentiation. A good example of a differentiation antigen is the TL antigen, which is present only on thymocytes. While the differentiation antigens affect only a certain specialized group of cells, the genes to be discussed in this chapter determine molecules or traits that affect the development of the whole animal. Probably, there is more than one genetic system that functions in the regulation of embryonal morphogenesis, but the *T-t* system in mice has been most extensively studied. There is no indication that this system affects immune function, although it has been suggested that it is evolutionarily and structurally related to the MHC, which, in turn, plays a crucial role in many immunologic phenomena (Chapter 19).

THE *T-t* SYSTEM OF MICE

The relationship between the *T-t* system and the *H-2* complex is apparent from several observations. Both systems are located on the same chromosome in close proximity. Both are highly polymorphic, and their molecular products seem to have similar structures. There is a striking temporal relationship in the ontogenic appearance of the two systems; the T-t products are expressed in the early stages of embryogenesis, and upon their repression, the H-2 products become expressed. All these similarities may be purely coincidental, but, unless proven otherwise, the concept that both systems originate from a common ancestral gene cannot be dismissed. In fact, some authors suggest that the *H-2* complex is not only functionally related to the *T-t* system, but the former may be an integral part of the latter.

24.1 Genetics of the *T-t* Complex

The *T-t* complex is located on murine chromosome 17 centromerically to the *H-2* complex (Fig. 24.1). Its size is still undefined, and, therefore, it is impossible to determine the exact distance between the two complexes. The problem is further compounded by the fact that the frequency of recombination between these two complexes apparently is influenced by certain alleles at the *T-t* complex. The suppression of recombination is probably responsible for the strong linkage disequilibrium between the *T-t* and *H-2* complex found in wild mice (Section 24.7). Studies in laboratory mice suggest that the centromeric end of the *T-t* complex is about 2 cM from the centromere and about 12–14 cM from the *H-2K* locus of the *H-2* complex.

The original interpretation of the *T-t* complex was that it consists of a single locus with multiple alleles, some of which are dominant (*T*) and others recessive (*t*). The putative alleles seemed to exert a pleiotropic effect resulting in a wide variety of combinations of several phenotypic traits that make up the so-called **t syndrome**. The characteristics that comprise the t syndrome include alteration of tail length, distorted segregation of the alleles of the *T-t* complex, disturbed recombination frequency within and between the *T-t* and *H-2* complexes, impaired viability of the embryos, and male sterility. However, the subsequent finding of recombination within the *T-t* complex necessitated a reevaluation of the rather simplistic concept and the proposition of an alternative model.

According to this new concept, the *T-t* complex consists of a cluster of genes that are

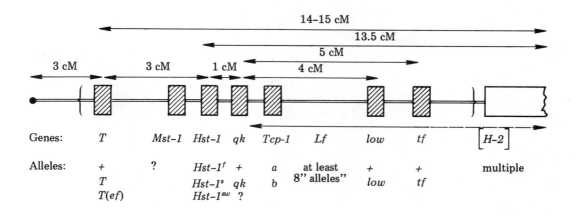

FIG. 24.1. Proposed genetic organization of the *T-t* complex ({ }) located between centromere (●) and the *H-2* complex [***H-2***]. Following genes are marked: ***T*** that has numerous alleles that include wild type (+), several brachury mutants (***T***), and several T expression factors [***T(ef)***]; male sterility (***Mst-1***); hybrid sterility (***Hst-1***) with two or three alleles; quaking (***qk***) with wild type (+) and mutant (***qk***) alleles; lethality factor (***Lf***) representing specific deletions associated with 8 complementation groups of *t* factors; low transmission (***low***) with wild (+) and mutant (***low***) alleles; tufted (***tf***) with wild type (+) and mutant (***tf***) alleles, *t* complex protein (***Tep-1***) with two alleles (*a*) that determines acidic and (*b*) that determines basic form of the protein found on the surface of the testicular cells. Various combinations of alleles at loci indicated form over one hundred *t* haplotypes. Distances between genes given in cM are compiled from various data and are not definite. For details, see text.

closely linked to each other (Fig. 24.1). More recent data, however, suggest that it is more appropriate to consider the *T-t* complex as a relatively large (approximately 1% of the total nuclear DNA stretch of the DNA rather than as a family of related genes. Within this stretch of DNA, occasionally referred to as **tDNA**, at least three distinct genes have been proposed: *T, Lf*, and *LS*, with alleles determining the length of the tail or expressivity of the *T* alleles, viability of embryos, and male sterility, respectively. The *Lf* seems to be an ill-defined segment of chromosome rather than a single gene. In addition to these three genes, many other genes are probably located within the complex or in its vicinity, but their exact position and their role, if any, in the determination of the t syndrome are not known. A multigenic concept of the *T-t* complex requires certain changes in nomenclature. The *T* and *t* loci must become the *T-t* complex and, accordingly, the *t* alleles or factors become *t* haplotypes.* Furthermore, the still

---

*The terms *t* factor and *t* haplotype will be used interchangeably in the following discussion.

often used representation of T and t as alleles of a single gene (T/t), should be abandoned in favor of the notation T-t to represent the linkage of two or more genes.

24.2 T Locus and the T Alleles

The T locus is believed to be at the centromeric end of the T-t complex. It carries a polymorphic gene determining tail length. Several distinct alleles have been identified at the T locus. Normal tail length is determined by the wild allele designated as $+$ and is found in most laboratory mice. The short tail (brachury) is determined by the remaining alleles that developed spontaneously or represent radiation mutants, designated T, T^h, T^{hg}, T^c, T^j, T^{J2}, T^{orl}, T^{or2}, T^{or3} and T^{orl}. All these alleles are dominant over the wild allele; therefore, the $T/+$ heterozygotes will have a short tail. The degree of expression of the T alleles, however, depends on the alleles at some other locus or loci (see below); shortening of the tail caused by a given T allele varies over a broad range. In some strains, e.g., C3H, a T allele results in the lack of only a few terminal vertebrae, whereas in other strains carrying the same T allele, e.g., B10, the entire tail may be missing. Homozygosity for any T allele is lethal, and all such individuals will die at approximately 10.5 days of embryogenesis. Because of the lethality of the T alleles, they are maintained in laboratory stocks only by breeding in a **balanced lethal system** in which $T/+$ heterozygotes are mated in each generation. Such a mating results in three classes of animals—T/T, which are never born, since they die as 10- to 11-day-old-embryos; $T/+$ which have a short tail and can be used for breeding the next generation; and $+/+$, which have a normal tail and are excluded from further breeding. At present, several inbred strains carrying various T alleles are maintained by this type of breeding [B10.T, B10.T(6R), B6.T^{J2}, and BALB.T^j].

   The expression of a given T allele is modified by the action of the other allele at the T locus on the homologous chromosome. The latter allele, referred to as the **T expression factor** [$T(ef)$ or t^T], by itself does not affect the development of the tail. However, it modifies the effect caused by the T allele present on the homologous chromosome. The effect of various $T(ef)$ alleles ranges between two extremes. Some $T(ef)$ alleles suppress the expression of T alleles— thus, the individual has a tail of normal length in spite of carrying a T allele. Other $T(ef)$ alleles have no detectable effect, and mice bearing the T allele express various degrees of tail shortening. Still other $T(ef)$ alleles enhance the effect of the T allele, which results in the total absence of a tail (anury). It seems that in the wild population of mice the frequencies of the suppressing and enhancing $T(ef)$ alleles are similar.

24.3 Lf "Locus" and Its Alleles

The Lf (lethality factor) locus is probably a large segment of the chromosome (t^{lethal}) encompassing as much as 15 cM rather than a single locus. The structural basis for the lethal effect of the Lf gene remains a total mystery. On the basis of data obtained with laboratory mice it has been speculated that deletions (mutations), either physical or functional, of various segments of the T-t complex may produce a lethal effect and mimic the effect of the Lf gene. If this is the case, then the Lf locus or gene would be a misnomer, and the different Lf "alleles" would, in fact, represent deletions of various parts of the T-t complex. Naturally, in such a case, the position of the Lf "gene" cannot be determined, since it would vary depending on the position of the deletions. Recent studies have shown clearly that the Lf of various T-t haplotypes are not allelic and map at different positions along the large segment of chromosome 17. Interestingly, in some t haplotypes of wild mice, the Lf factors were found on the right side of the H-2 complex, thus including the H-2 complex in the t haplotype. At least in one T-t haplotype (t^{w32}) two distinct Lf factors were identified and mapped at a distance of about 4.5 cM from each other.

24.4 LS Factor and Other Genes that Affect Male Fertility

The existence of the LS factor was proposed to account for the sterility of males carrying certain haplotypes of the T-t complex. The LS factor appears as a single gene, but its position within the T-t complex remains unknown. The LS factor is clearly distinct from other genes that also affect fertility. The male sterility (Mst-1) gene was identified in the vicinity of the H-2 complex during studies of mice heterozygous for the so-called T6 translocation (Section 2.7). The hybrid sterility (Hst-1) gene was originally demonstrated in some wild mice that, upon crossing with inbred strains, produced progeny containing males that were either sterile or fertile. Since male hybrids that result from crossing of such wild mice with B10, BALB, DBA/2, or AKR strains were sterile and hybrids between the wild mouse males and females of C3H, CBA or I strains were fertile, it appears that Hst-1 must have at least two alleles, Hst-1^s and Hst-1^f, that are carried by corresponding strains. Whether the allele of wild mice (Hst-1^{sw}) is identical with that of inbred strains (Hst-1^s) has not been determined. Subsequent studies have shown that the Hst-1 gene maps within the T-t complex and is separable from the Mst-1 gene. In contrast to the LS factor that appears as a single gene, the effect of the Hst-1 gene is the result of the epistatic interaction of at least three independently segregating genes. Finally, there is a gene called quaking (qk) whose recessive allele causes abnormal myelination in both sexes and arrested spermatogenesis in males. It is speculated that qk is simultaneously involved in the differentiation of both germ cells and neuroectoderm, thereby explaining its apparently pleiotropic effect.

24.5 The t Factors or t Haplotypes

The t factors were originally considered to be recessive alleles at the T locus, and the alternative terminology, t alleles, is the heritage of the original concept. Since then, it has been revealed that t factors represent a set of alleles at several loci within the T-t complex, and thus they should be considered as t haplotypes that include LS and Lf factors as well as Mst-1, Hst-1, qk, and probably some other genes (Fig. 24.1). As mentioned earlier, t factors may also be viewed as a large segment or t DNA of the murine chromosome 17 and being composed of multiple genes of which only some are responsible for the phenotypic effect known as the t syndrome, whereas other genes are only incidentally located within the limits of the T-t complex and do not contribute to the t syndrome. Presently, over 100 different t factors or haplotypes are known and all of them are recessive. Therefore, $t/+$ animals will not differ phenotypically from normal $+/+$ individuals, but t/t animals will display different characteristics of the so-called t syndrome. On the basis of one of those characteristics—viability—the following three types of t factors are distinguished: **lethal, semilethal,** and **viable** (Table 24.1).

Lethal t factors cause the death of all t/t homozygotes in the early stages of embryogenesis. Semilethal factors result in the death of some and the survival of other homozygotes. Depending on the particular semilethal factor, viability of homozygotes ranges from 2 to 50 percent. The viable factors permit the survival of all t/t homozygotes. Since the mechanism of the lethality remains unknown it is subject to many speculations. Assuming that Lf is a component of a t factor, the lethality of this t factor could be caused by the physical or functional deletion of a segment of that t factor. The deleted segment would correspond to the Lf gene. Since the deletion may occur at different locations in the T-t complex, the 50 known lethal t factors can be divided into eight complementation groups (Table 24.2). The t factors that belong to a given group are lethal regardless of whether they are present in a homozygote (t^x/t^x) or heterozygote (t^x/t^{x1}).* Lethality is due to deletion of the same or overlapping segments in all t factors of a given group. The factors belonging to two different complementation groups permit the survival of heterozygotes, since the deletion in each factor has occurred at a different location within the T-t complex—hence the part deleted in one factor is still present in the other factor and vice versa. However, one has to remember that complementation between groups almost always is incomplete. For example, among heterozygotes carrying t haplotypes of the t^0 and t^{12} groups, 80 percent mortality may still be observed. The cause of the incompleteness of complementation remains obscure. The t factors of a given complementation group are characterized by a precise time of death of embryos and typical pathological changes accompanying the death (Section 24.6). The t haplotype determines several phenotypic features that constitute the t syndrome.

24.6 The t Syndrome

There are several distinct symptoms (Table 24.3) of the t syndrome, and they will be briefly discussed below.

Alteration of the expression of the T alleles refers to the finding, mentioned earlier, that $T(ef)$ alleles may either suppress or enhance the expression of the T allele. Since $T(ef)$ is a part of the t factor, different t factors exert different effects on the T phenotype. For example, the t^{h7} factor suppresses the T allele and mice have normal tails, whereas the t^0 or t^3 factors enhance the expression of the T allele and the animals are tailless. Some of the t factors, e.g., t^{h18}, have neither a suppressive nor enhancing effect, and in animals carrying such factors the length of tail is determined exclusively by the T allele and possibly some background genes. In the presence of $+/+$ homozygosity at the T locus, all t factors determine a normal tail. The only exception to that rule is the t^{AE5} factor, which in homozygotes determines a short tail.

Another feature of the t syndrome is distortion of the segregation (transmission) of the T alleles. Under normal circumstances, lethal t factors are maintained in the laboratory by a balanced lethal system in which either $t/+$ heterozygotes or t^x/t^y heterozygotes carrying t factors

---

*The superscripts x and $x1$ denote two different lethal t factors belonging to the same group.

TABLE 24.1. Groups of t Factors and Their Phenotypic Effects

Group	Members	Tail [T(ef)]	Transmission	Recombination	Sterility (Hst?)	Lethality (Lf)
Lethal	See Table 24.2	NT,ST, or T	N or I	N,S, or E	+	+
Semilethal	$t^{w2},t^{w8},t^{w36},t^{219}$	T	I	S	+	Late Stages
Viable	$t^3,t^8,t^{13},t^{25},t^{28},t^{34},$	T	N or D	N	−	−
	$t^{38},t^{46},t^{52},t^{h26},t^{w19},$					
	$t^{w82},t^{w84},t^{w86},t^{w88},$					
	$t^{w90},t^{w91},t^{w92},t^{AE5}$					

NT = normal tail.
ST = short tail.
T = tailless.
I = increased.
D = decreased.
S = suppressed.
E = enhanced.
N = normal.

belonging to different complementation groups are bred. According to Mendelian principles, the progeny of the $(t/+ \times t/+)$ or $(t/+ \times +/+)$ crosses should consist of 50 percent $t/+$ heterozygotes. The segregation of t factors is demonstrable by their effect on the expression of cosegregating T alleles. Indeed, the expected proportion of heterozygotes is found among progeny when the female parent is $t/+$. However, when the $t/+$ heterozygote is the male parent, the expected segregation ratio is often significantly distorted. The type and degree of distortion vary among the different t factors. It is proposed that distortion is controlled by a specific factor called A, but its location within the t haplotype has not been established. In fact, it seems that the A factor, similarly to the Lf, has a variable position. The available data suggest that at least

TABLE 24.2. Complementation Groups of the Lethal t Factors

Complementation Group	Members	Embryonal Stage Affected	Death at Day
t^{12}	t^{w32}	Morula	3
t^{0*}	$t^6,t^{30},t^{h7},t^{h13},t^{h16},t^{h17},t^{h18},t^{h20},t^{w4}$	Inner cell mass	5½
t^{wPa}	—	?	
t^{w5}	$t^{w6},t^{w10},t^{w11},t^{w13},t^{w14},t^{w15},t^{w16},t^{w17},t^{w37},t^{w38},t^{w39},t^{w41},t^{w46},$ $t^{w47},t^{w74},t^{w75},t^{w80},t^{w81},t^{w93},t^{w94},t^{w97}$	Egg cylinder	5
t^{w73}	—	Implantation	5–6
t^9	t^4,t^{w18},t^{w30}	Primitive streak	7½–9
t^{Lub}	—	?	
t^{w1}	$t^{w3},t^{w12},t^{w20},t^{w21},t^{w71},t^{w72}$	Neural tube	9–21

*t^0 is identical with t^1 factor.

TABLE 24.3. Major characteristics of the t Syndrome

Symptoms	Putative Gene or Factor	Phenotype	t Factor
Altered expression of T allele	$T(ef)$ or t^T	Normal tail	Lethal
		Short tail	Lethal
		Lack of tail	Lethal, semilethal, or viable
Altered transmission of t and T	A	Normal transmission	Viable
		High transmission	Lethal or semilethal
		Low transmission	Viable
	$low(Lr)$	Low Transmission of T	
Altered recombination frequency	?	Normal	Lethal or viable
		Suppressed	Lethal or semilethal
		Enhanced	Lethal
Lethality	Lf	Death at specific stage of embryogenesis (see Table 24.2)	Lethal or semilethal
Male sterility	LS $Hst(?)$ $Mst(?)$ $Tcp-1$	Total sterility	Lethal or semilethal

three distinct factors located in different parts of the T-t complex are involved in the determination of the distortion.

Some t factors are transmitted to the progeny with a frequency higher than 50 percent, whereas other factors are transmitted with a frequency lower than 50 percent. The two distortions are referred to as a **high** or **low transmission ratio**. A high transmission ratio results in 59 to 99 percent of the progeny receiving the parental t factor, whereas a low transmission ratio leads to only 17 to 43 percent of the offspring receiving the t factor. The transmission ratio varies among different t factors, between different males carrying a given t factor (between-male heterogeneity), and among different litters of a given male (within-male heterogeneity). Notably, lethal and semilethal t factors produce high transmission ratios, whereas the viable factors tend to produce low transmission ratios. The high transmission ratio of lethal and semilethal t factors results in the maintenance of a high frequency of these lethal alleles in wild populations of mice (Section 24.7). It is proposed that this rather unexpected situation is due to the fact that reproductive advantages conferred by the t factors outweigh the lethal effect resulting from occasional homozygosity for these factors.

Finding a distortion in transmission raised the question concerning the stage at which such a distortion occurs. Since an equal number of t and $+$ spermatozoa develop and the litter sizes in reciprocal crosses are the same, it could be concluded that the distortion is not due to abnormal meiosis or the selective death of embryos. Thus, the distortion apparently occurs between meiosis and fertilization and probably is the result of properties of t-carrying spermatozoa. Indeed, shortening the time between insemination and fertilization from the normal eight hours to three hours, at least in some instances, lowers the high transmission ratio.

However, because this effect is variable and often not reproducible, the mechanism of distortion still remains poorly understood.

The transmission of *T* alles by *T/+* males is affected by a distinct gene called *low* (formerly *Lr*). The gene has at least two alleles, wild (+) and *low*. The wild allele permits the normal transmission of *T* alleles to 50 percent of the progeny of a *T/+* male. The *low* allele causes transmission to only 12 to 20 percent of the offspring of a *T/+* male. The latter allele also seems to suppress slightly the recombination ratio (see below). Interestingly, the lowering of transmission and recombination occurs only in *low/+* heterozygotes, wheres *low/low* homozygotes are not different from +/+ homozygotes. Furthermore, the *low* allele abrogates the effect of *t* factors on transmission.

Originally, alteration of recombination frequency was believed to be associated only with some lethal *t* factors that in *//t* heterozygotes suppressed the frequency of crossing-over in the centromeric portion of chromosome 17. However, according to more current views, essentially all *t* factors suppress the recombination frequency although the length of the chromosomal segment affected by the suppression varies considerably. On the basis of the size of the chromosomal segment in which suppression is demonstrable, one can distinguish two types of *t* haplotypes. The *t* haplotypes that suppress recombination along the entire segment that includes the *T* locus and the *H-2* complex are referred to as **complete *t* haplotypes**. In contrast, *t* haplotypes in which suppression affects only a certain portion of the above segment are called **partial *t* haplotypes**. The partial *t* haplotypes are derived by recombination between complete *t* and wild-type + haplotype. Recombination results in the formation of two partial *t* haplotypes each composed of a portion of the parental *t* haplotype and a portion of the parental wild-type + haplotype. The partial *t* haplotype seems to suppress recombination only along the segment that corresponds to the portion derived from the complete t haplotype, whereas no suppression is observed along the portion derived from the wild-type + haplotype. This correlation between the suppression effect and the origin of the genetic material supports the idea that suppression itself is a basic characteristic of the *T-t* complex and not the result of a particular gene(s). To put it differently, one may say that in each case the extent of the chromosome affected by suppression defines the extent of the *T-t* complex or the length of the *t DNA*. Phenotypically the suppression may result in false estimates of linkage strength between the genes on the left side of the *H-2* complex.

The mechanism responsible for the suppression of recombination has not been completely defined. However, the presently available data are consistent with the concept that pronounced structural differences between the DNA sequences of the wild type DNA and the *t DNA* result in insufficient homology between the two haplotypes. Insufficient homology interferes with the basic mechanism of crossing-over. This interesting concept finds strong support in observations that in *t/t* heterozygotes carrying two complete t haplotypes, the recombination frequency is normal along the entire complex; whereas in *t/t* heterozygotes carrying one complete and one partial haplotype or two partial haplotypes, the crossing-over frequency within the segment heterozygous for *t DNA* is normal but suppressed within the segment heterozygous for t and wild-type DNA. The source of the structural differences between *t DNA* and wild-type DNA remains unknown; multiple rearrangements, inversions, unequal recombinations, deletions, or any combination of the above may be the culprits. There are speculations that the suppression of recombination may represent a mechanism that counteracts the spread of lethal factors in the population and prevents the formation of new *t* factors. The formation of new *t* factors has been demonstrated in the laboratory. Interestingly, the new factors are formed by recombination between two known *t* factors or between *t* factor and wild-type (+) haplotype; most commonly the new factors belong to a viable group. No formation of *t* from the two + alleles or reversion of *t* to + has been observed.

Perhaps the most pronounced symptom of the *t* syndrome is the serious disturbance of early embryogenesis. Such a disturbance leads to the death of the embryo at a particular stage of development. The lethality of different *t* factors is ascribed to a so-called *Lf* "gene," which is believed to represent a "deletion" within the *T-t* complex. As mentioned earlier, lethal factors are subdivided into eight complementation groups. All the factors belonging to a given group have an identical, or nearly identical, deletion. Therefore, an animal carrying two *t* factors that belong to the same group will not survive because it lacks the same segment in both chromosomes. Furthermore, because each group has the same or a similar deletion, death occurs at a strictly defined stage of development and is accompanied by a specific set of symptoms. Table 24.2 summarizes the effect of *t* factors belonging to different complementation groups. In addition to a lethal factor, some semilethal *t* factors that allow survival of some but not all embryos may affect embryonal development, usually in later stages. Interestingly, most of the *t* factors appear to act on specific differentiation steps of the neuroectoderm.

Most of the lethal and semilethal factors result in varying degrees and various types of sterility of males carrying these factors. Sterility is believed to be the result of the putative *LS* factor (see above), but, most likely, other genes discussed earlier contribute significantly to the actual phenotypic effect. There are five distinct types of sterility associated with different *t* haplotypes. Male heterozygotes carrying two different lethal *t* factors produce spermatoza that have abnormal morphology and defective motility, rendering these mice totally sterile. The impaired motility may be responsible for difficulties in traversing the uterotubal junction; but, in addition, entrapment of spermatozoa by coagulation of sperm fluid may contribute to the sterility. Homozygosity for semilethal *t* factors results in abnormal spermatogenesis and spermiogenesis leading to **aspermia** and total sterility. A similar effect was observed in t^{AE5}/t^{AE5} viable homozygotes, though sterility was only partial since a certain number of spermatozoa were still produced. Heterozygotes carrying one semilethal and one viable factor are partially sterile, but the mechanism has not been clarified. Finally, heterozygotes carrying the T^{orl} allele together with the t^0 or t^{12} lethal factors are partially sterile.

The biologic significance of male sterility is not fully realized. However, it is often speculated that, on the one hand, male sterility may prevent spreading of the lethal factors in the population, while, on the other hand, sterility of hybrids (see *Hst-1*) may preclude the reconvergence of two new emerging subspecies and/or species.

24.7 The *t* Factors in Wild Mice

When several samples of wild mice were tested, the presence of various lethal *t* factors was demonstrated in half of such samples. In fact, since many of the samples were relatively small (fewer than 10 mice), the estimated frequency of *t* factor may be too low. In those populations that contained t factors, their frequency was found to be 0.175 with the most frequent being factors from t^{w5} and t^{w1} complementation groups. This surprisingly high frequency of t factors poses the question of their biologic role. One possibility being considered is that some t factors, by suppressing recombination around and within the *H-2* complex, preserve the integrity of this segment of chromosome. This concept finds support in the observation of linkage disequilibrium between *T-t* and certain *H-2* complexes. In the random population, more than 20 t haplotypes were associated with merely 4 *H-2* haplotypes.

Moreover, with very few exceptions, different t haplotypes that belong to the same complementation group were found to be associated with a single or very few and almost identical *H-2* haplotypes. The limited polymorphism of the *H-2* complex among the t-carrying mice as opposed to the extreme polymorphism of this complex among the remaining mice (Chapter 16) suggests an evolutionary relationship between the two systems. One plausible interpretation is that all t haplotypes developed from a small number of ancestral haplotypes with each ancestral haplotype being associated with a particular *H-2* haplotype and, thus, giving rise to one complementation group. The ancestral t haplotype and all t haplotypes subsequently derived from it remain associated with the original *H-2* haplotype probably owing to inheritance of the *T-t* and *H-2* complexes as a block or a **supergene**. This joint inheritance most likely is caused by the suppression of crossing-over within the *T-t* complex and between this complex and the *H-2*. As a result, a given variant of the supergene is perpetuated unchanged for a long time. The biologic significance of the conservation of the supergene remains unknown. Some studies suggest that any given t factor introduced to a given population by a single animal will initially increase in frequency, but ultimately will be eliminated by genetic drift (Section 1.8).

24.8 Molecular Products of the *T-t* Complex

Only preliminary data are presently available on the putative molecular products of the *T-t* complex. These products appear to be present on embryonic cells, spermatocytes, spermatozoa, and cells of the undifferentiated F9 teratocarcinoma. In the early studies both alloantibodies and xenonantibodies were produced by immunization of $+/+$ animals with either F9 cells or spermatozoa from animals carrying a T allele and/or t factor. Such antibodies were cytotoxic for spermatozoa and affected the early stages of embryogenesis in vitro. These antibodies precipitated molecules of molecular weight 40,000 and 12,000 from a homogenate of F9 teratocarcinoma cells. The size of these molecules suggests that they are similar to class I MHC antigens, with the smaller molecule being analogous to β_2-microglobulin.

Subsequent studies seem to point out that the antigen isolated from the F9 teratocarcinoma is not a product of the gene specifically associated with the *T-t* complex. On the other hand, a protein designated as **p63/6.9** has been recently isolated from testicular cells as well as the F9 tumor. This protein appears to be associated with the external surface of the cells but is not integrated into the cell membrane. Two electrophoretic variants of p63/6.9 are distinguished and called basic and acidic. The two variants are determined by alleles of a gene located in the central portion of the *T-t* complex. The gene is called *t complex protein-1* (*Tcp-1*). The $Tcp-1^b$ allele, which determines the basic form of protein, is found in all wild-type haplotypes. On the other hand, the $Tcp-1^a$ allele, which encodes the acidic form of protein is found in all complete t haplotypes. It has been suggested that the $Tcp-1^a$ allele and its product are responsible for alterations of spermatogenesis and spermiogenesis and the subsequent sterility associated with the t syndrome. Interestingly, in some cases of partial t haplotypes, the two $Tcp-1$ alleles are present on the same chromosome suggesting that such haplotypes developed by unequal crossing-over.

The biologic role of the T-t complex is far from clear. Perhaps the most intriguing concept proposes that the wild allele $(+)$ at the T-t complex determines a set of molecules responsible for cell-cell interactions that underlies **embryonic induction** and differentiation. The molecules should be detectable serologically on spermatozoa and embryonal cells at a particular stage of development. The antigenic determinants of the products have been identified as carbohydrate side chains of cell-surface glycoproteins. It is unknown whether various t factors encode several different glycosyltransferases or variants of the protein backbone, which serve as "substrate" for a single transferase. Various T-t haplotypes would represent mutations that result in the production of a faulty interaction among specific cell groups and subsequently in abnormal morphogenesis. Some of the defective molecules may result in the death of either all cells or a specific group of embryonal cells. In fact, death at a precise time was observed in vitro when the tissues of embryos carrying various t haplotypes were cultured.

Similarity of the complexity, polymorphism, and chemistry of the putative products, in addition to the chromosomal localization of their genes, led to the speculation that the T-t and H-2 complexes developed from a common ancestral gene that controlled primitive cell-cell interactions. As evolution progressed, the T-t complex became restricted to morphogenesis, whereas the H-2 complex became specifically engaged in controlling cell-cell interactions of lymphoid cells. Although this concept is quite appealing and intriguing, all similarities may be coincidental and many more data are needed to support it.

THE GROWTH AND REPRODUCTION COMPLEX (*Grc*) OF THE RAT

The discovery of the T-t complex in mice and its role in embryogenesis stimulated a search for similar gene complexes in other species. This search so far has brought clear-cut results only in the closely related species—the rat. The growth and reproduction complex (*Grc*) of the rat was found to be linked to the *Rt1* complex and shown to have several interesting features. It must be emphasized that it is still premature to consider *Grc* a true homologue of the T-t complex.

The *Grc* was first described in the $RT1^l$ homozygous B1 strain. This strain is characterized by small body size and strikingly small testes. Since in a segregating population the two characteristics could occasionally be separated from the *RT1* complex and from each other, it was postulated that *Grc* consists of at least two genes: a *dw-3* (dwarfism) gene* that determines body size and an *f* (fertility) gene that determines the size of testes and, hence, spermatogenesis. The *f* gene may, in fact, consist of a cluster of discrete genes, since, in some recombinants, the size of the testes was intermediate, suggesting that such recombinants acquired some mutant (small size) and some wild type (normal size) alleles. The relationship between the genes of the

---

*There are two other genes, *dw-1* and *dw-2*, affecting body size of rats.

Grc and the *RT1* is shown in Fig. 24.2. The allele that produces a dwarf body and the allele for small testes are both recessive. Homozygosity for these recessive alleles not only leads to small body size and a defect in fertility but also to diminished survival of the homozygotes of both sexes. Interestingly, it has been suggested that the genes in the *Grc* suppress the recombination rate—a feature shared withi the *T-t* complex of mice. However, to arrive at a definite conclusion one needs further studies; the available data should be interpreted cautiously.

The phenotypic effect of the *Grc* does not seem to be mediated by the endocrine system, since there is no detectable deficiency of gonadotropin or steroids. Neither are there gross karyotypic abnormalities, though by the Giemsa banding technique a subtle change was observed in chromosome 3. However, since the chromosomal localization of the *RT1* complex is unknown, it is impossible to relate these changes to the *Grc*, which is linked to the *RT1*.

Virtually nothing is known about the product(s) of the *Grc* genes. Preliminary studies in this direction show that the rat sperm contains an autoantigen that is present in variable amounts in different strains and absent from *Grc* heterozygous animals. Whether this antigen is related to the Grc product remains to be seen.

There are two other genetic systems affecting embryogenesis in the rat. One of these is linked to *RT1* and influences susceptibility to cleft palate induced by cortisone. The second bears a remarkable similarity to the *T-t* system of mice since it causes shortening of the tail and death of homozygous embryos, but it is not linked to *RT1*.

GENETIC DETERMINATION OF SPINA BIFIDA IN MAN

It could be expected that if there is an analogue of the *T-t* complex in man, it might be associated with a defect in development of the vertebral column. One relatively common defect is called **spina bifida** and is characterized by the improper junction of the vertebral arches. Until now, only a single study concerning the genetic determination of spina bifida has been reported. In a large family consisting of 200 members, spina bifida appeared to be associated with HLA phenotypes (A2-B12 and A2-B18) with a recombination frequency of about 27 percent. Inasmuch as these findings are highly suggestive, many more studies will be required before a claim of a human *T-t* complex can be made.

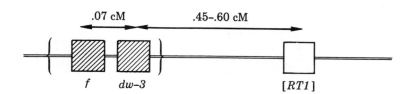

FIG. 24.2. Proposed structure of the rat growth and reproduction complex *Grc*: *f* = fertility; *dw-3* = dwarfism; [*RT1*] = major histocompatibility complex. Distances are marked in cM.

25 / *Antigens of Neoplastic Cells and Tumor Immunity*

The antigens found on neoplastic cells occupy a special place among the cell-surface molecules. Early attempts to transplant allogeneic tumor cells led to the discovery of the ordinary alloantigens and subsequently to the elucidation of their role in many biologic processes. Therefore, it seems quite appropriate to close this section of the book with a brief discussion of the antigens of neoplastic cells. Before beginning the discussion, however, it is necessary to define the basic terms to be used. Although the antigens found on neoplastic cells comprise a quite heterogeneous population of molecules, for the sake of brevity all will be referred to as **tumor antigens** (TA), a term that is not intended to imply that such antigens and their expression are necessarily either the cause or the result of neoplastic transformation.

Within the broad category of tumor antigens, the following two classes are often distinguished: (1) **tumor-specific antigens** (TSA) are those expressed only on neoplastic cells and not on any normal cells; the TL.4 antigen demonstrable on some leukemias but never on normal thymocytes is a good example of TSA; (2) **tumor-associated antigens** (TAA) include those found on neoplastic cells as well as on some normal cells of the tumor host; in some instances, TAA may actually reflect a quantitative change in the expression of otherwise normal alloantigens. In either of the two classes, a subclass called **tumor-specific transplantation antigens** or **tumor-associated transplantation antigens** (TSTA or TATA) is described occasionally to accommodate those antigens that are present on the cell membrane of neoplastic cells and that can elicit an immune response resulting in rejection of the grafted tumor.

In many instances, tumor antigens have been detected on lymphoid tumors, but this should not be construed as support for a thesis that they are exclusively associated with this type of neoplasia. In fact, unique tumor antigens have also been found on various carcinomas as well as on certain sarcomas. The leukemias of mice, being most amenable to experimental analysis, have been the most extensively studied, but the information gleaned from this analysis most likely applies to other animal species and to other types of tumors. Although some observations suggested the presence of tumor-specific antigens in man, these data still require confirmation. However, it must be emphasized that despite an extensive search no human tumor-specific antigen has been unequivocally identified.

DETECTION OF TUMOR ANTIGENS

Two principal methods are used for the detection of tumor antigens. On the one hand are serologic methods, based on analysis employing antibodies directed to the TA. On the other hand are cellular methods, recently introduced to the arsenal of the tumor immunologists, that assess cell-mediated responses elicited by tumor antigens. The serologic methods consist of cytotoxic and immunofluorescence tests that employ sera presumably containing antibodies specific for the tumor antigens. In these tests, the effect of antibodies to normal antigens must be eliminated either by immunization in a syngeneic combination or by prior absorption of the serum with normal cells. Unfortunately, the former approach often failed in the past and potent antisera could only be produced to tumor antigens that are exceptionally immunogenic. Several antisera containing natural antibodies to TA have been identified recently and have been instrumental in defining the antigens characteristic for certain virus-induced leukemias.

After the discovery and partial characterization of serologically detectable TA, it became possible to investigate the cell-mediated immune responses elicited by these antigens. These cell-mediated responses are believed to be an important component of the defense mechanism against neoplasia. The studies, in turn, led to the discovery of a unique set of cells, the natural killer (NK) cells, which are vested with the capability of destroying syngeneic or autologous tumor cells. All these studies evolved into the highly specialized and complex field of tumor immunology. It would be ludicrous to attempt a comprehensive presentation of the field. Nevertheless, a brief overview of tumor immunity cannot be avoided when discussing the topic of tumor antigens. Thus, a discription of various tumor antigens will be followed by a concise description of the cellular and humoral immune processes involved in tumor immunity.

Tumor antigens can be divided into two broad categories on the basis of their genetic determination. One category consists of molecules determined by genes that are unrelated to oncogenic agents (viruses or chemical carcinogens). The products of these genes are expressed on the normal cells at some stage of the development of such cells, but their expression is modified significantly when the neoplastic process sets in. The antigens of this category are often unique for a given tumor. Even similar tumors that developed in different individuals belonging to the same inbred strain may have remarkably distinct antigens. The second category consists of molecules determined by genes actually belonging to the **oncogenic viruses**. These genes become incorporated into the mammalian genome and may be expressed in both neoplastic and certain normal cells or exclusively in cells that have undergone neoplastic transformation. These antigens usually are similar when expressed in different tumors that developed in individuals belonging to different inbred strains. Because molecules encoded by both categories may be expressed simultaneously in any given neoplastic cell, these molecules have become the markers of neoplastic cells. The entire set of molecules expressed by a given tumor forms the **antigenic profile** of that particular tumor.

EXPRESSION OF NORMAL CELL SURFACE ALLOANTIGENS ON NEOPLASTIC CELLS

Two murine antigens, H-2 and TL, and two human antigens, HLA and CEA (carcinoembryonic antigen), are known to have altered expression on tumor cells. The normal genetic determination and phenotypic expression of the murine antigens have been extensively discussed in the preceding chapters (Chapter 16 and Section 22.1). Therefore, only alterations in expression that are characteristic for tumor cells will be discussed here.

25.1 MHC Antigens of Neoplastic Cells

Of the three classes of H-2 molecules, class I molecules appear to be the most affected by neoplastic transformation and, in addition, are involved in restriction of the antitumor responses. On the other hand, class II molecules seem to be of importance in the generation of antitumor immunity, but their involvement in the formation of tumor antigens has yet to be demonstrated. There seem to be two distinct, but not mutually exclusive, tumor-related phenomena in which class I molecules participate: association with oncogenic viral antigens and altered expression.

It has been repeatedly demonstrated that class I molecules are often physically associated with the immunogenic moiety specific for a given tumor. It has been observed that antibodies to class I molecules inhibit the destruction of the neoplastic cells by cytotoxic cells directed against the tumor cells. Furthermore, while redistributing the class I molecules on the cell surface (patching or capping), such antibodies simultaneously redistribute the viral antigens characteristic for a given tumor. Conversely, specific antiviral antibodies often redistribute not only viral antigens but also normal class I molecules. Additional evidence for the close association between class I molecules and the viral antigens was the finding that a deletion of chromosome 17, i.e., deletion of the entire *H-2* complex, significantly decreased either production or expression of the viral antigen by the tumor cells. The association between class I molecules and the viruses that induce neoplastic transformation is not fully clarified. One possible mechanism is that viral particles become physically linked to the class I molecules and form an immunogenic complex that, in turn, induces cell-mediated immunity. The response induced is MHC restricted since the T_c effector cells, to inflict specific damage on tumor cells, must recognize both virus and class I molecule(s) (Section 19.8). An obvious extension of this concept is that a given virus may preferentially associate with a given class I molecule or even its specific allelic variant. Indeed, in some instances, such a selective association has been demonstrated, as in the case of the **Friend leukemia virus**, which associates with H-2D^b but not H-2K^b molecules. The possibility cannot be ruled out that class II molecules may also be involved in this type of association. In fact, it has been observed that in some cases the resistance to a given tumor is associated with class II molecules, perhaps owing to the effect these molecules have on the generation of those T_h cells that enhance the subsequent response mediated by the T_c cells. It is still a matter of speculation whether the association between virus and class I molecules imparts structural alteration(s) upon the latter.

Since the original observation in the 1970s, several authors have reported that a pronounced alteration of the expression of H-2 molecules is demonstrable in certain tumors. This alteration was shown to consist of two types of changes: some class I molecules expressed on normal cells were not expressed on neoplastic cells (deletion), whereas some other class I molecules that were absent from normal cells of a given individual appeared on the neoplastic cells of that individual (addition). The molecules, absent from normal cells but expressed on neoplastic cells, are often referred to as **illegitimate** or **alien antigens**. Several mechanisms, possibly responsible for deletion and addition of the class I molecules, have been considered. The nongenetic mechanisms could involve masking or alteration of the normal class I antigens in such a way that these antigens either become undetectable (deletion) or simulate allelic variants (addition). The genetic mechanisms might involve the expression of viral molecules that could either mimic class I molecules (addition) or inhibit expression of normal molecules (deletion). Alternatively, the oncogenic agent (virus or carcinogen) could cause a mutation of structural *H-2* genes or of regulatory genes. Presently, the last possibility is favored by many researchers even though it still requires firm experimental support.

The concept that ascribes the deletion and/or addition of MHC molecules in tumor cells to an alteration of the putative regulatory genes requires the following two basic assumptions:

(1) the genome of a normal cell carries multiple copies of class I genes; different copies encode products presently considered to be determined by alleles at a single locus; and (2) there is a stable regulatory mechanism that, under normal conditions, permits the expression of only one such copy and simultaneously prevents the expression of all others. This fascinating and unorthodox concept of MHC genetics still awaits systematic exploration.

As much as one may ponder over the soundness of multiple interpretations of observed phenomena, the facts themselves cannot be ignored. This is especially true in light of the finding that alteration of the expression of the MHC molecules may have a profound effect on the antitumor response. For example, the **Gross virus** is capable of associating with only some allelic class I molecules. Deletion of these particular molecules precludes this association and adversely affects the development of an immune response to the virus or virus-related tumor antigens. On the other hand, addition of a new class I molecule provides a new restrictive element for the recognition of the tumor antigens.

Studies concerned with the alteration of HLA antigens on human tumors are still preliminary. Nevertheless, a great deal of information has been amassed. Although some of the alterations are similar to those reported in mice, striking differences are noted. Analysis of a wide variety of carcinomas revealed that many of these tumors display altered expression of class II molecules. The alteration may consist of an increased or decreased concentration of these molecules or reflect a conversion of cells from Ia^- to Ia^+ or vice versa. The class II molecules found in tumor cells do not appear to be different from those found in normal cells, but in some instances the β chain is significantly smaller. A special case of a human tumor is represented by the **hydatiform mole**—a chorion-derived neoplasm of women. The tumor cells express only paternal HLA antigens; it remains to be elucidated why these antigens, foreign to the tumor host, do not elicit an allograft reaction that results in rejection of the tumor. The physical association of an antigen with β_2-microglobulin in melanoma cells is considered an indication that these antigens may be altered HLA molecules.

25.2 TL Antigens of Neoplastic Cells

Because the *Tla* complex has been discussed in detail earlier (Section 22.1), it will suffice to recall that TL antigens are expressed only on thymocytes of those strains that are TL^+ and not on any cells of strains that are TL^-. However, the lack of expression of TL antigens in TL^- strains does not mean that such strains carry silent *Tla* alleles; the T cell leukemias of these strains often, but not always, express TL antigens. In fact, the leukemic cells of TL^+ strains may also express some antigens not detectable on their normal thymocytes (Table 22.2). One of the six known TL antigens, TL-4, is expressed only on leukemic cells and never on normal thymocytes. Therefore, the TL-4 antigen comes closest to the definition of a tumor-specific antigen because it has never been detected in any normal tissue. The anomalous expression of the TL antigens on leukemic cells has ben attributed to an alteration of regulatory genes. The alteration could be analogous to that proposed as an explanation for the appearance of alien H-2 antigens on neoplastic cells.

25.3 Carcinoembryonic Antigen (CEA) in Man

This antigen has probably been the most extensively studied tumor antigen in man since its detection has certain, though limited, diagnostic and prognostic value. The antigen is normally expressed on embryonic cells of entodermal origin; however, it is found only in very low concentration on normal adult cells. The antigen expressed on adult cells seems to be the source of minute quantities (2.5–12.5 ng/ml) of CEA found in the sera of healthy people. The expression of this antigen in a variety of tumors, as well as during nonmalignant inflammatory diseases of the lung, liver, and gastrointestinal tract, is correlated with an increased serum level of CEA frequently associated with these diseases. The genetic determination of CEA remains unknown since no allelic variations have been detected so far. It is speculated that the putative *CEA* gene is expressed predominantly during embryogenesis, especially by the entodermal cells that produce CEA molecules and to a smaller extent by the normal colonic cells that produce a moiety, presumably identical to CEA, found in **normal colonic washings** and called NCW. A malignant transformation may reactivate the *CEA* gene. Interestingly, it was found that the quantities of CEA and HLA molecules on a given cell are inversely related even though the two antigens are physically independent of each other. It has been speculated that the decreased concentration of HLA in CEA$^+$ cells may influence subsequent antitumor responses. It has been proposed that the *CEA* gene developed by duplication of an ancestral gene with one copy determining the CEA and the other copy diverging into gene(s) coding for the CEA-related antigens called **normal cross-reactive antigen** (NCA) and **tumor extracted antigen** (TEX). The gene encoding CEA-related antigens seems to be continuously expressed in neutrophils. Because a large population of these cells is indigenous to the normal lung and spleen, the NCA and TEX moieties are conveniently available and extractable from these organs.

CEA has been isolated and purified from liver metastases of colonic adenocarcinoma and from colonic washings. Chemical analysis has shown the antigen to be a glycoprotein (molecular weight 175,000–200,000) consisting of 40 to 50 percent protein (molecular weight 72,000) and 50 to 60 percent carbohydrate. The protein portion has a high content of asparagine, glutamine, serine, threonine, proline, and leucine but, characteristically, no methionine. The N terminal sequence of CEA has been determined for several residues. Since the deglycosylated CEA molecule retains about 85 percent of the antigenic activity of native CEA, it is reasonable to assume that most antigenic determinants are formed by the protein, whereas some may be associated with the carbohydrate portion. Each CEA molecule has 60 to 80 carbohydrate chains composed, on the average, of 10 monosaccharides. Chemical analysis of the CEA-related molecules (NCA and TEX) has shown that they are also glycoproteins in which the protein part has a molecular weight of 72,000, while the carbohydrate part has a molecular weight of 28,000 and consists of 30 chains, each with about 7 monosaccharides. Amino acid sequence analysis carried out so far has revealed a substitution at position 21 where NCA and TEX have alanine and CEA has valine. Other characteristics of NCA and TEX include the presence of methionine and changes in Asp-X-Thr(Ser) sequences required for glycosylations. There are several other CEA-related molecules extracted from either normal or neoplastic tissue; however, their structures have not been extensively studied but may be identical with either NCA [normal glycoprotein (NGP), CEA-associated protein (CEX), colonic-carcinoembryonic antigen 2 (CCEA-2)] or TEX [Colon carcinoma antigen III (CCAA III), β external protein (β_E)].

25.4 Ca Antigens

Recently, two glycoproteins (m.w. 35,000 and 39,000) have been described and designated **Ca antigens**. Initially these glycoproteins were demonstrable only on cells from malignant tumors of many human organs but not on cells of benign tumors or on normal cells of the corresponding organs. More important, the Ca antigens were shown to be present on hybrid cells that resulted from the artificial fusion of neoplastic and normal cells, provided that the hybrid cells displayed functional and morphologic features of malignancy. In contrast, the identical hybrid cells that appeared to be nonmalignant did not express Ca antigens. This observation was construed as an argument in favor of the concept that Ca antigens are the long sought for human tumor specific antigens. However, molecules that bound antibodies specific for Ca antigens were also found on normal epithelial cells of the Fallopian tubes and urinary tract. Thus, it is more likely that Ca antigens are in fact differentiate antigens expressed preferentially on malignant neoplastic cells but also present on normal cells that are in a particular developmental stage. In this respect the Ca antigens are similar to CEA molecules and must be classified as tumor associated antigens.

ANTIGENS OF ONCOGENIC VIRUSES AND THEIR EXPRESSION ON MURINE TUMOR CELLS

A viral etiology has been firmly established for many leukemias induced in mice by inoculating either cell-free material obtained from tumors or isolated viruses. The proteins and glycoproteins determined by the viral genome are actually incorporated into the cell membrane of the cells that either carry latent virus or are undergoing neoplastic transformation. With this in mind, viral antigens can be considered as tumor-associated antigens. To understand the nature of these antigens, a brief description of **murine leukemia viruses** (MuLV) is provided.

25.5 Structure and Classification of the MuLV

All MuLV belong to the type C murine RNA viruses (Fig. 25.1). The most common among these are the Gross virus (GV) and Friend virus (FV); the latter may be present in two variants—lymphatic leukemia virus (LLV) and spleen focus-forming virus (SFFV). Typically, these viruses contain a central **nucleoid core** that is composed of viral RNA and RNA-dependent DNA polymerase (reverse transcriptase) surrounded by protein **capsomeres**. The core and capsomeres form the **capsid**, which, in turn, is surrounded by a bilayer membrane **envelope** that is

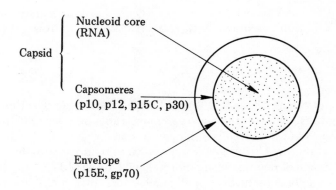

FIG. 25.1. Simplified scheme of the structure of the type C murine leukemia virus (MuLV).

derived from the eukaryotic host cell and is impregnated with viral glycoproteins and proteins. The components of the virus are encoded in the viral genome, which has three distinct regions: *pol*, determining the polymerase; *gag*, determining at least four distinct capsomere proteins (p10, p12, p15C, and p30); and *env*, coding for two glycoproteins (gp 69 and 71)* and one protein (p15E) of the envelope (Fig. 25.2). The viral proteins differ structurally and antigenically from each other; in addition, they differ among viruses found in various mammalian species (group-specific antigens) and among viruses of a given species (type-specific antigens). The classification of viruses according to their host range is determined primarily by the extremely polymorphic gp70 molecules, which most likely mediate the attachment of virus to the membrane of cells to be infected. The classification of the MuLV is based on several overlapping criteria and, accordingly, is far from being firmly established. A brief summary of the current classification is given in Table 25.1.

25.6 Expression of MuLV and Genetic Control of Leukemogenesis

Host cells may become infected by either endogenous or exogenous viruses. After infection, viral RNA is transcribed into DNA by reverse transcriptase; the DNA may be incorporated into the genome of an infected cell. Incorporation is random and often multiple copies of DNA (up to 50) become inserted into a cell's genome. The number of viral genomes of ecotropic MuLV (Table 25.1) incorporated into a host cell determines the rate of leukemia. Mice of strains that carry multiple copies in their cells (AKR, C58) have a high rate of leukemia (100 percent at one year of age), whereas strains carrying a single copy (BALB) have a low rate (<10 percent after one year). Notably, only part of the viral genome becomes incorporated in some strains (NZB, 129); mice of these strains only occasionally develop leukemias. The virus may be transmitted horizontally, by spreading from infected cells to adjacent cells, or vertically, by passing it from

---

*It is often referred to as a single glycoprotein gp70.

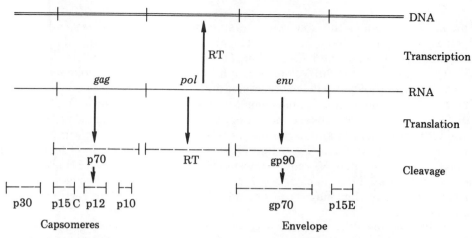

FIG. 25.2. Genome of the typical MuLV and its translation (**bottom part**) and transcription by reverse transcriptase (**RT**).

an infected cell to its progeny. In some strains, viral DNA may become inserted into the host's germ cells and be transmitted vertically from one generation to the other. The viral genome integrated in this manner represents a special category of structural genes responsible for the genetic transmission of MuLV or their components. At present, several such genes have been identified: *Akv-1, Akv-2, Akv-p, C3fv-1, Rjv-1, Gv-1,* and *Gv-2.* In many instances, two or more genes are required for the expression of a given MuLV; the presence of a single gene, e.g., only *Akv-1,* is insufficient for the virus expression. Furthermore, the expression of MuLV determined by the genes listed above and/or leukemogenesis caused by these MuLV is influenced by several other genes.

TABLE 25.1. Classification of MuLV According to Different Criteria

Host Range	RNA Structure	Antigenic Structure

Ecotropic (only in mice)
  B-tropic (in BALB/c
  strain)
  N-tropic (in NIH-Swiss)
  NB-tropic
  (in either strain)
		Class I

Xenotropic (predominantly other species)	MuLV-X$^\alpha$ (rat, rabbit, mouse strains AKR and BALB/c) MuLV-X$^\beta$ (man, primates, mouse strains NZB and NIH-Swiss)	Class II
Amphotropic (wild mice and other species)		

Among these genes, the following deserve special attention. Friend virus-induced leukemogenesis is affected by four *Fv* genes. The *Fv-1* gene has been mapped into chromosome 4 and has two alleles—*Fv-1^b* and *Fv-1^n*. The *Fv-1^b* (formerly *Fv-1^r*) allele is dominant and suppresses the expression of MuLV, hence resulting in a low rate of leukemia. On the other hand, the *Fv-1^n* (formerly *Fv-1^s*) allele is recessive and permits a high rate of MuLV expression.

The *Fv-2* gene maps into chromosome 9 and also has two alleles, *Fv-2^r* and *Fv-2^s*; the former allele is recessive and determines resistance to certain variants of leukemia virus, whereas the latter is dominant and determines susceptibility to infection with the same virus.

Two other genes, *Fv-3* and *Fv-4*, that affect susceptibility to Friend leukemia have no chromosomal position assigned. Moreover, the spontaneous recovery from Friend virus-induced leukemia is controlled by three genes, *Rfv-1, Rfv-2,* and *Rfv-3*. The first two genes were mapped into chromosome 17, and they may represent class I H-2 molecules that restrict antivirus cell-mediated responses.

The leukemia caused by Gross virus (GV) is affected by the *Rgv-1* gene, which has been mapped to, or in the close vicinity of, the *H-2* complex. Assuming that the *Rgv-1* gene is a part of the *H-2* complex, it likely has multiple alleles, some determining resistance and others susceptibility to GV. However, resistance requires the presence of a resistance allele at still another locus, *Rgv-2*, with unknown location.

There are several other genes that influence the expression of MuLV and the development of leukemias. Unfortunately, the effect of these genes is still poorly defined.

Once incorporated into the murine genome, the viral genome may remain silent until neoplastic transformation sets in. The neoplastic process may be intitiated by infection of the cell with an exogenous virus or by activation of the endogenous virus. Alternatively, the viral genome may be actively transcribed even in the absence of overt neoplastic changes. In this case, the products of the *gag* and *env* genes of the active viral genome are incorporated into the host cell membrane and behave like ordinary cell-surface antigens. Presently, several MuLV antigens identified in mice are known to be expressed either on normal and neoplastic or only on neoplastic cells.

25.7 Gross Cell-Surface Antigen (GCSA)

This antigen is present predominantly on the normal lymphoid cells of strains that have a high incidence of leukemia (AKR, C58, NZB), but it may be detected also in some strains with a low incidence of leukemia. Its expression is contingent upon active replication of the MuLV. The antigenic determinants are associated with the four capsid proteins. The antigen can be shed from cells that contain actively replicating virus and may be detected in the serum as **Gross soluble antigen** (GSA). The expression of the GCSA depends on the alleles of the *Fv-1* gene, the *Fv-1^n* allele permits and the *Fv-1^b* prevents expression of GCSA. In F1 hybrids, expression is determined by the dominant *Fv-1^b* allele. GCSA encoded by the genome of xenotropic MuLV is called Xen GCSA. The degree of Xen GCSA expression on thymus and spleen cells of a mouse strain appears to be a predictable characteristic of that particular strain. Accordingly, some strains have high expression in both thymus and spleen, other strains have low expression in both organs, and still other strains have low expression in the thymus but high in the spleen. The gene determining Xen GCSA seems to be located on chromosome 4, about 7 cM from the *Fv-1* gene.

25.8 Gross Antigen of Linkage Group IX (G_{IX})

This antigen is present only on the thymocytes of certain strains of mice; however, it was reported recently that G_{IX} can also be detected in serum, sperm, and seminal fluid. Strains that are GCSA$^+$ (see above) also express the G_{IX} antigen on splenic lymphocytes.

The G_{IX} antigen is determined by two independent genes—*Gv-1* and *Gv-2*—each having two alleles. In the mouse strain studied initially, the *Gv-1* gene was mapped into chromosome 17, about 36 cM to the right of the *H-2* complex. However, in another strain the *Gv-1* gene mapped into chromosome 4. These seemingly contradictory findings can be reconciled by postulating that the *Gv-1* gene in different strains is on different chromosomes. Such an unorthodox concept is actually quite plausible in light of the concept that the *Gv-1* gene represents a segment of viral genome incorporated into the murine genome. It is feasible that in two different strains the viral genome was incorporated into two different chromosomes. The *Gv-1* gene has two codominant alleles—*Gv-1^a* and *Gv-1^b*—with the former determining the presence and the latter the absence of the G_{IX} antigen. The *Gv-2* gene has been assigned to chromosome 7 and has two alleles—*Gv-2^a* and *Gv-2^b*; the *Gv-2^a* permits expression, whereas the *Gv-2^b* precludes expression, of the G_{IX} antigen encoded by the *Gv-1^a* allele.

The *Gv* genes affect the expression of the G_{IX} antigen that is identical with the gp70 component of the Gross virus. The molecule shows the features of both ecotropic and xenotropic MuLV, suggesting that the actual structural gene represents a recombinant between the two types of the virus. The precedent for this concept is the finding that MCF 247* MuLV, which displays dual tropic properties, codes for the G_{IX} antigen; infection with MCF 247 virus results in the expression of the G_{IX} antigen in otherwise G_{IX}^- mice. The antigen is detectable by xenogenic (rat) and natural alloantibodies. Four distinct phenotypes, differing from each other by the quantity of G_{IX} antigen, have been identified. The phenotypes are designated G_{IX}^- (no detectable antigen), G_{IX}^1 (⅓ expression), G_{IX}^2 (⅔ expression), and G_{IX}^3 (full expression of the antigen). The four phenotypes correspond to the combination of the four *Gv* alleles; there is no association between expressivity and a particular H-2 phenotype. In contrast to GCSA$^-$, expression of the G_{IX} antigen does not require active replication of the virus. The cells of G_{IX} strains can be converted into G_{IX}^+ after in vitro or in vivo infection with N-tropic MuLV. Interestingly, anti-G_{IX} serum causes decreased expression of the antigen. This indicates that G_{IX} antigen is subject to antigenic modulation (Section 22.2).

25.9 Other G Antigens

At least three other viral antigens have been found in leukemias and normal thymocytes. The $G_{(RADA1)}$ antigen was identified on normal thymocytes and on radiation-induced leukemias of the

---

*Mink cell focus (MCF) virus is characterized by the ability to infect mink lung cells in vitro.

A strain. Its identification became possible when a serum with natural antibodies was found. The G(ERLD) was found in a similar way with natural antibodies identified in a normal serum. The latter G antigen is present on normal thymocytes and radiation leukemias of A and B6 strains and on spontaneous leukemias of AKR mice. The G(AKSL2) is present on normal thymocytes and on the leukemia cells of the AKR strain. All three antigens apparently are related to the Gross virus but, at the same time, are antigenically distinct from each other and from G_{IX} antigen (Table 25.2).

25.10 X-1 Antigen

This antigen seems to be unrelated to the Gross virus, but the fact that leukemias of the X-1$^-$ strains are X-1$^+$ places the antigen in the same general category of tumor-specific antigens. The antigen was detected on the cells of the radiation leukemia of BALB mice (RL♂1). It elicits cytotoxic antibodies in (B6 × BALB/c) F1 hybrids but not in the BALB mice. The responsiveness of the hybrid but not of the parents probably depends on the *Rgv-1* gene, contributed by the B6 parent, which determines immune responsiveness to the virus and, thus, resistance to infection. Using cytotoxic antibodies, investigators demonstrated that the antigen is also present on normal cells of certain strains (AKR, C58, NZB, 129) but in extremely low concentration.

25.11 Mammary Tumor Viruses

The murine mammary tumor viruses (MTV) are type B RNA viruses characterized by an eccentrically located core. In contrast to MuLV, the MTV capsomeres contain only three proteins, p10, p14, and p28, and the envelope contains two glycoproteins, gp36 and gp52. Essentially, all mice have an MTV genome incorporated into their cellular DNA: the genome is in the form of at least two structural genes—*Mtv-1* and *Mtv-2*—which are vertically transmitted.

TABLE 25.2. Gross Virus Leukemia Antigens

Strain	Cells	Antigen				
		GCSA	G_{IX}	G(RADA1)	G(ERLD)	G(AKSL2)
A	Thymocytes	−	+	−	+	−
	Leukemia*	−	+	+	+	−
B6	Thymocytes	−	−	−	+	−
	Leukemia*	−	−	−	+	−
C58	Thymocytes	+	+	?	?	?
	Leukemia*	+	+	?	?	?
AKR	Thymocytes	+	+	+	+	+
	Leukemia*	+	+	+	+	+

*Some leukemias.

The genes have up to 40 copies in mammary cells but only a few copies in other cells. The *Mtv-1* gene was identified in C3H mice and mapped into chromosome 7; the *Mtv-2* gene was described in GR mice, but its chromosome position is unknown. The expression of either gene depends on various factors that include some undefined genes.

In addition to endogenous MTV determined by *Mtv* genes, there are many exogenous mammary tumor viruses that can be divided into several types (Table 25.3). The suckling mice become infected with exogenous virus via mother's milk—hence the MTV are sometimes referred to as milk factors. The infection can be prevented by foster feeding of animals by females devoid of MTV. Foster-fed animals are identified by the letter *f* after the symbol of the strain, e.g., C3H$_f$. Upon infection, the viral genome becomes incorporated into the DNA of mammary cells that are capable of proliferating. Development of the tumor (adenocarcinoma) proceeds through two consecutive stages—**preneoplastic**, characterized by formation of hyperplastic alveolar nodules, and **neoplastic**, with all the characteristics of a neoplastic transformation. The incidence of the tumor depends on several factors such as antitumor response, hormonal activity, amount of virus produced, and genetic makeup of an individual in which the tumor develops. Interestingly, the incidence also depends on whether the infecting virus is endogenous or exogenous.

PHENOMENA UNDERLYING IMMUNE RESPONSES AGAINST SYNGENEIC TUMORS

Initially, it was suggested that the immune system, at least in part, evolved as a defense mechanism directed against endogenously arising tumor cells. Taken to the extreme, this concept proposed that all immune functions are evolutionary products of the mechanism(s) directed against neoplastic cells, i.e., cells that represent altered-self. If this concept is tenable, the mechanism would involve various lymphoid cells capable of both recognizing tumor antigens and subsequently differentiating into either T_c or T_h cells, with the latter amplifying either T_c or T_{DTH} or B cells. These different cells would contribute to the general phenomenon of **immune surveillance**, which is responsible for the abrogation or retardation of the growth of deviant

TABLE 25.3. Major Types of Exogenous MTV and Their Origins

MTV Type	Synonym*	Strain of Origin
L	Nodule-inducing	C3H$_f$*, A$_f$
ML		BL
O		BALB/c
P	Mühlbock virus	GR*, DD
PS		RIII
S	Bittner virus	A, C3H*, DBA
W		Wild
X		O2O

*For the virus obtained from the mouse strain indicated by an asterisk.

cells. Innumerable studies in the field have generated a large body of data from which emerges a comprehensive, albeit incomplete, picture of the mechanism underlying resistance to tumors. By now, there is little doubt that the mechanism involves a wide variety of immune phenomena. The discussion below is not intended to be an exhaustive review of tumor immunology but merely a framework for more in-depth perusal of the literature by an interested reader.

25.12 Natural Cell-Mediated Cytotoxicity

The phenomenon of natural cytotoxicity appears to present the first line of defense against tumors. It is mediated by a unique population of lymphoid cells, called natural killer (NK) cells, identified in mice, rats, and humans.

The two basic features of NK cells are that they are present in the lymphoid and hemopoietic organs of an individual *before* the individual is exposed to a particular tumor antigen and that they are capable of lysing specifically tumor cells without prior immunization. In contrast to ordinary cytotoxic cells (T_c), NK cells not only are induced by interferon, but their contact with or exposure to an antigen does not result in typical immunologic memory. Studies aimed at the characterization of NK cells are impeded by their extremely low concentration (about 1 to 2 percent of all murine splenic cells), by an apparent heterogeneity of the NK population, and by the paucity of their surface markers.

There is little doubt that NK cells belong to a special category of lymphoid cells, a category that is distinct from T and B cells as well as from macrophages (Table 25.4). Although the distinction is based primarily on the distribution of various cell surface markers, distribution is not always clear-cut. Generally, NK cells are nonadherent, nonphagocytic, and radioresistant. These cells morphologically resemble **large granular lymphocytes** (LGL). Although upon separation of a mixed population of murine or human lymphoid cells the NK activity is associated with the LGL-rich fraction, it is impossible to determine whether NK cells are identical with the LGL or merely represent a contamination of the LGL fraction.

The absence of mIg and Lyb-2 in NK cells clearly distinguishes them from B cells, and the absence of Mph-1 differentiates them from macrophages. However, the distinction between NK and T cells is far from definitive. With the possible exception of NK-1 (Section 22.21), none of the known cell surface markers is strictly restricted to either NK or T cells. For example, the characteristic T cell marker Thy-1 has been demonstrated on about 50 percent of NK cells, especially those found in athymic mice, though admittedly in relatively low concentration. Other T cell markers—Lyt-1, Lyt-2,3, Qa-2,3—are also found on some NK cells. Considering the biologic function of NK cells, their distinction from T_c cells appears to be of primary importance. In contrast to T_c cells, the NK cells have a low concentration of Thy-1 molecules, are not restricted in target cell killing by class I molecules of MHC, do not react against PHA-induced blasts, and do not bind to lectin from *Vicia villosa* that specifically combines with the N-acetylgalactosamine residue found on T cells.

The difficulties in fully characterizing NK cells are further compounded by the fact that among NK cells several distinct types can be distinguished. Apparently, NK cells can be subdivided into Thy-1$^+$ and Thy-1$^-$ or Qa-2$^+$ and Qa-2$^-$ subsets; however, it is not clear whether

TABLE 25.4. Comparison of Cell Surface Markers Expressed on Various Immunologically Active Cells

Cell Surface Marker	NK Cells	T_c Cells	T_h Cells	B Cells	Mϕ
Thy-1	±(50)*	+(100)	+(100)	−	−
Lyt-1	± (28)	−	+	−	−
Lyt-2,3	−	+	−	−	−
Lyt-4(Ly-5)	+(80–100)	+	+ (?)	−	−
Qa-1	+(?)	−	−	−	−
Qa-2,3	+(50)	−	+	−	−
Qa-4,5	+(80–100)	−	−	−	−
mIg	−	−	−	+(~100)	−
Ia	−	−	±(?)	+(~100)	+(?)
Lyb-2	−	−	−	+	−
Mph-1	−	−	−	−	+
NK-1	+(80–100)	−	−	−	−
Asialo-GM1	+	±	−	−	−

*Numbers in parentheses indicate percentage of cells expressing a given marker.

TABLE 25.5. Comparison of Distinct Subsets of Murine NK Cells

Characteristic	NK_s	NK_L
Target tumor	Nonlymphoid solid tumors	Lymphoid tumors and leukemias
Time of maximum activity	24 hours	4 hours
Appearance	At birth	3 to 4 weeks
Level	Constant up to 24 months	Declining after 6 months
In vitro behavior	Maintained	Disappear
Cell surface markers		
MHC molecules	±	+
Thy-1	−	+ (50)[a]
Lyt-4(Ly-5)	−	+(80–100)
Qa-2,3	±	+ (50)
Qa-4,5	−	+(80–100)
Asialo-GM1	±	+
Ly-11	−	+
NK-1	−	+(80–100)
Activity inhibited by:	D-mannose D-galactose	Broad spectrum of monosugars
Effect of bg^b mutation	Normal number	Decreased number

[a]The number in parentheses represents the percentage of NK cells expressing a given marker.

[b]*bg* (beige) is a murine mutant affecting lysosomes and analogous to Chédiak-Higashi disease in man.

these subsets functionally correspond to each other or overlap. Additional subsets of NK cells may be distinguished on the basis of the presence or absence of the Lyt-1 marker.

Recently, a subdivision of NK cells into two subsets—NK_S and NK_L—was proposed on the basis of the tumor target to which their activity is directed (Table 25.5). The NK_S cells, which probably are identical to the **natural cytotoxic** (NC) cells described by some other authors, are active against solid nonlymphoid tumors, whereas NK_L cells display activity against both lymphoid tumors and leukemias. Among the NK_L, a further subdivision can be made according to the effect exerted by ^{89}Sr, a bone-seeking isotope that leads to the destruction of bone marrow. After treatment with ^{89}Sr, NK_L active against certain tumors are eliminated, whereas NK_L active against other tumors are preserved. The relationship between the two subsets has not been clarified. Several observations are consistent with the idea that the NK_S subset represents a less mature population that, under proper conditions, may differentiate into NK_L.

However, the observation that NK_L cells disappear during in vitro culture and that the remaining NK_S cells probably give rise to cells of a new type (NK_C) that are distinct from NK_L does not support the concept of a direct relationship existing between NK_S and NK_L. Also, the fact that there are striking differences in strain distribution of NK_S and NK_L cells is inconsistent with the direct developmental link between the two subsets.

Studies carried out so far indicate that NK_S and NK_L are under polygenic control, possibly exerted by partially different sets of genes. Still, both subsets of cells are influenced by genes linked to the *H-2D* locus as well as by genes in the non-*H-2* background. The genetic determination of a high number of NK cells is dominant, and in some cases intergenic complementation can be observed. Such complementation results in a high number of NK cells in the F1 hybrids of two strains, each displaying a low number of NK cells. Several genes influencing NK cells have been identified—e.g., the *nu* gene responsible for the absence of a thymus, the *lpr* gene determining lymphoproliferation, and the *If-1* and *If-2* genes encoding interferon; all are associated with a high number of NK. Conversely, the *mi* gene responsible for osteoporoesis, the *bg* gene affecting lysosomes, and the *ob* gene causing obesity are related to a low number of NK. The genetic control of NK appears to be extremely complex and is still poorly understood.

Equally poorly understood is the mechanism underlying the antitumor activity of NK cells. Arguments have been made in favor of the concept that NK activity reflects the **antibody-dependent cell-mediated cytotoxicity** (ADCC) mediated by so-called **killer** (K) **cells** (Fig. 25.3). Accordingly to this concept, K cells become NK cells after binding with an appropriate antibody via the Fc receptor. To support this concept, authors cite features shared by NK and K cells. Indeed, both types of cells do appear at about the same stage of ontogenesis, have similar strain distribution, express similar cell surface markers, are induced by interferon, and are inhibited by prostaglandins. Furthermore, in some instances K cells are inhibited or adsorbed by the same tumor that is attacked by NK cells. However, to accept the concept of identity of NK and K cells, one must demonstrate that activity of both cells requires the presence of antibodies and Fc receptors. Experimental studies have shown that, in contradistinction to K cells, NK cells do not require antibodies or Fc receptors for their activity. Moreover, in these studies NK activity remained unchanged in the absence of B cells and antibodies (e.g., in agammaglobulinemia) or after removal of Fc receptors (by modulation),

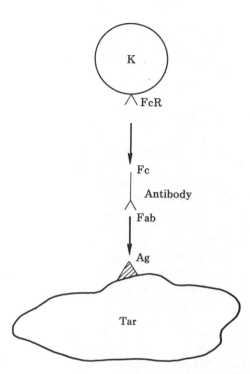

FIG. 25.3. Antibody-dependent cell-mediated cytotoxicity (ADCC) by killer (**K**) cell, which interacts via Fc receptor (**FcR**) with **Fc** portion of an antibody molecule specific for cell surface antigen (**Ag**) of the target cell (**Tar**).

whereas under all these conditions K cell activity was either significantly decreased or totally abrogated. Further indications that distinct mechanisms govern NK and K cells come from the observation that in cancer and chronic lymphocytic leukemia patients the NK activity is decreased or absent while K activity is fully expressed. Conversely, in patients with agammaglobulinemia, NK activity is normal while K activity is decreased or absent.

Recently, on the basis of observations that NK cells can be inhibited by simple sugars, it was proposed that NK cells recognize carbohydrate antigens by lectinlike receptors rather than via Fc receptors. Even accepting that NK and K cells possess different receptors, the actual cytotoxicity may be mediated by a similar mechanism, e.g., lysosomal enzymes. This is supported by several similarities in NK and K effects—metabolic and temperature dependence, effect of Ca^{++} ions, inducibility by interferon, and similar kinetics.

The discovery of the phenomenon of natural cytotoxicity, which is independent of conventional T cells, permits one to obviate the major objection raised against the concept of immune surveillance, which attributed the monitoring of tumor growth to T cells. According to the original version of immune surveillance, one expected that athymic mice should have an increased frequency of spontaneous tumors and that they should be extremely susceptible to oncogenesis. However, the actual observations were in total disagreement with these expectations. The extraordinary resistance of athymic mice can be easily explained by the phenomenon of natural cytotoxicity, since high levels of NK activity were found in the spleens of these mice.

25.13 Induced Cell-Mediated Cytotoxicity

Contrary to natural cytotoxicity, induced cytotoxicity requires prior exposure to the tumor antigens and is mediated by conventional T cells. In most, but not all, instances, the tumor antigen is recognized in the context of or in association with class I MHC molecules; the activity of the induced T_c cells is MHC restricted. This restriction, however, may not be absolute because upon prolonged exposure of the T_c to target cell, the original restriction becomes significantly less stringent. The presentation of the antigen may be accomplished directly by the tumor cells or with the help of macrophages that process and present the tumor antigens.

As in the case with any cell-mediated response, T_c cells have the phenotype Lyt-2,3$^+$ and their generation may be amplified by the Ly-1$^+$ T_h cells. Interestingly, in some models only T_h cells (Lyt-1$^+$) were induced, and these cells were capable of conferring in vivo resistance to the tumor. The final outcome of the activities of T_h and T_c cells may be modified further by the involvement of T_s cells (Lyt-2,3$^+$, I-J$^+$), which interact primarily with the T_h but probably, in some instances, may directly affect the T_c cells. The frequent involvement of T_s cells makes the antitumor responses relatively weak, but they may be significantly enhanced by the elimination of the T_s with the help of anti-I-J sera. The actual mechanism of the lysis of tumor cells by T_c cells remains poorly understood. Besides direct lysis by the T_c, there are indications that T-derived factors may activate macrophages, providing them with the so-called **macrophage arming factor** (MAF) and, thus, enabling these macrophages to lyse tumor cells.

The cell-mediated response to tumor antigens may be unspecifically potentiated by a variety of factors such as immunization with BCG or by the action of genes influencing responsiveness. There have been many attempts to manipulate the cell-mediated responses to combat syngeneic tumors. One of the more interesting models is an attempt to employ the GVHR potential to destroy the leukemic cells of a host. Unfortunately, although the reaction decreases the recurrence of the leukemia, it also inflicts injury upon normal host cells. A considerable amount of study is still needed to separate pure **graft-versus-leukemia** (GVL) reactivity from the GVHR effect.

25.14 Humoral Responses to Tumors

Although many tumor antigens are relatively poor immunogens and induce rather insignificant responses, tumor-specific antibodies have been convincingly demonstrated in some models. The induction of such antibodies seems to be mediated by mechanisms not drastically different from those underlying conventional responses. In some instances, the responses appear to be under genetic control resembling the Ir phenomenon (Section 19.2). Once produced, antibodies may affect tumor cells in a variety of ways.

For example, binding of antibodies to tumor antigens may, in the presence of complement, lead to the lysis of the tumor cells. Indeed, based on such an assumption, total inhibition of a murine T cell leukemia was accomplished. Moreover, in the absence of complement, antibodies bound to the tumor cells may create a target for K cells, which, by virtue of Fc receptors, bind with the Fc portion of these antibodies cause the lysis of the tumor cells. Since lysis is preceded by binding of antibodies and the subsequent involvement of K cells, the ensuing death of the tumor cells is referred to as ADCC (Section 25. 12). However, it is important to consider that under certain conditions binding of antibodies to tumor cells may not result in cell death. Instead, antibodies may cover antigenic determinants, thus preventing their recognition by NK and/or T_c and, as a consequence, protecting the tumor cells from immune attack. Such antibodies, rather than being protective for the host, protect the tumor cells and accordingly enhance survival of the cells.

Although studies on tumor immunity began almost a century ago, only recently has a semblance of the cohesive picture emerged in regard to the role and mechanism of the immune processes that affect the development and growth of neoplastic cells. Historically, studies of tumor transplants laid the groundwork of modern immunogenetics. Because one of the many aims of science has always been to organize and systemize knowledge and phenomena so that true relations can be seen, immunogenetics has evolved as a discipline. Unequivocally, it has earned its current status of respectability. Predictably, uncovering the secrets of inheritance by relating historical events to present and emerging knowledge will provide the basic framework for detailed studies of tumor immunity. Accordingly, the debt of immunogeneticists to the pioneers of immunology will be paid, at least in part.

VI / *Suggested Supplementary Reading*

The following list of publications has been compiled to provide the reader with a source of specific references. It predominantly consists of the most recent textbooks, monographs, reviews, and some selected original papers. Each publication listed has an extensive list of references that may be useful for the reader who desires to pursue in depth some topics discussed in the preceding section.

Ades, E. W., Zwerner, R. K., Acton, R. T., Balch, C. M., Isolation and partial characterization of the human homologue of Thy-1. J. Exp. Med. **151**: 400–406, 1980.

Ashall, F., Bramwell, M. E., Harris, H., A new marker for human cancer cells. 1. The Ca antigen and the Ca antibody. Lancet **ii**: 1–6, 1982.

Bona, C. A., *Idiotypes and Lymphocytes*. Academic Press, New York, London, Toronto, Sydney, San Francisco, 1981.

Cantor, H., Gershon, R. K., Immunological circuits: cellular composition. Fed. Proc. **38**: 2058–2064, 1979.

Cudkowicz, G., Landy, M., Shearer, G. M. (eds.), *Natural Resistance Systems against Foreign Cells, Tumors, and Microbes*. Academic Press, New York, San Francisco, London, 1978.

Demant, P., Roos, M. H., Molecular heterogeneity of D-end products detected by anti-H-2.28 sera. I. A molecule similar to Qa-2, detected in the BALB/cBy but not in the BALB/c.*H-2^{dm1}* mutant. Immunogenetics **15**: 461–466, 1982.

Fougereau, M., Dausset, J., *Immunology 80*, Progress in Immunology IV (3 volumes). Academic Press, London, New York, 1980.

Fudenberg, H. H., Pink, J. R. L., Wang, An-Chuan, Douglas, S. D., *Basic Immunogenetics*. Oxford University Press, New York, 1978.

Goding, J. W., Shen, F-W., Structure of the murine plasma cell alloantigen PC-1: Comparison with the receptor for transferrin. J. Immunol. **129**: 2636–2640, 1982.

Hammerling, G. J., Hammerling, U., Kearney, J. F. (eds). *Monoclonal antibodies and T-cell hybridomas*. Elsevier/North Holland, Amsterdam, 1981.

Heberman, R. B., Natural killer (NK) cells and their possible roles in resistance against disease. Clin. Immunol. Rev. **1**: 1–65, 1981.

Herberman, R. B. (ed.), *Natural Cell-Mediated Immunity against Tumors.* Academic Press, New York, London, Toronto, Sydney, San Francisco, 1980.

Hildeman, W. H. (ed.), *Frontiers in Immunogenetics.* Elsevier/North-Holland, New York, Amsterdam, Oxford, 1981.

Hildeman, W. H., Clark, E. A., Raison, R. L., *Comprehensive Immunogenetics.* Elsevier/North-Holland, New York, 1981.

Janeway, C. A., Cone, R. E., Rosenstein, R. W., T cell receptors. Immunol. Today **3**: 83–86, 1982.

Janeway, C. A., Helper T cell interactions. Fed. Proc. **38**: 2071–2074, 1979.

Katz, D. H. (ed.), *Monoclonal antibodies and T cell products.* CRC Press, Boca Raton, 1982.

Katz, D. H., *Lymphocyte Differentiation Recognition and Regulation.* Academic Press, New York, San Francisco, London, 1977.

Kennard, J., Meruelo, D., A new murine lymphocyte alloantigen, Ly21.1, mapping to the seventh chromosome. Immunogenetics **15**: 239–250, 1982.

Klein, J., *Biology of the Mouse Histocompatibility-2 Complex.* Springer-Verlag, New York, Heidelberg, Berlin, 1975.

Loor, F., Roelant, G. E. (eds.), *B and T Cells in Immune Recognition.* John Wiley, Chichester, England, 1977.

Loveland, B. E., McKenzie, I. F. C., Which T cells cause graft rejection? Transplantation **33**: 217–220, 1982.

McKenzie, I. F. C., Potter, T., Murine lymphocyte surface antigens. Adv. Immunol. **27**: 179–338, 1979.

Potter, T. A., McKenzie, I. F. C., Identification of new murine lymphocyte alloantigens: Antisera prepared between C57L, 129 and related strains define new loci. Immunogenetics **12**: 351–369, 1981.

Reinherz, E. L., Schlossman, S. F., The characterization and function of human immunoregulatory T lymphocyte subsets. Immunol. Today **2**: 69–75, 1981.

Reisfeld, R. A., Ferrone, S. (eds.), *Current Trends in Histocompatibility.* Plenum Press, New York, London, 1981.

Rola-Pleszczynski, M., Sirois, P. (eds.), *Immunopharmacology.* Elsevier/North Holland, New York, Amsterdam, 1981.

Schrader, J. W., Battye, F., Scollay, R., Expression of Thy-1 antigen is not limited to T cells in cultures of mouse hemopoietic cells. Proc Nat Acad Sci **79**: 4161–4165, 1982.

Sell, S., *Cancer Markers. Diagnostic and Developmental Significance.* Humana Press, Clifton, New Jersey, 1980.

Silver, L. M., Genetic organization of the mouse *t* complex. Cell **27**: 239–240, 1981.

Silver, L. M., Genomic analysis of the *H-2* complex region associated with mouse *t* haplotypes. Cell **29**: 961–968, 1982.

Silver, M., White, M., A gene product of the mouse *t* complex with chemical properties of a cell surface-associated component of the extracellular matrix. Develop. Biol. **91**: 423–430, 1982.

Silvers, W. K., Gasser, D. L., Eicher, E. M., H-Y antigen, serologically detectable male antigen and sex determination. Cell **28**: 439–440, 1982.

Simon, M. M., Eichman, K., T cell subsets participating in the generation of cytotoxic T cells. Springer Semin. Immunopath. **2**: 39–62, 1980.

Simpson, E., The role of H-Y as a minor transplantation antigen. Immunol. Today **3**: 97–106, 1982.

Snell, G. D., Dausset, J., Nathenson, S., *Histocompatibility*. Academic Press, New York, San Francisco, London, 1976.

Steinmuller, D., Tayler, J. D., Waddick, K. G., Burlingham, W. T., Epidermal alloantigen and the survival of mouse skin allografts. Transplantation **33**: 308–313, 1982.

Steinmuller, D., Wachtel, S. S., Transplantation biology and immunogenetics of murine skin-specific (Sk) alloantigens. Transplant. Proc. **12**: 100–108, 1980.

Stutman, O., Intrathymic and extrathymic T cell maturation. Immunol. Rev. **42**: 138–184, 1978.

Swain, S. L., Dutton, R. W., Mouse T-lymphocyte subpopulations: Relationship between function and Lyt antigen phenotype. Immunol. Today, **1**: 61–65, 1980.

Torrigiani, G., Bell, R. (eds.), *Immunological Recognition and Effector Mechanisms in Infectious Disease*. Schwabe & Company, Basel, 1981.

Wachtel, S. S., *H-Y Antigen and the Biology of Sex Determination*. Grune & Stratton, New York, 1982.

Williams, A. F., Gagnon, J. Neuronal cell Thy-1 glocoprotein: Homology with immunoglobulin. Science **216**: 696–703, 1982.

Zaleski, M. B., Abeyounis, C. J., Kano, K. (eds.), *Immunobiology of the Major Histocompatibility Complex*. S. Karger, Basel, 1981.

Index

All abbreviations and letter symbols are arranged alphabetically before the listing of the full-word entries within a given letter. Bold face page numbers indicate the position of the definition of the term and/or its extensive discussion. The letters t or f following the page number indicate that the entry is cited in a table or figure, respectively. More than one table or figure on a given page is indicated by a corresponding double letter. When the entry appears simultaneously in a table or figure and in the text on a given page, the number of this page is shown in parentheses. When the entry is discussed continuously rather than incidentally, on several consecutive pages, only the first and last pages are given and separated by a hyphen.